Audiology
Practice Management

Audiology Practice Management

Edited by

Holly Hosford-Dunn, Ph.D.
President
Tucson Audiology Institute, Inc.
Managing Member
Arizona Audiology Network, LLC
Tucson, Arizona

Ross J. Roeser, Ph.D.
Professor and Director
Callier Center for Communication Disorders
School of Human Development
University of Texas at Dallas
Dallas, Texas

Michael Valente, Ph.D.
Professor of Clinical Otolaryngology
Division of Audiology
Department of Otolaryngology–Head and Neck Surgery
Washington University School of Medicine
St. Louis, Missouri

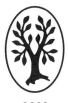

2000
Thieme
New York • Stuttgart

Thieme New York
333 Seventh Avenue
New York, NY 10001

Audiology: Practice Management
Holly Hosford-Dunn, Ph.D.
Ross J. Roeser, Ph.D.
Michael Valente, Ph.D.

Senior Medical Editor: Andrea Seils
Editorial Director: Avé McCracken
Editorial Assistant: Thomas Soper
Director, Production and Manufacturing: Anne Vinnicombe
Senior Production Editor: Eric L. Gladstone
Marketing Director: Phyllis Gold
Sales Manager: Ross Lumpkin
Chief Financial Officer: Seth S. Fishman
President: Brian D. Scanlan
Cover Designer: Kevin Kall
Compositor: V&M Graphics, Inc.
Printer: Maple-Vail

Library of Congress Cataloging-in-Publication Data

Audiology : practice management / edited by Holly Hosford-Dunn, Ross J. Roeser,
Michael Valente.
      p. ; cm.
   Includes bibliographical references and index.
   ISBN 0-86577-858-2—ISBN 3131164115
   1. Audiology—Practice.   I. Title: Audiology practice management.   II. Hosford-Dunn,
Holly.   III. Roeser, Ross J.   IV. Valente, Michael.
   [DNLM: 1. Audiology—organization & administration.   2. Practice Management,
Medical. WV 270 A912 2000]
   RF291 .A93 2000
   617.8'0068—dc21   99-050353

Important note: Medical knowledge is ever-changing. As new research and clinical experience broaden our knowledge, changes in treatment and drug therapy may be required. The authors and editors of the material herein have consulted sources believed to be reliable in their efforts to provide information that is complete and in accord with the standards accepted at the time of publication. However, in view of the possibility of human error by the authors, editors, or publisher of the work herein, or changes in medical knowledge, neither the authors, editors, publisher, nor any other party who has been involved in the preparation of this work, warrants that the information contained herein is in every respect accurate or complete, and they are not responsible for any errors or omissions or for the results obtained from use of such information. Readers are encouraged to confirm the information contained herein with other sources. For example, readers are advised to check the product information sheet included in the package of each drug they plan to administer to be certain that the information contained in this publication is accurate and that changes have not been made in the recommended dose or in the contraindications for administration. This recommendation is of particular importance in connection with new or infrequently used drugs.

Some of the product names, patents, and registered designs referred to in this book are in fact registered trademarks or proprietary names even though specific reference to this fact is not always made in the text. Therefore, the appearance of a name without designation as proprietary is not to be construed as a representation by the publisher that it is in the public domain.

Printed in the United States of America

5   4   3   2   1

TNY ISBN 0-86577-858-2

GTV ISBN 3-13-116411-5

Contents

Principles of Practice Management

Applications in Practice Management

Clinical Applications

Business Applications

Computer Applications

Future Directions

Appendices

Preface

This book on the topic of practice management in audiology is one in a series of three texts prepared to represent the breadth of knowledge covering the multi-faceted profession of audiology in a manner that has not been attempted before. The companion books to this volume are titled **Diagnosis** and **Treatment.** In total, the three books provide a total of 73 chapters covering material on the range of subjects and current knowledge audiologists must have to practice effectively. Because many of the chapters in the three books relate to each other, our readers are encouraged to have all three of them in their libraries, so that the broad scope of the profession of audiology is made available to them.

A unique feature of all three books is the insertion of highlighted boxes (pearls, pitfalls, special considerations, and controversial points) in strategic locations. These boxes emphasize key points authors are making and expand important concepts that are presented.

The 21 chapters in this book cover or touch on all aspects of audiology practice management. In the first chapter, we define practice management and discuss how it applies to the provision of audiology services. Chapters 2 through 8 present basic and advanced information on fundamental principles of practice management, as they apply to audiology, including: professional education, professional ethics, quality control, principles of outcome measurement, human resource management, marketing principles, and fundamentals of private practice.

Clinical audiology practical topics are reviewed in Chapters 9 through 12. The diverse topics include: interpretation and application of professional Codes of Ethics in audiology, clinical report writing and presentation, infection control, and cerumen management.

Chapters 13 through 18 address a wide variety of business issues including: selecting and designing office space, preparing a business plan, selecting a business type, managerial and financial accounting, functioning in managed care environments, and responding to managed care contracting requests for proposals.

Computer technology comprises the final applications section. Chapters 19 and 20 provide extensive explorations of hardware structures and software applications for teaching and administering audiology services. Finally, in Chapter 21, diverse insights into the future of audiology practice management are provided by three leaders from audiology, business, and manufacturing.

The three of us were brought together by Ms. Andrea Seils, Senior Medical Editor at Thieme Medical Publishers, Inc. During the birthing stage of the project Andrea encouraged us to think progressively—out of the box. She reminded us repeatedly to shed our traditional thinking and concentrate on the new developments that have taken place in audiology in recent years and that will occur in the next 5 to 10 years. With Andrea's encouragement and guidance, each of us set out what some would have considered to be the impossible—to develop a series of three cutting-edge books that would cover the entire profession of audiology **in a period of less than 2 years.** Not only did we accomplish our goal, but as evidenced by the comprehensive nature of the material covered in the three books, we exceeded our expectations! We thank Andrea for her support throughout this 2-year project.

The authors who were willing to contribute to this book series have provided outstanding material that will assist audiologists in-training and practicing audiologists in their quest for the most up-to-date information on the areas that are covered. We thank them for their diligence in following our guidelines for preparing their manuscripts and their promptness in following our demanding schedule.

The consideration of our families for their endurance and patience with us throughout the duration of the project must be recognized. Our spouses and children understood our mission when we were away at editorial meetings; they were patient when we stayed up late at night and awoke in the wee hours of the morning to eke out a few more paragraphs; they tolerated the countless hours we were away from them. Without their support and encouragement we would never have finished our books in the timeframe we did.

Finally, each of us thanks our readers for their support of this book series. We would welcome comments and suggestions on this book, as well as the other two books in the series. Our email addresses are below.

Holly Hosford-Dunn – *tucsonaud@aol.com*
Ross J. Roeser – *roeser@callier.utdallas.edu*
Michael Valente – *valentem@msnotes.wustl.edu*

Acknowledgments

The editors of this book series, Ross J. Roeser, Ph.D., Michael Valente, Ph.D., and Holly Hosford-Dunn, Ph.D., would like to extend their deepest gratitude to the following companies and manufacturers who, through the generosity of their financial support, helped defray the costs incurred by our hard-working authors in the development of their contributions.

Beltone Electronics
Oticon
Siemens
Sonus USA, Inc.
Starkey Labs
Widex Hearing Aid Company

Contributors

Harvey B. Abrams, Ph.D.
Chief, Audiology and Speech Pathology Service
VA Medical Center
Bay Pines, FL

Aukse E. Bankaitis, Ph.D.
Director of Audiology
Department of Otolaryngology–Head and Neck Surgery
St. Louis University Medical Center
St. Louis, MO

Joseph P. Barimo, M.S., M.B.A., CCC-SLP
Director of Budgets and Planning
Fischler Graduate School of Education
Nova Southeastern University
Sunrise, FL

Darcy Benson, M.S.
California Hearing Center
San Mateo, CA

James A. Benson
Vice President
Albuquerque Hearing Associates
Albuquerque, NM

Teresa M. Clark, M.S.
California Hearing Center
San Mateo, CA

David R. Cunningham, Ph.D.
Audiology Section, Division of Communicative Disorders
Department of Surgery
University of Louisville School of Medicine
Louisville, KY

Robert R. de Jonge, Ph.D.
Department of Communication Disorders
Central Missouri State University
Warrensburgh, MO

T. Newell Decker, Ph.D.
Professor of Audiology
Department of Special Education and
Communication Disorders
University of Nebraska-Lincoln
Lincoln, NE

Daniel R. Dunn, M.B.A., HIS
One Point Support
Tucson, AZ

Gilbert S. Fox, III, LUTCF, M.B.A.
South Central Financial Associates
Nashville, TN

Barry A. Freeman, Ph.D.
Program Dean
Department of Communication Sciences and Disorders
Nova Southeastern University
Fort Lauderdale, FL

Alan Freint, M.D.
North Shore Ear, Nose and Throat
Highland Park, IL

Stephen Gonzenbach, Ed.D.
New York VA Medical Center
New York, NY

Gail Gudmundsen, M.A.
Advanced Hearing Systems, Inc.
Elk Grove Village, IL

Earl R. Harford, Ph.D.
Director of University Services
Starkey Labs
Eden Prairie, MN

Joseph W. Helmick, Ph.D.
Professor
Department of Communication Sciences and Disorders
Texas Christian University
Fort Worth, TX

Theresa Hnath-Chisolm, Ph.D.
Associate Professor
Department of Communication Sciences and Disorders
University of South Florida
Tampa, FL

Holly Hosford-Dunn, Ph.D.
President
Tucson Audiology Institute, Inc.
Managing Member
Arizona Audiology Network, LLC
Tucson, AZ

James F. Jerger, Ph.D.
Distinguished Scholar in Residence
Department of Communication Sciences and Disorders
University of Texas at Dallas
Richardson, TX

Karen C. Johnson, Ph.D.
Audiology Section, Division of Communicative Disorders
University of Louisville School of Medicine
Louisville, KY

Gyl A. Kasewurm, M.A., F.A.A.A.
President
Professional Hearing Services, Ltd.
St. Joseph, MI

Robert J. Kemp, M.B.A.
Oaktree Products, Inc.
Chesterfield, MO

Lars Kolind
Chairman
National Competency Council
Copenhagen, Denmark

Jodell Newman-Ryan, M.S.
Associate Professor of Audiology
Department of Communication Disorders
Northern Illinois University
Dekalb, IL

Paul M. Pessis, M.S.
North Shore Ear, Nose and Throat
Highland Park, IL

Ross J. Roeser, Ph.D.
Professor and Director
Callier Center for Communication Disorders
School of Human Development
University of Texas at Dallas
Dallas, TX

Wayne J. Staab, Ph.D.
President
Dr. Wayne J. Staab and Associates
Phoenix, AZ

Marjorie D. Skafte
Editorial Director
The Hearing Review
Duluth, MN

Michael Valente, Ph.D.
Professor of Clinical Otolaryngology
Division of Audiology
Department of Otolaryngology–Head and Neck Surgery
Washington University School of Medicine
St. Louis, MO

Phillip L. Wilson, Ph.D.
Head of Audiology
Callier Center for Communication Disorders
Faculty Associate
University of Texas at Dallas
Dallas, TX

Ian M. Windmill, Ph.D.
Associate Professor and Director of Audiology
Department of Surgery
University of Louisville School of Medicine
Louisville, KY

Michael K. Wynne, Ph.D.
Associate Professor
Department of Otolaryngology–Head and Neck Surgery
Indiana University School of Medicine
Indianapolis, IN

David A. Zapala, Ph.D.
Chief of Audiology
University of Tennessee Hearing and Balance Center
Methodist Healthcare
Memphis Hospitals
Memphis, TN

Chapter 1

What Is Practice Management?

Holly Hosford-Dunn, Ross J. Roeser, and Michael Valente

Outline

The chapters in this book explore practice management and its application to audiology service delivery. Publication of this volume marks a departure from previous comprehensive, handbook-type audiology texts, which do not treat practice management as a special topic, if at all. Consistent with recent, dramatic changes in the profession of audiology, the volumes in this series recognize that today's audiologist must be supported by a training triumvirate of diagnostics, treatment, and practice management. Diagnostic audiology and treatment have been addressed in numerous texts and are fairly well differentiated in most readers' minds, but "practice management" conjures up disparate and confusing images for most audiologists on the basis of their individual experiences or lack of experience. The first purpose of this text is to arrive at useful definitions of practice management.

DEFINING PRACTICE MANAGEMENT

Operational Definition

Audiology is diversifying so rapidly that it is sometimes difficult to recognize the kinship between audiology services performed in one environment versus another or to acknowledge that the audiologists performing the different services are products of the same discipline. It is not even clear *where* and *how* audiologists work because survey methods cannot stay abreast of rapid shifts in audiologists' professional alliances, workplace environments, and workforce employment.

PEARL

Today's audiologists work in private practices, hospitals, physicians' offices, or in *newly developing environments.*

The situation is manifest in Figures 1–1A and 1–1B, depicting 1997 U.S. audiology work settings. Figure 1–1A is an unscientific composite of three surveys (Chermak et al, 1998; Kirkwood, 1998a; Martin et al, 1998). Overall, audiologists appear to be fairly evenly distributed into private practice, hospital, and physician office work settings. The distribution is not so even in Figure 1–1B, although the data underscore the observations that about one third of the audiologists are in private practice settings, with hospital and physician offices offering the other two primary employment opportunities. According to Figure 1–1B, more audiologists are employed in "other" environments than in any of the remaining "traditional" employment categories. Operationally, the safest conclusion seems to be that today's audiologists are practicing in private practices, hospitals, physicians' offices, or in newly developing environments.

It is clear from Figures 1–1A and 1–1B that most audiologists will work in, direct, or develop one or more hearing healthcare organizations at some time in their careers. Whatever the name given, these audiologists are performing practice management. As seen in the 1990s, some audiologists will feel comfortable working in supporting positions in traditional settings, whereas other audiologists will push the envelope by bringing strong entrepreneurial forces into practice environments.

Audiology: Practice Management. Edited by Hosford-Dunn, Roeser, and Valente. Thieme Medical Publishers, Inc., New York © 2000

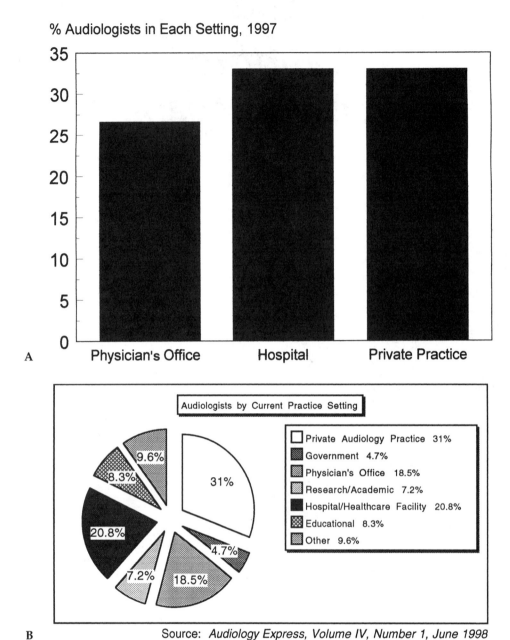

% Audiologists in Each Setting, 1997

A

Audiologists by Current Practice Setting

Private Audiology Practice 31%
Government 4.7%
Physician's Office 18.5%
Research/Academic 7.2%
Hospital/Healthcare Facility 20.8%
Educational 8.3%
Other 9.6%

B   Source: *Audiology Express, Volume IV, Number 1, June 1998*

Figure 1–1   Estimates of workforce distribution of audiologists in the United States. **(A)** Audiologists' work settings according to combined data from three 1997 surveys. (From Chermak et al, 1998; Kirkwood, 1998a,b; and Martin et al, 1998.) **(B)** Work settings of members of the American Academy of Audiology in 1997. (From *Audiology Express*, 4 [1998], with permission.)

In the present milieu many different ways exist to deliver the tests and services for which audiologists are trained: just as audiologists are unique, so are the organizations they comprise. As examples, hearing health organizations are now categorized according to *quantitative* measures such as plant or staff size, marketing efforts, service delivery models, treatment outcomes, financial success, staff turnover, staff credentials, and so on. *Qualitatively,* these same organizations work hard to differentiate themselves by developing objectives and values that define their varying "cultures" (Collins & Porras, 1997) as shown by the example in Table 1–1.

Despite the intentional diversity, these organizations share a common trait: they are all audiology *practices* that must conform to legal and ethical constraints. Audiologists who participate in or direct these practices must produce in line with organizational objectives; must uphold organizational values and encourage similar action by their colleagues; and must ensure that individual and organizational efforts are ethical and legal according to state, federal, or professional organization dictates. This formidable array of "musts" is the operational definition of practice management in audiology (Table 1–2).

TABLE 1–1   Example of values and objectives for an audiology organization

> **Purpose:** To maintain or improve the quality of our patients' lives by optimizing their communication ability
>
> **Core Values**
>
> - Expecting personal best: honest, diligent, always learning
> - Teamwork and loyalty
> - Our only job is customer service
> - Dignity and respect for our patients and each other

Operational definitions are based on observation and are helpful in identifying things: "We know it when we see it." But operational definitions yield little information about the underlying structures and theories that explain how something came to be and how it functions: "What is it?" "How does it work?" Answering these questions requires formal definitions of practice and management.

TABLE 1–2   Operational definition of audiology practice management

> Audiologists must produce in line with organizational objectives, uphold organizational values, encourage similar action by their colleagues, and ensure that their individual and organizational efforts are ethical and legal.

Formal Definitions

What Is a "Practice?"

A practice is a professional organization. Organizations do not have to be professional and can come in all shapes and sizes. Most audiologists work for one organization, belong to several, and interact with many more: universities, audiology clinics, private practices, book clubs, homeowners' associations, alumni groups, ASHA, AAA, ADA, Rotary, the IRS, a church, and so on. All successful organizations, regardless of how they differ, do a few basic things (Stoner & Wankel, 1986):

- **Accomplish objectives:** Organizations use human and other resources to achieve goals that would be difficult or impossible to achieve by individuals acting alone.
- **Preserve knowledge:** Organizations keep records, communicate information, and expand knowledge by developing new or better ways of doing things.
- **Provide vocations and avocations:** Organizations offer ways of making a living and/or pursuing an area of interest, often serving as a source of personal satisfaction and self-fulfillment.

Audiology practices of all types and sizes satisfy the generic criteria of an organization: set objectives, maintain patient and business records, employ people, and provide settings in which those people can realize personal and professional achievements. More specifically, audiology practices belong to an exclusive subset of *professional organizations*, along with accounting, medical, legal, and other practices that employ specially licensed and/or credentialed staff. Professional organizations function with special privileges carved out by law (e.g., the right to perform specific procedures and bill for them) and likewise are subject to special scrutiny according to laws and ethical oaths (Silverman, 1999).

> ### SPECIAL CONSIDERATION
> **Professional organizations have special privileges and are subject to special scrutiny.**

What Is "Management?"

In the classic business definition, management is an internal process for achieving organizational objectives:

> Management is the process of planning, organizing, leading, and controlling the efforts of organization members and of using all other organizational resources to achieve stated organizational goals. (Stoner & Wankel, p. 4)

The internal management process is important for maintaining a business, but Drucker (1986) envisions *management as a dynamic entity* that is more applicable to professional organizations such as audiology practices. Drucker's management model functions in three arenas internal and external to the practice (see Fig. 1–2):

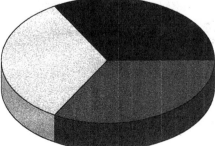

Business Objectives

Human Organization

Public Interest

Figure 1–2   Three dimensions of audiology practice management.

i. *In the business:* Monitoring performance and producing economic results in line with organizational goals.

ii. *In the human organization:* Using governance, values, and relationships of power and responsibility to develop, pay, and organize people for productivity.

iii. *In the dimension of public interest:* Developing and using policies to affect business impact on society and the community (Drucker, 1986).

A Dynamic, Three-Dimensional Model of Audiology Practice Management

To complete the definitions, the operational definition of audiology practice management at the beginning of this section can be deconstructed into its component parts, using the formal definitions of practices as organizations and management as a dynamic, three-dimensional entity:

i. *In the business:* Audiologists must produce in line with organizational objectives.

ii. *In the human organization:* Audiologists must uphold organizational values and encourage similar action by coworkers in the practice.

iii. *In the dimension of public interest:* Audiologists must ensure that their individual and organizational efforts are ethical, legal, and positively influence the impact of audiology on society and the community.

This definition leads to important conclusions about successful audiologists, who must use many skills in practice that were not acquired in graduate school. These audiologists function simultaneously on several organizational levels. *They are all managers.** It is easy to see why Drucker calls this type of management an "entity." For audiology practices, the management entity is the audiologists, all of whom must manage in the business, in the human organization, and with the public interest in mind.

Practice Management Is a Balancing Act

The constant attention to three management dimensions also makes it easy to understand why Drucker calls this type of management entity "dynamic." Those who have worked in busy clinics or private practices may feel more comfortable describing the dynamic as a three-ring circus. By this analogy, practice management is a balancing act in which managers keep a number of balls in the air all the time. Good managers do not hesitate to introduce new and different balls to their mix and do not hold on to outmoded balls just because they are in the air. At the same time, they are careful

---

PEARL

Good managers master the never-ending balancing act by virtue of learned competencies and training.

---

*Chial (1998) lists a practical inventory of managerial attributes for audiologists. That list is reproduced in Chapter 6 in this volume.

to maintain a balanced mix of balls so that business, human, and public objectives are all well represented. It is a challenging job that never stops—there are always new balls, sometimes many more balls than before, and the balls often appear in groups that threaten to topple the delicate balance of business, human, and public interests. Like other skilled performers, good managers master this never-ending balancing act by virtue of learned competencies and training.

The motivation of this chapter and others in this volume is to explore and develop principles and applications that help audiologists learn to manage according to the objectives of the three-dimensional model of audiology practice management.

IS PRACTICE MANAGEMENT NECESSARY?

The short answer is "Yes." Practice management is necessary everywhere in the audiology profession, all the time. The operational and formal definitions evoke an ideal image of audiology practices as entities that function both as profit-making businesses and community resources by virtue of competent, caring audiologists who exercise solid management and business skills on a daily basis. Simplistically, this image suggests that all audiology practices should function in about the same way, with little need for discussion as to what is "right" or "best." After all, audiologists are trained in accredited institutions with a prescribed curriculum, profitability is an easy concept to grasp, and audiology services improve societal problems. What could be more straightforward than getting paid to provide services that help people hear better? Who needs a manager to do that?

Realistically, the simplistic ideal does not begin to account for the organizational differences and disagreements that currently exist in audiology. Without active management, these differences and disagreements could become problems for individual practices or for the profession as a whole. One obvious difference already mentioned is the employment data in Figures 1–1A and 1–1B. Private practice emerged as the dominant employment mode in the 1990s, shifting the profession's emphasis away from diagnostic testing and toward hearing aid dispensing. The shift produced many positive changes for the profession and for individual practices, but its repercussions include internecine and external quarrels. Universal agreement does not exist that this shift is in accord with the goals of the audiology profession (see Chapter 26 in *Diagnosis*). Individual practices assume more businesslike profiles when selling hearing aids, perhaps to the detriment of professional standing and ethical footing (see discussion of ethics in this volume in Chapters 3 and 9). Turf disputes surface because dispensing practices must compete with nonaudiology providers for hearing aid sales (Kirkwood, 1998a) and with physicians for the "entry point" of hearing care in health systems (Yaremchuk et al, 1990). Practice management must address these disagreements as they arise.

Among private practices, another obvious difference causing conflict is that audiologists do not all practice in the same kind of organization. Practices differ by objectives, personnel, markets served, and autonomy. The employment situation in audiology is so fluid that no business organizational type is dominant. At the time of this writing, new types of business organizations are appearing almost out of nowhere, employing audiologists in ways that no one envisioned just 10 years ago (Kirkwood, 1998b; Practice Builder Association, 1999). Professional and education organizations are in a similar state of flux, differing in their objectives but all vying for audiologists' membership or enrollment. The success or failure of organizations, from the smallest independent practice to the largest professional association, hinges on how competently the organizations are managed over time.

Natural Evolutions and Revolutions

Northern (1998b) calls this the "natural evolution" of organizations. As he and also Jerger (1998) comment, organizations begin to fragment if they fail to serve all their component parts. From a management perspective, the balancing act fails and new organizations (and managers) step in to fill the void. These natural evolutions are continuous and occur at all levels of the profession and within individual practices. The evolutions are reflected by changes in the employment settings in which audiologists chose to practice (see Figs. 1–1A and 1–1B), the journals read, the schools attended, the professional memberships renewed or dropped, the topics of continuing education selected, and so forth. The natural evolutions influence the three dimensions of audiology practice management by effecting many professional changes, including audiology training requirements, certification options, scope of practice, professional associations, professional autonomy, and work settings (Audiology Express!, 1998; Radcliffe, 1998).

PITFALL

Without active management, natural frictions disrupt individual practices and the profession as a whole.

Like a three-ring circus, natural evolutions are occurring simultaneously in areas outside of audiology (Jones, 1997). These external evolutions affect the internal workings of the audiology profession. Technological advances are already eroding audiology's diagnostic "turf" (Northern, 1998a). Other external changes stem from consumer demands that have prompted the emergence of managed care healthcare delivery services and the creation of the Americans with Disabilities Act. With these external changes come new questions and challenges to audiology practices (e.g., What services are provided? To whom are they provided? How are services provided? In what setting are they provided?) (Baquis, 1998). These external changes also introduce people with different backgrounds into the audiology profession, often in controlling positions. For example, audiology service delivery in managed care environments is often controlled and reviewed by employees of the managed care organization rather than employees of the audiology practice(s). Such supervisory personnel may have backgrounds in accounting, management, medical, or even sales, but rarely are they audiologists (Danhauer, 1998). In all cases these external changes affect the three-dimensional balance of business, human interest, and public interest. In the balancing act analogy these changes are like new and different balls that either replace or are added to those already in the air. Whether external changes are good or bad for an audiology organization, depends on how well and how quickly management integrates the changes and resumes the balancing act at a new equilibrium point.

Occasionally, natural evolutions produce so many internal and external changes that a revolution occurs. At such times, professions and organizations must seriously consider redefining business objectives and human organization objectives in ways that affect the public they market and serve. If consideration prompts action, a revolution occurs. For individual practices, revolutions can be as simple as moving the practice from a hospital setting to a retail mall or as complicated as forming an independent practice association with former competitors. For the profession, revolutions can be as small as the change in educational guidelines shown in the Appendix, or as large as the creation of AAA or the Au.D. Going back to the balancing act analogy, these are the times when practice managers pull all the balls out of the air and start new acts with different balls, or they drop the balls and yield to new managers with different acts.

Frictions Create Dynamic Tensions

New or unmet needs are the stimuli for change, which produces natural evolutions and revolutions in organizations. In the physical universe movement from one position to another creates friction, and the same is true of change in organizations. Audiology evolutions and revolutions are generating new needs in the three dimensions of practice management and spawning frictions of all types:

i. *In the business:* Business objectives are commandeering a larger role as audiologists become more entrepreneurial, hearing aid sales increase, and competitive pressures grow. "Needs of the business" may clash with "patient-first" professional motives.

ii. *In the human organization:* Audiologists assume more professional responsibility as they move to a rehabilitation emphasis, as the audiology scope of practice expands, and as audiology becomes the entry point for hearing healthcare. At the same time managed care controls may reduce professional autonomy and severely limit scope of services and professional "creative" time.

iii. *In the dimension of public interest:* As business practices become a greater part of the profile of audiology, the professional becomes much more susceptible to the impositions of legal and regulatory bodies and, thereby, loses considerable autonomy. (Paraphrased from Chapter 3 in this volume.)

These frictions even affect how audiologists perceive themselves and what they do. For instance, the increased penetration of managed care (Berkowitz, 1998) with emerging state consumer protection laws has stimulated strong interest in measuring outcomes of audiology services, especially hearing aid treatment intervention. The emphasis on treatment has produced observable changes in the way audiologists define themselves as professionals, such as the new classification title "Diagnostic Audiology *and Rehabilitation*" (italics added) in the 10th edition of the *International Classification of Disease System* (American Speech-Language-Hearing Association, 1997). In this milieu one practice manager states that audiologists are in the "business of changing behavior," whereas another states that audiologists are in the "business of data collection."* Both audiologists are correct in the sense that amplification use should result in positive behavioral changes that should be documented by outcome measures, but what a difference in outlook when organizational objectives *(fitting hearing aids on persons with hearing loss)* are expressed through the eyes of the human organization *(business of changing behavior)* versus those of the public interest *(business of data collection)*. The dichotomy does not signify that one outlook is more "right" than the other. In fact, both outlooks are necessary to manage the practice (as is the unstated outlook that hearing aid fittings must produce profit). The reason for the difference in statements has to do with who is judging audiology competencies. Audiologists *measure* changes in patients' behaviors to satisfy treatment goals that are set internally (human organization dimension). Practices *collect data* on treatment changes to satisfy intervention criteria that are set externally by legal or regulatory agencies. Figures 1–3 and 1–4 offer tangible evidence that this type of identity confusion is causing real friction in the audiology profession. According to a large industry survey in 1997 (Kirkwood, 1998a), 52% of the audiologists worked in environments penetrated by managed care, where at least 1 in 10 patients had managed care benefits (Fig. 1–3). Only 13% of the audiologists reported a "positive attitude" toward managed care (Fig. 1–4).

CONTROVERSIAL POINT

Are audiologists in the business of changing behavior or in the business of data collection?

Frictions are always frustrating, especially in the trenches of individual practices, where audiologists are running their businesses day to day, working diligently to provide excellent services, staying abreast of the technology curve, and keeping up with changes in the practice and the profession. Not everyone can or will maintain this level of effort, so the playing field is not level. As a result, one of the biggest sources of friction in the profession stems from resistance to change by practitioners who cannot or will not invest the effort to evolve.[†]

But, frictions are not necessarily bad. They identify potential problems and highlight areas that need improvement. Frictions prompt discourse that, at its best, results in a dynamic tension that maintains a forward momentum for audiology practices and the profession. Without friction, the status quo prevails and the organization languishes while more dynamic organizations step in to fill the void. Back to the balancing act analogy, the performer must always "top" the act with something new and more daring to keep the audience's attention and goodwill. If the act is dull and repetitious, it fails, and the audience goes in search of a better act. Good practice managers understand this analogy and welcome frictions as a means of improving their practices in the eyes of their patients, their personnel and their bankers. Examples of issues that cause friction

and discussion of how they are handled by practice management are discussed later in the chapter.

This section of this chapter posed the question "Is Practice Management Necessary?" It concludes as it began, with a definite "Yes." Audiology is changing rapidly in response to internal and external pressures. In some cases the changes follow a course of natural evolution as organizations move to accommodate new technologies, new constituents, and demands of the economy and the workforce.[‡] Managers are necessary to weigh these changes against the three-dimensional practice management model and decide how and when to adopt the changes for the good of the practices or other organizations. This is the classic balancing act that makes management worth its keep.

In a few cases change is so rapid or draconian that bedrock positions shift, with revolution as the outcome. One need only peruse the first two volumes of this trilogy to realize that evolution culminating in revolution is standard operating procedure for diagnostic audiology and hearing aid dispensing over the last decade. These are exhilarating, exciting times, but they are also the times that try audiologists' souls, not to mention their practices and associations. These are the times when good practice management is the difference between life and death of any organization; when the balancing act can no longer sustain, it is management's job to land the organization on the "right" side of revolution. This is the ringmaster role of management that makes it absolutely necessary to the survival and fitness of our practices and our professional organizations.

HOW DOES PRACTICE MANAGEMENT WORK?

Many management experts exist and many books are dedicated solely to analysis of management processes. As editors and audiologists, we do not pretend to know as much about management as these experts, nor is this chapter intended to compete with books written by these experts. Therefore the following discussion is practical in nature, eschewing management theories in favor of personal experiences and examples from the audiology profession. Audiologists who are interested in the history of management and synopses of management theories are referred to Chapter 20 in Hosford-Dunn et al (1995).

It Takes Common Sense

As trivial as it sounds, exercising common sense is arguably the single most important part of practice management. "Common sense" is hardly an academic or intellectual construct, so the ensuing brief discussion is intended only to entertain and lightly instruct.

Our culture is replete with aphorisms for every occasion that serve as rules to live by for those who aim to achieve wealth, harmony, and respect in their lives. It should come as

---

*Both quotes are real and published, but their authorship is left anonymous in this discussion to "protect the innocent."
[†]See Skafte's comments on this issue in Chapter 21.

[‡]Audiologists who favor acronyms can refer to these as PEST (political, economic, social, and technological) issues.

Managed Care Penetration of Audiology Services

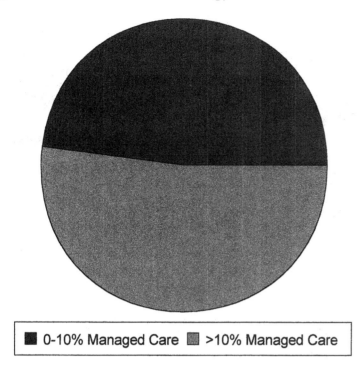

■ 0-10% Managed Care ▨ >10% Managed Care

Figure 1–3 Managed care penetration of audiology services in the United States in 1997, showing that 48% of audiologists worked in unpenetrated settings (less than 1:10 ratio of managed care services to private pay or indemnity insurance) and 52% of audiologists worked in penetrated settings (more than 1:10 ratio). (Data estimated from Kirkwood [1999].)

no surprise that these same aphorisms apply in the three-dimensional model of practice management. Interestingly, most adages are opposed by equally true-sounding aphorisms (e.g., "absence makes the heart grow fonder" versus "out of sight, out of mind"), so "managing" to live a well-balanced life requires the knack of selecting the right aphorism for every occasion. The same is true in practice management, which must always balance needs of the business against those of the staff and patients. In the three-dimensional model the business structure requires attention to detail ("the devil is in the details") but not to the point that the overview is lost ("can't see the forest for the trees"). It also requires financial

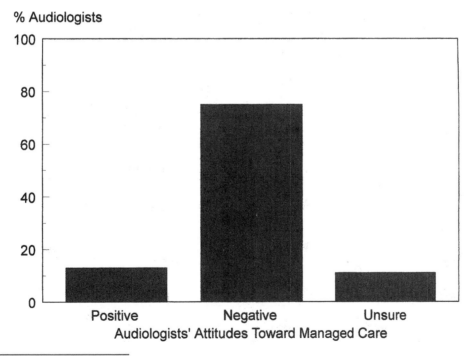

Figure 1–4 Attitude of audiologists surveyed in Figure 1–3 toward managed care. (Data estimated from Kirkwood [1999].)

control ("a penny saved is a penny earned") but not beyond reason ("penny wise and pound foolish"). In the human structure one of management's jobs is to inspire efficiency and productivity ("a stitch in time saves nine") but not to the point of diminishing returns ("haste makes waste"). In the public interest domain the need to take care of patients (golden rule) must be balanced by the need to keep the business viable ("charity begins at home"). Although slightly tongue-in-cheek, these examples underscore the point that practice management is always a balancing act that "works" by making context-sensitive decisions in which a course of action is chosen on the basis of all the information available.

Good practice management is also guided by common organizational pledges ("semper fi"; "loyal, faithful, and true"; ". . . help other people and obey the law of the pack") that give common sense advice on how to live with and inspire groups of people. The Rotarian's "Four-Way Test" in Table 1–3 is a fairly elaborate and very useful pledge for practice managers, touching on all three dimensions of the practice management model.

TABLE 1–3 The Four-Way Test from Rotary International

The Four-Way Test of the things we think, say, or do:
First . . . Is it the Truth?
Second . . . Is it Fair to all concerned?
Third . . . Will it Build Goodwill and better *friendships*?
Fourth . . . Will it be Beneficial to all concerned?
Rotary International

The Rotary pledge stresses that the four-way test applies not only to what is done but, also to what is said and thought as well. This is an important, commonsensical point for practice management, but one that is easy to overlook in day-to-day practice management. In an audiology practice words must match deeds at all levels or patients and staff will perceive mixed messages. If management states that patients are important or that staff members are empowered to make management decisions, then *all* practice policies and *all* staff actions must reflect those statements. In today's jargon, this is what is meant by "walking the walk and talking the talk."*

Getting the Act Together

Common sense is particularly important during the formative stage of a business. The following sequential steps are prescribed for starting or redirecting a practice (Hosford-Dunn et al, 1995):

 I. Define the business
    A. Who are the primary and secondary customers?
    B. How are the customers reached?
    C. What do the customers value?

 II. Develop a vision of the organization (mission statement and practice philosophy)
    A. Write the purpose
    B. Write the core values
 III. Identify *strengths, weaknesses, opportunities,* and *threats* (SWOT)
 IV. Write specific and measurable goals and objectives
 V. Set strategies outlining plans for achieving goals and objectives
 VI. Specify tactics for what will be done by whom and by when to meet objectives

If one follows these steps in the prescribed order, it becomes clear that practice management is an entity that always exists *before* creation of the organization that it will subsequently manage. Recall that Drucker envisions practice management as a dynamic entity and this is an example of why it is dynamic: It plans and creates what it will manage. Of course, not all groups follow the prescribed steps and not all practice management is dynamic. Organizations can come into being by accident, without any planning. In such cases practice management is a passive pastiche, pasted on as an afterthought. Internal frictions are likely to abound in these chaotic organizations.

Taking the Act on the Road: Using Frictions as Stepping Stones

In a well-run organization the SWOT analysis in Step III of the previous section is the first of many times that practice management brushes up against frictions of one type or another. As stated earlier, good practice managers welcome frictions as a means of improving practices in the eyes of patients, personnel, and bankers. This section looks at a few of the "frictions" (Table 1–4) and examines how they are handled in the three-dimensional, dynamic practice management model.

What Is Known versus What Is Implemented

In this friction the practice management decision is complicated by too much information rather than not enough information. Researchers and academicians frequently complain, with some justification, that clinicians do not use all the information and resources at their disposal to diagnose or treat patients with hearing loss. For instance, it is *known* from clinical research that multifrequency acoustic immitance yields more diagnostic information than conventional acoustic immitance (see Chapter 17 *Diagnosis*), yet multifrequency immitance is rarely *implemented* in clinical practice (Martin et al, 1998). This is so for a variety of reasons. Implementation requires replacing existing equipment with new equipment that is more expensive; it also may be larger and less portable. Practicing audiologists are used to single frequency immitance and many do not understand or feel comfortable interpreting results of multifrequency immitance. Depending on the patient population, the additional diagnostic information may be more or less helpful to the clinician. But, given the *known* benefits of multifrequency immitance, it is likely that it will become the test of choice when it is packaged for ease of

---

*Refer to Chapter 4 in this volume for a more complete discussion of this topic.

TABLE 1–4 Some practice management issues

Examples of Dynamic Tensions in Audiology Practices	
What is *taught*	What is *practiced*
What is *known*	What is *implemented*
What is *complete*	What is *allowed*
What is *desirable*	What is *available*
What is *recommended*	What is *affordable or reimbursed*
What is a *right*	What is a *privilege*
What is an *organizational need*	What is a *patient need*
What is *necessary*	What is *sufficient*
Practices that are *ethical*	Practices that are *unethical*
Outcome measures for *counseling*	Data for *utilization review*

service delivery (i.e., automated, quick, compact) and interpretation (e.g., automated diagnostic categories).

Here is how the three-dimensional management model works in this example:

i. *In the business:* The organizational objective is to include acoustic immitance as part of every comprehensive audiometry evaluation in a cost-effective manner. Multifrequency immitance equipment will not be purchased for this purpose unless proven cost-effective.

ii. *In the human organization:* The audiologists who perform acoustic immitance tests want equipment that is accessible, rapid, reliable, and results oriented. Management needs input from the audiologists after they have had an opportunity to test drive the multifrequency immitance equipment in the clinic and compare it with their present equipment. If the audiologists' responses are mixed, management may enter into dialog with the equipment manufacturer or supplier to resolve ergonomic issues.

iii. *In the dimension of public interest:* The organization is aware that multifrequency acoustic immitance affords better diagnostic information in some cases. The first step is to estimate differences in diagnostic outcomes for a representative patient sample that would accrue if single tone immitance were replaced by multifrequency immitance in the clinical protocol. If outcome differences are deemed clinically significant, the next step is to make the case to consumers of care in an attempt to influence reimbursement decisions.

Management's role is to balance the public interest information gleaned from the public interest analyses against business objectives and audiologists' needs and develop an equation in which estimated value to consumers and projected revenue to the business exceed the financial and human costs of new equipment (e.g., purchase price, physical placement and access, training time, test administration time, test interpretation time). A key aspect of dynamic practice management in this example is that it works proactively rather than reactively. The final steps in the human organiza-

tion and public interest analyses call for management to use clinical data to influence equipment manufacturing and payors' reimbursement rates. These proactive stances illustrate how practice management works by turning frictions into dynamic tensions that serve to improve and advance the organization in all three dimensions.

SPECIAL CONSIDERATION

A key aspect of dynamic practice management is that it works proactively rather than reactively. Practice management "works" by working all the time, before the practice is even a reality and long after patients have gone home.

Other Issues that Cause Friction

Some of the issues in Table 1–4 have already been discussed or alluded to in other contexts. For example, in the previous acoustic immitance example, potential exists for future friction if clinical data support the use of multifrequency immitance but managed care refuses to reimburse for that service at a higher rate *(friction between what is recommended and what is reimbursed; between what is complete and what is allowed)*. If that friction arises, it begs the question of whether the better test should be administered to patients even if they cannot pay for it *(friction between healthcare as a right and healthcare as a privilege)*. The audiologists may have concerns that reflect their graduate training in immitance testing *(friction between what was taught and what is practiced)*. Suppose the clinical data support the use of multifrequency immitance but the equipment is too expensive to purchase *(friction between what is needed and what is available; friction between organizational needs and patient needs)*? Suppose that a hearing aid manufacturer whose products are not used in the practice offers to purchase the immitance equipment for the practice in return for a minimum of 10 hearing aid orders a month (*friction between what is ethical and what is unethical*)? Is there friction if the same offer is made by a manufacturer whose products are dispensed regularly in the practice and that is considered a "partner" of the practice (Iskowitz, 1998)?

The list goes on and on, even for simple diagnostic examples. One can only imagine the list attached to controversial hearing aid fitting approaches. Frictions and subfrictions abound, and practice management must anticipate the frictions by using SWOT analyses and making informed decisions that consistently land the practice on the most satisfactory, or least objectionable, side of every question.* Practice management "works" by working all the time before the practice is even a reality and long after patients have gone home. For practice management, it begins before it starts. As for ending, to quote Yogi Berra, "It's not over till it's over." Practice management may not be rocket science, it may be harder.

MANAGEMENT COMPETENCIES AND TRAINING

Practice management does *not* always work. Numerous examples of failed management decisions causing organizational setbacks or even demise exist. Practice management does not work in the absence of management competencies. In almost every case management competencies are not innate but are acquired by training.

In What?

One reason that practice management fails has to do with limitations in today's graduate education programs and practicum settings for audiology (Geffner, 1997). As Silverman (1999) aptly puts it, "A number of issues affect the management of communicative disorders and tend to be considered superficially—if at all—in the disorder-oriented courses in speech-language pathology and audiology curriculums." (p. ix) This refrain is addressed head-on in Chapter 2, where Harford reviews and critiques *Professional Education in Audiology*. Few graduate programs offer courses in practice management, but this is changing as Au.D. programs become more widespread. As to what competencies such courses should teach, the ASHA published curriculum guidelines that identify six areas of knowledge and skill (American Speech-Language-Hearing Association, 1995):

- Basic management
- Service planning
- Practice, business, and government rules
- Computers and office automation
- Quality improvement issues
- Risk management and professional liability

The ASHA "Guidelines for Education in Practice Management" is reproduced in the Appendix. At the time of this

writing, few graduate training programs have adopted the recommended guidelines into their curricula. Moreover, demonstrated competency in these areas is not required for ASHA certification in audiology. In the authors' opinion this is an oversight that has grave implications for the viability of audiology as an autonomous profession. It is a good example of how *not* to manage.

The need for guidelines in daily practice has prompted preparation of several protocol manuals for audiology service delivery (see American Speech-Language-Hearing Association, 1993; Joint Audiology Committee Statement on Overview of Audiologic Services, in preparation; Margolis, 1997); but none of these manuals directly addresses the competency areas identified previously in the ASHA Guidelines for practice management.

PITFALL

Practice management does not work in the absence of management competencies.

By Whom?

Another example of how *not* to manage is for audiologists to attempt to practice without seeking some business and management training on their own. The scenario is familiar, if not encouraging. Audiologists with good professional skills open practices without first preparing a sufficient business case. The practices flounder or fail for a variety of reasons, usually related to high overhead, poor organizational skills, poor tax planning, or inadequate or inappropriate marketing. Here, balance in the three-dimensional practice management model is sorely lacking in the business organization sector.

Alternately, some practices flourish, either because of sheer luck or because the audiologist possesses innate business acumen. New problems are likely to arise in start-up practices that experience early success, and this has to do with an imbalance in the human organization. As the practice grows, additional audiologists are hired to handle the workload and increase the bottom line. Many good audiologists with good business heads do not have good people-handling skills. If these audiologists function as owners and practice managers, they run a real danger of disturbing the delicate balance of practice management by diminishing the importance of the human organization. The typical result is high staff turnover with concomitant increases in staff training costs and decreases in productivity. This is not an indictment of audiologists, but a general observation that human resource management is a rare and highly valuable skill in any organization.

Some audiologists handle the obstacle by staying small, rationalizing that the only way to get things done right is to do it themselves. Three practice management problems exist with this approach—one for each of the three practice management dimensions. In the business organization growth and profit are limited to the productivity of one audiologist who must try to see new patients while caring for an ever-growing backlog of patients requiring follow-up care. In the human organization the only asset is the lone audiologist, who runs the risk of burnout as the practice tries to grow in

---

*For an example of a complete SWOT analysis of private practice and managed care, see Hosford-Dunn (1999).

spite of itself. In the public interest dimension continuity of services to patients depends on the health, age, and motivation of the audiologist. This is negative practice management in action: business trends show negative growth over time; the value of the practice sans audiologist is low or nil, so it dies when the audiologist does, leaving patients in the lurch.

All the preceding scenarios are reasons why audiologists must acquire some practice management training and competencies. Some training opportunities are present within the profession. Continuing education offerings and publications on practice management topics are offered by state associations, AAA, ADA, and ASHA (AAA, 1999; Geier, 1997; Hosford-Dunn et al, 1994; Marion et al, 1999), hearing industries, and hearing publications (Bronkesh, 1998; Kochkin, 1993; Kochkin & Strom, 1997), audiology clinics, and audiology independent professional associations. The AAA website (www/audiology.org) contains practice management information (e.g., AAA Physicians Referral Task Force). At least one audiology independent professional association offers individualized practice management tools for private practice audiologists (Hosford-Dunn & Katz, 1997; Katz & Hosford-Dunn, 1997). This textbook and one other (Hosford-Dunn et al, 1995) are devoted entirely to practice management education for audiologists.

A readily available option for gaining practice management proficiency is to journey beyond the profession for management training. The chapters in this book underscore the necessity of this approach at this time. Even though most of the chapters are written by audiologists, their topics are rarely addressed in audiology graduate curricula offerings and their references rarely come from the refereed journals of the profession. A few of the chapters had to be "outsourced" to nonaudiologists with special expertise in a particular aspect of practice management (e.g., chapters 3, 5, and 15). It is also not an oversight that two of the three authors of the "Futures" chapter in this volume are not audiologists. In the same vein not all audiologists can or want to upgrade to an Au.D., but certainly all audiologists can search out training by enrolling in accounting, business, or computer classes offered by the Small Business Administration, by local colleges, or universities. Most of the latter also offer distance learning opportunities (Losak, 1998). In addition, a number of businesses offer seminar training in practice management issues (e.g., Fred Pryor Seminars; Survival Strategies; Practice Builder Association; Dale Carnegie).

Yet another option is to go outside the profession to obtain a management team. Pro and con arguments exist as to whether this approach yields good or bad management of audiology organizations. The arguments are best framed with reference to the three-dimensional model of practice management. On the pro side, outside managers have competencies that lend themselves to efficiencies within the business organization and the human organization. These managers are trained in how to manage businesses and human resources to achieve organizational objectives and optimize productivity. Large audiology practices and professional organizations that employ office managers or management teams with MBAs endorse this approach wholeheartedly (see Kieserman, 1996). Practices of all sizes that outsource some jobs (e.g., payroll accounting, computer support, marketing) acknowledge the usefulness of the approach without embracing it totally.

On the con side the competencies of nonaudiology managers usually do not include an appreciation of the "patient-first" training that distinguishes audiology, dentistry, medicine, and so on as health-related professions. Outside managers have difficulty balancing the three-dimensional practice model because their training and past experience do not recognize the public interest dimension as an equal player. When one part of the triumvirate is diminished, all parts are affected and the balancing act may fail. In this instance the outside management rightly perceives a fiduciary duty to the organization (e.g., private practice owner, corporate shareholders, elected officials) and translates this duty into business objectives that audiologists are expected to meet by their daily actions and productivity (emphasis on business organization and directives to human organization). Just as rightfully, the audiologists perceived a fiduciary duty to their patients first and the business second (emphasis on public interest dimension before business organization).*

PEARL
Human resource management is a rare and highly valuable skill in any organization.

This is a classic case of two rights making a wrong. When business objectives are set by outside managers without sufficient regard for professional objectives, conflict arises and balance is lost in the practice. The human organization is pulled in two directions and may experience a breakdown, either because a patient-first attitude prevails over management's demand for productivity or because audiologists subsume professional responsibility to business demands. Either way, loss of balance places both practitioners and organizations at risk: in the former, because the business no longer turns a profit; in the latter, because day-to-day operations may not endure ethical or legal scrutiny. All scenarios point to a failure of practice management.

PRINCIPLES THAT PROVIDE STRUCTURE

As editors of the third volume in this series, we identified certain refrains that caused confusion, consternation, and occasional hostility for the authors, who are themselves competent audiologists trying to grapple with various aspects of "practice" and "management." In most instances the frictions in Table 1–4 derive from discussions that surfaced as the authors prepared various chapters. Their efforts are consistent with one purpose of this volume, which is to respond to these nagging refrains with infusions of structured information, much of it integrated from sources outside the discipline and profession of audiology.

These refrains were closely coupled to a call for guiding principles for managing our practices. The volumes are neatly divided into "Principles" and "Applications on Diagnosis and Treatment" sections, and this was the intended

---

*See Chapter 6 of this volume for a fuller discussion of this concept.

plan for the Practice Management volume. However, the superficial and near-random consideration of management issues in graduate training noted earlier makes it very difficult to arrive at a set of principles governing these issues, and some readers may take issue with our efforts to categorize chapters. Those authors who agreed to write chapters for the "Principles" section of this volume were exploring new territory or bringing new order to old ground without getting stuck in existing ruts. The latter is exemplified by Helmick's chapter on ethics in this volume, which acknowledges that ethics are not absolute or unchangeable but represent guiding principles to enhance the impact of our practices and our profession on society. Much new ground is covered in complementary chapters by Abrams and his associates, in which we are introduced to the related principles of "Quality: The Controlling Principle of Practice Management" and "Outcome Measures: The Audiologic Difference."

Another refrain is that audiologists have little exposure to other disciplines whose principles form the very core of the business aspects of audiology practices. Many audiologists may find that statement almost nonsensical: How can another discipline form the core of an audiology practice? Chapters in the "Principles" section by Zapala ("Human Resource Management") and Staab ("Marketing Principles") pull together structured principles from public policy, business management, and marketing. These compelling chapters convincingly show that audiologists are not the first managers to encounter thorny personnel issues, discover mentoring, perform needs assessments, or collect and analyze data. It is a humbling and exhilarating experience to realize that audiologists can tap into cohesive theories and well-done research in disciplines much larger and older than audiology, rather than dealing with such issues piecemeal and superficially.

A closely related refrain from the private practice sector is that audiologists do not have practicum experience in technical, business, and management applications. How can they know what they do not know? The routine in the past was to find out by stumbling on an issue in practice. Once again, the de facto treatment was superficial and contributed little to a knowledge base because we usually hoped it was a one-time encounter and rarely communicated our fleeting knowledge to others. The final chapter in the "Principles" section by Clark and Benson is a remarkably condensed look at the broad range of "Private Practice Issues" that can and do arise, many of which are highlighted as "Pearls," "Pitfalls," "Special Considerations," and "Controversial Points." The chapter is necessarily short on principles, but it belongs in this section because it makes the important point that private practitioners must wear "many hats." Consistent with that principle, this chapter serves as a jumping off point—pointing to the remaining sections that are organized according to practice applications.

APPLYING STRUCTURE TO PRACTICES

The "Clinical Applications" section is composed of four chapters addressing issues that arise in most audiology practices. "Ethics in Professional Practice" by Newman-Ryan and Decker reviews general principles of ethical behavior manifest in ASHA and AAA Codes of Ethics. The authors use

thought-provoking, sometimes controversial case studies to show how the Codes are enforced. "Preparing the Clinical Report" by Gonzenbach looks at a variety of approaches to documentation of patient interactions. "Infection Control" (Kemp and Bankaitis) and "Cerumen Management" (Roeser and Wilson) educate readers on characteristics of cerumen and principles of infection, respectively, and proceed to describe clinical procedures for both. The "Clinical Applications" chapter grouping is editorially interesting because it illustrates the uneven development of different aspects of audiology practice management and the resulting tensions: some things that are done are well documented but controversial (i.e., cerumen management); some are universally accepted to the point that they are de facto principles (i.e., infection control); some aspects enjoy the status of organizational principles but are not universally agreed on (i.e., ethics); some are so commonplace that they are taken for granted, even though little consensus exists as to how they should be done (i.e., clinical reporting).

CONTROVERSIAL POINT

Audiology practice management is not consistent. Some activities are well documented but controversial; other activities are done so often they are taken for granted, even though little consensus exists as to how they should be done.

The "Business Applications" section contains six chapters covering a wide range of topics that at first glance seem to bear little or no relation to one another. This is essentially correct and serves to underscore the "many hats" principle of Clark and Benson. The section begins with Windmill, Cunningham, and Johnson's discussion of the physical plant ("Designing an Audiology Practice"). Chapters by Kasewurm ("The Business Plan and Practice Accounting") and Dunn ("Managerial Accounting for Daily and Long-Term Practice Success") provide lively discussions of normally deadly topics. Freeman, Barimo, and Fox follow up with a high-level discussion of "Financial Management of Audiology Practices and Clinics." The last two chapters in this section address the topic of the 1990s: managed care. In "Managed Care and Reimbursement" Pessis and Freint offer guidelines for working in managed care environments and close their chapter with an interesting practicum section. But what if the practice is not "in" managed care—how does one establish dialogue with and secure business from a managed care organization? Benson and Gudmundsen address these complicated questions in a chapter with a necessarily long title: "Proposing Audiology Services and Responding to Requests for Proposals for Managed Care Contracting."

The final applications section, "Computer Applications," divides along hardware ("Basic Computer Principles") and software applications ("Computer Applications for Audiology and Dispensing") in extremely comprehensive chapters written by Wynne and de Jonge, respectively. These chapters aim to simultaneously offer in-depth education and practical tips for almost every conceivable audiology application. It is axiomatic that practice management requires office automation, and these two important chapters should be frequently referenced when reading other chapters in this book. As editors, we know of no comparable computer discussion in the audiology literature.

CONCLUSIONS

This volume ends in the same manner as did the first two volumes, with several authors bravely predicting the future—of practice management in this case. Given the friction between ideal practice management and the current realities, it comes as no surprise that predictions vary widely in their optimism and scope. Dr. James Jerger foresees continued difficulty, growing pains, and the danger of professional diminishment as audiology departs from traditional mooring in diagnostic audiology and moves toward a more retail presence. Conversely, Marjorie Skafte of *The Hearing Review,* sees a long and fruitful history in the move of audiologists toward hearing aid dispensing and applauds the profession's efforts to gain business expertise. Dr. Lars Kolind, past president of Oticon International, foresees increasing alliance between audiologists and manufacturers, resulting in better product distribution, more "audiologic" approaches to designing products that meet the needs of persons with hearing loss, and development of hearing devices that are unlike anything previously encountered in the hearing care field. It is a fitting end

to a set of books that mark the end of one century and the beginning of a new one.

Looking toward the future in 1995, Hosford-Dunn et al commented and predicted in a chapter entitled *Audiologists as Managers:*

> The old-fashioned scope of management to control and monitor is being replaced with new requirements to motivate, train, support, and lead. As audiologists learn and implement modern management concepts, the profession has an opportunity to improve the level of service to patients and become a more vigorous entry point into the healthcare system. (p. 480)

The fact that an entire volume of an audiology handbook is now dedicated to teaching and implementing practice management marks an important step toward incorporating a forward-thinking mode of audiologists as managers into audiology training programs and practices. As editors, we have worked closely with all the authors who contributed to the Practical Management volume and have come to believe that the three-dimensional model of practice management is not only exciting and inspirational, but is "doable" on the basis of the teachings of this volume. By learning to be managers and by managing practices well, audiologists have the potential to enhance all aspects of the profession: improve service delivery, empower practitioners, raise profitability, expand market visibility, and increase the satisfaction of both providers and patients.

Appendix
Guidelines for Education in Practice Management

Education in Audiology Practice Management

Ad Hoc Committee on Practice Management in Audiology

The Guidelines for Education in Practice Management were prepared by the American Speech-Language-Hearing Association (ASHA) Ad Hoc Committee on Practice Management in Audiology and approved by the ASHA Executive Board (EGB 2-94) and 1994 Legislative Council (LC 8-94). Members of the committee who prepared the guidelines include Holly Hosford-Dunn, chair; Jane H. Baxter; Evelyn Cherow, ex officio; Alan L. Desmond; Gary Jacobson; Jean L. Johnson; and Patty F. Martin. Diane L. Eger, vice president for professional practices (1991–93), served as monitoring vice president. These guidelines are an official statement of ASHA. They provide guidance on the use of specific practice procedures but are not official standards of the Association.

Specific Competency Areas in Practice Management

These areas are directly related to practice management and are suggested for inclusion in a model curriculum for a graduate level course in practice management in audiology. They are considered the minimum requirements for providing an adequate base of knowledge for managing a practice. Students should be encouraged to take additional classes in cognate areas such as accounting and marketing. Persons managing or directing audiology services should demonstrate knowledge of, and skills in, the following areas:

I. Basic Management, including:
   A. Preparation of feasibility studies, market surveys, business plans
   B. Account management, budgeting, billing & collections
   C. Knowledge of financial reports (balance sheet, income statement)
   D. Human resource management/staff recruiting
   E. Knowledge of healthcare models (e.g., PPO, HMO, fee for service, sliding scale)
   F. Marketing
   G. Contracts and negotiations
   H. Financial planning/retirement plans

II. Service Planning
   A. Physical plant
      1. Site selection
      2. Equipment selection
      3. Leasing space and/or equipment
      4. Automation
   B. Service structure
      1. Record keeping
      2. Establishing referral networks
      3. Scheduling patients
      4. Fee setting

III. Practice, Business, and Government Rules
   A. Americans with Disabilities Act (ADA) accessibility considerations
   B. Federal employment laws
   C. Accreditation requirements (e.g., Joint Commission on Accreditation of Healthcare Organizations [JCAHO], ASHA Professional Services Board [PSB], Commission on Accreditation of Rehabilitation Facilities [CARF])
   D. Antitrust regulations
   E. Business entities: tax implication and government reporting regulations
   F. Requirements for nonprofit status
   G. Ethical codes of practice
   H. Licensing requirements

IV. Computers and Office Automation
   A. Diagnostic applications
   B. Data storage/access
   C. Tracking patient outcomes and consumer satisfaction
   D. Professional correspondence
   E. Scheduling and billing
   F. Marketing applications

V. Quality Improvement Issues
   A. Personnel/leadership training
   B. Client satisfaction/functional assessment
   C. Supervision
   D. Multicultural issues
   E. Professionalism (interactions with competitors, colleagues, associates, agencies)

VI. Risk Management and Professional Liability

    A. Insurance

    B. Best practice guidelines and preferred practice patterns

    C. Malpractice trends in the profession

    D. Infection control requirements

American Speech-Language-Hearing Association. (1995). Guidelines for Education in Audiology Practice Management. *ASHA,* 37 (Suppl. 14); 20.

REFERENCES

American Academy of Audiology. (1999). Practice manage instructional course descriptions. In: *11th Annual Convention and Exposition Registration Program.* (pp. 84–89). Alexandria, VA: AAA.

American Speech-Language-Hearing Association. (1993). Preferred practice patterns for the professions of speech-language pathology and audiology. *ASHA, 35* (Suppl. 3); 1–102.

American Speech-Language-Hearing Association. (1995). Guidelines for Education in Audiology Practice Management. *ASHA, 37* (Suppl. 14); 20.

American Speech-Language-Hearing Association. (1997). 1997 Year in Review—Audiology. *ASHA, 39;*4.

Audiology Express! (1998). Opinion survey on the Doctor of Audiology. IV(1);1–6.

Baquis, D. (1998). A primer on hearing assistance technology and the ADA: Public policy and the ADA. *The Hearing Review, 5*(6);38–40.

Berkowitz, A.O. (1998). U.S. managed care penetration. *The Hearing Review, 5*(10);28–32.

Bronkesh, S.J. (1998). Handling complaints. *Audiology Today, 10*(6);14.

Chermak, G.D., Traynham, W.A., Seikel, J.A., & Musiek, F.E. (1998). Professional education and assessment practices in central auditory processing. *JAAA, 9*(6);452–465.

Collins, J.C., & Porras, J.I. (1997). *Built to last.* New York: HarperCollins.

Danhauer, J. (1998). Who are those major multi-office audiology groups moving in on us, and—is this town big enough for the both of us? *Audiology Today, 10*(2);47–51.

Drucker, P.F. (1986). *The practice of management.* New York: Harper & Row.

Geffner, D. (1997). Graduate programs face realities of health care. *Advance for Speech-Language Pathologists & Audiologists,* August 25, (p. 4).

Geier, K. (1997). *The handbook of self-assessment and verification measures of communication performance.* Academy of Dispensing Audiologists.

Hosford-Dunn, H. (1999). What does managed care want? There's good news and bad news! *Audiology Today, 11*(1);21–23.

Hosford-Dunn, H., Baxter, J., Desmond, A., Jacobson, G., Johnson, J., Martin, P., & Cherow, E. (Eds.) (1994). *Development and management of audiology practices.* Rockville, MD: ASHA.

Hosford-Dunn, H.L., Dunn, D.R., & Harford, E.R. (1995). *Audiology business and practice management.* San Diego, CA: Singular Publishing Group.

Hosford-Dunn, H.L., & Katz, K.R. (1997). *Employees' policy and procedures guide.* Tucson, AZ: Arizona Audiology Network, LLC.

Iskowitz, M. (1998). Manufacturers as partners. *Advance for Speech-Language Pathologists and Audiologists, January 26* (pp. 13–15, 29).

Jerger, J. (1998). It's time to break free! *Audiology Today, 10*(6);11.

Joint Audiology Committee Statement on Overview of Audiologic Services. (In press.)

Jones, D.J. (1997). Editorial: Let's join the consumer revolution. *American Journal of Medical Quality, 12*(3);141–142.

Katz, K.R., & Hosford-Dunn, H.L. (1997). *Preparing a response for a request for proposal for audiology services and hearing aid dispensing for managed care.* Tucson, AZ: Arizona Audiology Network, LLC.

Kieserman, R. (1996). Hiring administrator can benefit practice. *Advance for Speech-Language Pathologists and Audiologists,* September 30, (p. 3).

Kirkwood, D. (1998a). In survey, dispensers report growth, express views on professional issues. *The Hearing Journal, 51*(3);21–30.

Kirkwood, D. (1998b). The corporatization of dispensing: Is it the wave of the future? *The Hearing Journal, 51*(8);25–36.

Kochkin, S. (1993). MarkeTrak III identifies key factors in determining customer satisfaction. *The Hearing Journal, 46*(8);39–44.

Kochkin, S., & Strom, D.E., (Eds.) (1997). *High performance hearing solutions* (Vol. I.). Supplement to the Hearing Review, (pp. 28–31).

Losak, J. (1998). Hearing the call of distance learning. *Audiology Today, 10*(5);19.

Margolis, R.H. (1997). *Audiology clinical protocols.* Needham Heights, MA: Allyn & Bacon.

Marion, M.W., Burkart, B., Dunn, J., Freeman, B., Goldstein, M., & Rybarski, M. (1999). Responding to the age wave and marketing audiology services to the primary care physician. In: *11th AAA Convention and Exposition Registration Program* (p. 38). Alexandria, VA: AAA.

Martin, F.N., Champlin, C.A., & Chambers, J.A. (1998). Seventh Survey of Audiometric Practices in the United States. *JAAA, 9*(2);95–104.

Northern, J.L. (1998a). Technology marches on! *Audiology Today, 10*(1);4.

Northern, J.L. (1998b). Untying the ties that bind. *Audiology Today, 10*(5);7.

Practice Builder Association. (1999). Update: The rapid changes in hearing care. Research Report #98-273, Market Research Division, (pp. 1–14).

Radcliffe, D. (1998). Scope of practice. It's more than turf wars. *The Hearing Journal, 51*(10);23–34.

Silverman, F.H. (1999). *Professional issues in speech-language pathology and audiology.* Boston: Allyn & Bacon.

Stoner, J.A.F., & Wankel, C. (1986). *Management* (3rd ed.). Englewood Cliffs, NJ: Prentice-Hall.

Yaremchuk, K., Schmidt, J., & Dickson, L. (1998). *Hearing For Hospital Medical Journal, 38*(1);13–15.

Chapter 2

Professional Education in Audiology

Earl R. Harford

Outline

The first people graduated from a university with a specialty in audiology in the late 1940s. The content of the curriculum of these early graduates was weighted in speech correction, as it was called then, and speech science. Other areas of study were anatomy and physiology of the ear and vocal mechanism, acoustics, psychoacoustics, pathological conditions of the ear, medical/surgical treatment of the ear, and psychology. The courses specific to applied audiology were limited to audiometry and aural rehabilitation, which included lip-

reading, auditory training, and hearing aids. Compared with today's standards, the curriculum offered these early audiologists was basically the same as that of the speech pathologists with a smattering of audiology. In fact, most of the course registrations were composed of both speech pathology and audiology students. This is understandable because the substance to teach in this young discipline was limited and very few students were interested in audiology. Nearly all audiological subject matter was borrowed from other disciplines. Independent study and dissertations, of course, involved some aspect of hearing.

Most of the small number of audiologists who completed a university program by 1950 held the Ph.D.; very few terminated with a master's degree. Most of the Ph.D. graduates joined the speech pathology faculties of other universities to teach a limited number of courses, develop an audiology curriculum, or conduct research on the auditory system. A few actually started audiology and speech pathology graduate programs from scratch.

After a decade of expansion, the curricula undergirding the discipline of audiology settled into a status quo in the mid 1960s. The objective of this chapter is to provide some insight into the history of the education of audiologists, the current status, and some projections for the future.

SPECIAL CONSIDERATION

After more than 30 years of quiescence, the preparation of audiologists is now undergoing a major reawakening and is on the threshold of a new era of educational development largely because of the emergence of a professional doctorate, called the Au.D., and a move to require a doctorate as the entry-level degree to practice audiology.

IN THE BEGINNING

"Audiology"

Let us first investigate the origin of the use of the word *audiology*. Although hearing aid dealers, Trainor and Hargrave claimed they used the term *audiology* starting about 1939 (Berger, 1976), it did not come into popular use until several years later. In fact, about 1940, the John Kirby Sextet recorded

17

a musical selection entitled, "Audiology"(J. Curran, 1998, personal communication). So, the word had been in use, but not as a descriptor of an academic discipline. It was during World War II, however, when Raymond Carhart, Ph.D., and Norton Canfield, M.D., coined the term to describe the services being provided military personnel with hearing loss in an Aural Rehabilitation Center at Deshon Army Hospital in Butler, Pennsylvania (Shambaugh & Carhart, 1951). Soon the term spread to other military aural rehabilitation centers, where similar personnel were offering the same kinds of services. Thus the term audiologist came into popular use.

PEARL

The word *audiologist* emerged to designate a person with a university degree who tested hearing and provided rehabilitative services for hard-of-hearing individuals. It seemed appropriate to find a label to differentiate university graduates who served the hard-of-hearing population from educators of teachers of the deaf.

The Seeds Are Planted

The discipline of audiology is now barely 50 years old. The seeds of audiology were planted during World War II, when a handful of army and navy technicians, college professors, otolaryngologists, psychologists, and teachers of the deaf realized they had provided a unique and valuable service to military personnel with hearing loss in three Army Aural Rehabilitation Centers and at the Philadelphia Naval Hospital. The technicians were mainly enlisted personnel who were trained on the job to do pure tone audiometric tests, take ear impressions, inventory demonstration hearing aids, and other rather routine jobs. The college professors were trained in speech pathology and speech science. Some of them had already had experience in their university speech clinics serving persons with impaired hearing, especially those whose speech was affected by a hearing loss. The psychologists were helpful not only in providing counseling for those who were having difficulty accepting and adjusting to their hearing loss but also in dealing with military personnel who manifested pseudohypacousis. The otolaryngologists and teachers of the deaf were the only team members who could claim extensive experience serving individuals with hearing loss. None had ever had direct experience selecting and fitting hearing aids. No hearing aid dealers were represented on these rehabilitation teams; they were considered to be commercial sales people and not professional rehabilitators.

The pure tone audiometer was a rather crude device in the mid 1940s. The tuning fork was the most popular tool for testing hearing. The standard reference level for normal hearing was first established in 1951 with the publication of the American Standards Association norm. The audiometers themselves were unstable, and calibration instruments were scarce.

Consequently, test-retest reliability was tenuous at best. No standard reference levels existed for bone conduction and no artificial mastoid existed, so only qualitative information could be gained from this measurement. Speech audiometry was in its infancy. Some early research on the application of speech intelligibility word lists was conducted during this period at Deshon General Hospital Aural Rehabilitation Center in cooperation with the Harvard Psychoacoustic Laboratory, where Hallowell Davis was director.

The services for veterans with impaired hearing at Deshon were under the direction of Raymond Carhart, who considered himself a speech scientist; his doctoral dissertation was on a functional aspect of the larynx. Carhart went to Deshon as a civilian from his faculty post at Northwestern University, but soon after his arrival, he received a commission as captain in the army (L. Doerfler, 1998, personal communication). Over the next two decades, he would have a profound influence on the educational course of audiology.

PEARL

Because of his pioneering work, both in establishing the foundation of the discipline of audiology and also the first graduate program in this specialty at Northwestern University, Carhart is recognized as the "Father of Audiology."

By the end of World War II, more than 3000 service personnel had been served by these rehabilitation centers with a significant degree of success. As the war ended, the personnel who served in these centers returned to civilian life, a few returning to a university faculty or private practice and some actually enrolled as students to study this new discipline now being called audiology. Those who returned to a university campus designed a course or two that served as supplements to the speech pathology major (e.g., a survey course about hearing and hearing disorders, and an aural rehabilitation course). In the rare case in which an actual curriculum in audiology was developed, such as at Northwestern University, more extensive course offerings began to emerge: acoustics, anatomy and physiology of the hearing mechanism, hearing disorders, audiometry, aural rehabilitation, hearing aids, conservation of hearing, and clinical practice. Because a relative dearth of subject matter and limited faculty existed, all early graduates with a primary interest in audiology had a degree in speech *and* hearing, with a major in audiology.

Because audiology did not have its own professional degree, requirements for the Ph.D. and master's degree were set forth by the university's graduate school. The master's degree usually required a thesis, and the Ph.D. required a reading knowledge of one or two foreign languages and an extensive research project, the dissertation. In due time, the composition of the master's degree would be determined and monitored by the American Speech and Hearing Association (ASHA). The Ph.D. was designed to prepare the recipient as a teacher/investigator. In the early years of audiology, this did not pose a problem because most holders of the Ph.D.

found employment on a university faculty. Thus they benefited from the scientific rigors of the Ph.D. curriculum and preparation because they were expected to do research, publish, and teach. Also, most people who got a Ph.D. first obtained the masters, which was weighted toward clinical practice. By the time a person got to the Ph.D. level of study he or she had experienced substantial clinical exposure, considering the state of the art at that time.

By the mid to late 1950s, it became obvious that not all graduates with a Ph.D. preferred to seek a university faculty post. Indeed, some wanted to locate in a hospital, clinic, rehabilitation center, or the like. These students had a problem reconciling the time, energy, and expense in learning German or some other language and spending a year or more on a research project if they never intended to be teacher/investigators. They wanted to have more clinical training, but because of the demanding Ph.D. curriculum, time did not allow deviation from the typical Ph.D. requirements. Instead, there seemed to be a certain amount of pride in the fact that audiologists could hold either the distinguished scholarly Ph.D. or a Master of Arts or Science. Some of the pioneers of audiology believed that a professional degree,* such as a Doctor of Audiology, would degrade the prestige of the profession. They preferred to look on audiology as a research-based academic discipline composed of scholars and investigators. They believed that as long as the student had a good knowledge of audiology, clinical service was something that could be learned on the job. Moreover, the existence of hearing clinics at universities was justified on the basis of obtaining research data and gaining more knowledge about the process of hearing rather than to provide locations for obtaining clinical experience.

CONTROVERSIAL POINT

Despite this obvious trend toward clinical practice and away from a research career, little concern was expressed by faculty and leaders of the audiology movement about the need for a proprietary professional degree for audiology.

In fact, some of these pioneers were careful to avoid the word *training* when discussing the preparation of audiologists, associating this term with something that was done in a trade school, not in a graduate program in a university. Later, however, the word *training* did creep into the vernacular

---

*An important difference exists between a professional degree and the traditional academic degree. The academic degree is established in a traditional university structure, and the requirements are set forth by a representation of faculty from several different disciplines. The professional degree is established by a specific discipline and the requirements are set forth by that discipline alone, following general guidelines of the university or institution awarding the degree. A professional degree may be awarded by a college or school not associated from a university.

of audiology, perhaps because some federal grants used the term and successful grantsmanship was more important than tradition.

SPECIAL CONSIDERATION

For a realistic appreciation of the issues being faced today concerning a professional doctorate, it is important to understand that the founders of audiology graduate programs intended for the discipline to be composed of academically educated scholars rather than professionally trained practitioners. They did not wish to have audiology viewed by their colleagues in academia as a skill-oriented discipline.

The issue of a professional degree for audiology was first discussed and debated formally at a conference sponsored by ASHA in Highland Park, Illinois, in 1963. The conclusion was that the profession did not need a professional degree but that the Ed.D. could be substituted to lessen some of the requirements for the Ph.D., thereby allowing more time for clinical practice. The Ed.D. is not considered a professional degree as such; but it does *not* have the same research requirements as the Ph.D., which is held up as the most scholarly degree offered by a university anywhere in the world. Today, however, one would have to view this status of the Ph.D. more as perception than fact. For whatever reasons, events over the following 30 years proved that the Ed.D. did not serve as a viable alternative to the Ph.D. because very few audiologists chose to pursue that degree.

Complicating the issue was the fact that most departments of speech and hearing were located in a school of speech, college of arts and science, college of liberal arts, school of education, or the like. Graduate degree programs in these academic-based segments of a university structure fall under the aegis of the graduate school and typically do not offer a professional degree (i.e., M.D., D.D.S., LL.D., O.D., R.N., and a multitude of others). Professional degrees are usually offered by professional schools and colleges within the university community or in an institution separate from a university.

The First "Real" Audiologists

The first person in the United States to earn a Ph.D. in audiology was John Keys in 1947 (L. Doerfler,1998, personal communication). After completion of his program at Northwestern University, he went to the University of Oklahoma and established a graduate program in audiology. A year later, Leo Doerfler earned his doctorate from Northwestern and went to the University of Pittsburgh Medical School. Other pioneering graduates of the late 1940s and early 1950s from Northwestern and elsewhere were John Gaeth, Francis Sonday, Don Markle, Frank Lassman, Harriet Haskins, Leo DeCarlo, Moe Bergman, Freeman McConnell, and others. DeCarlo set up the audiology program at Syracuse University and Bergman at Hunter College in New York. In the mid 1950s the Bill Wilkerson Hearing and Speech Center was built from the ground up in Nashville, Tennessee, under Freeman McConnell's direction and became the largest such facility in the United States. This Center served as the nucleus for the Division of Hearing and Speech Sciences undergraduate and graduate programs at Vanderbilt University and Peabody College, which McConnell started in the early 1950s. Other universities to offer degree programs in audiology in the late 1940s and early 1950s included, but were not limited to, University of Wisconsin, University of Minnesota, Syracuse University, University of Southern California, and Brooklyn College.

The only graduate program in audiology, *separate from speech pathology,* was established in 1965 at Wayne State University Medical School under the direction of John Gaeth. This program remained an autonomous Department of Audiology within the Medical School until 1995 when it joined speech pathology in the College of Sciences. All other programs awarding a degree in audiology in the United States were and are associated with another discipline, typically speech pathology.

Suffice it to say that the evaluation of hearing loss was limited when audiology got started in the late 1940s and early 1950s. Hearing tests consisted of air and bone conduction pure tone audiometry, speech reception threshold, and speech discrimination tests, using spondaic word lists and W-22s, and the Doerfler-Stewart test for malingering. Galvanic skin response or electrodermal audiometry was being used in a small number of Veterans Administration (VA) Clinics starting in the late l940s, but not in general use. All tests were done under earphones, and speech was delivered through loudspeakers and earphones. No standard reference level was established for bone conduction and the calibration for sound field was yet to be established. It was considered unethical and unnecessary to do an otoscopic examination, even to inspect for cerumen because almost all patients were referred by a physician, usually an otolaryngologist. Furthermore, the audiologist had no test that involved placing anything in a patient's earcanal, so cerumen was not expected to be a problem as a rule. Audiologists did not take ear impressions because they sent patients to hearing aid dealers for hearing aids, so the dealers made the impressions. Emphasis was on remediation, specifically on the selection and use of amplification, lipreading, and auditory training.

A small number of early students of audiology terminated with a master's degree and took positions on the staffs of hospitals, community speech clinics, schools for the deaf, ENT offices, and VA clinics. Some individuals went to work as audiologists with a bachelor's degree in speech and hearing because no barriers (e.g., licensing, registration) existed for working as an audiologist with the bachelor's degree.

Early Degree Programs

During the first full decade after the end of World War II, the seeds of audiology were scattered across the country in university programs of speech pathology by a handful of pioneers who earned doctoral degrees in audiology. These people had to develop their own curricula, no doubt

> ## SPECIAL CONSIDERATION
>
> Some hearing aid dealers referred to themselves as audiologists, and their society, *The National Society of Hearing Aid Audiologists,* offered certification as a "hearing aid audiologist." This state of affairs would end, but it took many years and required legal challenges in various courts for the hearing aid dealers to stop using the term *audiologist.*

patterned after their own doctoral programs. Textbooks on the subject of hearing were limited to the classic *Hearing, Its Psychology and Physiology* by S.S. Stevens and H. Davis, published in 1938, and *Clinical Audiometry* by C.C. Bunch, published in 1943. The first text that specifically addressed the subject of audiology was *Hearing and Deafness: A Guide for Laymen,* edited by Hallowell Davis and published in 1947. *Hearing Tests and Hearing Instruments* by L. Watson and T. Tolan came next in 1949. Even though this book contained valuable information about hearing aids, audiometers, and hearing tests that could not be found elsewhere, it was not a popular text among the audiology community. Although Thomas Tolan was a physician, Lee Watson was the president of a hearing aid company. Even though Watson was a Rhodes scholar, this did not seem to matter because he was associated with the commercial hearing aid sector and this did not sit well with the professors of audiology in those days. Audiologists remained at arm's length with the hearing aid business, except possibly the acoustic engineers who worked for some companies. Consequently, writings by anyone from the hearing aid industry did not find their way into the curricula of audiology during these formative years of the discipline.

Princeton University Professor of Psychology, Ernest Glen Wever, published his classic text, *Theory of Hearing,* in 1949. This text became the foundation for the study of the physiology of hearing for this small group of budding audiologists. In 1952, another experimental psychologist, Ira Hirsh, published *Measurement of Hearing,* which quickly became a constant companion of students of audiology. A year later, in 1953, Harvey Fletcher's book, *Speech and Hearing in Communication,* appeared and provided some valuable information on speech perception, acoustics, and psychoacoustics. The first textbook written by an audiologist for students of audiology was Hayes Newby's *Audiology,* published in 1958. This book competed with subsequent editions of *Hearing and Deafness,* now coauthored by Davis and S. Richard Silverman. These texts were used extensively for courses entitled "Introduction to Audiology" in practically all university programs.

With the exception of these few texts, practically all readings involved journal articles for at least the first 10 to 15 years that audiology was taught in universities. For example, one of the favorite course assignments was to have students abstract *all* articles on hearing, hearing aids, and hearing disorders for 5 years from a journal that was assigned to them by the professor. This consisted mainly of articles written by physicians in medical journals, acousticians, or experimental psychologists in the *Journal of the Acoustical Society of America,* or educators of the deaf in *Volta Review* and other periodicals. The hearing aid trade journals were not considered scholarly reading at that time. Thus articles in these periodicals were not assigned. Publications by audiologists were scarce because there were not very many audiologists to write them. However, a growing number of articles appeared in the foreign journals, where audiology was beginning to develop through a medical model, but the quality of translation into English and rigor of research left something to be desired. Most of the foreign authors were not trained researchers. Each student in the class would mimeograph or "ditto" process (purple "ink" on white paper that often rubbed off on one's hands) and exchange their copies with other members of the class. Photocopy machines were not available and personal computers came much later. Actually, this technique proved quite effective for bringing the students up to date on the literature. Of course, each student's final collection of abstracts was a hodgepodge of uncategorized subjects, but that did not seem to bother the students.

Those who wrote master's theses or doctoral dissertations will remember laboriously copying by hand on 3 × 5 cards pages of reference articles from library sources. Anything on the subject of hearing in those days was novel and a welcome addition to the student's knowledge of the subject. Practically everything about hearing was new business in those days because researchers during earlier times did not have the advantage of electronic technology to study the auditory system.

Source of Students

An ongoing speech pathology department would hire a junior faculty member to teach an introductory course in hearing and hearing disorders and perhaps an aural rehabilitation course for the students in speech pathology. In due time, some of these students would express a special interest in pursuing audiology in more depth and to the extent of a major. From this humble beginning would come more course offerings and clinical services for persons with impaired hearing in the university speech and hearing clinic. Most students came, and continue to come, from speech-language pathology, but a small number of students declared a major in audiology after starting in another discipline of study such as education of the deaf, general speech, special education, theater or dramatic arts, and psychology.

PEARL

Most audiology degree programs started as an outgrowth of one or two courses in a speech pathology curriculum.

The Supporters

During these formative years of the education of audiologists, the founders of degree programs received special support from colleagues in speech pathology, otolaryngology, and the Bureau of Veterans Affairs. Speech pathologists and speech scientists provided a "home" in academia for this upstart discipline. They gave audiology faculty financial support; offices; a space to teach, see patients and do research; a shared student recruiting mechanism; exchange of teaching assignments; and an established identity on campus.

Otolaryngologists practicing in the same community as the university or on the faculty of the university's medical school would give lectures and provide practicum sites for the students. ENT physicians often collaborated on research with audiology faculty, publishing under joint authorship. Clearly, many otolaryngologists were eager to see this field develop and provide future trained technical support personnel for their private practices without the need to train a nurse or hire and train a technician to do hearing tests. For ENTs associated with medical schools, audiology would yield future researchers and publication collaborators. On a national and international level, audiologists began to appear on professional and scientific programs and as faculty at ENT regional and national conventions. No question exists that otolaryngology promoted and fostered this fledgling profession in its formative years.

The VA played an important role in development from the earliest days of audiology. Not only did the VA serve as a stable employer, but it also played a role in setting a precedent for clinical conduct, salaries, and level of competency for the clinical practice of audiology. These factors had a decided influence on the curricula offered by the small number of degree programs in the 1950s and later. Most of the advisors to the Chief of Audiology for the VA were selected from audiology degree programs. Therefore most of those who advised and set the standards for the VA were in a position to teach the standards they set themselves.

SPECIAL CONSIDERATION

Even at present, the VA is playing a significant role in facilitating the movement to a mandatory professional doctorate as an entry-level degree to practice audiology (see section on "Distance Learning").

THE DIE IS CAST

As audiology was beginning to emerge as an identifiable discipline, the closest colleagues to those who had chosen this field of endeavor were speech pathologists and speech scientists. This was natural because audiology aligned itself on campus with speech pathology rather than otolaryngology or education of the deaf, which were the other established professions serving persons with hearing disorders at that time. As stated earlier, the speech pathologists provided the audiologists a convenient academic home, which fostered this close relationship. The audiologists taught courses on hearing and hearing impairment and enriched the clinical speech pathology services by evaluating the hearing of persons with a speech and/or language disorder. Both parties needed each other: speech pathologists belonged to a professional and learned national society called the American Speech Correction Association. This association took that name in 1934, having previously been called the American Society for the Study of Disorders of Speech (1927) and American Academy of Speech Correction (1925). Before that, speech correctionists were members of The National Association of Teachers of Speech. Because of a growing lack of common interest and identity with their colleagues in public address, speech arts, and debate, the speech correctionists left that society and formed their own. By 1947, the governing body of the American Speech Correction Association convinced the small number of "audiologists" to join their organization. They would change the name to the American Speech and Hearing Association and give the audiologists freedom to set their own destiny (Doerfler, 1991). Consequently, the audiologists did not start their own society, but instead joined their colleagues, the speech pathologists. At the time, it seemed the most expedient and logical thing to do and it served audiology well for many years. The current name, American Speech-Language-Hearing Association, was adopted in 1978, but the acronym ASHA has been retained.

Examining Boards and Standards

In 1959 the ASHA established the American Board of Examiners in Speech Pathology and Audiology (ABESPA). One of the fundamental missions of ASHA was to ensure that speech and hearing services to the public were of the highest quality. This board provided ASHA with the mechanism by which the goal could most likely be achieved. Subsequently, this body has been named the Boards of Examiners in Speech Pathology and Audiology (BESPA). BESPA consists of three boards: the Clinical Certification Board (CCB) that certifies practitioners, the Professional Services Board (PSB) that accredits institutions and organizations that provide professional services, and the Educational Standards Board (ESB) that accredits academic departments of universities and colleges that train speech pathologists and audiologists. This latter is now entitled the Council on Academic Accreditation in Audiology and Speech-Language Pathology or CAA. The purpose of ESB, and now CAA, is to accredit master's degree programs in speech and/or audiology, but it does not have jurisdiction over doctoral programs.

It was through the power and influence of ESB that the die was cast for the composition of the curriculum for the education and training of audiologists since the early 1960s. It may be noteworthy to mention here that the composition of these boards was heavily weighted by academics: those who were responsible for the speech pathology, speech science, and audiology teaching and curricula at various universities and colleges. Also, some of the founders were able to call on the experiences they had in the military aural rehabilitation centers during World War II. Little or no input came to these bodies from otolaryngologists, educators of the deaf, or hearing aid dealers, who at this time had more experience with the hard-of-hearing population than any other specialists in this country. Consequently, the speech pathology model was used when constructing the academic standards for audiology.

Certification

In the 1950s two levels of certification were awarded by ASHA to individual audiologists: basic and advanced. These were modeled after the speech correctionists' requirements. Basic

certification required that one must hold a bachelor's degree in speech correction or audiology or both, in which case there was a dual certification. Basic certification was rather easy to achieve, mainly by presentation of credentials and possibly a simple written examination. Advanced certification was much more stringent, requiring a master's degree and the successful completion of a 1-day written examination and an intensive oral examination administered by persons who were not from the faculty of the institution awarding the degree. In the early 1960s, these two levels of certification were collapsed into a single certification and all those with basic were "grandfathered" into a new single level but not without a great deal of furor from the holders of the advanced certificates.

Since the early 1960s, eligibility for full membership in ASHA requires at least a master's degree or equivalent with major emphasis in audiology "or a master's degree and evidence of active research, interest, and performance in the field of human communication"(Newby, 1964). This latter provision was for researchers and administrators who did not have an interest or perhaps training to provide clinical services for persons with hearing loss. To be *certifiable,* one had to earn the master's degree in audiology from an ASHA-accredited university or college and meet the following requirements: (1) a minimum of 60 semester hours of course work, which could include undergraduate studies, with at least 18 semester hours in courses that provided fundamental information applicable to the normal development and use of speech, hearing, and language, and (2) at least 42 semester hours in courses that provided information about the training in the management of speech, hearing, and language disorders and supplementary information. The major portion of this course work had to be in the area of audiology. Also required for certification in the early 1960s was the completion of 275 clock hours of supervised direct clinical experience as part of the training program awarding the degree (later changed to 350 hours). Each applicant had to pass a national examination monitored by an independent testing service. A final requirement was one academic year (9 months) of full-time "satisfactory" professional experience after completion of the degree program (Newby, 1964). This later became known as the "Clinical Fellowship Year" or CFY. After the applicant had satisfied these requirements, he or she was awarded the Certificate of Clinical Competence in Audiology or CCC-A.

The intent of ASHA was to require that all individuals employed as audiologists hold certification by ASHA. The leaders of the association believed that this was the best and most logical way to ensure quality audiological care for the hearing challenged. This seemed reasonable at the time because no other safeguards were built into the system to provide such protection of the public. State licensure was on the horizon, but not yet in effect in any state. ASHA had a Code of Ethics, and if an audiologist was found to violate any provisions of the Code, he or she could lose certification. This did happen in a number of instances, especially when the prohibition against the "sale or promotion of products related to their profession"(i.e., hearing aids) was violated.

State Licensing and Registration

ASHA believed that licensing was unnecessary because it already had certification of members, a Code of Ethics, and accreditation of professional service institutions and organizations. ASHA's position did not impress the Florida State Legislature because the state had no control over the performance and actions of audiologists and speech pathologists.

CONTROVERSIAL POINT

After months of debate and opposition from ASHA, Florida became the first state to enact a licensing law for audiologists and speech pathologists in 1969. The leaders of ASHA believed that licensure would impose unrealistic control and restrains on the practice of audiology and speech pathology.

This was the beginning of state licensing and registration of audiologists. Today, nearly all states have some type of legislation that sets forth the provisions for the practice of audiology. Most state laws use the framework of the ASHA requirements for membership and certification to define eligibility to practice, but no state *requires* membership in ASHA to be licensed. What these regulations do, however, is reinforce the content of the curriculum set forth by ASHA that an audiologist must take to meet the provisions of licensure. Even though the states can dictate who can and who cannot practice audiology within their state, ASHA is the body that determines the content of the training of audiologists.

CONTROVERSIAL POINT

An audiologist does not need to be a member of ASHA or hold certification by ASHA to be eligible for state licensure, but the audiologist must be able to document the *equivalency* of ASHA certification.

THE INTERVENING YEARS

Throughout the 1960s and 1970s, the profession of audiology grew steadily, from just a few hundred to more than 5000. Most audiologists were employed in some capacity in a health care environment. Some were in an educational setting, such as the public schools and schools for the deaf, but most were in hospital clinics; ENT offices; VA clinics; and community, college, and university speech and hearing clinics. By far, most audiologists were providing services directly to the hearing impaired. Only a small percentage were teacher/investigators.

Scope of Practice

The scope of practice of audiology was also increasing rapidly with emphasis on tests and measurements but not on rehabilitation. Hard-of-hearing patients wanted a quick solution to their hearing problem through wearable amplification and were resistant to multiclinic visits to learn lipreading and take auditory training. On the other hand, special auditory tests to aid in the differential diagnosis of auditory disorders were gaining great popularity among the ENT, pediatric, and neurological communities. Industrial audiology was becoming popular as a result of the Occupational Safety and Health Act of 1970 (Olishifski & Harford, 1975). Pediatric audiology was gaining popularity because of improved testing techniques and the increase in the number of audiologists to serve the preschool and school-age population.

This increase in scope of practice along with the overwhelming number of graduates going into hearing health care provided impetus to reevaluate the educational requirements for the master's degree. In the 1950s one could satisfy requirements in about a year beyond an undergraduate degree in speech and hearing, which often included a master's thesis, but now it was becoming difficult to achieve in less than 18 months. Some universities increased their program of study to five to six semesters or seven to eight quarters, which is about 18 to 24 months. ASHA increased the requirement for clock hours of direct patient experience from 275 to 325 hours plus 25 hours of observation.

Government Support

Large sums of federal moneys were being pumped into programs for the health care system for the disadvantaged. Audiological services were frequently included in these programs. Audiologists were in short supply in the early 1960s, so several federal agencies appropriated substantial sums of money to support students pursuing a degree in communicative disorders, including audiology. This support came in the form of traineeships, fellowships, assistantships, and scholarships. Some of the agencies providing these funds were the Federal Children's Bureau, U.S. Office of Education, Rehabilitation Services Administration, the VA, and the Bureau of Indian Affairs. The National Institutes of Health and a small number of private foundations were also funding audiology programs. Most of these moneys were used to support students in a terminal master's program. The availability of financial support for graduate study enticed scores of students to pursue a master's degree in audiology.

The Role of ASHA

Starting in the mid-1950s, soon after Kenneth O. Johnson became the Executive Secretary of the American Speech and Hearing Association, a steady increase occurred in the control and monitoring of academic programs for speech pathology and audiology. Johnson was an audiologist recruited by ASHA from a VA position in San Francisco, California. He was the first full-time paid Executive Secretary of the

---

PEARL

Throughout the 1960s a very strong trend developed that set the educational course for audiology to this day. The message sent was *if you want to be a clinical audiologist, you need a master's degree and money is available to do this. If you want to be a professor or researcher, you must get a Ph.D., but funds are more difficult to get.* Consequently, the profession of audiology became flooded with master's level audiologists, most of whom were engaged heavily in hearing testing and audiological evaluations.

Association. The number of universities offering graduate degrees in audiology climbed steadily until reaching a peak of some 115 programs in the 1980s. Many of these programs had less than five students. Such audiology programs were sustained by speech-language pathology enrollments.

With this growth came dozens on dozens of reports, guidelines, committees, task forces, conferences, and the like, designed to promulgate recommendations and standards for the education and training of audiologists. Committees and working groups established standards and guidelines on how to test hearing, how to screen infants, how to calibrate audiometric instruments, how to supervise students, how to select hearing aids, how to provide audiology services in the schools, and how to evaluate preferred practice patterns and quality assurance, just to name a few. Over a period of 30 years ASHA defined the education of audiologists, set standards of practice, set a code of ethics for professional conduct, and served as the national voice of audiology in legislative and political circles at every level.

PEARL

No doubt exists that ASHA played the most critical and fundamental role in the evolution of the discipline of audiology. For 30 years, educational standards, eligibility for membership in ASHA, and requirements for clinical certification from ASHA remained essentially unchanged.

Because the ASHA Code of Ethics prohibited the dispensing of hearing aids for profit, only a few audiologists were involved in private practice. It was impossible to survive as an independent practitioner doing only hearing tests and evaluations. Audiologists employed by the VA were, in fact, fitting and dispensing hearing aids that were included in veterans' benefits, but they were in the minority.

Recall that in the beginning, most persons entering the field of audiology held the Ph.D. Only the minority terminated with a master's degree. Starting in the early-to-mid-1960s, this situation reversed to where most audiologists in this country had 1½ to 2 years of graduate school and hold

either the Master of Arts or Master of Science degree. During these intervening years of the 1960s and 1970s, nearly all audiologists were employees. Only a small fraction were self-employed in a private practice that typically was some form of industrial hearing conservation service. A great many audiologists found themselves in a technical-type situation, where they were spending their days doing a variety of routine and perhaps special hearing tests and routing the results to an otolaryngologist to interpret to the patient. Salaries were low and the dropout rate was high. Saying this another way, throughout the 1960s and 1970s, a large number of audiologists in this country were providing audiological diagnostic test services for members of the medical profession, not for persons with abnormal hearing. That is, patients consulted physicians for help with their hearing, not audiologists, unless they were referred to a hearing clinic by a physician.

PITFALL

From the earliest days of audiology it was considered inappropriate, if not unethical, for an audiologist to serve a patient who had not first been examined by a physician. This remains a standard in some quarters for the clinical practice of audiology in the United States.

The National Council of Graduate Programs in Speech Pathology and Audiology

Independent of ASHA, the Council of Graduate Programs was established in the 1960s. This organization, composed of chairpersons of speech and hearing programs, maintained a vigilance on the curricula of speech pathology and audiology, discussed weaknesses and prospective improvements, and made recommendations to ASHA. The work of this council, which continues today, is aimed primarily at master's degree programs and it focuses heavily on clinical practicum and professional experiences of the students. This council is composed primarily of members of ASHA, and in some cases the same persons who sit on boards and committees of ASHA. Thus in some respects, they were talking to themselves.

CONTROVERSIAL POINT

Because most chairpersons of speech and hearing programs are speech-pathology educated, audiology is not well represented by this theoretically independent advisory board.

THE LATER YEARS

Scope of Practice

In 1978, ASHA was forced by a U.S. Supreme Court decision involving a professional society of engineers to change its Code of Ethics. Before this time the code had prohibited

ASHA members from engaging in the sale of products related to their profession. For audiologists, the change in the Code meant that they could sell hearing aids without fear of retribution from ASHA. This event would have a profound effect on the future education and training of audiologists, but it would take years to be realized.

By 1979, about 900 audiologists were selling hearing aids and by the end of the 1980s the number had reached 5000, or half of all hearing aid dispensers in the United States (Skafte, 1990). Indeed, the profession of audiology was now becoming a profession of both diagnosticians *and* rehabilitators of hearing loss.

PEARL

By the end of the 1980s the profession of audiology was quickly changing from a field heavily composed of salaried (diagnostic) test-oriented persons under direct or tacit control and supervision of the medical profession to a corps of independent practitioners providing rehabilitative services *directly* to persons with hearing loss.

During the same time this shift to hearing aid dispensing was taking place, a steady and impressive improvement was occurring in technology applicable to audiology. Auditory brain stem response measurements were gaining popularity in newborn intensive care units and for screening for suspected space-occupying lesions and demyelinating diseases. Immitance measurement was gaining great popularity in the basic audiological evaluation. Real-ear or probe microphone instrumentation and techniques were introduced and well received for measuring the performance of hearing aids in situ. More recently, otoacoustic emissions were introduced for the early identification of hearing loss in babies and other purposes. These technological advances enhanced the effectiveness of audiology for certain applications and broadened the scope of practice, but the greatest impact on the profession came from the hearing aid-dispensing sector.

Dispensing hearing aids made it possible for scores of audiologists to enter private practice and make a decent living. Dispensing hearing aids was profitable enough to allow an audiologist to operate and maintain an independent practice, and many elected to take that course. By 1990, a significant number of audiologists in private practice were dispensing hearing aids, and the number continued to grow at an impressive rate. Operating a private practice required new knowledge and skills to be competent and competitive. For example, audiologists quickly learned that they needed to take responsibility for dealing with cerumen, a skill that was not taught in graduate school. Infection control in the practice of audiology took on important significance. Business and practice management issues became important to understand and follow, including compliance with local and federal rules and regulations. Managed healthcare was taking charge in many communities and gaining momentum with every passing day. None of these needed areas of modern practice were included in the audiology curriculum.

By this time, most audiologists completing their graduate programs were finding employment in a healthcare setting (i.e., ENT practices, hospitals, medical schools and medical centers, pediatric facilities, and the like). Even though ASHA published survey results showing that most audiologists were in a medical setting, most audiology graduate programs continued to use the academically based education model rather than a professional training model.

SPECIAL CONSIDERATION

Students at the master's level were not being trained as healthcare providers. Stated another way, students in training for audiology were being left far behind by the fast-moving developments in the workaday world. It was time to reevaluate the current educational model for audiologists.

The Professional Degree

Toward the end of the 1980s and beginning of 1990s, there was a ground swell of support for a professional doctorate by rank and file audiologists throughout the United States. Surveys were conducted by the Academy of Dispensing Audiologists (ADA) and ASHA that overwhelmingly supported the need for such a degree. This was especially evident to audiologists who were hiring students just completing their programs and entering their clinical fellowship year.

SPECIAL CONSIDERATION

The scope of practice of audiology had increased to the extent that it was virtually impossible to prepare persons by means of a master's degree program to possess the knowledge and skills required to practice modern audiology, even at an entry level. The education and training model designed for the 1970s simply was inadequate for the 1990s.

The Au.D. seemed to catch on quickly as the designator for the professional degree that was being proposed. The proposed course of study and residency would take about 4 years beyond the bachelor's degree. The intent was to abolish the master's degree. An example of an Au.D. program contrasted with a master's degree program can be found near the end of this chapter.

The professional doctorate is in no way intended to replace the Ph.D. Although the first 3 years of both an Au.D. and Ph.D. curriculum may be quite similar in course offerings and content, the last year will be very different. Whereas the Au.D. student enters a clinical residency in the fourth year, the Ph.D. student embarks on a research project culminating in a doctoral dissertation. Also, during the first 3 years, the Au.D. student engages in more clinical activities, whereas the Ph.D. student is involved with course work and other projects outside the audiology program. The Ph.D. degree must be preserved for those students entering the field of audiology who wish to pursue a research, and possibly teaching, career, and most importantly to continue to advance the scientific basis of contemporary audiology.

The Impact of Academies of Audiology

The impetus for a change in the education of audiologists came from the Academy of Dispensing Audiologists (ADA), a professional organization founded in 1977 and composed mainly of audiologists in private practice. Underscoring this voice was the Audiology Foundation of America (AFA), an independent nonprofit organization committed to the establishment of a professional degree in Audiology (the Au.D.), led by David Goldstein of Purdue University.

During the early years, the ADA devoted much of its energies to promoting hearing aid dispensing by audiologists. By the mid to late 1980s, ADA became a vocal advocate for a professional doctorate in audiology. This group of private practitioners was keenly aware of the new role of audiologists in our society, the need to expand and enrich the preparation of audiologists, and the importance of a professional doctor designation for the practitioner in the highly competitive health care system.

It was just about this time (1988) that the seeds were planted for the founding of the American Academy of Audiology (AAA). The rationale for the founding of a society of audiologists, separate from ASHA, was to have: "a national organization run by and for Audiologists; an organization uniquely sensitive to the professional issues, and the professional concerns affecting all audiologists" (Jerger, 1998). As AAA took shape, one of its objectives was the adoption of a professional doctorate as the entry level degree for the practice of audiology.

PEARL

The 1988 Mission Statement of the fledgling AAA read as follows: "The aim of the Academy shall be to promote the public good by advancing the highest professional standards for the diagnosis, habitation, rehabilitation, and research in hearing and its disorders".

In 1991 the AAA published a position paper strongly endorsing the concept of a professional doctorate in audiology as the appropriate entry-level degree for the practice of audiology. It stated that the specific purpose of a professional doctorate is to prepare highly skilled practitioners and that it should be designated as the Au.D. (doctor of audiology) to differentiate it from the research-oriented Ph.D. Excerpts from this position paper delineate further objectives of a professional doctorate.

. . . there is major emphasis on the clinical learning experience. Although the professional doctorate in audiology (Au.D.) is not a

research-oriented degree, it is imperative that student practitioners be familiar with the scientific and research literature that undergirds audiology, have the knowledge and skills requisite to evaluate and interpret the audiological and related research literature, and be able to synthesize and apply pertinent research knowledge to the problems of clinical practice.

Ideally, Au.D. degree programs should be organized and implemented within sponsoring institutions, such as colleges and universities, that will provide for an independent school and faculty and should be constituted similar in nature to the degree programs which grant doctorates to other professions, such as dentistry, medicine, optometry, veterinary medicine, etc. Traditional graduate programs are structured to grant academic doctorates rather than professional doctorates. Consequently, Au.D. programs should be administered whenever possible independent of existing graduate school programs. They should be practitioner and patient-service driven, i.e., the basic orientation of the training programs should be to facilitate the development of the highest level of audiological skills in the student-practitioner, with concomitant emphasis on delivery of superior audiological services to the patient." (Berlin et al, 1991).

This proposal goes on to recommend that the student receive between 2500 and 3000 hours of clinical experience with an extensive variety of cases and preceptors. Emphasis should be on course work in the early portion of the proposed 4-year program beyond the bachelor's degree level with a steady increase in clinical learning experiences after the first year, culminating in a full-time residency during the fourth year.

The AAA grew very rapidly, signifying the need that audiologists felt for more identity and control of their destiny, not the least of which was the education and training of future audiologists. By the end of 1988 the membership was about 1800, and by the end of 1997 the ranks had increased to nearly 7000 members, which was about two thirds of the practicing audiologists in the United States.

Many audiologists shifted their allegiance and support from ASHA to AAA. They recognized AAA as more sensitive to their needs and that through AAA they would have a more direct voice in shaping the course of audiology. Many audiologists believed that ASHA did not allow them to have their own identity. The speech-language pathology membership of ASHA outnumbers audiologists by a margin of more than 7 to 1. Audiologists are far outnumbered in the Legislative Council, which is the main governing body of the association.

Only after several years of debate and pressure from AAA, ADA, and AFA, did ASHA set time lines for the doctorate to be effective. Initially, ASHA set 2007 as the first year when a doctorate was required for an audiologist to be eligible for membership. Later, they changed this date to the year 2012. Regardless of the delayed timing, ASHA's position is that the Au.D. must be earned through a bona fide university system. That is, persons seeking the Au.D. must return to campus or earn their Au.D. through distance learning or some other means that is officially sanctioned by an accredited university.

Opposition to the Professional Degree
ASHA

In 1992 (LC4-92) the Legislative Council of ASHA supported "the *concept* of doctoral degrees as the entry level academic credentials for the practice of audiology" (Annon., 1993).

Again in 1993 (LC44-93) the council supported "the professional doctorate as the entry-level credential for the practice of audiology" (Annon, 1994). In both years these were "watered down" versions of the original resolutions put to the floor of the Legislative Council for discussion and ultimate approval. Many audiologists believed this endorsement of "concept" was simply to placate the audiologists and really did not represent true support and commitment on the part of ASHA. The audiologists wanted the council to set deadlines for the requirement of the professional doctorate. This did not come until the fall of 1997.

Since the earliest days, ASHA has been the only body authorized to accredit degree programs in audiology and certify the competence of audiologists (CCC-A). Consequently to elevate the requirements to practice audiology to a doctoral level, it would be helpful to have the endorsement and support of ASHA to transfer this authority to another accreditation and certification body. Also, one must recognize that audiologists from the academic arena continue to have a strong influence on the direction of ASHA. Recall that most departments offering graduate degrees in audiology are in academically based schools that do not award professional degrees. Furthermore, in many universities no mechanism exists for moving the audiology program into a school (e.g., medical school) in which a professional degree can be awarded. Another major concern underlying the resistance to move audiology to a professional doctoral level is the loss of students who may resist committing to the additional years and expense of training. This concern even poses a threat to the total loss of a degree program including faculty jobs. Therefore it is understandable that considerable resistance to the professional doctorate has come from many faculty in academia, especially those with only a few students, which represents most of the more than 110 university programs.

Another problem has to do with money and control. As audiologists flocked to the AAA, many simultaneously withdrew membership from ASHA, even though they continue to pay a fee to retain their certification. ASHA had to feel this decrease in the membership of audiologists in their income revenue. Furthermore, if ASHA gave up its accreditation and certification control of audiology, that organization would stand to lose even more money, amounting to millions of dollars. In response to losing audiology membership, ASHA has responded in recent years by establishing a journal dedicated to audiology (*American Journal of Audiology*); a Vice President of Audiology; publishing an audiology newsletter periodically; and other provisions to demonstrate a sensitivity to audiologists' needs. Despite these efforts, the gap between ASHA and AAA seems to be widening.*

Some Practicing Audiologists

A significant number of audiologists at the master's level, especially those working for ENT specialists, either feel threatened by a requirement to hold a doctoral degree or believe that it is

---

*Apropos to the current situation between ASHA and AAA, it seems appropriate to quote an excerpt from Raymond Carhart's ASHA presidential speech that he presented at the ASHA National Convention in Cincinnati, Ohio, on November 20, 1957, entitled, "The Personal Need for Professional Unity."

It is the loneliness which men feel as they live each day amid people whose work-a-day interests are unlike their own that causes the myriad of organizations characterizing our culture. One may scoff at some of the organizations he sees on the social scene, but these organizations will survive as long as they supply emotional havens to their members.

As a corollary to this last observation is the fact that an organization tends to sub-divide as the field it serves becomes more diversified, as it adds specialization's. The history of the American Speech and Hearing Association supplies an excellent example of this trend. The older members of ASHA will remember the progression of events. The early years were spent essentially as a minority group within the household of the National Association of Teachers of Speech, which has since become the Speech Association of America. Almost all ASHA members had received their training in departments of Speech and the majority felt their prime affiliation to this field as it was traditionally defined in the academic world. They were, however, beginning to find their interests deviating from those of their colleagues in public address and in the speech arts. They were beginning to evolve the traditions, the substantive subject matter, and the distinctive professional activities of an independent specialty. The fact was not appreciated by most of the leaders of NATS. Only the minority conceived that the area of communicative disorders was more than a subordinate specialty of Speech. To be sure, ASHA was given encouragement to organize its own convention programs and to produce its own journal. The point is that many people in NATS believe that ASHSA's problems of growth could be adequately solved by integrating its evolving fields into the contemporary boundaries of academic Speech. (Carhart, 1958).

I have to conclude from these words of Carhart that he had a vision for the direction of audiology more than 40 years ago. I believe he was sending a message to his colleagues in audiology from the podium that day in 1957, but perhaps we were suffering from the very impairment we were dedicated to try to correct.

unnecessary. They are unwilling to return to a university campus and assume the expense and time commitment to get a higher degree. The *Hearing Journal* (Kirkwood, 1998) published the results of a survey conducted in 1997. One of the questions asked was: "Do you think the Au.D. should become the minimum educational requirement for new audiologists?"

CONTROVERSIAL POINT

Whereas 69% of the audiologists in private practice think the Au.D. should become the minimum educational requirement for new audiologists, only 31% of those working in the M.D's office agree. Apparently, some working for the M.D. simply do not understand the significance of the issues and see what they do as a *job* rather than a *professional career*. Therefore they do not identify with the long-term implications of a professional doctorate in audiology.

Otolaryngologists

The otolaryngology community has not supported audiology moving to a professional doctorate for obvious reasons. They tend to see doctors of audiology disrupting their patient flow by taking referrals directly from primary care physicians, which currently is a major source of referrals for otolaryngologists. Some ENTs have expressed concern that future audiologists actually will prescribe some medications and treating some disorders of the ear that properly belong in their domain, such as cerumen removal and external otitis. Management of cerumen had always been perceived by medical doctors as in the purview of the medical profession. Fueling their concern is a large surge in the number of audiologists managing cerumen since the first reports of this practice were published in 1991 by Ross Roeser and Carl Crandell, both audiologists (Roeser & Crandell, 1991). In addition, both ASHA and AAA have included cerumen management in their scopes of practice for audiologists.

Nevertheless, it will be interesting to note how otolaryngology handles the role that audiology will ultimately hold in the health care system as the professional doctorate and higher level of training become the standards for the profession.

SPECIAL CONSIDERATION

Even though otolaryngology has not supported the Au.D., it apparently has not been effective in any opposition movement, perhaps because it has other bigger problems with the managed care movement.

The Current Master's Degree in Audiology

To qualify for ASHA certification, all graduate course work and clinical practicum must be initiated and completed at an institution with a program accredited by the ASHA

Council on Academic Accreditation in Audiology and Speech-Language Pathology. As previously discussed, because CAA specifies the courses and practicum that a degree program must offer, it is evident that ASHA controls the education and training of audiologists, not the universities and colleges. Establishing rigid standards and curricula quashes a university's potential to offer creative and innovative programming and to shift easily with changes in the scope of practice. At least this seems to be one of the principal reasons why the master's level audiology programs have failed to keep pace with changes in the scope of practice over the past 25 to 30 years.

If one is interested in learning what is required to obtain a Master of Arts or Master of Science degree in audiology, contact ASHA or the institution of interest. The information from both sources should be virtually identical. The following information contains a general framework of the more specific requirements.

Academic Course Work (75 Semester Hours)

Seventy five (75) semester credit hours that reflect a well-integrated program of study dealing with (1) the biological/physical sciences and mathematics; (2) the behavioral and/or social sciences, including normal aspects of human behavior and communication; and (3) the nature, prevention, evaluation, and treatment of speech, language, hearing, and related disorders. Some course work must address issues pertaining to normal and abnormal human development and behavior across the life span and to culturally diverse populations.

Basic Science Course Work

At least 27 of the 75 semester credit hours must be in basic science course work. These hours may be earned at the graduate or undergraduate level with certain restrictions.

Professional Course Work

At least 36 of the 75 semester credit hours must be in professional course work. At least 30 of the 36 semester hours must be in courses for which graduate credit was received, and at least 21 of those 30 credit hours must be in the area of audiology. (These 30 hours represent an increase of 3 semester credit hours in the past 30 years.) At least 6 of the 36 semester credit hours of professional course work must be in speech-language pathology.

The remaining 12 semester hours, of the total 75, may be distributed between basic science and professional subjects.

Supervised Clinical Observation and Clinical Practicum

Each student is required to log a specified number of patient contact hours under close supervision by an audiologist who holds a current certificate of clinical competence (CCC-A). The total minimum number of hours is 375, broken down as follows:

Twenty five (25) clock hours of supervised observation that concerns the evaluation and treatment of children and adults with disorders of speech, language, or hearing. Videotapes may be used.

Three hundred and fifty (350) hours of direct supervised clinical practicum involves direct time spent in actual evaluation or treatment of patients with communication disorders. At least 250 of the 350 clock hours must be completed with patients with a known or suspected hearing disorder. At least 250 hours in audiology must be completed at the graduate level. These hours must be initiated and completed in a CAA accredited program. These hours must be broken down as follows: at least 40 hours testing the hearing of children and adults, and at least 10 of these hours must be with one of these age groups. At least 80 hours involved in the selection and use of amplification for children and adults, and again, a minimum of 10 hours must be spent with one of these age categories. Finally, at least 20 hours must be spent in the treatment of hearing disorders in children and adults.

Summarizing practicum requirements, to be eligible for certification by ASHA, at the time of this publication, a person must present documentation of 250 clock hours of supervised contact providing diagnostic and treatment services to patients of various ages with a hearing disorder. An additional 100 hours *could* be spent providing services to patients with speech-language disorders. Finally, 25 hours need to be spent observing services provided to persons with a speech, language, and/or hearing disorder. This represents an increase of 75 clock hours in the past 35 years.

New Educational Standards for Certification
American Speech-Language-Hearing Association

During the period of 1996 and 1997, the ASHA Council on Professional Standards in Speech-Language Pathology and Audiology studied the level of professional education in audiology in relation to the scope of practice of the profession. This council ultimately proposed new educational and training standards that were approved by the Legislative Council of ASHA. These can be summarized as follows (changes are noted in italic print).

Persons who apply for certification after December 31, 2006, must be able to document a minimum of 75 semester credit hours of *postbaccalaureate* courses addressing the knowledge and skills pertinent to the field of audiology culminating in a doctoral *or other recognized graduate degree*. The requirement for a *doctoral degree* is mandated for persons who apply for certification after December 31, 2011. The program of study must include a practicum experience that is equivalent to a minimum of *12 months* of full-time supervised experience.

American Academy of Audiology

In 1988 AAA established the Audiology Board Certification (ABC) program to: "provide recognition to those audiologists whose knowledge base and clinical skills were consistent with professionally established standards and who advance their knowledge, skills and abilities through advanced training" (Annon, 1997). ABC has specific entry level requirements and *mandatory* continuing education activities for recertification every 3 years. Administration of the ABC is carried out by the American Board of Audiology (ABA), an independent certifying body for the American Academy of Audiology. The ABA is composed of seven persons: five are audiologists who are audiology board certified and elected by the ABA certified audiologists to represent various audiology practice settings, one is an appointed public member, and the other is appointed to represent the AAA Board of Directors. Audiology board certification is available to all audiologists regardless of membership in any professional organization. At the time of this writing, an audiologist needs to have a postbachelor's degree in audiology from a regionally accredited university program, pass an audiology specialty area test administered by the Educational Testing Service, complete 1400 hours or 1 year of full-time professional practice, and agree to comply with the ABA Code of Ethics.

PEARL
An audiologist need not be a member of any professional organization to be board certified. Recertification every 3 years requires 45 hours of continuing education activities that meet the guidelines of the AAA Continuing Education Programs.

These programs are divided into two categories: *Category A* (a minimum of 30 contact hours) is (1) conferences, short courses, workshops, and seminars sponsored by AAA; (2) journal or computer-based instructional programs that require an examination; and (3) other distance learning activities that require an examination.

Category B (a maximum of 15 contact hours) is (1) conferences, instructional courses, seminars, or workshops conducted by non-AAA continuing education providers; (2) participation in professional activities such as service on boards, committees, or task forces (maximum of 5 contact hours); (3) authoring or publication of an audiology-related article, chapter, book, or other educational material for the profession (maximum of 5 contact hours); and (4) teaching activities such as academic instruction, supervision, presentation at a professional meeting, and other instructional programs (maximum of 5 contact hours).

The AAA ABC differs from ASHA certification (CCC-A) in four major respects. *First,* ABC does not require that the applicant be a member of *any* professional organization. In contrast, to hold the CCC-A, the audiologist must be a member of ASHA. *Second,* ABC does not specify the content of the applicant's degree program. Emphasis is placed on passing the national examination and not the courses the applicant takes in college. *Third,* ABC wants documentation of 1400 hours or 1 year of full-time professional practice. ASHA requires as little as 1080 hours. *Fourth,* ABC requires a mandatory continuing education program requiring recertification every 3 years with documentation of CE credits. ASHA does not have a mandatory CE program but does require an annual fee to keep the certification active. As this new ABC process develops in the months ahead, it should serve as a viable alternative to the CCC-A issued by ASHA. Time will tell. At the time of this writing, ASHA had threatened AAA with litigation, claiming that AAA copied ASHA's certification requirements (Northern, 1998).

The Au.D. Degree

Baylor College of Medicine

In 1993 the first Au.D. program was established by James Jerger at the Baylor College of Medicine in Houston, Texas. Jerger is the founder of AAA and a lifelong, highly respected researcher and contributor to the body of knowledge in audiology. This Au.D. program created considerable excitement and encouragement among those in the audiology community who were working hard to promote the Au.D. The setting for such a degree program in the college of medicine seemed ideal. Students had access to a rich source of clinical opportunities in the large, culturally diverse metropolitan area surrounding Baylor and the faculty and staff were of the highest quality. It seemed that Jerger was in a unique position to establish a model Au.D. program for future emulation.

The first group of students entered the program in January 1994 and were awarded their Au.D. in May of 1996. Drs. Tabitha Parent, Amy Wilson, and Kimber Gallagher were the first persons in the world to earn an Au.D. But in early 1997 Dr. Jerger announced, with regret, that it was necessary to phase out the Au.D. program at Baylor. The medical school setting dictated overlapping curricula for Au.D. and M.D. students. Yet the undergraduate and pre-Au.D. graduate preparation of the Au.D. students was not comparable or competitive with those students who had completed premed programs. The Baylor College of Medicine refused a double standard for the Au.D. students. Dr. Jerger and his group tried to recruit from applicant pools other than speech-language pathology, but with little success. Thus the decision was made to phase out the program over a period of time to ensure that students already enrolled in the program could complete their Au.D. degrees.

Central Michigan University

Soon after the Baylor program started, Central Michigan University (CMU) in Mt. Pleasant, Michigan, initiated an Au.D. program under the direction of Gerald Church. The Au.D. program at CMU is a 4-year postbaccalaureate program with course work distributed among the following topic areas:

Basic science underlying audiology: 15 credit hours
Disorders/assessment: 24 credit hours
Management: 24 credit hours
Research: 15 credit hours
Clinical practicum: 37 credit hours
TOTAL: 115 credit (semester) hours

The first 2 years of study are devoted to mastery of the audiological knowledge base and basic clinical skills. In the final 2 years of the program, students work with practicing audiologists in a variety of clinical experiences designed to evolve in scope and complexity.

Each student must pass a comprehensive examination before beginning the third year of study. Before a student is allowed to begin the fourth year of clinical residency, he or she must have successfully initiated a doctoral research project that must be completed before graduation.

The Au.D. degree at CMU is awarded on successful completion of course work, clinical practica, a comprehensive examination, a doctoral research project, and clinical residency requirements. The residency can be used to satisfy the clinical fellowship year required by ASHA, if the Au.D. student elects to obtain ASHA certification.

To date, the Au.D. program at Central Michigan University has been very successful. The CMU program consistently receives an abundant number of good quality applicants and has no problem filling quotas for classes. At the time of writing (1998), there are now 10 full-time faculty, 6 with a Ph.D. and 4 with a master's degree. All 10 hold ASHA certification and are Fellows of the American Academy of Audiology. The program is a separate division of the Department of Communicative Disorders, so it is self-directing and independent of speech-language pathology. Plans are under way at the time of this writing for the Au.D. program to establish its own School of Audiology. Even though CMU is located in a semirural location, it does maintain a fairly large and well-equipped audiology clinic. More importantly, they have successfully located a variety of outstanding professional settings in Michigan and other parts of the country for their students to do their residencies. The Au.D. students at Central Michigan University will accumulate 1800 to 2000 hours of supervised professional experience *before* they are awarded their degree.

Consequently, CMU and other universities that now offer Au.D. programs are using a combination of guideposts to develop an effective degree program, including: (a) the AAA Position Paper mentioned earlier (Berlin et al, 1991); (b) ASHA certification requirements; (c) the Baylor program; (d) established Ph.D. programs; and (e) input from practicing audiologists. More specific guidelines may be forthcoming for Au.D. programs. The competencies of the graduates and their performance on national examinations should attest to the effectiveness of the programs.

> **PITFALL**
>
> Because of the way in which the training programs for the Au.D. have evolved, no standard curriculum exists.

Table 2–1 contrasts a typical current Master of Arts program with the CMU Au.D. program in semester hours.

Inherent in the Au.D. curriculum is emphasis on clinical practice for hearing health care providers. Many of the CMU faculty are themselves service providers and teach the students concurrently. Before entering their residency in the third year, each student accumulates about 500 hours of supervised clinical practice.

At the time of this writing, other universities have Au.D. programs in operation or have received authorization to start. These include Ball State University, Nova Southeastern University, University of Louisville, Washington State University, University of Florida, and Gallaudet University. Several others are in the process of preparing a proposal for their university review panels.

The Au.D. National Standards Council

In 1994 James Jerger convened a group of about 30 audiologists from various settings throughout the country to study and pre-

TABLE 2–1   Semester hours required for a typical M.A. program and for an Au.D. program

Basic Science	
M.A.	*Au.D.*
Calibration	Calibration
Hearing science	Hearing science
	Anatomy/physiology
	Neuoanatomy
	Speech science
Hours = 6	Hours = 15
Disorders/Assessment	
M.A.	*Au.D.*
Disorders	Disorders
Speech auiometry	Speech audiomety
Pediatrics	Pediatrics
Diagnostics	Diagnostics
	Diagnostics II
AEP/ENG	AEP
	AEP II
	ENG
Hours = 15	Hours = 24
Management	
M.A.	*Au.D.*
Industrial	Industrial
Amplification	Amplification
	Amplification II
Rehabilitation	Educational rehabilitation
	Adult rehabilitation
	Sign language
	Psychosocial
	Professional issues
Hours = 9	Hours = 24
Research	
M.A.	*Au.D.*
Statistics	Statistics
Independent project	Project design
	Project analysis
Hours = 6	Hours = 15
Practicum	
M.A.	*Au.D.*
Hours = 7	Hours = 37
Total hours = 43	Total hours = 115

to advocate the professional doctorate. Beginning in the early 1990s, the AFA wanted quick change in requirements and became impatient, probably justifiably, with the slow pace of ASHA. Consequently, this foundation moved forward with a plan, and then a mechanism, for obtaining the Au.D. designation by way of "earned entitlement." Recognizing that scores of audiologists with master's degrees provide competent hearing health care in a variety of settings every day, it was assumed these people have earned, through experience, the equivalent of what is being proposed as the additional training experiences for new Au.D. students. Thus if an audiologist has had a minimum of 5 years of full-time employment after completion of a master's degree in audiology, he or she can submit documentation of these experiences to a review panel. The panel will decide what additional, if any, experiences and/or course work must be gained to be allowed to use the Au.D. designation after his or her name.

Practically every state has a deceptive trade law that forbids one to cause confusion or misunderstanding as to the sponsorship, approval, or certification of services. Several states have a "Use of Degree Law" that forbids the use of the term "Dr." or any other term if it is not accurate or earned from an accredited institution. For example, New York's law states: "No person shall append to his name any letters signifying a degree unless the degree is received from an approved college or university" (Ford, 1997).

CONTROVERSIAL POINT

The AFA mechanism for obtaining the Au.D. title has received staunch opposition from both ASHA and AAA. Both organizations believe that the use of earned entitlement would degrade the value of an earned Au.D. from an accredited university and place the reputation of audiology at risk in the mind of the public, other healthcare professionals, insurance carriers, and legislative bodies. In short, it could do the profession far more harm than good. Nevertheless, the AFA movement continues at the time of this writing.

pare a document that might serve as a model resource for Au.D. accrediting bodies. This group was referred to as *The AuD National Standards Council.* The document was developed by six writing groups. Each group approached its task by asking, "What are the minimal standards that all Au.D. programs must meet?" It was recognized that some, indeed many, programs will exceed these standards. The goal was to delineate minimal standards basic to the successful operation of any Au.D. training program. A copy of this document appears in the Appendix along with the names and affiliations of the members of the council.

Earned Entitlement

The AAA movement notwithstanding, the Audiology Foundation of America (AFA) has been the most aggressive group

Distance Learning

A major concern surrounding the move to a professional doctorate is the large number of audiologists with a master's degree. Many of these people have been in practice for several years, have families, financial commitments, and are established in a community. They are not willing to relocate to a place where they can pursue an Au.D. The cost of relocating would be prohibitive for many and the number of universities awarding the degree is very limited. As a consequence, some feasible and cost-effective alternative is needed to accommodate a significant number of audiologists who will want to earn an Au.D. Earned entitlement, described earlier, is not a viable alternative for many audiologists probably because of the legal implications involved in using the title without being awarded the degree from an accredited university. Also, many audiologists are opposed, in principle, to using a title that could be construed by the public as having been awarded by a university.

In April 1997 the Joint Service/Veterans Affairs Au.D. Steering Committee, through the Henry M. Jackson Foundation for the Advancement of Military Medicine, released a request for proposal (RFP) to all institutions that offer a graduate degree in audiology. The foundation is a nonprofit organization that facilitates medical education and research initiatives. The committee's goal was to create an opportunity for audiologists employed by the federal government to earn a doctoral degree while still on the job. The request stipulated that the proposals must be (1) accessible, (2) affordable, and (3) reasonable. That is, the program should be available no matter where the audiologist is located geographically, affordable, and not redundant if the audiologist can "pass" certain requirements on the basis of experience and past academic record.

Several good proposals were submitted from the 120 colleges and universities that received the RFP. Central Michigan University and Vanderbilt University filed a joint proposal and in the spring of 1998 received the award of $250,000 to develop and provide a distance learning Au.D. degree program. The degree program is offered primarily through the Internet and supplemented with workshops and face-to-face seminars. The seminars are offered in conjunction with annual meetings of AAA, ASHA, and the Military Audiology Short Course. The program is offered to audiologists without regard to their employment location, whether employed by the federal government or in the private sector. The first students are expected to be admitted in September 1999. The program is designed to be self-paced, accessible to the student's convenience, and completed in 1 to 2½ years. It is estimated to cost up to $8000 for government employees and up to $12,000 for audiologists in the private sector for the 36 credit hours required for the degree. To start, the program will accept about 1000 students with 40 to 50 in a class. Applications are reviewed by an admissions committee and each applicant is assigned an advisor to assist in designing a course of study commensurate with the needs of the applicant. Table 2–2 is a summary of the admission and degree requirements of this Central Michigan University/Vanderbilt University Au.D. distance learning program.

The Hearing Aid Manufacturer's Role

This chapter would be incomplete without citing the role of the hearing aid manufacturers in the education of audiologists. By the early 1970s, several hearing aid manufacturers began to hold product information presentations, seminars, facility tours, and other efforts to inform and educate audiologists to new hearing aid technology. Before this time random efforts were made by some manufacturers to update audiologists but not to the extent that was evident in the 1970s. Even though audiologists did not sell hearing aids at this time, they did do hearing aid evaluations and make referral to hearing aid dealers. Manufacturers realized that it was in their best

TABLE 2–2 Admission and degree requirements for an Au.D. program

Admission Requirements

Master's degree in audiology with a minimum of 3.0 GPA in audiology graduate work

CCC-A or state licensure (or the equivalency for Canadian audiologists) and 5 years of professional audiological experience beyond the master's degree (including the CFY)

Three letters of recommendation that attest to the individual's background, employment and employment setting, a resume that highlights the applicant's academic preparation, career, and continuing education activities

Non-English-speaking applicants must score a minimum of 600 on the TOEFL.

Degree Requirements

Core sequence (21 credit hours)
    Advanced amplification for the hearing-impaired (3 credit hours)
    Advanced electrophysiological techniques in audiology (3 credit hours)
    Psychosocial aspects of hearing loss (3 credit hours)
    Doctoral project (12 credit hours)
Electives (minimum of 15 credit hours)
    Developed jointly between the student and his or her advisory committee (required credits may be more on review of the student's previous graduate course work)
Comprehensive examination
Capstone experience
Most audiologists are required to complete 36 credit hours to qualify for the Au.D. Nine of the 36 hours are in a core sequence taken by every student; 12 of the hours are independent study. After completion of 24 credit hours and before enrolling for more than 3 hours of Capstone experience, students must pass comprehensive examinations in the following content areas: auditory and vestibular systems; speech and hearing science; auditory and vestibular disorders; medical management; diagnostic audiology; habilitative/rehabilitative audiology; clinical professional issues; and case studies (Annon., 1998; Konkle, 1998).

interest to educate the audiologists in hopes that better knowledge of their products would lead to more referrals. By the mid 1970s, it was common practice for several manufacturers to organize nationwide seminars, study tours, special open house sessions during regional and national conventions attended by audiologists, and domestic and foreign trips with programs on hearing aids and other audiological topics.

After ASHA lifted the ban on dispensing hearing aids by audiologists in 1978, the hearing aid manufacturers increased their efforts to educate audiologists. Now, manufacturers viewed audiologists as a new corps of dispensers, and it became more important than in the past to help them understand the function and application of their products. Thus by the beginning of the 1980s, hearing aid manufacturers were devoting much of their time, money, and efforts to the education of audiologists. Regardless of the motives of the manufacturers, there was no other source where audiologists could get the information they needed to enter the hearing aid dispensing arena. Audiologists who started selling hearing aids as part of their professional role in the hearing health care system learned that it was essential to establish and to maintain a relationship with manufacturers to remain current with hearing aid technology.

CONTROVERSIAL POINT

Some audiologists, especially those not dispensing hearing aids and those in academia, took a dim view of the efforts by hearing aid manufacturers to educate audiologists, characterizing them as commercial ventures driven by sales-motivated self-interests.

Throughout the 1980s and 1990s, hearing aid manufacturers, especially the larger more financially secure companies, hired audiologists in increasing numbers and, as a consequence, established more professional educational formats for the practicing audiology community, thus shifting from a sales-oriented to a more genuine educational approach. Simultaneously, hearing aid technology and methods of verification, office management tools, and special instrumentation became increasingly more sophisticated and required teachers with knowledge commensurate with these advancements. The manufacturers were learning that the sale of their products had to be based more on technical knowledge than salesmanship, as it had been in years past. It was a new era for the sale of hearing aids. By the mid-1990s, some manufacturers were spending significant sums of money on the education of audiologists. Furthermore, a few manufacturers made large contributions to the Au.D. initiative through the AFA which routed these funds to defray the expenses of Au.D. students. They also donated generously to the Henry M. Jackson Foundation for the Advancement of Military Medicine which provided seed money to start a distance learning Au.D. degree program and the American Academy of Audiology. For several years, two manufacturers (Starkey Labs and Siemens) paid for professional and scientific journals to be sent to all graduate students of audiology.

Other efforts included, but were not limited to, providing equipment to university programs to teach students hearing aid modification techniques, real-ear measurements, and otoscopic examinations. Starkey Labs commissioned Michael Hawke, M.D., and Andrew McComb, M.B., to prepare a book, entitled *Diseases of the Ear.* This same manufacturer purchased and distributed several copies of the book, *Probe*

Microphone Measurements, by Mueller, Hawkins, and Northern, and distributed these books free or for a nominal cost to scores of audiologists and students.

Over a period of several decades, many manufacturers have supported state, regional, and national professional meetings; conventions; continuing education activities; and the like. They also support, through generous advertising, most audiology publications and purchase exhibit space at national and smaller meetings and conventions. Without question, hearing aid manufacturers have played a significant role in the education of audiologists for decades and their role in this respect is certain to increase in the years ahead. The hearing aid manufacturing industry recognizes that the better trained and more knowledgeable professionals are about their products, the greater will be the sale of these products with fewer returns for credit. Thus more persons with impaired hearing will receive assistance from hearing aids.

Audiological Specialties

Following the natural evolutionary path of most professions, audiology has definitely branched off into some identifiable specializations that have their own body of knowledge and skills. Undergirding each specialization is a core of common knowledge that all audiologists should have to practice their profession. It seems inevitable that the day will come when there will be specialty boards within the structure of the forthcoming ABC. These boards will probably have their own process of certification above and beyond the regular ABC.

Some audiologists have chosen a certain area of practice that requires special knowledge and skills. Following are some of these potential areas of professional specialized services:

Audiological diagnostics with adults
Audiological diagnostics with children
Industrial audiology
Hearing aid selection, fitting, and dispensing
Aural rehabilitation with adults
Aural rehabilitation with children
Public and private school audiological services
Electrophysiology/intraoperative monitoring
Vestibularology

CONCLUSIONS

A specialized curriculum for the study of audiology, leading to a graduate degree, started in the mid 1940s. The course of study was modeled after the already established degree in speech pathology. For the first 50 years most students terminated with a master's degree and located in a health care professional environment. The curriculum and credentialing of audiologists was determined, controlled, and monitored by the American Speech-Language-Hearing Association, even though states introduced licensing or registration laws. Starting in the late 1970s, audiologists began to dispense hearing aids and assume responsibility for the rehabilitative management of the patients they serve. This represented a major shift in the role of the audiologist who, heretofore, had been engaged mainly in the role of a diagnostician, supplying test data to the medical profession.

Hearing aid dispensing also made the private practice of audiology financially feasible. Thus many audiologists established their own private practice and became independent healthcare providers.

Not only did the scope of practice of audiology change and increase, so did the technology undergirding the profession. By 1990, it started to be obvious that the growth of knowledge and skills being required to provide competent services for the hearing impaired was not being met by the audiology degree programs across the country. Practicing audiologists and newly formed audiology academies and an audiology foundation began to pressure ASHA to upgrade requirements for certification, which in turn would impact curricula and practicum requirements to practice audiology. Inherent in the expansion of the preparation of audiologists was the need for a professional doctoral degree called the

Au.D. or Doctor of Audiology. Following the lead of Baylor College of Medicine, a couple of other universities introduced an Au.D program. The first three persons graduated with an Au.D. in May of 1996.

After 7 years of surveys, discussion, conferences, and confrontations, the issue of a professional degree as an entry level requirement to practice audiology came to fruition. In 1997 the ASHA Legislative Council passed a resolution mandating an upgrade in the requirements for certification effective January 1, 2007, and a doctorate degree as a basic requirement for certification effective January 1, 2012. Distance learning opportunities are becoming available to practicing audiologists with a master's degree who wish to earn an Au.D. It is anticipated that by the year 2015 virtually all audiologists practicing in this country will have a doctoral degree and that a large number of them will hold a specialized board certification.

Appendix
Proposed Minimal Standards for Au.D. Programs

prepared by
The Au.D. National Standards Council
November, 1995

The Au.D. National Standards Council (TANSC) was organized in 1994 with the aim of developing a document summarizing minimal standards for programs proposing to offer the Au.D. degree. The goal has been to develop a document that can serve as a model resource for accrediting bodies.

The present document was developed by six writing groups. Each group approached its task by asking, "what are the minimal standards that all Au.D. programs must meet?" It is understood that some, indeed many, programs will exceed these standards. The aim here has been to delineate minimal standards basic to the successful operation of any Au.D. training program.

Successive iterations of the complete document were circulated to the chairs of writing groups, who in turn circulated them to individual members of their group for feedback on the entire document. After these comments had been collected the document was re-edited to take into account, as much as possible, the reactions of each responding person. This entire process was carried out three times. In addition, members of the council commented individually at various times over the period of more than one year in which the document was in process of preparation.

Inevitably, this set of standards represents a compromise between the recommendations of those who feel it is important to spell out precise details of every aspect of Au.D. programs and those who feel that only broad guidelines should be specified, the details of implementation being left to the discretion of the individual program. Editing such a compromise document has been an extremely challenging undertaking, calling for a steady course between the Scylla of micromanagement and the Charybdis of *laissez faire*. Yet we are confident that the importance of establishing standards transcends individual positions at either extreme of the philosophical spectrum.

For further information about The Au.D. National Standards Council (TANSC) and/or the development of this document, please contact:

James Jerger, Ph.D.
2612 Prairie Creek Drive East
Richardson, TX 75080-2679
Phone: (972) 664-9123
Fax: (972) 668-1827
e-mail: jjerger@bcm.tmc.edu

INTRODUCTION

The Au.D. program is a four-year course of full time study including both academic and practicum components. It is a new model for the education of audiological practitioners stressing the integration of classroom and clinical learning across a broad spectrum of specialties and environments. The present document is divided into five sections, each concerned with a specific aspect of Au.D. training. It is not the purpose of this document to dictate what shall be the immutable constituents of Au.D. training. The goal is simply to provide accrediting and other interested bodies with the minimal requirements that responsible members of the profession regard as basic to any Au.D. program. These recommended minimal requirements are organized under five headings as follows: Facilities, Curriculum, Faculty & Staff, Patient Populations, and Student Qualifications.

FACILITIES

Essential Technology

Programs Applying for accreditation under these standards shall demonstrate that students will have the necessary didactic instruction in, and practical hands-on experience with, state-of-the-art instrumentation in the following areas: amplification; rehabilitation; electrophysiology; electroacoustics; and other basic diagnostic audiological technology. This standard requires that programs have, in-house, diagnostic and rehabilitative hardware, software, and the necessary physical environment for utilizing such technology.

Educational Facilities

Programs proposing to offer the Au.D. degree must be housed in an academic institution of higher education capable of providing a strong program in communication sciences and disorders and providing the critical elements of all academic programs, including libraries, laboratories, access to academic advising, teaching space and modern teaching methodologies including telecommunications, media resources, computer facilities, tutoring, etc. The institution must be regionally accredited by one of the nationally recognized accreditation bodies (e.g., SACS).

Clinical Facilities

Programs applying for accreditation under these standards must demonstrate that students will receive clinical instruction and experience within at least the following four types of clinical environment: (1) hospital or other medical setting; (2) autonomous private practice setting; (3) educational setting; and (4) rehabilitation setting. It is recognized that some institutions may house more than one of these types of facilities in the same physical plant; however, the intent of this standard is that students will have the opportunity to develop an awareness of and entry level competence to work in the unique practice environments found in each of these settings. Clinical facilities can be provided entirely by the didactic training program or partially contained in affiliated programs.

Clinical facilities supporting Au.D. training may be part of a consortium of unique experts, linked together electronically for teleconferencing or through travel and support grants to facilitate diverse and specialized learning experiences for students that might not be accessible in any one location. Alternatively, specialty areas (e.g., hearing aids, auditory brain stem response, otoacoustic emissions) could be developed at distant sites providing special clinical training internships.

Supervision

Students must be supervised during their practicum experience. Supervisors must be licensed to practice audiology by the state in which the institution is located, or, if there is no licensure in that state, must have earned nationally recognized certification, or its equivalent. Institutions must assure on-site supervision. Although direct supervision may vary according to student level or nature of the patient, the supervisor must review all patient reports completed by the student on a regular basis.

Scope of Clinical Facilities

The program must ensure that facilities provide students the opportunity to receive training across the following range of clinical activities relating to adults, children and infants:

1. Comprehensive Audiologic Assessment
2. Electrophysiologic Assessment
3. Hearing Screening
4. Vestibular Assessment
5. Amplification
6. Implantable Devices
7. Audiologic Rehabilitation

CURRICULUM

Introduction

The following program description is based on a semester system with a full time load defined as 12 credit hours per semester and the four-year program divided into 12 semesters (8 regular, 4 summer). Seven semesters of full time work are devoted to the academic component and five semesters are devoted to the practicum component. Academic course work and practica may be completed concurrently or the practicum may follow the academic component, provided that the program provides the minimum requirements.

Academic Course Work

A total of 84 semester hours of academic course work must be completed (7 semesters, 12 credits per semester). The 84 credits must be distributed among the major content areas listed in Table 2A–1. Additional course work beyond the minimum requirements presented here is encouraged. Training programs may adopt requirements that are more stringent than these minimum requirements.

The minimum required semester hours for the major content areas is provided in Table 2A–1. *All* of the topic areas listed under each major category must be covered in the academic course work. The organization of the topic areas into courses is left to the discretion of the program.

Of the 84 required semester hours, a minimum of 63 hours must be completed in the six major content areas and electives listed in Table 2A–1. The minimum number of hours that must be completed in each content area is also shown in Table 2A–1. The remaining 21 semester hours must be distributed among the major content areas with a maximum of nine hours in the elective category. More elective hours are encouraged but cannot be counted toward the 84 semester-hour minimum requirement.

The academic course work must be completed at the host institution. Course work completed at another institution may be transferred only when pre-approved by the host institution. For students with previous educational experiences, specific requirements may be waived if they demonstrate knowledge in a particular content area by written examination. Waiving academic requirements without a written examination should not be permitted.

Practicum

A total of 2500 practicum contact hours is required. Only experiences that provide direct contact with a patient can be used to satisfy the practicum requirements. It is recognized that there will be additional time for preparation, review of results, report writing, electroacoustic evaluation, and calibration that are required in the practicum experience. Although these activities are of critical importance, for purposes of defining minimum requirements, only patient-contact hours are specified.

The practicum component represents five semesters of full time study with 33.3 hours per week devoted to patient contact, to result in a total of 2500 practicum hours (5 semesters × 15 weeks × 33.3 hours = 2500). The practicum can be distributed throughout the four-year course of study. However, it is recommended that some academic course work precede practicum in each area. It is important that academic and practicum components be coordinated to provide consistency and continuity to the program.

The assignment of semester hours to practicum experiences is done at the program's discretion. These credit hours do not count toward the 84 semester hour academic credit hour minimum.

Each patient visit may include a variety of practicum experiences, such as case history, pure tone audiometry, hearing

TABLE 2A–1 Academic course work

Content Area	Minimum Semester Hours

ANATOMY & PHYSIOLOGY
   Embryology and Development
   General Head & Neck (including the speech mechanism)
   Neuroanatomy and Neurophysiology
   Anatomy & Physiology of the Auditory and Vestibular Systems
	6

PATHOLOGIES
   General Head & Neck
   Syndromes
   Diseases of the Auditory System
   Diseases of the Vestibular System
	3

BASIC AREAS
   Electronics
   Acoustics
   Hearing Science
   Speech Science
   Statistics
   Language Development
   Human Development and Cognition
   Research Methods
	18

MEASUREMENT
   Psychophysics
   Electrophysiologic Measurement
   Measurement of Auditory Function
   Measurement of Vestibular Function
   Instrumentation and Calibration
   Noise Measurement and Control
   Assessment of Disability/Handicap
	15

HABILITATION & REHABILITATION
   Amplification for the Hearing-Impaired
      (including hearing aids and
      assistive listening devices)
   Manual Communication
   Remedial Communication Strategies
   Hearing Conservation
   Educational Audiology
   Counseling
   Implantable Devices
	15

RELATED AREAS
   Clinic Administration and Management
   Clinical Otolaryngology
   Clinical Pharmacology
   Clinical and Professional Issues
   Clinical Psychology
   Neuropsychology
   Ethics in Healthcare Delivery
   Gerontology
   Computer Science
	6

aid assessment, and electrophysiologic assessment. The total time of the visit shall be divided among the various practicum activities listed in Table 2A–2 based on the proportion of time spent in each of the activities.

Of the 2500 required practicum hours, 1850 must be in the activities in Table 2A–2. The minimum number of practicum hours that must be completed in each activity are also listed in Table 2A–2. The remaining 650 practicum hours must be dis-

TABLE 2A–2 Clinical practicum

Activity	Hours
Case History, interview	100
Basic and advanced assessment methods	
(including pure tone audiometry, speech audiometry, and handicap assessment)	400
Physiologic assessment methods	
Acoustic immittance measurement (tympanometry and acoustic reflex measurement)	100
Electrophysiologic assessment (auditory brain stem response, middle latency, late and event-related auditory evoked potentials, electrocochleography, intraoperative auditory monitoring)	250
Otoacoustic emissions	100
Evaluation of the vestibular system	150
Hearing aid and other ALD assessment and fitting	350
Implantable Devices (evaluation of candidacy, programming, habilitation and rehabilitation)	100
Hearing Screening	100

tributed among the listed activities. At least 600 of the 2500 practicum hours must be completed with pediatric patients.

The student's role in the assessment and management of patients will systematically expand and develop during the Au.D. program. That is, the student will begin as an observer, progress to an assistant, then to an experienced clinician, and culminate as a semi-independent provider of services and care.

PATIENT POPULATIONS

Background Information

Access to and direct contact with sizable and diverse patient populations is an essential component of Au.D. education and training. The student can develop clinical skills only by practicing audiology with actual patients requiring audiologic services. The Au.D. student must encounter patient populations that, minimally: 1) are varied in age, ranging from newborn infants to elderly adults; 2) are varied in ethnicity; 3) include outpatients and inpatients; 4) span a broad spectrum of pathologies; and 5) are undergoing all clinical procedures encompassed within the audiologist's scope of practice.

Au.D. programs must have access to patients managed with a wide variety of diagnostic procedures, rehabilitative methods, and patient database management systems, representing contemporary clinical practice. Students need exposure to patients spanning various audiologic, social, and cultural spectra.

Recommended Minimum Standard

Within the Au.D. program, the student must have multiple direct contacts with each of the patient populations relevant to the scope of practice of audiology. Minimally, these patient populations include, but are not limited to:

1. Neonates and infants, including well babies and those at risk for hearing impairment.

2. Infants and young children with communicatively significant hearing impairment, including those with multiple disabilities and traditionally "difficult-to-test" audiologically. Both assessment and coordinated multi-faceted management should be included.

3. Preschool and/or school age children undergoing comprehensive audiologic assessment for suspected central auditory processing disorder (CAPD) and requiring audiologic, educational, and speech-language management.

4. Adults with confirmed otologic pathology, including those undergoing pre- and postoperative audiologic assessment.

5. Adults with communicatively significant hearing impairment who are candidates for amplification and other audiologic management strategies.

6. Adults with vestibular and balance disorders undergoing comprehensive electrophysiologic assessment and requiring medical, surgical, or rehabilitative management.

7. Adults with neurotologic and/or neurologic disease undergoing diagnostic audiologic assessment.

8. Adults with senescent auditory disorders.

SPECIAL CONSIDERATION

Au.D. programs without access to sizable special populations (e.g., neonatal and pediatric) must have established arrangements for pre-approved off-site sponsors with clearly identified faculty and adequate patient populations, or collaborative or consortium arrangements with other Au.D. programs with populations sufficient to support the training requirements of students.

STUDENT QUALIFICATIONS

Undergraduate Preparation

The student must have earned a baccalaureate degree from an accredited institution. It is recommended that students should have successfully completed:

1. A core science curriculum including:
Two semesters of Biology, with labs
Two semesters of Chemistry, with labs
Two semesters of Physics, with labs

2. Two semesters of college level Math from the areas of algebra, geometry, trigonometry, calculus.

3. Two semesters of English including grammar and composition.

4. Course work in:
Normal Language Development
Anatomy for Speech and Hearing
Linguistic Factors in Speech Perception

Additional Requirements

Additional requirements for admission to an Au.D. program should be assumed by each institution, i.e., GRE score, GPA cutoffs, letters of recommendation, etc. so long as the minimal standards for entrance to graduate study at the institution are met.

Undergraduate Programs

Universities should be encouraged to develop pre-Au.D. programs at the undergraduate level similar to other pre-professional programs (e.g., pre-med, pre-law).

APPENDIX

COMPOSITION OF TANSC WRITING GROUPS

I. Academic Facilities

Rick Talbott, Chair	University of Central Florida
Diane Brewer	George Washington University
Carol Flexer	University of Akron
Susan Jerger	Baylor College of Medicine
Jerry Northern	University of Colorado

II. Clinical Facilities

Allen Boysen, Chair	Department of Veterans Affairs
Charles Berlin	LSU Medical Center
James Hall, III	Vanderbilt University
Earl Harford	Starkey Labs
Gary Jacobson	Henry Ford Hospital
Tom Littman	Texas Childrens Hospital
Brad Stach	California Ear Institute

III. Curriculum

Robert Margolis, Chair	University of Minnesota
Sue Erdman	University of Maryland-Balt. County
David Fabry	Mayo Clinic
James Lynn	University of Akron
William Rintelmann	Wayne State University
Richard Wilson	VAMC, Mountain Home, TN

IV. Faculty Staff

Deborah Hayes, Chair and	Denver Childrens Hospital
Lucille Beck	VA Medical Center, Washington, D.C.
Fred Bess	Vanderbilt University
Gerald Church	Central Michigan University
Laura Wilber	Northwestern University

V. Patient Populations

James Hall III, Chair	Vanderbilt University
Charles Berlin	LSU Medical Center
Sharon Fujikawa	University of California, Irvine
Deborah Hayes	Denver Childrens Hospital
Robert Keith	University of Cincinnati
Frank Musiek	Dartmouth-Hitchcock Med Ctr
Jerry Northern	University of Colorado

VI. Student Qualifications

Linda Hood, Chair	LSU Medical Center
Gerald Church	Central Michigan University
Gary Jacobson	Henry Ford Hospital
Laszlo Stein	Northwestern University
Laura Wilber	Northwestern University
Michael Dennis	University of Oklahoma

REFERENCES

ANNON. (1993). Professional education in audiology. *ASHA, 35(3)*;34.

ANNON. (1994). Professional education in audiology. *ASHA, 36(3)*;31.

ANNON. (1997). *Audiology Express, 3(3)*;1–3.

ANNON. (1998). Au.D. distance-learning program. *Audiology Today, 10(3)*;22.

BERGER, K.W. (1976). Geneology of the words "audiology" and "audiologist." *Journal of the American Audiological Society 2(1)*;38–44.

BERLIN, C., CURRAN, J., NORDSTROM, P., & SYFERT, G. (1991). Position paper. The American Academy of Audiology and the professional doctorate (Au.D.). *Audiology Today, 3(4)*;10–12.

CARHART, R. (1958). The personal need for professional unity. *Journal of Speech and Hearing Disorders, 23(1)*;6–7.

DAVIS, H. (1960). Audiometry. In: H. Davis, & S.R. Silverman (Eds.), *Hearing and deafness* (Rev. ed.) (p. 216). New York: Holt, Rinehart and Winston.

DOERFLER, L. (1991). Remembering how it all began. Audiology CO-OP *Newsletter, 3*;3.

FORD, M. (1997). Law and regulations relating to the use of degrees and degree designators. *9(5)*;27,29, 31.

JERGER, J. (1998). Letter of invitation to attend a discussion for a national society of audiology, December 1, 1987. *Audiology Today, 7 (Special Issue)*.

KIRKWOOD, D.H. (1998). In survey, dispensers report growth, express views on professional issues. *Hearing Journal, 51(3)*;22

KONKLE, D. (1998). Joint services initiate distance learning Au.D. program. *Hearing Review, 5(6)*;53.

NEWBY, H. (1964). The profession of audiology. In: *Audiology* (2nd ed.) (p. 361). New York: Appleton-Century-Crofts.

NORTHERN, J. (1998). ASHA threatens action against AAA over audiology board certification program. *Audiology Today, 10(3)*;9.

OLISHIFSKI, J., & HARFORD, E. (Eds.) (1975). Occupational safety and health act of 1970. *Industrial noise and hearing conservation* (p. 863). Chicago: National Safety Council.

ROESER, R., & CRANDELL, C. (1991). The audiologist's responsibility in cerumen management. *ASHA, 33(1)*;51–53.

SHAMBAUGH, G.E., & CARHART, R. (1951). Contributions of audiology to fenestration surgery. *Archives of Otolaryngology, 54*;699.

SKAFTE, M.D. (1990). Fifty years of hearing healthcare. *Hearing Instruments, 41(9)*;96.

Chapter 3

Professional Ethics and Audiology

Joseph W. Helmick

Outline

Ethics, as a branch of philosophy, has been studied and professed for hundreds of years. It is a discipline that seeks to describe values in the context of societal norms and expectations. The ancient Greeks viewed ethics as life choices—goals to be attained and situations to be avoided—in pursuit of the "telos," which is the chief good of life. Enarson (1991) remarks "The domain of ethics is the domain of human choice with respect to values" (p. 3). Thus ethics represents the enactment of a recognized and accepted value system and not merely the representation of "personal taste . . . or passing fads" Enarson (1991, p. 3–4). Unfortunately, public attention to ethics has been driven to a high level of visibility, largely through reports in the media about ethical misconduct. Ethical controversies in politics, academia, business, and the professions appear with an uncomfortable degree of periodicity in all media forms. One of the results has been a growing public perception that ethical values and conduct are at an all-time low.

In the past ethical conduct within professions has not been viewed with the same degree of concern as exists today. In fact, Stromberg (1990) notes that "it is hard to recall a time when there was such pervasive skepticism about professional ethics" (p.15). In the face of such pervasive public skepticism

all professions, including audiology, are painted with the same brush when incidents of professional misconduct are unveiled. Society has always held higher expectations for conduct in the professions than it has for the trades or for business. In the context of a society that has grown increasingly concerned about professional ethics, it is useful to understand what distinguishes a profession from a trade or a business.

CHARACTERISTICS OF A PROFESSION

A distinction between a profession and a trade or business can be made, in general terms, by examining the origins of the words *trade* and *profession*. *Trade* comes from the Middle Low German and Old Saxon words for "trace" and "trail," respectively (*Webster's*, 1960, p. 1237). Thus a tradesman was literally a person who trod the trails and pathways selling his (or her?) goods. *Profession* is derived from the Latin word meaning a "declaration" (*Webster's*, 1960). Someone who belonged to a profession declared (or more literally professed) certain beliefs, values, or truths. A professional, therefore, is one who is "engaged in, or worthy of the high standards of, a profession" (*Webster's*, 1960, p. 1437).

From these definitions another distinction between trades (businesses) and professions also emerges. Members of a trade come together not only out of mutual interest but also to promote economic gain. By contrast, a profession is committed to a set of ideals and values, such as serving others, that is considered to be higher than those of the marketplace (Stromberg, 1990). On the basis of the objectives of economic gain and service to others only, audiology, at least dispensing audiology, seems to be both a profession and a trade.

But a profession is characterized by more than the objectives of affirming values and providing services. Professions are distinguished from other groups by the following:

1. They possess a highly specialized body of knowledge and skills that require extensive preparation and experience for mastery.

2. They set their own standards and, thereby, control the entry of individuals to the profession.

3. They define a scope of practice and conduct tasks within that scope of practice without supervision.

4. They establish and enforce levels of conduct for members that are higher than those required of others.

5. They serve the public good.

Audiology: Practice Management. Edited by Hosford-Dunn, Roeser, and Valente. Thieme Medical Publishers, Inc., New York © 2000

As a consequence of these characteristics, professions are subject to less social control than trades or businesses. Professions also tend to enjoy a higher level of prestige because they are viewed as value-oriented service providers as opposed to profit takers. That is, they act for the welfare of others and are both self-regulating and self-disciplinary (DeGeorge, 1986). By contrast, the popular view of business is that it is more directed to self-interest, in the form of economic gain, than it is to serving others and that it tends to be less involved in self-regulation and self-discipline. Thus social institutions at the local, state, and national levels impose more restrictions on businesses than on professions and view businesses as less value oriented than professions.

This is not to suggest that professionals are only value-affirming and not profit-oriented or that members of the business community always seek profits, are only self-serving, and have no concern for values. Such is simply not the case. Because professions and business each pursue somewhat different primary objectives, however, they adhere to differing sets of values or, ethical principles. Thus the terms *professional ethics* and *business ethics* serve to distinguish the different objective-drawn value sets of these two groups.

ETHICS AND ETHICAL CODES

Some Brief Definitions

A number of different ethical value sets exist, at least as represented by terms such as professional ethics, business ethics, and personal ethics. Subsets even occur within professional ethics, such as medical and legal ethics, to name two. As the terms imply, each designator occupies some limited, although not necessarily exclusive, position on a broader spectrum known as ethics.

An examination of differing definitions of ethics reveals that ethics, both as a discipline of study and as a factor of conduct, is fundamentally an issue of social values. For example, DeGeorge (1986) states that "Ethics in general can be defined as a systematic attempt, through the use of reason, to make sense of our individual and social moral experience, in such a way as to determine the rules that ought to govern human conduct and the values worth pursuing in life" (p.15).

Clearly, DeGeorge views ethics as moral values that are derived from reason within a social context for the purpose of imposing restrictions on human conduct. A more pragmatic definition is that offered by Leo Strauss (1983) of the University of Chicago, who noted that ethics is the state wherein individuals "are willing and able to prefer the common interest to their private interests, to do what is noble and right because it is noble and right and for no other reason" (p. 36). That definition calls for an attitude, a belief, and a commitment in which altruism and the welfare of others are the beacon principles. The most utilitarian definition may be the one attributed to Mark Twain, who reportedly quipped, "Always do what is right. This will gratify some people and astonish the rest." Regardless of which definition one accepts, it is clear that ethics, while derived from the social codification of behaviors over time, lives within the heart and mind of the individual. Codes of ethics cannot engender such personal

traits of ethical conduct; they are merely the more public signposts that give direction to acceptable and unacceptable ethical behaviors.

PEARL

Ethical dilemmas force us to make choices between advancing the welfare of others and achieving personal gains.

American Speech-Language-Hearing Association and American Academy of Audiology Codes of Ethics

Of course, not everyone agrees on what "doing right" means exactly. Two people observing the same situation may disagree on whether some specific conduct was ethical or unethical. It is also the case that each person's internal standard for what is "noble and right" may not remain constant over time (Silverman, 1983). To resolve the variable of individual judgments about what is or is not right, professions have developed codes of ethics. So it is for the profession of audiology. In 1930 the American Society for the Study of Disorders of Speech adopted a set of "Principles of Ethics" (Paden, 1970). Of course, that original document has gone through several revisions, the most recent one issued in January 1994. Nevertheless, the ASHA Code of Ethics (1994) continues to serve as a guidepost that describes ethical conduct expectations for individuals within the audiology profession. More recently, the American Academy of Audiology has also issued a Code of Ethics specifically for the profession of audiology (AAA, 1991). The effect of a professional code of ethics is not only to describe what is "noble and right" for a variety of situations but, in so doing, to also impose restrictions and obligations on the professional activities of individuals.

As one examines the ethical codes of ASHA and AAA, it is apparent that they both seek to promote similar values—values that are characteristic of a profession. For example, both codes direct members to maintain high standards of competency and to not engage in conduct that would degrade the dignity of the profession. Each code requires that representation by members to the public not be false, deceptive, or misleading. Each code cites as its first and highest ethical principle the responsibility of members to direct their efforts to the "benefit" (AAA, 1991) and "welfare" (ASHA, 1994) of those they serve professionally. In these examples, as with all other stipulations in the ASHA and AAA ethical codes, the objective is to promote the public good, to put "common interests" above "private interests" (Strauss, 1983).

Characteristics of Professional Codes of Ethics

Professional codes, such as those advanced by ASHA and AAA, share three common characteristics. First, they describe in rather practical terms the values held by the profession. Because these values often appear in the form of normative statements, they also serve as a standard against which the professional conduct of members is to be evaluated (see Chapter 9). Second, they impose an obligation on the member to accept both the value and the practices inherent in the particular stipulations of the code. By accepting membership into the profession, members also accept the obligation to conduct their professional affairs in accordance with the norms delineated by the profession's code of ethics. Third, members accept responsibility for their professional conduct, including penalties imposed by the profession in instances of ethical misconduct. Members voluntarily accept the higher standards reflected in the professional code and, in turn, they are also held responsible for their professional conduct by the profession. In addition, society holds professionals responsible not only for following a high standard of professional conduct but of personal conduct as well. Professionals are expected to "set an example of proper conduct, and be above suspicion . . . not only to refrain from improper conduct but also to be known to refrain" from such conduct (DeGeorge, 1986, p. 339). The societal expectation that professionals avoid the appearance of improper conduct is not typically reflected in a code of ethics. Yet, this does not diminish societal expectations that professionals "be known to refrain" from improper conduct.

Ethics Versus the Law

However, this presents distinct challenges to both the professional and the profession. Regarding the professional, the challenge is a definitional one. That is, what constitutes improper ethical conduct as distinguished from issues of legal conduct? Clearly, ethical behavior is related to both morality and the law, yet it must also be distinguished from each of these matters in those instances where judgments relative to the appropriateness and acceptability of professional behavior (ethical conduct) are to be made. Ethical principles and practices need to stand on their own merit. To be sure, some breaches of ethics might be of such a character as to rise to the level of illegality. However, actions that may be judged to be unethical do not necessarily represent a violation of civil or criminal laws. For example, it may be unethical to take on so many patients that the overall quality of service is reduced, but case overload, in and of itself, is not illegal. Should the erosion of service quality result in malpractice, however, the issue becomes both an ethical and a legal matter. It is also the case that violations of the law are not necessarily ethical violations. Court actions taken against a person may not represent behaviors that are contrary to one or more of the stipulations in an ethical code. For example, although we may not condone someone cheating on his or her income tax, that is not a violation of the ASHA or AAA codes of ethics.

Ethics Versus Morality

Just as a relationship exists between ethics and the law, a relationship also exists between ethics and morality. Again, however, it is important to be able to distinguish between the two. Morality refers to a set of values that is broadly invested in all behaviors, professional, personal, and so forth. Oftentimes, those values are rooted in religious tenets and beliefs. Moral values are not set by the profession but rather by society. As such, all persons are expected to evidence some common set of values in their personal conduct. Values such as honesty and truthfulness, for example, are expected of everyone. Because professional ethics are norms that exist in addition to those of personal morality, society expects professionals

to be more than possessors of moral principles common to everyone. Professionals are also expected to be exemplars of and advocates for both moral and ethical principles. More tolerance is present in society for exaggerated product claims by a cosmetic manufacturer than for unsupported claims of benefit for medical services by a physician. The reasons for this are probably multiple. Certainly one reason is that society requires higher standards of both moral and ethical conduct from members of a profession than it does from business or corporate men and women. Thus when the choice is made to become a member of a profession, the obligation is to accept greater not lesser moral obligations (DeGeorge, 1986).

Professional Versus Personal Ethics

Still another area of similarity and contrast is that between professional and personal ethics. The latter is much more akin to individual moral issues. The former, on the other hand, speaks to standards set by a group for the conduct of its members. That is, of course, most appropriate. After all, the conduct of an individual, whether that be as a clinician, teacher, researcher, administrator, consultant, and so on, reflects not only on that person but also on the profession at large. The profession, therefore, not only has the *right* to set appropriate and acceptable standards of conduct but also, by definition, the *responsibility* to do so. That responsibility extends not just to individual members of the profession but to the persons served professionally. The professional conduct of any one member reflects on all members. The dignity and respect accorded to a profession is usually based on the public's contact with an individual member of that profession. As a group that provides a variety of professional services, those served expect value-positive conduct in the provision of those services. Thus professional groups set standards of conduct, in this case ethical conduct, both as guideposts for members and for the protection and well-being of consumers.

PROFESSIONS AS BUSINESS AND BUSINESS AS PROFESSIONS

In contemporary society the sharp distinctions between professions and business have become considerably blurred. Professions have added a business image to their self-profile. It is common for professionals to be engaged in private practice, to form partnerships and corporations, to competitively advertise, and to sell products and services. As professionals become increasingly engaged in these activities, they begin to take on much of the appearance of businesspersons. This incorporation of business characteristics, perhaps more than any other single event, has altered the professional profile of audiology. Audiologists fought long and hard for the opportunity to incorporate the dispensing of hearing aids into their professional scope of practice. It was a rightful pursuit that did much to enhance the quality of service available to those in need of assistive listening devices. At the same time, however, audiology moved dramatically from being a "pure" profession to being a hybrid of professional and business practices.

By the same token, businesses have made a conscious effort to increase the image of *professionalism* that is presented to the public. For example, many corporations, industries, and businesses have adopted codes of ethics. The content of the codes is often quite divergent. For example, some merely specify legal standards applicable to employees, others address specific issues of misconduct, such as bribery or theft, while still others focus heavily on practices that are or appear to be conflicts of interest (DeGeorge, 1986). For the most part, however, the focus of industry-specific codes of ethics is the establishment of standards of fair competition with considerably less attention, if any, given to advancing the welfare of consumers or promoting the public good.

Thus although professions look more like businesses and business has increased its public profile with an appeal to professionalism, they continue to distinguish themselves somewhat by their ultimate goals—service to others and economic gain. Nevertheless, as individual professions increasingly engage in the practice of business, they are meeting different and more complex ethical challenges. These ethical challenges are no less for the profession of audiology than they are for any other profession.

ETHICAL CHALLENGES

Ethical challenges to the audiology profession, or to any profession as it increasingly engages in business practices, come from forces both internal and external to the professions. Internal forces include (1) an expanding scope of practice and (2) advances in technology, both of which lead to (3) an altered professional role in healthcare delivery. External forces include (1) allowances and restrictions imposed by legal and regulatory bodies and (2) public perceptions and expectations.

Expanding Scope of Practice

Anyone who has been practicing audiology for more than 20 years has witnessed firsthand the remarkable expansion in the profession's scope of practice. With the landmark decision within ASHA to allow audiologists to engage in dispensing hearing aids for profit, the face of audiology was immediately, dramatically, and irrevocably changed. Arguably, no other single event so significantly influenced the profession of audiology. It affected not only the clinical practice of audiology but also the nature of research and professional preparation standards. Most importantly, however, it thrust the profession of audiology into the business arena. Now audiologists were faced with the challenge of potentially competing and conflicting objectives—service to others and personal economic gain.

PITFALL

A code of ethics is not limited to professional conduct in the clinical arena. It governs conduct in all practice settings, under all practice conditions, and with all individuals.

But product dispensing for profit also spawned other ethical challenges. Because audiologists, as sellers of a product, were now engaged with product manufacturers, and because both audiologists and manufacturers were seeking economic gains, serious issues of conflict of interest needed to be addressed. The issues for discussion were not the appropriateness of these two groups seeking economic gain. That, in and of itself, is decidedly not an ethical dilemma. Rather the dilemma for audiology derived from how to balance economic gain with the needs and interests of those individuals served professionally. Resnick (1992) addressed this dilemma effectively in noting that when the practice of audiology is viewed primarily as a business, "the atmosphere becomes suited for professional ethics to give way to self-interest" (p. 18). Achieving an appropriate balance between good business practices and ethical conduct is, to be certain, a significant but an achievable challenge.

Advances in Technology

Significant enhancements in instrumentation have also brought new ethical challenges. As the audiologist is presented with improved technology for assessing the auditory system, scope of practice challenges occur and issues of competency come to the fore.

Technological advances in instrumentation yielded the opportunity to measure responses to auditory stimuli at selective points along the neural pathways for hearing. Subsequently, another frontier, intraoperative auditory monitoring, was crossed. Cochlear implant surgery reflects still another change in scope of practice that is driven, at least in part, by improved technology. These are but a few of the scope of practice issues that can be linked to technological advances. They require that the profession of audiology actively consider the ethical implications of the ever-expanding scope of practice boundaries. Lane and Bahan (1998) argue that cochlear implant surgery in children has raised serious ethical issues. Some have argued that audiology is exceeding its defensible scope of practice boundaries. (J. Jerger, personal communication, Annual Meeting of the Texas Speech-Language-Hearing Association, Houston, TX, 1989.) Obviously, others could argue that the measurement of hearing along any dimension is appropriately the purview of audiology.

In the face of rapidly advancing technological changes, the more complex ethical issue is that of competency. As changes in technology push the limits of professional scope of practice, how are issues of competency to be addressed? To be certain, opportunities for continuing education (CE) experience are both available and used as new instrumentation and new clinical strategies are evolved. Is it sufficient, however, that the individual practitioner report participation in such activities as a standard of competency? Does the profession have a responsibility to establish competency standards that include not only an exposure to basic information (academic coursework) but also demonstrated abilities (supervised clinical practicum)? Does the sponsorship of CE programs in the use of new technology by instrument manufacturers create ethical challenges for both the professional and the profession? What is the ethical responsibility of personnel preparation programs as scope of practice and technological advances occur? How does the profession assure itself that individuals will not engage in these new clinical arenas using recently developed instrumentation in the absence of appropriate training and demonstrated competency? Each of these is an ethically provocative situation that requires some level of consideration within the audiology profession. The resolution will reflect the degree to which audiology retains its primary identity as a profession or moves still closer to being recognized as a specialized business.

Altered Professional Role

An expanding scope of practice and advances in instrumental technology inextricably lead to an alteration in the audiologist's professional role. Now the boundaries between audiology and other professions (medicine, for example) must be reexamined and perhaps reset. In this particular instance, significant concerns may exist for the autonomy of the audiologist to set appropriate boundaries. But what of the public's understanding of the role of the audiologist in hearing healthcare? Does it become even less clear, and, if so, does that lead to any ethical concerns?

SPECIAL CONSIDERATION

Judicial responses by the profession to ethical misconduct are expected. The more salient professional concern, however, should be to advance the higher values expected of and consistent with the privilege of being a profession. To do this requires more of a profession than the *thou shalls* and *thou shall nots* that comprise a code of ethics.

As private practice in audiology has increased, the profession takes on more of the characteristics of a business enterprise. One of the unfortunate concomitants has been increased reports of fraudulent billing. Certainly, this ethical misconduct (and illegal act) is not peculiar to audiology. In fact, the public is much more aware of fraudulent behavior in the medical profession than in the audiology profession. But this does not relieve any profession from examining the causes of such ethical transgressions and taking appropriate action when they occur. Judicial responses by the profession to ethical misconduct are expected. The more salient professional concern, however, should be to advance the higher values expected of and consistent with the privilege of being a profession. To do this requires more of a profession than the *thou shalls* and *thou shall nots* that comprise a code of ethics. It requires that a profession aggressively promote the values of service to others as a primary professional characteristic and objective. Arguments and practices that place economic gain before the welfare of those served professionally can significantly erode the professional role of the audiologist and the image of the audiology profession.

Impact of Legal and Regulatory Bodies

As discussed earlier, professions are granted greater autonomy by society than are the trades or businesses. This does not mean that professions are immune to regulation by socially constituted bodies of authority. States, for example, have a long history in the regulation of professions through licensing.

However, even here, the individual profession has been the primary source for determining the nature and extent of the state's licensing act. This occurs because the state does not possess the specialized knowledge base of the profession and, therefore, must accede to the profession for the development of most of the licensing provision. Thus although the state enacts and enforces the licensing of professions, it depends on the profession to help construct the licensure law. This most certainly preserves a high degree of autonomy for the profession.

Again, by way of contrast, businesses are less autonomous in that states and the federal government set far more restrictions on business and do so with considerably less participation from the business community. Yet the state's interest in regulating businesses is the same as its interests in licensing professions—the welfare and protection of its citizenry.

As business practices become a greater part of the profile of a given profession, including the audiology profession, that profession becomes much more susceptible to the impositions of legal and regulatory bodies and, thereby, loses considerable autonomy. A part of the loss might be the opportunity both to set standards and to engage in the self-regulation of its members. To be certain, the nature of the primary ethical principles would also be dramatically changed.

Public Perceptions and Expectations

At a time when professions were less like businesses than they are today, the public's perception of professions and their expectations for the conduct of professionals was rather clear. As professions became increasingly more businesslike and as the media reported more and more incidents of scientific and professional misconduct, public perceptions and expectations also changed. It is probably true that societal values change somewhat with each new generation. Therefore each generation conceivably has a somewhat different perspective of ethics and ethical conduct.

Contemporary society seems to perceive that ethical values within the professions are not so much changed as they are weakened or absent (Schwartz, 1990). The climate is one of pessimism and mistrust, accompanied by an increased consumerism that demands explanations and justifications from professionals for both the nature of services provided and the costs of those services. Audiologists, like other professionals, are confronted with public perceptions and expectations that require them to be more accountable, and that ask for and even demand tangible evidence of ethical conduct. Truly, the age of accountability has become firmly entrenched.

THE PRACTICE OF ETHICS

Concepts of ethical conduct in professional practice, as in the practice of audiology, focus largely on matters associated with clinical practice. Yet, as with most professions, the practice of audiology is invested in a much broader array of activities, including teaching, research, and administration. Each of these practice arenas is marked by a particular set of contextual characteristics and each involves different constituent groups (i.e., people who are the recipients of the professional service or services provided). Regardless of the variability of characteristics across practice arenas, a common bond is to be found in the first ethical principle of both the ASHA and AAA Code of Ethics, which is to give highest consideration to the welfare of persons served professionally. This ethical principle is first not only in order of appearance but also in order of guidance for ethical decision making. Thus the determination as to whether professional conduct is ethical or not must take into consideration the particular set of variables and values associated with the nature of the service and its impact on related constituent groups. To make such a determination, the professional practitioner (the audiologist) must ask and answer at least two fundamental questions. First, "Who are the persons I serve professionally?" Second, "How do I go about fulfilling my responsibility to each of these individual groups?"

PEARL

The ASHA regularly publishes "Issues in Ethics" statements, which provide detailed interpretations of individual elements of the Code of Ethics.

Teaching

Audiology professionals working in colleges and universities are expected to engage in multiple professional roles. Because of this, a response to the question "Who are the persons I serve professionally?" creates a veritable laundry list of constituent groups. As classroom teachers, of course, the clear answer is students. However, because teaching also occurs in the clinical laboratory, the response in that context must be not only students but also patients and their families. Thus audiologists in their professional roles as teachers must be concerned with multiple groups as recipients of their services.

A review of the literature reveals very little information regarding ethical conduct (or misconduct) in teaching. The available references address related matters such as how to teach ethics to students in communication sciences and disorders (Gonzalez & Coleman, 1994; Pannbacker et al, 1993) or how universities at large must recognize that an institutional need to be concerned with ethical issues exists (Counelis, 1993; Enarson, 1991). Despite the limited research attention, however, teaching, as with any other practice arena, presents the practitioner with ethical dilemmas. A few common scenarios will serve to exemplify ethical dilemmas in teaching. (NOTE: For a broad set of scenarios reflecting ethical dilemmas in teaching and a variety of other professional circumstances, see Pannbacker et al, 1996.)

- The instructor of a course uses a book that he or she has written as a required text for the course.
- After enrolling in a course, students fail to receive a complete or comprehensive syllabus.
- Students in a doctoral program receive teaching assistantships that provide tuition and a monthly stipend. As a condition of their financial aid, they are assigned full and independent responsibility for teaching a course or a laboratory.
- At the end of the academic term, the clinical instructor and student meet to review the final clinical report for an adult

in the department's aural rehabilitation program. The report, approved by the instructor, recommends that the patient return for service even though the clinical documentation reveals no substantial gains and the prognosis for improvement is quite poor.

These examples are not meant to infer that the conduct of the professional is inherently unethical. Rather, they pose circumstances in which relatively "private" considerations may be in conflict with the "welfare of those served professionally." Whose interest is "held paramount" forms a critical basis for judgments regarding ethical conduct in each situation.

Research

No doubt exists that research endeavors have come under greater scrutiny in the recent past than in any other time in history. Anecdotal incidents of scientific misconduct in the media have driven public awareness and public concern to an all time high. Government funding agencies have instituted enforcement programs designed to uncover scientific fraud and to punish the responsible researcher. Congress assumed an unprecedented role in the determination of what types of research would be eligible for federal funding. Colleges and universities carefully reviewed their institutional policies relative to academic fraud and amended them as needed or created official statements where none had existed. Like codes of ethics, institutional policies offer statements of principles regarding scientific or academic misconduct. Unlike ethical codes, however, they also tend to include statements about possible penalties should misconduct charges be substantiated. Typically, however, institutional policy statements do not address other involved individuals (e.g., students) or their rights and responsibilities. In other words the array of possible constituent groups is not included in policy statements. What are those possible constituent groups? They include, of course, the subjects of a study but may also include students, funding entities, professional colleagues, and the profession at large. This latter group is certainly affected by any public awareness of misconduct by one of its members.

In the professional practice arena of research, intentional misrepresentation of data is the most obvious and most frequently occurring example of ethical misconduct. Deliberate falsification of credentials, especially as they may argue successfully for funding a researcher's project, is also not uncommon. Other circumstances exist that are not so obvious and require careful consideration of both the involved constituent groups and the characteristics of the research endeavor. Some examples, again, may serve to illustrate these issues:

- A graduate student successfully completes a thesis or dissertation under the direction of a faculty mentor. Although the mentor offered the basic idea behind the research, he or she did not directly conduct the research project. As a matter of policy in this situation, the mentor's name appears as a coauthor on the resultant publication:
- A researcher receives funding from an "outside" agency for a particular project. At the end of the project period it is determined that some funds remain. Although not specifically identified in the approved budget, the researcher uses

the unexpended funds to present the results of the research at a professional conference.

Like ethically laden circumstances in other practice arenas, the research audiologist must confront conflicting interests between and among involved constituent groups and the values inherent in the conduct of scientific inquiry. Problem identification is relatively simple. Problem resolution, on the other hand, is not so simple.

Administration

Professionals who practice in the area of administration arguably confront some of the more complex and impactful ethical circumstances. This is largely due to the expanded sphere of influence that administrators have. The decisions and actions of an administrator affect available resources, opportunities for individuals and groups, public perception about the agency or institution and the individuals who work there, along with a host of other possibilities. The range of constituent groups (those served professionally) can be totally inclusive. They may include patients, colleagues in the same profession, colleagues in other professions, students, families, and the public at large. It is difficult to imagine a professional setting in which administrators do not confront most if not all of the preceding constituent groups.

Likewise, the circumstances an administrator confronts can be equally complex in terms of the ethical issues that may be involved. This requires that the individual be familiar with all of the applicable organizational policies and practices and related legal and institutional employment prescriptions and proscriptions. In many respects the professional who practices as an administrator has ultimate local responsibility for the identification and adjudication of ethical matters, including his or her own professional conduct. What are some of the example ethical scenarios that confront the audiologist administrator?

- Income from third-party funding is critical to the growing operational budget of the institution or agency. Audiological assessments that determine normal acuity are not funded because they do not represent an abnormal condition. To avoid reductions in personnel or operating budget, the administrator advances a policy whereby tests showing normal acuity will be billed under a code acceptable to the third-party payer.

- An individual in the organization provides competent services but is not well liked by his or her co-workers. In fact, the organizational climate is perceived by those co-workers to be strained because of their working relationships with that individual. In a merit-based system for determining salary adjustments, the administrator rates this individual last on the list of employees and recommends only a marginal salary increase.

These example scenarios again evidence the fact that ethical issues are complex, often involve conflicts of interest, and require careful deliberation to arrive at adequate and appropriate resolutions. They demand much of the individuals involved and usually offer alternatives that may not be acceptable to everyone. The determining question, as Levy and Mishkin (1990) suggest, is "In whose best interest is it anyway?"

Promulgating Professional Ethics

In the preamble the ASHA Code of Ethics states that ethical principles are "affirmative obligations" to be observed in all areas of professional endeavor. That obligation has a special meaning to the practitioners of today. After all, they are the ones responsible for developing the ethical consciousness of the next generation of professional audiologists. Whether it be by direct and formal instruction (such as in a college or university training program), by indirect teaching (such as in the advice and counsel given to new colleagues), or by the example of one's own professional (and personal?) conduct, currently practicing audiologists are responsible for the ethical consciousness of the next generation of professionals and through them to future publics who will be served by them professionally. It is clear that how audiologists deal with ethical issues in their several professional contexts and roles today will significantly shape the image of the profession tomorrow. That is a challenge worth meeting.

SPECIAL CONSIDERATION

The primary characteristics of a profession (i.e., self-regulation and self-discipline) are but derivatives of more fundamental characteristics, those of self-analysis and self-correction.

CHALLENGES FOR THE FUTURE

The increasing number and complexities of ethical challenges facing audiology and other professions, coupled with a rise in public distrust, tend to paint a rather negative picture of current circumstances and the opportunities to alter those circumstances. But the history of audiology would suggest otherwise.

Professions like audiology that remain in a dynamic, as opposed to a static, state not only possess the solutions to the ethical dilemmas that confront them but also hold the key to their own future. The primary characteristics of a profession (i.e., self-regulation and self-discipline) are but derivatives of more fundamental characteristics, those of self-analysis and self-correction. A profession that is willing and able to critically examine itself in the context of contemporary social values, practices, and expectations will be responsive to emerging ethical challenges. The challenges to the audiology profession are easily specified. To cite but a few, they include issues such as the following:

- Ensuring competency in the context of an expanding scope of practice.
- Creating a balance between service to others and the legitimate pursuit of economic gain.
- Identifying and establishing guidelines for conflict of interest issues in all practice environments.
- Ensuring the continuity of ethical principles and practices into the future.

However, the specific challenges are only iterations of a broader challenge, that being the degree to which the *profession* of audiology is merged with the *business* of audiology.

Professions and businesses pursue different primary objectives and, as a consequence, accept different ethical norms.

Audiologists as individuals and audiology as a profession must make a choice. It is certainly not a choice between mutually exclusive options because the profession of audiology has already included the business of audiology in its recognizable profile. Rather, as Harford (1991) points out, the choice is one of prioritization. Will the choice be to give first priority to matters of business and individual profit and secondarily to the provision of competent and comprehensive services dictated by patient needs? Or will the higher values demanded of audiologists as professionals supersede the private interest of economic gain? The contrast is one of focus. Where professions and professionals focus on the welfare of the individual, "the market is an impersonal mechanism" (Powers & Vogel, 1980, p. 5).

By retaining the classical traits that embody a profession while adopting those business practices that stand highest on the value continuum, audiology can continue to successfully balance the competing objectives of service to others and economic gain. Much is to be retained by audiology holding itself to the higher ethical values and practices that characterize a profession. Much is to be lost by sacrificing those values in favor of becoming more of a business than a profession. Achieving a balance in both professional and business ethics is probably not enough. Audiology should continue to conduct itself first and foremost as a profession, placing business values in a secondary position. To strive for equity in professionalism and good business practices will likely not retain the valued position reserved solely for the professions. Audiology must remain primarily a profession in its values and its practice so as to retain the privilege of autonomy and self-regulation afforded to it. By doing so it will ensure its continuation as a vital profession with a distinguished place in the competent delivery of services to those in need.

REFERENCES

AMERICAN ACADEMY OF AUDIOLOGY. (1991). *Code of ethics*. Houston: American Academy of Audiology.

AMERICAN SPEECH-LANGUAGE-HEARING ASSOCIATION. (1994). Code of ethics. *ASHA, 36* (March, Suppl. 13); 1–2.

COUNELIS, J.S. (1993). Toward empirical studies on university ethics. *Journal of Higher Education, 64* (January/February);74–92.

DEGEORGE, R.T. (1986). *Business ethics* (2nd ed.). New York: Macmillan.

ENARSON, H.L. (1991). Ethics for University Administrators, *Academic Administrators Retreat*. Blacksburgh, VA: Virginia Polytechnic Institute and State University.

GONZALEZ, L.S., & COLEMAN, R.O. (1994). Students prefer case study approach. *ASHA, 36* (August); 47–48.

HARFORD, E. (1991). What they didn't teach you about hearing aid dispensing in your own Private practice. *Audiology Today* (September/October); 29–31.

LANE, H., & BAHAN, B. (1998). Ethics of cochlear implantation in young children: A review and reply from a deaf-world perspective. *Otolaryngology–Head and Neck Surgery, 119* (October); 297–313.

LEVY, N.I., & MISHKIN, D.B. (1990). In whose best interest is it, anyway?—Solutions to ethical problems caused by influences outside the professional relationship. *Ethics Colloquium*. Rockville, MD: American Speech-Language-Hearing Association.

PADEN, E.P. (1970). *A history of the American Speech and Hearing Association 1925–1958*. Washington, DC: American Speech-Language-Hearing Association.

PANNBACKER, M., LASS, N.J., & MIDDLETON, G.F. (1993) Ethics education in speech-language-pathology and audiology training programs. *ASHA, 35* (April); 53–55.

PANNBACKER, M., MIDDLETON, G.F., & VEKOVIUS, G.T. (1996). *Ethical practices in speech-language pathology and audiology*. San Diego, CA: Singular Publishing Group.

POWERS, C.W., & VOGEL, D. (1980). *Ethics in the education of business managers*. Hastings-on-Hudson, NY: The Hastings Center.

RESNICK, D.M. (1992). Issues in ethics: Balancing the ethics of a business and a profession. *Audiology Today* (March/April); 18–20.

SCHWARTZ, A.E. (1990). Ethics of professional engineering. In: S.C. Goldsmith, & J.H. Ciuccio (Eds.), *Reflections on ethics*. Washington, DC: American Speech-Language-Hearing Association.

SILVERMAN, F.H. (1983). *Legal aspects of speech-language pathology and audiology*. Englewood Cliffs, NJ: Prentice-Hall.

STRAUSS, L. (1983). On classical political philosophy. In: T.L. Thorson (Ed.), *Plato: Totalitarian or democrat*. Englewood Cliffs, NJ: Prentice-Hall.

STROMBERG, C.D. (1990). Key legal issues in professional ethics. In: S.C. Goldsmith, & J.H. Ciuccio (Eds.), *Reflections on ethics*. Washington, DC: American Speech-Language-Hearing Association.

WEBSTER'S NEW TWENTIETH CENTURY DICTIONARY OF THE ENGLISH LANGUAGE. (1960). Unabridged (2nd ed.). New York: World Publishing Company.

Chapter 4

Quality: The Controlling Principle of Practice Management

Harvey B. Abrams

THE HEALTHCARE REVOLUTION—FROM A PROVIDER-DRIVEN TO A CONSUMER-DRIVEN INDUSTRY

Those of us born shortly after the Second World War, the "Baby Boomers," may recall a time when our family doctor made housecalls. Following the visit, it was customary for the full payment to be rendered immediately to the physician. Today, of course, it is rare for a doctor to provide treatment in the household and equally as rare for patients to pay for the entire cost of services directly to the provider. How our society has gotten to this point represents a revolution in healthcare that has occurred within a single generation. The reasons for this revolution and the societal dynamics that have shaped our healthcare system are many and complex. They include the changing role of women in American society, the increased sophistication of healthcare, the emergence of medical specialties, the increasing independence of nonphysician specialties, the increased number of healthcare providers, the demographic shifts of the American population (age, residence, income, distribution of wealth), the rising cost of healthcare, and the changing cultural precepts concerning aging and dying.

One constant that has persisted throughout these changes has been the continuing effort to improve the quality of the care we provide to our patients, manifest in a drive to improve diagnostic accuracy, treatment efficacy, involvement of the patient and family members in treatment decisions, and decreasing hospital lengths of stay. Just as healthcare in general has dramatically changed, so has the concept and measurement of quality. Quality, however, is only one of many dimensions of healthcare that has experienced significant change. To understand the revolution in the healthcare industry, it may help to understand the forces that "drive" healthcare decisions.

In the days when doctors made housecalls, the healthcare industry was "provider driven." The method of payment was fee-for-service, access was provider-controlled, costs were relatively unimportant, and the outcome of the healthcare episode was the elimination of disease. During the 1970s and 1980s, along with the widespread availability of health insurance, healthcare became "payer driven." The method of payment was based on new concepts such as diagnostic-related groups (DRGs) and relative value units (RVUs). Access was payer controlled, costs became very important, and the outcome of the episode was reduced costs. The healthcare reform initiative begun during President Clinton's first administration has shaped our present system which can be viewed as "consumer driven." The method of payment is largely based on a risk-adjusted capitation system; access is largely consumer choice; and the outcome is determined by measurements of functional status, quality of life, and consumer satisfaction.

The dimension of "quality" has also been influenced by the shift of healthcare from a supply-side to a demand-side industry. When the industry was provider controlled, quality was determined by accreditation and credentialing by an outside review agency or by a board within the hospital. During the payer-driven phase of healthcare, quality was determined by the institution's self-perception of quality through

Audiology: Practice Management. Edited by Hosford-Dunn, Roeser, and Valente. Thieme Medical Publishers, Inc., New York © 2000

quality assurance, and later, total quality indices. In a consumer-driven industry, treatment outcomes and measures of consumer satisfaction determine quality. Allthough the concept of "continuous quality improvement" (CQI) is associated with the payer-driven system, it is a concept that is totally appropriate in any type of healthcare setting or model. CQI extends beyond a mere measurement of the outcome of the healthcare episode to all processes and relationships that comprise and finally culminate in some change in the patient's health status.

This chapter will review the recent history of quality measures in healthcare, the principal concepts of CQI, how CQI is assessed, the emergence of customer service in the healthcare setting, and some examples of CQI in an audiology setting.

TOWARD A DESCRIPTION OF QUALITY

In the book *Zen and the Art of Motorcycle Maintenance* (Pirsig, 1984) the narrator, Phaedrus, is eventually driven insane in his attempt to define "quality." Early in his intellectual journey, Phaedrus recognizes that "Quality is a characteristic of thought and statement that is recognized by a nonthinking process. Because definitions are a product of rigid, formal thinking, quality cannot be defined." (Pirsig, 1984, p. 206). Yet Phaedrus understands, as we all do, that although we may not be able to absolutely define "quality," we can recognize it when we see, hear, feel, or experience it. What is it about a piece of music, a painting, a piece of furniture, or an automobile that determines its quality? Can we recognize quality in the service we receive at a shop in the mall, an auto repair shop, a hospital, an audiology clinic?

I think most of us will agree that we can recognize quality in the goods and services we receive but that the perception of quality is personal and individualized, or a "characteristic of thought" as Phaedrus observed. To avoid Phaedrus' fate, I will not attempt to define "quality," but instead I will attempt to describe it in the narrow arena of healthcare. Just to add an extra measure of safety, I will use the work of others to present a working definition of "quality."

The Quality Measurement and Management Project (QMMP) is a hospital industry-sponsored initiative to develop quality monitoring and management tools of choice for hospitals. In a 1989 publication (James, 1989) QMMP described healthcare quality as, representing ". . . an individual's subjective evaluation of an output and the personal interactions that take place as the output is delivered to the individual. It is rooted in that individual's *expectations*, which depend upon the individual's past experiences and individual needs. Quality evaluations therefore arise from, and are part of, an individual's value system. As a value system, quality expectations can be measured and changed through time and through education. They cannot be dictated." (James, 1989, p.2). I think Phaedrus would agree.

THE BUSINESS OF QUALITY IMPROVEMENT

The quality concepts and tools currently used in healthcare have their origins in business and specifically in manufacturing.

Perhaps the individual most commonly associated with conceptualizing and applying the concepts of quality to business is W. Edwards Deming. Deming, with advanced degrees in mathematics, engineering, and physics, is often credited with the emergence of postwar Japan into a global powerhouse whose products, particularly electronic and automotive, are synonymous with quality. Deming maintains that quality improvement requires a total commitment by everyone within the organization. He articulated his philosophy of quality management through his "Seven Deadly Diseases" of management (Table 4–1) and his famous "14 Points" (Deming, 1986):

1. *Create constancy of purpose for the improvement of product and service:* A business must develop a vision for itself that encourages innovation, puts resources into research and education, commits itself to the continuous improvement of services and products, and invests in the maintenance of equipment and other aids to improve production.

2. *Adopt the new philosophy:* All members of the organization must religiously reject negativism and the acceptance of errors.

3. *Cease dependence on mass inspection:* Businesses must reject the practice of inspecting products or services after they are produced. Quality is improved when processes are in place that eliminate errors in the first place.

4. *End the practice of awarding business on the basis of price tag:* The low bidder may not produce the best product. Find the best quality supplier and develop a long-term relationship to ensure the best quality at the best price.

5. *Improve constantly and forever the system of production and service:* Quality improvement is a lifelong commitment.

6. *Institute training:* Employees cannot expect to provide quality products or services if they have not been adequately trained in both their particular job and in the company's commitment to quality.

7. *Institute leadership:* Lead by example. Be a coach to your employees.

8. *Drive out fear:* Create an environment where the employees feel safe to question the ways things are done.

9. *Break down barriers between staff areas:* Create an environment of teamwork rather than competition among the departments within an organization.

10. *Eliminate slogans, exhortations, and targets for the workforce:* Let the workforce create their own slogans.

TABLE 4–1 Deming's Seven Deadly Diseases

1. Lack of constancy of purpose
2. Emphasis on short-term profits
3. Evaluation by performance, merit rating, or annual review of performance
4. Mobility of management
5. Running a company on visible figures alone
6. Excessive medical costs
7. Excessive costs of warranty, fueled by lawyers who work for contingency fees

11. *Eliminate numerical quotas:* Workers may feel pressured to meet production quotas at the expense of quality.
12. *Remove barriers to pride of workmanship:* Eliminate faulty equipment, defective materials, and counterproductive policies so employees can take pride in the work they accomplish.
13. *Institute a vigorous program of education and retraining:* When new methods are introduced, both management and non-management employees must be educated. Training should include statistical methodology and teamwork.
14. *Take action to accomplish the transformation:* It takes a dedicated team of top management with a well-defined action plan to lead the quality improvement initiative.

PEARL

All members of the organization must reject negativism and the acceptance of errors as just a part of doing business.

Another quality assurance engineer is J.M. Juran. Juran was also instrumental in creating a quality-conscious environment in Japan in the 1950s. Such corporations as AT&T, DuPont, and IBM embraced the "Juran Trilogy," which stressed the three elements of quality: quality planning, quality control, and quality assurance. Through his many years consulting with business, Juran identified the following eight factors that characterized successful organizations that had made a commitment to improved quality (Juran, 1988):

1. Senior managers personally led the quality process and served on a quality council as guides.
2. Managers applied quality improvement to businesses and traditional operational processes. These managers addressed internal and external customers.
3. The senior managers adopted mandated, annual quality improvement with a defined infrastructure that identified opportunities to improve and gave clear responsibility to do this.
4. The managers involved all those who affected the plan in the improvement process.
5. Managers used modern quality methods instead of empiricism in quality planning.
6. Managers trained all members of the management hierarchy in quality planning, quality control, and quality improvement.
7. Managers trained the workforce to participate actively in quality improvement.
8. Senior mangers included quality improvement in the strategic planning process.

SPECIAL CONSIDERATION

Creating change is how managers break through to new levels of performance; preventing change is how managers control the organization.—Juran

Philip Crosby is another quality improvement consultant who maintains that implementing quality is cost-effective.

Doing things right the first time avoids considerable expense associated with time, manpower, and resources associated with doing things wrong and having to fix it. Crosby is the architect of several quality-related programs for industry including the Quality Management Maturity Grid, Zero Defects (a method for eliminating errors instead of establishing a small but acceptable defect rate) *and* Do it Right the First Time; also the Quality Improvement Process that involves 14 steps that, according to Crosby, can turn any business around (Crosby, 1979):

1. Management commitment
2. Quality improvement team
3. Quality measurements
4. Cost of quality evaluations
5. Quality awareness
6. Corrective action
7. Establish an ad hoc committee for the zero defects program
8. Supervisor training
9. Zero defects day
10. Goal setting
11. Error cause removal
12. Recognition
13. Quality councils
14. Do it over again

PEARL

A goal of CQI is to do the right things and do things right the first time.

THE HEALTHCARE QUALITY EVOLUTION: FROM QUALITY CONTROL TO CONTINUOUS QUALITY IMPROVEMENT

The evolution of quality assessment methods in healthcare has taken about 30 years to reach the point where we now find ourselves. This process is not a linear one in which one concept is discarded as the next is embraced. Rather, it is a building process in which the building blocks of each concept or program create the foundation for the next.

Quality Control: Conformance to Specifications

Audiologists are familiar with quality control issues as they apply to the measurements of hearing aids. For example, ANSI 3.2 (1996) specifies the operating characteristics of hearing aids. The inherent "quality" of a hearing instrument can be determined by measuring the hearing aid on receipt of the instrument from the manufacturer and comparing the results to the published specifications to determine whether the hearing aid meets "specs." Such measurements allow us to make assumptions regarding the quality of the device, although they tell us nothing about the effect of the device on treatment outcome. Similarly, audiologists can measure the "quality" of equipment and the testing environment by ensuring that they meet published specifications for calibration and ambient noise levels. Again, adherence to such standards ensures a certain level of quality but does not ensure a positive treatment outcome. Adherence to standards, however, may eliminate many variables that decrease the opportunities for patient satisfaction and positive outcome.

Quality Assurance

The origin of quality assurance in healthcare can be traced to the beginning of the twentieth century with the establishment of minimum standards and on-site inspections of hospitals through the American College of Surgeons. The Joint Commission later assumed the responsibility of inspections and standards development for the Accreditation of Hospitals (JCAH). The Commission was created as a private, not-for-profit organization composed of representatives from large professional associations representing physicians, dentists, and hospitals and was charged with developing standards and accrediting hospitals through a voluntary survey. Accreditation by the JCAH became critical after the creation of Medicare regulations that determined that only accredited hospitals could be reimbursed through the Medicare program. It was not until the 1980s, however, that the Commission's standards first began to focus on quality assurance by requiring hospital departments to identify problems through chart audits.

CONTROVERSIAL POINT

It is questionable whether quality can be "assured." Quality can be measured, evaluated, compromised, and improved, but not likely guaranteed.

In 1986, the organization changed its name to the Joint Commission for the Accreditation of Healthcare Organizations (JCAHO) to reflect the need to establish quality care in all settings where healthcare is provided, including long-term care facilities, rehabilitation units, and outpatient departments. Extending the concept of quality beyond equipment, the JCAHO established standards for each department of the hospital to include standards for leadership, care of patients, training, records, documentation, safety, facility management, and so on. In addition, the Commission established specific criteria to assist healthcare organizations in determining whether they were meeting the standards, and if not, what they needed to do to comply.

Some of the standards that directly affect audiology services in a hospital setting include assessment of patients, care of the patient, performance improvement, and patient and family education (JCAHO, 1997). The process through which the JCAHO hoped healthcare organizations would be able to identify real or potential problems and improve healthcare quality was called the 10-step monitoring and evaluation process (Table 4–2).

SPECIAL CONSIDERATION

"[Quality] is the degree to which patient care services increase the probability of desired patient outcomes and reduce the probability of undesired outcomes given the current state of knowledge."
—JCAHO Definition of Quality

TABLE 4–2   JCAHO's 10-step monitoring and evaluation process

1. Assign responsibility
2. Delineate scope of care
3. Identify important aspects of care
4. Identify indicators
5. Establish thresholds for evaluation improvement
6. Collect and organize data
7. Evaluate care
8. Take action to improve care
9. Access actions and document
10. Communicate information improvement

The 10-step program was designed to identify processes that were high volume, high risk, or problem prone; establish some threshold beyond which action would be taken to determine what went wrong; and fix the problem so that performance would remain below that threshold. Each department within the healthcare facility was responsible for identifying processes for review and for establishing thresholds before action was taken. As in manufacturing, this approach to healthcare quality is a *detection* approach (Fig. 4–1) that relies on the inspection or examination of services after they have been completed. Often specific individuals (supervisors, managers) are assigned the responsibility of quality assurance through inspection or data review. These inspectors act as screens to ensure a reasonable level of quality.

The Costs of Detection

High quality can be achieved through the detection approach of quality assurance but only at a high cost. Because problems must be identified to drive an improvement effort, inspectors need to wait before action is taken. Some of the costs associated with the detection approach are:

• Waste
• Time lost for the customer and the department
• New or additional material required to repair the problem
• Delay in service delivery
• Inspection costs
• Customer dissatisfaction

The Detection Approach

Process → Service/Product → Inspection

Pass → **Customer**

Fail → **Waste**

"Do It Again"

Figure 4–1   The detection approach to quality assurance. (From Abrams & Siferd [1994], with permission.)

Case 1:   Detection approach to quality improvement

The owner of a busy multioffice audiology practice in a large metropolitan area in the southwest established a threshold that 90% of all hearing aids will be delivered to the patients within 14 calendar days of the audiological examination. Once a month, the owner would review all records to determine whether the threshold had been surpassed. During most months, the performance level was acceptable with about 91 to 94% of instruments delivered within an acceptable time frame. During those periods when performance fell to less than 90%, no specific reason (office, clinician, manufacturer, etc.) could be identified.

- What are the costs associated with this approach?
- Is 90% an acceptable criterion? Why not 85%, 95%, 100%?
- Is 14 days an acceptable criterion?
- How can performance improve if the threshold is rarely crossed?
- Is the owner necessarily the best individual to make these measurements? Should others be involved?
- How can opportunities for improvements be identified using this approach?

How does this approach maximize patient satisfaction?

Continuous Quality Improvement: The Prevention Approach

The concept of CQI assumes that a process or outcome can always be improved. In contrast to QA that relies on repeated measures to determine whether performance is meeting some predetermined threshold, CQI encourages a preventive approach to identifying and eliminating problems (Fig. 4–2). CQI strives to set the bar higher (move the threshold) by improving efficiencies, decreasing costs, improving patient satisfaction, reducing morbidity, reducing lengths of stay, and so on *before* the product or service is delivered to the customer. Detecting product or service problems is no longer the responsibility of an inspector but rather the responsibility of each individual participating in the process. Costs are associated with the prevention approach, however, and these include the following:

- Measurement and analysis
- Quality training

PEARL

Doing it right is better than doing it fast.

These costs can be considered "investment" dollars because continuously increasing quality will ultimately result in less waste and improved patient satisfaction.

The essence of CQI is illustrated in Table 4–3. Satisfying the patient should be the unifying principle of everyone in the department. Elimination of waste can be accomplished through a number of means, including simplification of processes, elimination of duplication, introduction of new technologies, and implementation and expansion of training. The culture must encourage the participation of everyone in the organization. Inherent in this culture is an environment of respect and trust. Chances are, the people who have the solutions are the ones performing the functions. Constructive change and innovation are possible only in an environment of trust. Improving products or systems must be based on data

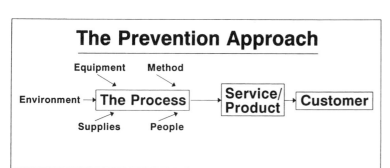

Figure 4–2   The prevention approach to quality assurance. (From Abrams & Siferd [1994], with permission.)

TABLE 4–3   The essence of CQI

- Obsession with satisfying customers
- Obsession with eliminating waste
- A culture which encourages ethical, open, respectful and participative behavior
- Formal systems based on data and continuous improvement

From Abrams and Siferd (1994), with permission.

gathered through a formalized approach. This approach should include a clear statement of what needs to be changed and why, how the process is to be changed, how the effects of the change will be measured, and how success will be determined. Decision by assumption cannot succeed.

As discussed earlier, Deming, Juran, and Crosby came out of manufacturing industries, not healthcare. However, the same principles taught by these individuals have been proven to work in the healthcare environment. Donald Berwick has adapted industry's quality improvement lessons to healthcare (Berwick et al, 1990).

Berwick's "lessons" are listed in Table 4–4. Both quality assurance and quality improvement are essential to the success of a business organization. A comparison of the two is illustrated in Table 4–5.

THE INTEGRATION OF CONTINUOUS QUALITY IMPROVEMENT

Up to this point, I have reviewed the general concepts and philosophies of quality improvement as it applies to organizations in general and to healthcare facilities in particular. The overall purpose of improved quality is to improve patient outcome. CQI provides us with a process to examine the way we perform care and determine ways of improving that care. In fact, CQI requires the integration of information from many sources within the organization. The most important

of these are utilization management, risk management, safety, and infection control (Fig. 4–3).

TABLE 4–4   Berwick's 10 key lessons for quality improvement

1. Quality improvement tools can work in healthcare.
2. Cross-functional teams are valuable in improving healthcare processes.
3. Data useful for quality improvements abound in healthcare.
4. Quality improvement methods are fun to use.
5. Costs of poor quality are high and savings are in reach.
6. Involving doctors is difficult.
7. Training needs arise early.
8. Nonclinical processes draw early attention.
9. Healthcare organizations may need a broader definition of quality.
10. In healthcare, as in industry, the fate of quality improvement is first of all in the hands of leaders.

Utilization Management

Utilization management in healthcare can be defined as "... a series of actions to produce a quality healthcare product in a cost-effective manner while contributing to the overall goals of an institution" (Koch & Fairly, 1993, p.73). Utilization management is critical in identifying those products and services that result in excessive cost and inefficient delivery of healthcare. Utilization review examines such things as the appropriateness of admissions, length of stay, use of resources such as laboratory tests and pharmaceuticals, duplication of services, and discharge planning.

Utilization review has been driven, in large part, by the creation of a prospective payment system (PPS) through the development of DRGs. DRGs were developed as a means of grouping patients by lengths of stay, and hence, resources

TABLE 4–5   Quality assurance versus quality improvement

Quality Assurance	Quality Improvement
Inspection oriented (detection)	Planning oriented (prevention)
Reactive	Proactive
Correction of special causes (individual, machine, etc.)	Correction of common causes (systems)
Responsibility of few	Responsibility of many
Narrow focus	Cross-functional
Leadership may not be vested	Leadership actively leading
Problem solving by authority	Problem solving by employees at all levels

Reprinted, with permission, from Koch and Fairly (1993).

Case 2: Prevention approach to quality improvement

In response to periodic patient complaints and increasing competition in the community, the owner in Case 1 determines that the existing 14-day time frame for delivering hearing aids is no longer appropriate. The owner appreciates the complexity of the business and the many separate processes that culminate in the final delivery of the hearing aid. She appoints a team consisting of the appointment clerk, an audiologist, and the business manager to review all processes involved and recommend improvements that will decrease the delivery time to no more than 7 calendar days.

- What are the advantages of appointing a team to identify solutions as opposed to having the owner of the practice develop solutions?
- How can this approach prevent problems from occurring as opposed to detecting them after the fact?
- How can this approach maximize patient satisfaction?
- Might the team benefit from training in CQI techniques?
- What should the role of the owner be as the team analyzes the processes and develops recommendations?
- What should the role of the remaining staff be during this process?

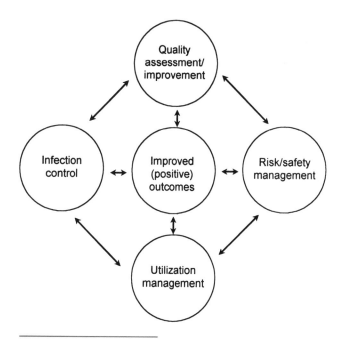

Figure 4–3   Integrated quality improvement model. (Reprinted with permission from Koch & Fairly [1993].)

TABLE 4–6   DRG considerations

- Principal diagnosis
- Principal procedure
- Complications
- Comorbidities
- Age

consumed (Table 4–6). Medicare and private health insurance companies used the DRG system to base its payment to hospitals. Before the PPS system, Medicare would reimburse hospitals on a fee-for-service basis. No incentive was present for physicians or hospitals to control costs because those costs would be reimbursed through Medicare or private health insurance. A "capitated" system that reimburses hospitals a specific amount as a function of diagnosis, regardless of resources consumed, dramatically changed the way the healthcare industry operates. Naturally, the hospitals were under great pressure to examine utilization to ensure that they were not expending more resources than they were recovering. By examining and controlling resources consumed, the hospital could hope not only to recover costs, but also perhaps to make a profit.

Utilization Review Techniques

Several ways exist to analyze utilization management activities as follows.

Prospective review determines the anticipated resources required before treatment. Insurance companies exercise this type of review to determine the appropriateness for admission for a particular type of disorder. Often, third-party payers will deny coverage for an inpatient procedure requiring admission to a hospital if the same procedure can be performed on an outpatient basis. Healthcare facilities perform prospective review to determine the ability of a patient to pay for the proposed treatment.

Concurrent review is performed at the time of or within 24 hours of admission to determine the appropriateness of the admission and the anticipated resources required. The facility determines the need for continued stay on the basis of specific criteria as determined by clinical guidelines or by the condition of the patient at the time of review.

Retrospective review takes place after the patient is discharged. The facility can determine the entire costs of the admission episode retrospectively to determine whether criteria for admission, continued stay, use of resources, and practice patterns were appropriate and consistent with the facility's criteria.

Focused reviews concentrate on specific issues that may be of particular concern to the facility, such as length of stay; readmission within 72 hours; infection rates; blood use; use of ancillary services; and so on. These reviews may be targeted as a result of an internal review (CQI initiative) or an external review (e.g., peer review, JCAHO inspection).

Utilization Management Criteria

The criteria used to determine the appropriateness of care and resource utilization issues is the responsibility of the healthcare facility (Tables 4–7 and 4–8). Increasingly, however, representatives of specific medical specialties are developing these criteria. The criteria may be based on the diagnosis of the patient, severity of the illness, the length of stay, or normative or empirically determined data. The development of clinically oriented algorithms, clinical pathways, and practice guidelines, discussed later in this chapter, is providing new ways for facilities to determine whether they are meeting established criteria. Utilization reviews or CQI initiatives may be triggered by comparing a facility's procedures against published algorithms, pathways, or guidelines.

**TABLE 4–7 Utilization management activities—
outpatient setting**

Assessment
Continuity of care per illness
Patient/family ability to follow plan
Postdischarge needs

Reprinted, with permission, from Koch and Fairly (1993).

TABLE 4–8 Utilization management activities—acute care

Assessment
Admissions
Level of care
Resource use
Need for continued stay
Discharge
Evaluation
Overutilization
Underutilization
Inefficiencies
Lack of cost restraint
Intervention
Problems adversely affecting cost and quality
Discharge planning
Identifying needs after patient leaves hospital

Reprinted, with permission, from Koch and Fairly (1993).

Risk Management

No industry exists in which the cost of error is so extreme as healthcare. The patient's quality of life, and indeed life itself, is jeopardized when processes fail in a healthcare setting. The reputation of practitioners and the hospital are at stake, and the economic costs to patient, provider, and facility can be enormous. Indeed, the economic survival of healthcare facilities rests largely on its ability to provide a safe environment.

Risk management is the process of making and carrying out decisions that will minimize the adverse effects of accidental losses on an organization (Koch & Fairly, 1993). The driving forces behind the risk management movement emerged primarily in the 1970s and 1980s. These forces included the rising number of malpractice claims, inflated jury awards for malpractice, increasing premiums among healthcare providers, and the growing tendency to hold the healthcare facility (and its stockholders—private or public) legally responsible for the

actions of its staff. Attempts to limit liability payments at state levels have been largely unsuccessful.

Today, the audiological community is fortunate that malpractice claims are relatively few, the awards are not astronomical, and the malpractice premiums remain reasonable. Historically, our work has not involved disorders for which risky, invasive procedures pose a significant risk of harm to the patient. However, our scope of practice has widened significantly in recent years with the inclusion of cerumen management, deep canal impression techniques, intraoperative monitoring, and early identification of hearing loss. These expanded procedures and services create opportunities for serious mistakes and expose the audiologists and the employers to substantial economic liabilities. Opportunities for economic exposure are associated not only with acts of commission, such as a perforated tympanic membrane after an ear impression, but also with acts of omission, such as neglecting to perform an appropriate diagnostic test or failing to advise patients on the dangers of ingesting batteries.

Risk management and loss avoidance involves a number of discrete steps as follows (Table 4–9).

TABLE 4–9 Risk management decision process

• Identify potential exposures.
• Examine alternative risk management techniques.
• Select the apparently best alternative risk management technique.
• Implement the chosen risk management technique.
• Monitor the results of the chosen technique.

Adapted from Koch and Fairly (1993).

Identify exposures to accidental loss: Examine your scope of practice. What services or procedures are provided that pose a risk to the patient? Recall that risk not only involves potential physical harm to the patient but also the potential effects of misdiagnosis. For example, failing to properly diagnose hearing loss in an infant may result in significant speech and language delay and associated "pain and suffering" on the part of the child and parents. High-risk procedures may include cerumen management, deep canal impressions, intraoperative monitoring, electrocochleography, electronystagmography, and neonatal testing.

Examine alternative risk management techniques associated with these exposures: As examples: Are there techniques to reduce injury associated with deep canal impression such as improved illumination, video-otoscopy, vented blocks, lubricated blocks, high-viscosity impression material, training, and powered syringes? Are methods available to improve the accuracy of diagnosing hearing loss in a neonate population? Are otoacoustic emissions (OAEs) the test of choice or should the clinician use a battery approach including OAEs, evoked potentials, and middle ear immittance measures? Are transtympanic electrodes always necessary for measuring the action and summating potentials, or can earcanal electrodes be used with reduced risk at the expense of waveform morphology?

Select the best risk management technique: The "best" technique is determined by deciding which technique or techniques provide the best result, in terms of accuracy and efficiency, with the least risk. This is not an easy process, sometimes requiring a cost/benefit analysis where cost is the additional expense associated with reducing risk and benefit is defined as the savings realized by avoiding the financial consequences of risk. An organization may be willing to accept the possibility of an infrequent and less severe loss (in terms of claims) than invest heavily in equipment or personnel to eliminate loss exposure. More often, the "best techniques" are being defined by professional organizations in the form of practice guidelines. These guidelines are often based on current research and represent the "state of the art" for a particular diagnosis or procedure. Some state legislatures have passed laws that protect a practitioner from litigation as long as that person was following current clinical guidelines for that episode of care. At the time of this writing, no specific published practice guidelines are associated with the practice of audiology.

Implement the chosen risk management technique(s): Once a decision is made to implement a different protocol to minimize loss exposure, it is important that everyone responsible for delivering audiology services is informed of the change, educated in the new technique(s) if necessary, informed of the implementation date, and held accountable for implementing the techniques.

Monitor the results of the chosen technique(s): After implementation of the best technique(s), it is important to establish a monitoring program to ensure that the desired effect has taken place and at the cost anticipated. For example, if the audiology department has decided to purchase a video-otoscope to minimize claims resulting from perforated tympanic membranes and earcanal hematomas, it is critical to determine whether the costs associated with the equipment, training, and implementation have, in fact, reduced the number and severity of claims associated with deep canal impressions. Although videootoscopy may significantly reduce loss exposure, it is possible that the same results may have been accomplished at a greatly reduced cost with the use of relatively inexpensive vented oto-blocks.

In addition to the establishment of formalized risk management programs by an employer, the individual audiologist has a responsibility to minimize risks to the patient (adapted from Koch & Fairly, 1993) as follows:

1. Familiarize yourself with those standards and laws that govern the practice of audiology.
2. Know the policies of your facility and your scope of practice as outlined in your job description.
3. Take responsibility for the education and skills required to perform your particular responsibilities, including new or unfamiliar procedures.

Safety

A quality work environment is a safe environment. Safety can be considered a subset of risk management in the sense that safety policies are put in place to reduce the risk of accidents incidental to the delivery of healthcare but are not necessarily associated with a particular clinical practice. Accidents are costly in terms of loss productivity, compensation payments, and the retraining of replacement staff. Examples of safety-related issues are listed in Table 4–10 and include electrical

TABLE 4–10   Workplace safety concerns

- Electrical safety
- Hazardous materials
- Spills
- Workplace violence
- Needle sticks
- Work-related injuries
- Work-related exposures (noise, chemicals)
- Equipment maintenance

safety; the handling and disposal of hazardous materials; spills; needle sticks; maintenance of medical equipment; patient-on-patient, patient-on-staff, and staff-on-staff violence; work-related injuries; and work-related hazardous exposures including noise.

The Occupational Safety and Health Administration (OSHA) regulates safety in the workplace, and it is the responsibility of the employer to ensure that all applicable laws and regulations are being followed. These include the education of staff, the monitoring of hazards, the provision and maintenance of safety equipment, the health monitoring of employees, and the maintenance of records.

JCAHO requires the presence of a safety officer and the establishment of a safety committee to include representatives from administration, clerical and support services, and safety experts. JCAHO considers risk management and safety to be integral components of a continuous quality improvement program.

Infection Control

Quality management in the healthcare setting requires an uncompromising commitment to infection control. Perhaps no single issue has focused the attention of healthcare workers on infection control as has acquired immune deficiency syndrome (AIDS) and the human immunodeficiency virus (HIV). In fact, the risk of infection is much greater to the patient than to the healthcare worker.

Nosocomial infections: Nosocomial infections are those that occur as a result of hospitalization. Nosocomial infections include pneumonia, bloodstream infections, surgical wound infections, and urinary tract infections typically associated with long-term catheter use. The fact that patients are ill and often immunocompromised when they enter the hospital, that they are in an environment with other individuals who are ill, and that they have had invasive procedures performed on them are all factors that place hospitalized patients at risk for infection. Patients who contract to nosocomial infections tend to stay longer and require greater resources increasing the cost of care and jeopardizing a satisfactory outcome.

JCAHO requires the presence of an infection control program to include written policies and procedures for collecting and analyzing data. The healthcare facility must have a multi-disciplinary committee in place to deal with infection control issues. CQI methodology provides an outstanding system for identifying, analyzing, improving processes, and ultimately decreasing the rates of infection.

Although much of the preceding discussion is directed toward a hospital-based audiology program, the issues of risk management, safety, and infection control are no less critical for the community-based clinic or private practitioner. In fact, smaller practices are more financially vulnerable than hospitals, where a certain amount of litigation is considered part of the cost of doing business. A serious injury to a patient or the spread of an infectious disease could jeopardize the survival of a small practice. Smaller practices do not have the advantage of in-house experts and departments devoted to patient safety and infection control; nor are nonhospital-based clinics subjected to periodic reviews by organizations such as JCAHO, which tend to focus an organization's attention on risk management issues. Expert assistance is available to the small practice, however. Many companies that provide business or employer insurance, particularly for healthcare–related businesses, will provide risk management experts to evaluate the practice and determine the potential for accidents, work-related injuries, and spread of infectious diseases.

IMPLEMENTING CONTINUOUS QUALITY IMPROVEMENT

One way quality-related issues are addressed in an organization is through trial and error. Unfortunately, because the causes of and solutions to organizational problems are usually complex, this approach tends to address only the superficial and obvious and fails to resolve the underlying causes of problems. Improvements may occur, but such improvements are not systematic and are rarely continual. Also, because such approaches often are imposed on the employees by management, the employees have no vested interest in the "solution" and may be at best unenthusiastic and at worst noncompliant, essentially sabotaging the effort even if the proposed solution is a reasonable one. FOCUS-PDCA provides a strategy that is systematic, involves employees in the process, and permits continuing improvement.

PITFALL
When implementing quality improvement, existing organizational structures may need to be modified or the development of parallel structures could upset the existing distribution of power throughout the organization and create conflict.

FOCUS-PDCA

FOCUS-PDCA is a method of quality improvement that uses a systematic approach to analyzing and improving processes. The FOCUS phase of the method is designed to build a knowledge base concerning the process to be improved, including an understanding of how the process is presently operating, what the objective is, and sources of variation between the existing and desired outcomes. The PDCA phase represents a learning cycle where a plan is conceived, executed, and the results compared with the predicted outcomes with modifications added. Taken together, FOCUS-PDCA is a

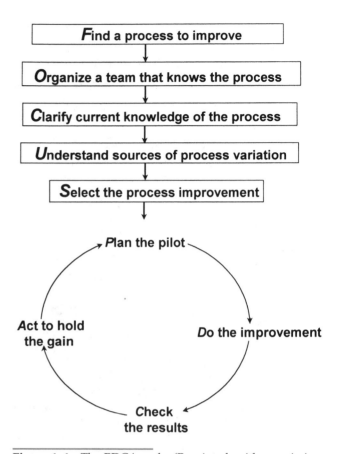

Figure 4–4 The PDCA cycle. (Reprinted, with permission, from Gift, R.G. & Kinney, C.F. (Eds.) (1996). *Today's management methods: A guide for the healthcare executive.* American Hospital Publishing. All rights reserved.)

nine-step process, with each step resulting in sets of data, a plan, or a decision as illustrated in Fig. 4–4.

PITFALL
FOCUS-PDCA can become an end in itself and replace effective decision making by management even when the cause and solution of a problem are evident.

Step 1: Find a Process to Improve

The purpose of the *F* step is to identify a process to improve and to articulate to the employees and management why this is an important process, how it will affect customers, how the process currently performs, and what the objective of the improvement will be. Identifying a process to improve can come from many different sources (Table 4–11).

Customer feedback: Information from patients in the form of compliments *and* complaints, or through satisfaction surveys can reveal the things an organization is doing well and important deficiencies and opportunities for improvement.

TABLE 4–11 Methods for finding a process to improve

- Customer feedback
- Quality audits and assessments
- Customer needs analysis
- Benchmarking
- Peer review
- Clinical pathways
- Clinical algorithms

Quality audits and assessments: Audits and assessments provide an excellent way of identifying opportunities for improving quality. Usually, it is far preferable to identify these opportunities through self-assessment than through an external review where negative findings can jeopardize an institution's credentials and ability to deliver care and stay in business.

JCAHO provides specific standards against which to compare the organization's quality of care. A self-audit conducted through a mock survey before a JCAHO inspection can identify opportunities for improvement while correcting errors that might jeopardize the facility's accreditation.

The Commission on Accreditation of Rehabilitation Facilities (CARF) has established standards for rehabilitation programs and facilities. Specific standards exist for audiology and speech-language pathology services if they are provided as part of a Medical Rehabilitation Program. A review of these standards may reveal a process in need of improvement. The specific CARF standards for "Performance Improvement" are as follows (CARF, 1998):

- Documented evidence is available that the program uses the results of its analysis of outcomes information to establish areas for improvement.
- The results of analysis of outcomes information are disseminated to personnel within the organization.
- Personnel assist in the determination of why performance fell below acceptable levels and give input into an appropriate action plan to improve performance.
- The program prioritizes the items in the performance improvement plan on the basis of how the persons served will be affected.
- The program implements the performance improvement plan.
- The program demonstrates ongoing
  a. Measurement of performance
  b. Modification of the performance improvement plan as needed
  c. Communication with all levels of personnel regarding performance improvement
  d. Use of information gathered from
     1. Stakeholders
     2. Operational systems

PEARL

"The only performance standard is zero defects."
—Crosby

The American Speech-Language-Hearing Association (ASHA) has published standards for professional service programs in audiology and speech-language pathology (ASHA, 1995). Included in the standards are elements related to the mission, goals, and objectives of the program, the nature and quality of the program, quality improvement and program evaluation, administration, financial resources and management, human resources, the physical facilities and program environment, and equipment and materials. Interestingly, the Professional Services Board (PSB) of ASHA and CARF developed a joint accreditation process. When an audiology and speech-language pathology program is being reviewed as part of a CARF survey, the outcome of that survey will apply to both CARF and ASHA PSB accreditation. Similarly, CARF and JCAHO are involved in a cooperative accreditation initiative for medical rehabilitation programs eliminating the need for separate surveys.

The Malcolm Baldridge National Quality Award is presented to companies that have met the rigorous criteria established for this prestigious award. It was originally established to improve the global competitiveness of American for-profit industry but has recently been applied to not-for-profit and specifically healthcare institutions. The award involves a 7 point weighted criteria (National Institute of Standards and Technology, 1994):

1. Leadership (90 points)
2. Information and analysis (75 points)
3. Strategic planning (55 points)
4. Human resource development and management (140 points)
5. Process management (140 points)
6. Business results (250 points)
7. Customer focus and satisfaction (250 points)

As with other audits, the self-assessment, which is accomplished in preparation for the application and site visit, can provide very important diagnostic information to the organization for the purposes of quality improvement. Many states and large organizations have created their own version of the Baldridge award such as the Governor's Sterling Award in the state of Florida and the Secretary of Veterans Affairs Robert W. Carey Quality Award in the Department of Veterans Affairs.

Customer needs analysis is a formal, systematic exploration and analysis of customer expectations as driven by the customer's hierarchy of needs and described in the customer's own words (Young, 1996). Such an analysis can effectively reveal problems within the organization that are not necessarily apparent to the management or clinical staff. Identification of customer needs can be achieved through the use of the following several tools.

1. Focus group: A forum of customers who communicate their needs, expectations, concerns, and preferences to the organization. Often, the group dynamics allow for the exchange of information that might not otherwise be communicated in a survey or personal interview format.
2. Surveys: Questionnaires designed to solicit information concerning customer needs. It is important to provide open-ended questions so as not to limit the responses of the individual. Survey information can be collected through the mail or over the telephone.

PITFALL

Do not plan and develop strategic initiatives entirely on the results of a focus group. The group may not reflect the opinions of your market. Confirm focus group data with market surveys.

3. Personal interviews: Allows for greater flexibility for gathering information in terms of the time, location, or length of questioning. Some individuals may feel more comfortable and be more responsive in a one-on-one situation as opposed to a group situation.

Benchmarking: Another effective method of finding a process to improve is benchmarking. Benchmarking is a process of finding the best practices within the organization, community, or specialty and implementing them in your department or organization. Gift (1996) describes four types of benchmarking as follows:

1. Internal: This involves studying similar practices among different departments or individuals within the same organization. For example, an audiology department may want to benchmark its customer service practices against the radiology department, which has been recognized as a leader in customer service.

2. Competitive: This type of benchmarking involves comparing a process or function within an organization with that of a competitor in the community or with one who shares the same market.

3. Functional: This involves comparing a function within an organization with a similar function in an entirely different industry. For example, a hospital may benefit from benchmarking its admissions process against the reservations processes of hotels, airlines, or rental car companies.

4. Collaborative: This type of benchmarking involves collaborating with several organizations that provide the same services, identifying best practices within the group and then comparing and benchmarking these best practices against the best practices of external organizations.

PEARL

"Benchmarking stimulates innovation and creativity by helping the organization remove self-imposed barriers to greater performance." (Gift, 1996, p. 255.)

Peer review: Opportunities for improvement can be found by establishing a system of peer review. Such a system involves identifying an individual or group of individuals who are assigned the responsibility of reviewing specific processes within a department or organization. For clinical purposes, a peer review will likely involve a review of patient records to determine whether specifically established quality standards are met. For example, an audiology program may enlist the assistance of an audiologist working outside the organization to review a sample of records to determine whether accepted clinical practices have been followed for the appropriate referral of neonates for additional hearing testing. This method is particularly effective when a department consists of a small number of clinicians who may feel uncomfortable reviewing each others' work or if the department head has clinical responsibilities and a review of that person's work by individuals he or she supervises is awkward.

Clinical pathways: Clinical pathways are described as an optimum sequencing and timing of interventions of healthcare providers for a particular diagnosis or procedure designed to minimize delays and resource utilization and to maximize quality (Coffey et al, 1992). Such pathways are developed either by the facility or by professional associations. Often the services of specialties such as audiology are included within the clinical pathways of a particular diagnosis or procedure. For example, the timing of OAEs testing might be described in the clinical pathway for postnatal care in a hospital. If the audiology department is unable to consistently meet these guidelines, resulting in increased lengths of stay or discharge before the test, the process of providing OAE testing will have to be reviewed.

Clinical algorithms: Clinical algorithms are systematically developed statements to assist practitioner and patient decisions about appropriate healthcare for specific clinical circumstances (Agency for Healthcare Policy and Research, 1993). They provide clear, concise formulas and visual detail of the care plan. They can improve the quality of care and decrease costs by guiding clinicians toward standardization and clinically optimum, cost-effective strategies, and by facilitating valid measures of clinical process and outcomes (Kleeb, 1996). Clinical algorithms can be developed by the healthcare facility, but because they tend to involve specific diagnoses and treatment plans, they are often formulated by a task force and published by a professional association for use by practitioners. Using the previous example, a clinical algorithm may be developed for neonatal hearing testing and would include criteria for testing, pass/fail criteria, referral options, and follow-up requirements. The algorithm might be developed as a visual flow chart with decision trees indicating the direction of the process at any point. The algorithm may represent the "standard of care" for neonatal testing throughout the country against which the practice of any specific program can be compared. According to Kleeb (1996), algorithms provide the following benefits:

- They provide a method for involving clinicians in clinical quality improvement efforts and give them an opportunity to gain insight into previously unknown practice variation.
- They provide a method for scrutinizing clinical information, which allows for easy isolation of clinical decisions.
- They provide the foundation for problem identification and improvement opportunities.
- They provide a visual representation of the care plan and difficult decision-making processes for students.
- They reduce variation in practice and improve care through a series of step-by-step recommendations.
- They provide a forum for education, debate, and conflict resolution.
- They improve the morale of clinicians by demonstrating commitment to deliver the highest quality of clinical care possible.

Step 2: Organize a Team That Knows the Process

Once an opportunity for process improvement is found from one or more of the methods described in step 1, the purpose of the *O* step is to identify a group of people familiar with the process, bring them together, provide them with the necessary resources, and allow them to examine the problem and recommend specific actions to improve the process. Stolz (1996) describes the following actions involved in organizing the team:

- Ensure appropriate representation of all parts of the process between the boundaries named.
- Identify the process owner or the person with authority and responsibility for leading the improvement effort.
- Identify sources of technical or educational support, often a facilitator/advisor.
- Identify the leadership liaison responsible for helping align the improvement effort with other, often larger, organizational priorities and for securing necessary resources.
- Formulate a plan or road map for the improvement effort.
- Determine how those engaged in making improvement will work together, including roles, responsibilities, and expectations.
- Initiate methods to keep others in the organization informed of progress and to promote learning and buy-in.

An essential part of this step is to develop a charter describing the purpose of the team, goals, membership, meeting times, roles of the members, and "rules" for interaction to ensure a civil and constructive interchange of ideas. The charter is developed and agreed on by all members of the team.

Step 3: Clarify Current Knowledge of the Process

To improve a process, it is imperative that an accurate assessment be made of how the current process operates. The *C* step is designed to ensure that all members of the quality improvement team have a complete and shared understanding of the way things are currently being done. An effective tool for the *C* step is flowcharting. Flowcharting allows the members of the group to describe each step of the process as a logical and visual progression of events. Flowcharting may identify opportunities for immediate improvement such as eliminating obvious redundancies or unnecessary steps. If published clinical algorithms exist for this process, the group can identify where the current process deviates from accepted clinical practice. In the absence of published algorithms, the group will determine how the current flow needs to change to improve the quality of the process—a quicker return appointment for hearing aid fittings or a faster response rate to provide baseline examinations for patients on cochleotoxic drugs, for example.

Step 4: Understanding the Source of Variation in the Process

The improvement team cannot simply recommend changes to the existing process on the basis of what they assume will result in the greatest improvement. Implementing changes that may appear to be intuitively reasonable may, in practice, be counterproductive. The *U* step allows the team members to examine and understand the types and sources of variation in the process by studying the performance of the process over time and identifying which factors within the process have a strong influence on the outcome most important to the customer (Stolz, 1996). The following actions are recommended as part of this step (from Stolz, 1996):

- Reviewing customer requirements and judgments of quality.
- Gathering and analyzing data on process performance variation over time.
- Removing or incorporating special causes to make the process stable over time.
- Identifying, gathering, and analyzing data on factors within the system of common causes that have a significant influence on the process outcome.

As part of the data gathering, the group will need to agree on what and how the data will be measured, who will collect the data, and how long the data will be gathered.

Step 5: Select the Process Improvement

After analysis of the data in step 4, the *S* step requires the group members to list, prioritize, and select the changes most likely to result in a significant quality improvement. The choice of which change to select may not necessarily be based on effectiveness alone. The cost of implementing the change compared with the amount of predicted benefit should be considered as well. Costs may be associated with additional personnel, equipment, structural changes, overtime, contracting, and so on. After a decision concerning the planned changes, the group enters into the second phase of the quality improvement process—the PDCA cycle.

Step 6: Plan the Pilot

At this point in the process, the quality improvement team needs to plan how the changes identified in the above step will be implemented and how the effects of those changes will be measured. The actions associated with this step include (from Stolz, 1996) the following:

- What the change is in terms that are easily understood
- Who is responsible for implementation
- Who must be informed and/or trained
- Where the pilot test will be held
- When it will begin
- How long it will last
- What are the implementation requirements, such as communication, equipment, and training, and how will they be addressed.

PITFALL

Take care not to tackle processes that are too complex or beyond the control of the quality improvement team. This will lead to frustration and a reluctance to participate in future quality improvement efforts.

Step 7: Do the Improvement, Data Collection, and Analysis

This is the point at which the team implements their plan and measures the results. Actions associated with this step include (from Stolz, 1996) the following:

- Preparing workers and the work environment for the process change
- Implementing the change and conducting work accordingly
- Observing and documenting the effects of the change
- Observing for, documenting, and addressing, as appropriate, surprises or unforeseen circumstances such as failures or deficiencies in planning and implementation and changes in the organization that could affect the process under study.

Step 8: Check and Study the Results

The C step involves reviewing the results to see if the implemented change had the desired and anticipated effects. Actions included in this step involve comparing the outcome before the changes were implemented to those achieved after implementation. The team needs to understand the causes of any failures that may have occurred or, conversely, explain why outcomes exceeded the predicted results.

Step 9: Act to Hold the Gain and to Continue to Improve the Process

Recall that FOCUS-PDCA is a method for implementing *continuous* quality improvement. It is not enough to demonstrate that the implemented changes had a positive result. The team must take action to ensure that realized gains continue to occur and to examine methods to improve outcome even further. Actions associated with this step include (from Stolz, 1996) the following:

- Anchoring the benefit and extending the gain: Make changes to organization policies and procedures, implement training programs, develop a mechanism for monitoring the long-term effects of the change

- Acting to continue making improvements: Review the initial list of potential changes (step 5), implement another pilot study, find another process to improve
- Adapt the change: Modify the change if it appears that an improved outcome will result
- Abandon the change: Select another change from the list if the assumptions on which the predicted change were based proved to be in error.

Because the FOCUS-PDCA approach to CQI is data-intensive, analysis, decision making, and tracking are made easier when appropriate measurement tools are used (Table 4–12).

TABLE 4–12 FOCUS-PDCA tools

- Cause-and-effect diagrams: An illustration representing an identified problem (effect) and the possible contributing factors (causes).
- Flowcharts: A simple illustration of the steps involved in a process, usually represented chronologically
- Gantt charts: A timetable displaying action items, assignments, and time frames for completion.
- Pareto diagrams: A vertical bar graph developed through brainstorming or existing data to help identify those issues that represent the greatest problems associated with a process.
- Run charts: A line graph representing the occurrence of an event over time. Useful in monitoring the results of a new or modified procedure.
- Control charts: Similar to a run chart but with a statistically determined upper and/or lower limit to identify critical variations in a process.
- Scatter plots: A plot of data points often representing two variables that may help to identify relationships between those variables.
- Histogram: A bar chart that displays the frequency at which particular events occur.

CUSTOMER SERVICE

An audiology program that is committed to quality improvement is passionate and uncompromising in its commitment to customer service. The reader may recall that the customer satisfaction and service element of the Baldridge award was worth 250 points—tied for the most points of any of the seven criteria in the program. Industry recognizes the importance of customer service in a competitive marketplace where the customer has many choices and loyalty is no longer a motivating factor in the customer's purchasing decisions.

PEARL

Okyakusama wa kamisama desu.
—"The Customer is God."

What is customer service? We recognize good and poor service when we encounter it. We recognize it in the businesses we use and in the businesses we are in. Customer service is simply a measure of the degree of *caring* communicated by the people, processes, and environment in the organization, whether that organization consists of one person or 100,000 persons.

Who are your customers? Almost all businesses have both *internal* and *external* customers. Your internal customers are the people you report to in an organization or your business and the people who report to you. They are other members of the organization on whose support you depend—both administratively and clinically. External customers are the people who refer patients to you, the vendors you depend on, your banking and business associates, and, most importantly, your patients.

Critical Success Factors for Outstanding Customer Service

Customer Feedback and Information Management

Feedback and information from customers is designed to inform the organization of their customers' expectations and needs. These needs and expectations drive the identification of other organizational information needs that support improving customer service. One strategy that can improve an organization's ability to perform is to involve and listen to its customers through the types of customer feedback methods described earlier in this chapter. Good customer feedback and information management systems are used to support managerial, operational, financial, performance improvement, and clinical decision making (Table 4–13).

TABLE 4–13 Customer service: critical factors

- Customer feedback and information management
- Leadership
- Strategic planning
- Continuous improvement
- Empowerment and accountability
- Education, training, and staff development
- Reward and recognition
- Communication
- Patient-centered culture

Leadership

Leadership has overall responsibility for planning and directing an organization's activity. Leadership in this context refers to top and middle management such as department and section heads and supervisors. Middle managers are key individuals in achieving customer goals. A key responsibility of leadership is to use customer input and assessments to evaluate available resources and to set priorities. The leadership team must model their commitment to customer service and support staff in complying with customer requirements appropriately. The principal duty of leadership is to ensure that daily work is aligned with the organization's strategic direction and that all efforts remain patient centered.

The importance and responsibilities of leadership are not restricted to large organizations. The clinician-manager of a community clinic or clinician-owner of a private practice will likely succeed or fail on the basis of leadership skills. Small business owners and managers must be able to develop strategic and business plans; hire, reassign, counsel, reward, train, and terminate employees; develop networks within the community; make decisions regarding capital expenditures; communicate the values of the practice to internal and external customers; and serve as a model for the types of attitudes and behaviors expected of employees and business associates.

No matter how large or small the practice, the principal responsibility of leadership is to ensure that the patient remains at the center of all decisions.

> ### PITFALL
> Without the absolute, unwavering commitment from top management, CQI is doomed to eventual failure. Organization leaders must demonstrate this commitment through words, action, and resources.

Strategic Planning

Strategic planning includes using information derived from the community and customer feedback and information systems, as well as the organization's mission and vision. The resource deployment process involves how an organization allocates, aligns, and integrates major resources (e.g., human resources, capital, information, and technologies) into its strategies to meet its customer needs and expectations, goals and objectives, and mission. This convergence of an organization's major resources using a systems approach is essential to achieving sustainable performance improvements.

Process of Continuous Improvement

Customer-focused continuous improvement is a data-driven process planned by leadership to accomplish the strategic goals of the organization. It is achieved through teams of individuals who work day-to-day on the processes that produce the organization's services and products.

Empowerment and Accountability

Excellent organizations accomplish good customer service by allowing and encouraging all levels of staff to meet or exceed customer needs and expectations. It applies not only to direct customer interactions but to the day-to-day operation of processes. Successful *empowerment* of staff requires an understanding that they know what they can do, that they feel that their actions will be valued by their colleagues, and that they are supported by all levels of leadership within the organization. Table 4–14 summarizes the changes in management's role in an empowered environment. *Accountability* refers to the responsibility assumed by empowered employees. Successful organizations define and communicate customer service expectations to employees and ensure that those expectations are met through the establishment of customer service performance standards.

TABLE 4–14   Management's role changes in an empowered environment

From	To
Commander	Coach, facilitator
Controller	Leader
Individualist	Team builder
Internally competitive	Cooperative
Withholding	Open, explaining
Owner mentality	Trustee mentality

SPECIAL CONSIDERATION

Empowerment allows employees the freedom to act; it imposes on them the accountability for results.

Education, Training, and Staff Development

Education, training, and staff development are ongoing processes used to develop customer-focused knowledge, skills, and attitudes of employees. Organizations that are known for their excellent customer service are also known for investing substantial resources to ensure that staff is competent to do their job and are skilled in providing customer service.

Reward and Recognition

PEARL

Measure performance; reward results.

Reward and recognition systems are generally extrinsic methods developed by organizations to enhance employees' feeling of satisfaction with their work. It is important to realize, however, that an individual's job satisfaction is inherently grounded in his or her perception and feelings about work and the environment. The intrinsic rewards are more closely aligned with the culture and values of an organization than its formal reward and recognition systems. It is essential that formal reward and recognition processes and programs be aligned with both the values and strategic goals of a patient-centered culture. Reward systems that promote customer service ensure that performance ratings and bonuses are at least partially based on serving customers well. They also reward teams rather than individuals. Customer service organizations are characterized by a variety of creative methods of recognition that are clearly tied to meeting customer needs and expectations.

Communication

Customer-focused organizations have and use multiple methods of communicating with customers, stakeholders

SPECIAL CONSIDERATION

Although many organizations have reward and recognition systems, not all are constructed to recognize team vs. individual accomplishments. Because most quality improvement efforts involve a team approach, the organizational culture must adapt to reward team efforts.

PITFALL

Rewarding employees for actions that have occurred months ago is not as meaningful, effective, or reinforcing as rewarding individuals immediately.

(employees, vendors, business associates, etc.), the community, and each other. Both formal and informal methods of communication abound. Effective communication builds commitment, investment, and ownership toward the principles of customer service.

Patient-Centered Culture

Most importantly, organizations that are outstanding in customer service have a patient-centered culture. Culture refers to the way people interact, communicate, and behave based on a shared system of values, beliefs, mores, and attitudes. These organizations put patients'/customers' needs at the very center of what they do. They continuously and consistently adopt the patients' perspective. Their highest priority strategic goals come from identified customer needs and expectations. For instance, patients have identified continuity, coordination of care, and emotional support as areas that need improvement. This has led many organizations to implement a patient-centered primary care model. They focus on understanding a patient's experience with illness and healthcare. Everyone must be involved in making the culture a primary and legitimate expression of the organization's values by designing processes and services to meet customer needs and not employee or service needs.

BUILDING CUSTOMER LOYALTY

In a highly competitive environment where consumers are becoming more educated about the marketplace and will seek out the best service for the lowest cost, how can a business create an environment where the customer wants to return? As mentioned earlier, loyalty to a particular business (or hospital, clinic, private practice, etc.) is no longer a motivating factor driving consumer choice. Establishing a strategy for customer loyalty, however, should remain a high priority for any clinical practice. Returning "customers" are particularly critical for dispensing audiologists because a large percentage of hearing aids are dispensed to previous hearing aid users. Heil et al (1995) describe six challenges of revolutionary service that, if successfully met, will help an organization develop a loyal customer base by adding value to every aspect of the customer relationship.

Challenge 1—Make an Emotional Connection

Giving your customers a quality product or service at a fair price meets only your customers' minimum expectations. To develop loyalty, we have to make an emotional connection with our customers. That means bringing humanity back into the workplace, showing empathy, and providing a personal touch with every customer contact.

Challenge 2—Attack the Structures

Do our structures make sense to our customers? Do our policies, procedures, and decisions add value for our customers, or do they make it more difficult to do business with us? Current structures were designed to get current results. If we want dramatically different results tomorrow, we will have to redesign our structures.

Challenge 3—Align Structures with Words

Are we walking our talk? If not, the front line does not lie. Practices that undermine employees' efforts to build customer loyalty will make everyone cynical. Ensure that employees have been trained adequately, have enough information, and that all procedures exist to give customers the best service possible.

PEARL

"Only positive consequences encourage good future performance."—Kenneth Blanchard

---

Challenge 4—Know Your Customer

One size fits one. We must improve at understanding our customers, their preferences, needs, and their reasons for choosing to do business with us to personalize our relationship with them. What high-tech and low-tech methods can we use to gather customer data?

Challenge 5—Make Recovery Strategic

Relationships are tested when times are tough, not when everything is going smoothly. When we have made a mistake or a customer wants a customized product or service, it is our opportunity to demonstrate our true colors. Are our policies and procedures limiting or enhancing our abilities to recover from mistakes?

Challenge 6—Service is ReSelling

There is no more "old business." Whether we have had a customer relationship for 10 days or 10 years, every time that customer chooses to do business with us, he or she should be recognized for that choice. The business we get from now on is brand-new business. We need to change our focus from recruiting new customers to retaining the customers we already have.

Complaint Resolution

Heil and Tate (1995) describe the importance of recovering from mistakes. The techniques associated with this type of recovery are often referred to as complaint resolution (Table 4–15). Those organizations truly committed to customer service see complaints as a significant opportunity to improve processes and build customer loyalty. Some of the suggested techniques for complaint resolution are the following:

- *Remain calm:* Patients who are ill or in pain may have little tolerance for what they perceive as poor service. If you are the target of their anger or frustration, remain calm and do not become hostile or defensive. When you remain calm in the face of adversity, you exercise a critical interpersonal skill.

- *Stop, look, and listen:* Stop what you are doing, even if busy. Look at the person; make eye contact. Let him or her know you are engaged in the conversation. Listen to what is being said and communicate your empathy with facial expressions and occasional nods.

- *Accept anger:* Anger is a common expression of frustration. Allow the patient to ventilate the emotion.

- *Accept responsibility:* Do not immediately pass off a complaint by saying "That's not my department" even if the problem is not within your area of responsibility. In the patient's eyes, you are a representative of the organization that has caused a problem. Become an advocate for the patient, not the organization. Assist the patient with identifying the individual or office who will be most effective at resolving the complaint.

- *Refer:* Make certain that the person to whom you refer the patient is the appropriate individual. The patient's frustration will only grow if he or she finds out that they have been sent to the wrong place.

- *Ask questions:* Engage the patient in direct, open-ended questions that will assist you to define the specifics of the problem, for example, "What is the problem?" "Where did it happen?" What can I do to resolve this situation to your satisfaction?"

- *Restate:* If the situation is a complicated one, make sure you understand the problem by restating your interpretation of the events and asking for confirmation.

- *Respond:* Act quickly. A visual confirmation that you take the problem seriously by taking notes or making a phone call will reassure the patient that something is being done.

- *Agree:* Try to find something in the person's remark with which you agree. Emphasizing what you have in common, even if it is relatively unimportant, can eliminate an argument.

- *Develop solutions:* If a single solution to the problem is obvious, implement it. If you have the opportunity to develop several alternative solutions, allow the person to make a choice. The opportunity to choose a plan of action most suitable to one's needs invariably forces the individual to be reasonable.

- *Exceed expectations:* Do not promise anything you may not be able to deliver. Your effectiveness in handling complaints is based on honestly stating what can reasonably be done. Let the patient know what to expect and, whenever possible, exceed those expectations.

- *Personalize:* Introduce yourself to the patient and learn the person's name. For many, it is difficult to remain angry when you show you care enough about an individual to know his or her name.

- *Thank:* If possible, thank the patient for bringing the problem to your attention. Often the problem may be systemic and has caused problems in the past but has never been brought to your attention. Communicating an attitude that you sincerely appreciate knowing about problems will encourage the person to feel more satisfied about the way in which it is handled.

"Thank you for bringing this problem to my attention."

TABLE 4–15   Ten steps to successful complaint resolution

- Remain calm
- Personalize
- Stop, look, listen
- Accept anger
- Accept responsibility
- Respond
- Agree
- Restate
- Develop solutions
- Thank

Customer Service Self-Assessment

The following self-assessment may be helpful in identifying opportunities in your organization for improving customer service:

- Do you reward behavior in others that would further support customer service standards?

- Do you know how others view you and your behavior in relation to furthering effective customer service?

- How do you determine customer service expectations?

- Do you compare or benchmark yourselves to others?

- Do you view customer complaints as problems or opportunities for improvement?

- How does your organization make it easy for employees to solve problems?

- In what ways do you communicate and explain the mission, vision, and values of your organization to employees?

- What methods do you use to reinforce positive customer service?

- Are you measuring what you want repeated in your organization? Are you communicating these expectations to your employees?

- Do you set aside time each week to solicit feedback from patients, employees, and visitors?

- Do you "walk around" the department on a regular basis?

- Do you personally participate in employee orientation?

- Do you personally participate in CQI training?

- Are you or have you ever been a member of a process action or quality improvement team?

- Do you personally review summary data related to customer service? Can you name any actions taken recently as a result of such a review?

- Can you name a time recently when you have encouraged a staff member to "take a risk" or recognized one who did?

TREATMENT OUTCOME AS AN INDICATION OF QUALITY IMPROVEMENT

All of the concepts discussed to this point, from the integration of continuous quality principles to customer service, are designed to improve the outcome associated with the patient's episode of care. Managed care firms, insurers, government agencies, and our patients are justifiably demanding that our interventions make "meaningful differences." It is these meaningful differences that we commonly refer to as "treatment outcomes," and it is these outcomes that we can point to as the fruit of our CQI labors.

In an attempt to demonstrate effective treatment outcomes, the entire healthcare industry, including audiology, has developed an impressive array of outcome measures. Unfortunately, the proliferation of these tools has created confusion concerning the terminology and appropriate use of these instruments. The result is that we do not always measure what we think we are measuring. Audiologists are interested in assessing a number of outcomes. These include impairment, disability, handicap, activity limitations, participation restrictions, satisfaction, and quality of life. Although some of these terms are used (and misused) interchangeably, they do have distinct meanings and measuring instruments that are unique to that domain. Because of the complexities associated with the issue of outcome measures and the emerging importance of accountability in the profession, the topic of outcomes is addressed more completely in Chapter 5 in this volume.

CONCLUSIONS

In this chapter the concepts of quality improvement in a healthcare setting have been reviewed. The reason quality remains a controlling principle of practice management is that it is infused, knowingly or unknowingly, in every aspect of what we do as healthcare providers. From the moment we open our doors in the morning to the time we shut off the lights in the evening, the effectiveness of the care we provide to our patients is determined by the investment in quality we place in our planning, staff, resources, education, equipment, customer service, marketing, physical plant, and networking. Committing yourself and your practice to an ethic of excellence, however, will not be enough. You will need to discover ways to continue to improve the quality of your practice. And when you do, perhaps you will come to the same realization as Phaedrus at the end of his journey ". . . there is a feeling now, that was not here before, and it is not just on the surface of things, but penetrates all the way through: We've won it. It's going to get better now. You can sort of tell these things" (Pirsig, 1984, p. 412).

REFERENCES

ABRAMS, H.B., & SIFERD, S.T. (1994). Total quality improvement: The Department of Veterans Affairs audiology and speech pathology program. *Seminars in Hearing, 15*(4);277–287.

AGENCY FOR HEALTHCARE POLICY AND RESEARCH. (1993). *Clinical practice guideline development.* Rockville, MD: AHCPR.

AMERICAN NATIONAL STANDARDS INSTITUTE. (1996). *Specification of hearing aid characteristics (ANSI S3.22-1996).* New York: Acoustical Society of America.

ASHA. (1995). Standards for professional service programs in audiology and speech-language pathology. *ASHA Desk Reference* (Vol. 1) (1995 Ed.). Rockville, MD: American Speech-Language-Hearing Association.

BERWICK D.M., GODFREEY A.B., & ROESSNER, J. (1990). *Curing healthcare: Strategies for quality improvement.* San Fransisco: Jossey-Bass.

CARF. (1998). *1998 medical rehabilitation standards manual.* Tucson, AZ: CARF, The Rehabilitation Accreditation Commission.

COFFEY, R.J., RICHARDS, J.S., REMMERT, C.S., LEROY, S.S., SCHOVILLE, R.R., & BALDWIN, P.J. (1992). An introduction to critical paths. *Quality Management in Healthcare, 1*(1);45.

CROSBY, P.B. (1979). *Quality is free: The art of making quality certain.* New York: McGraw-Hill.

DEMING, W.E. (1986). *Out of the crisis.* Cambridge, MA: Massachusetts Institute of Technology, Center for Advanced Engineering Study.

GIFT, R.G. (1996). Benchmarking. In: R.G. Gift, & C.F. Kinney (Eds.), *Today's management methods* (pp. 245–261). Chicago: American Hospital Publishing.

HEIL, G., TATE, R., & PARKER, T. (1995). *Revolutionary service: Building customer loyalty one customer at a time.* Des Moines, IA: Excellence in Training Corp.

JAMES, B.C. (1989). *Quality management for healthcare delivery.* Chicago: The Hospital Research and Education Trust.

JOINT COMMISSION FOR THE ACCREDITATION OF HEALTHCARE ORGANIZATIONS. Update 4. (1997). *Comprehensive accreditation manual for hospitals: The official handbook.* Oakdale, IL: JCAHO.

JURAN, J.M. (1988). *Juran on planning for quality.* New York: The Free Press.

KLEEB, T. (1996). Pathways and algorithms. In: R.G. Gift, & C.F. Kinney (Eds.), *Today's management methods* (pp.187–207). Chicago: American Hospital Publishing.

KOCH, M.W., & WADE, T.M. (1993). *Integrated quality management.* St. Louis: Mosby–Year Book.

NATIONAL INSTITUTE OF STANDARDS AND TECHNOLOGY. (1994). 1995 Award criteria, Malcolm Baldridge national quality award. Gaithersburg, MD: NIST.

PIRSIG, R.M. (1984). *Zen and the art of motorcycle maintenance.* New York: William Morrow.

SCHIPPER, H., CLINCH, J., & POWELL, V. (1990). Definitions and conceptual issues. In: B. Spilker (Ed.), *Quality of life assessments in clinical trials* (pp. 11–24). New York: Raven.

STOLZ, P.K. (1996). FOCUS-PDCA. In: R.G. Gift, & C.F. Kinney (Eds.), *Today's management methods* (pp.223–244). Chicago: American Hospital Publishing.

WORLD HEALTH ORGANIZATION. (1980). *International classification of impairments, disabilities, and handicaps–A manual of classification relating to the consequences of disease.* Geneva.

YOUNG, J.O. (1996). Customer needs analysis. In: R.G. Gift, & C.F. Kinney (Eds.), *Today's management methods* (pp. 115–124). Chicago: American Hospital Publishing.

Chapter 5

Outcome Measures: The Audiologic Difference

Harvey B. Abrams and Theresa Hnath-Chisolm

"You got to be very careful if you don't know where you're going, because you might not get there."—Yogi Berra

This chapter represents, in part, the efforts of a Department of Veterans Affairs (VA) Audiology and Speech Pathology Service task force charged with the responsibility of developing hearing aid outcome measure guidelines for VA audiologists. More than $45,000,000 was spent in fiscal year 1998 for hearing aids and related supplies, not including the labor and administrative costs associated with the selection and fitting

of the more than 130,000 hearings aids dispensed to veteran patients that year. From a purely fiscal perspective, it is imperative that the VA demonstrates to American taxpayers that they are getting "their money's worth." It is equally critical that we demonstrate that we are fulfilling the VA's healthcare goals by providing the right care in the right way at the right time in the right place at the right cost each time. Outcome measures attempt to assess these objectives. Although originally drafted for the VA, the information in this chapter is equally applicable to all audiologists in all employment settings.

PEARL

Outcome measures refer to any clinical method or tool that can be used to evaluate a patient's status as a result of audiological intervention.

The general goal of outcomes measurement is to provide objective information to customers and to promote data-driven decision making by managers. In the context of this chapter, the term *outcome measures* refers to those methods and tools that can be used to evaluate a patient's status as a result of audiological intervention. Although the use of outcome measures is critical for all audiological services, the focus of this chapter will be on hearing aid selection and fitting. It is the hearing aid that will ultimately define the profession and discipline of audiology. Turner (1998) argues that by virtue of their education, research productivity, knowledge transfer, and clinical services, audiologists should be the recognized hearing aid expert. To truly claim the right to declare themselves as the hearing aid providers of choice, however, it is imperative that audiologists objectively document the benefits achieved as a result of their expertise.*

RATIONALE FOR HEARING AID OUTCOMES ASSESSMENT

We are firmly entrenched in an era of increasing accountability and shrinking healthcare resources. As a result, administrators, third-party payers, and our patients themselves are

---

*The interested reader is referred to the 1993 Carhart Memorial Lecture delivered by Dr. Earl Harford (Harford, 1993) to the annual meeting of the American Auditory Society. Dr. Harford delivered an eloquent and convincing case for the indispensable role of the hearing aid in the past, present, and future of audiology.

Audiology: Practice Management. Edited by Hosford-Dunn, Roeser, and Valente. Thieme Medical Publishers, Inc., New York © 2000

seeking evidence that our treatments make meaningful differences in our patients' lives. An impressive array of outcome measures is available for documenting the efficacy of intervention with hearing aid(s). These outcome measures can be used to perform an economic analysis of various hearing aid options. For example, to justify, economically, the selection of a digital as opposed to an analog circuit, the measured benefits with the more expensive (digital) option would need to increase in proportion to the additional costs to demonstrate cost-effectiveness. In addition to their use in economic evaluations of treatment options, outcome measures can be used for other purposes, such as (1) adjusting the hearing aid parameters; (2) counseling patients regarding expectations of benefit; and (3) documenting patient satisfaction.

SPECIAL CONSIDERATION

Outcomes are for all of your customers—patients, employer, families, insurers, co-workers, and accrediting organizations.

The choice of appropriate outcome measures depends on the establishment of clear goals for hearing aid intervention. This process can be facilitated by application of the World Health Organization (WHO) classification scheme for describing the consequences of health conditions (i.e., disorders and diseases). Initially, the WHO (1980) used the terms *impairment, disability,* and *handicap* to describe the multidimensional impact of a health condition. Recently, however, as a result of changes in healthcare practices and a new social understanding of disability, the WHO (1997) proposed revising the system. Although the term *impairment* remains, health condition consequences in the "disability" domain are now described in terms of *activity* limitations, while those in the "handicap" domain are described in terms of restrictions in *participation.* These differences in terminology are summarized in Table 5–1. The revised classification system also includes a consideration of "contextual factors." This concept was added to the model to highlight the fact that the disablement experienced by an individual with a given health condition will be influenced by both environmental and personal contextual factors. Environmental factors include social attitudes, architectural characteristics, legal and social structures, and so on, while personal factors allow for consideration of a person's gender, age, coping style, socioeconomic background, education, and other demographic variables. This new scheme involves not merely a change in terminology but a change in concept.

DEFINITIONS

Impairment is the effect of the disorder at the level of the body structure and function, *activity* at the level of the person, and *participation* at the societal level. When a hearing disorder results in changes in the auditory anatomy or functional aspects of audition, such as the ability to detect or localize sounds, then a *hearing impairment* is present. Presence of a hearing impairment, then, can result in *limitations of daily*

activities such as understanding of speech, which may adversely affect conversing at a restaurant, using the telephone, listening to a lecture, or watching television. Within certain societal contexts, these activity limitations might restrict *participation,* such as attending religious services or social gatherings. The individual might also have difficulty in aspects of job performance that require the use of a telephone that may ultimately lead to their resignation or termination. Finally, the individual may withdraw from participating in common social interactions. Unlike the domains of *impairment* and *activity limitations,* the domain of *participation restrictions* is highly influenced by environmental factors such as the presence of federal and local regulations pertaining to the disabled, the availability of assistive devices, community support for the rights of the disabled, architectural considerations, workplace accommodations, and transportation alternatives. When an enlightened community or place of business provides the appropriate accommodations, the impact on the individual's *participation* in society is minimized. However, when the presence of impairment leads to significant activity limitations and participation restrictions, then an individual's overall physical, mental, and social well-being may also be adversely affected. When this occurs, an individual is said to experience a reduction in his or her *health-related quality of life* (HQL; National Institutes of Health, 1997). Although "health-related quality of life" is not a specific domain within the WHO classification system, it is understood that HQL represents the sum of the effects of each of the domains described in Table 5–1.

It is generally accepted that activity limitations, participation restrictions, and consequent health-related quality of life are related to the magnitude and type of hearing loss. However, widespread clinical recognition shows that it is not possible to accurately predict the nature and extent of an individual's limitations and restrictions solely on the basis of audiometric data alone. Two persons with the same degree of impairment may have very different perceptions regarding their HQL (Testa & Simonson, 1996). Similarly, we cannot measure the effects of audiological intervention solely by its impact in the impairment domain. If this were the case, the provision of reasonably good audibility across a broad frequency range, without making average and loud speech uncomfortable, would be the *only* determinant of a successful hearing aid fitting. Because activity limitations and participation restrictions are significantly influenced by the individual's personality, communication needs, and the environment, as well as the degree of impairment, assurance of audibility at comfortable listening levels, unfortunately, does not guarantee an improvement in quality of life.

The Impairment Domain

On the basis of the WHO's classification scheme, hearing aid intervention can be conceived of as having several general goals. The first general goal is to alleviate, as much as possible, the *impairment* resulting from disorder or damage to the auditory system. As is well known, the primary *impairment* resulting from a conductive disorder is a decrease in the ability to detect sounds. When damage to the sensorineural mechanism is present, however, impairments in loudness perception, temporal resolution, and frequency resolution

TABLE 5–1   A comparison of the 1980 and 1997 World Health Organization (WHO) classification systems for impairment, disability, and handicap

WHO-1980 Domains	WHO-1997 Domains	Level of Functioning Affected	Characteristics
Impairment —abnormalities of body structure and appearance and organ system function, resulting from any cause.	Impairment —a loss or abnormality of body structure or of a physiological or psychological function.	At body level	Body function Body structure
Disability —restrictions or lack of ability to perform an activity in a manner or within the range considered normal for a human being.	Activities —the nature and extent of functioning at the level of the person. Activities may be limited in nature, duration, and quality.	At person level	Person's daily activities
Handicap —a disadvantage for a given individual resulting from an impairment or disability that limits or prevents the fulfillment of a role that is normal for that individual.	Participation —the nature and extent of a person's involvement in life situations in relation to impairments, activities, health conditions, and contextual factors. Participation may be restricted in nature, duration, and quality.	At societal level	Involvement in the situation

often accompany the impairment in detection. Although future technology may allow us to address frequency and temporal resolution impairments, current hearing aid technology provides the audiologist with the ability to address impairments of detection and loudness perception through the preselection of electroacoustic characteristics, while also considering the style of the instrument (e.g., behind-the-ear [BTE], in-the-ear [ITE], in-the-canal [ITC], and completely-in-the-canal [CIC]), the hearing aid arrangement (e.g., monaural, binaural, contralateral routing of signal(s) [CROS]), circuitry options (e.g., linear, output compression, wide dynamic range compression), and user options (e.g., t-coil, directional/omni-directional switching, multiple programs).

In current practice the selection of hearing aid parameters begins with obtaining data from a complete audiological evaluation. Standard audiometric data are often supplemented with information from additional perceptual measures, such

---

PEARL

Use outcome measures to modify the fitting and to determine the success of the fitting.

---

as loudness comfort and growth. In addition, relevant information may be obtained through informal discussions or formal assessment of an individual's self-perceived listening difficulties, needs, and concerns. To select an initial set of electroacoustic characteristics, these data are often applied to one of several available prescriptive approaches. The prescription defines several parameters including the frequency/gain response at one or more input levels, the OSPL-90, and additional characteristics such as crossover frequency between channels and dynamic/static characteristics of compression circuitry.*

Electroacoustic and other hearing aid parameters are typically selected to meet three specific goals: (1) make soft sounds audible; (2) make normal conversational speech comfortably loud and understandable; and (3) make loud sounds loud but tolerable. Outcome measures selected to demonstrate that these specific goals are achieved involve *verifying* that the electroacoustic and other hearing aid characteristics meet the objective criteria used in their preselection. Once it is determined that the electroacoustic and other characteristics of the hearing aid(s) are optimal for meeting the *impairment* level goals, we need to determine that general and specific goals set at the levels of *activity* and *participation* are also met. At these levels, the outcome measures selected will be used to *validate* that the use of hearing aid(s) makes meaningful differences (i.e., that the treatment is efficacious).

The Activity Domain

The general goal of hearing aid fitting at the *activity* level is to improve a patient's ability to understand speech and improve communication functioning. At present, outcome measures used to validate the efficacy of hearing aid intervention at this level include objective performance measures and subjective self-report measures of speech understanding and communication performance. It is important to keep in mind that as more sophisticated and nonlinear signal processing technologies are introduced in amplification systems, other types of outcome measures aimed at validating the efficacy of hearing aid intervention at the activity level may be seen in the audiology clinic. For example, it would not be unreasonable to include a measure of sound localization ability when evaluating multiple-microphone versus single-microphone technology. Indeed, techniques for addressing localization performance are currently available (Besing & Koehnke, 1995).

SPECIAL CONSIDERATION

The WHO dropped the domains "disability" and "handicap" from its revised classification document because of negative connotations associated with this terminology.

The Participation Domain

The measurement of *restrictions in participation* resulting from a hearing impairment and its consequent activity limitations is not a common focus in standard audiological testing protocols. We often infer this data, however, through the case histories we obtain from our patients. For example, patients may report seeking our services because they can no longer enjoy attending social gatherings or are having difficulty with communication at work. After hearing aid fitting, we may informally ask

our patients if they experience less difficulty in these or similar situations. Although this informal approach may satisfy us that we have accomplished our goals, more formal assessments allow for the quantification of successful outcomes at the level of *participation*. A variety of self-report measures that can be used for this purpose. Because the level of participation is highly influenced by the environmental factors described earlier, the audiologist may need to take a more active role in evaluating the social, occupational, and living environments in which the patient exists. As a result, the audiologist may become involved in the development of hearing accessibility programs for communities or groups of listeners with hearing impairments (Jennings & Head, 1994; Pichora-Fuller & Robertson, 1994). Such programs are designed to address the needs, wishes, and abilities of the listener within specific communication situations with specific communication partners in specific communication environments.

SPECIAL CONSIDERATION

A major change in the 1980 and 1997 WHO classifications is the inclusion of "contextual" factors (environment, law, accessibility, social attitudes, etc.) that have an impact on the patient's activities and participation.

Health-Related Quality of Life

We are also concerned that meeting our clinical objectives in the *impairment, activity,* and *participation* domains will result in measurable changes in self-perceived *HQL*. Although HQL measurement has received little clinical application among audiologists, it is a construct that is receiving increased attention in the research literature, including those studies aimed at demonstrating the efficacy of hearing aid intervention (Crandall, 1988; Jerger et al, 1996; Mulrow et al, 1990). Review of this literature provides information regarding available tools and approaches that can be adopted for use in our clinical protocols. The most clinically useful of these techniques involves the demonstration of successful treatment outcomes through self-report of improvements in perceived quality of life.

Satisfaction

Finally, no hearing aid fitting could be considered fully successful without demonstrating that the patient was *satisfied* with the device and services received. *Satisfaction* does not always correspond to significant or quantifiable changes in *impairment, activity limitations, participation,* or *HQL*. In addition to improvements in communication and real-world functioning, the domain of *satisfaction* involves the patient's relationship with service providers, the ease of access to services, and the influence of factors such as cosmetics, comfort, expectations, and perceived value. It is a construct that needs independent assessment.

The remainder of this chapter provides detailed discussion of clinically useful outcome measures that provide a means for demonstrating that in the clinical processes of selection, fitting, and counseling in the appropriate use of hearing

---

*Although not common in current clinical practice, technological advances may result in the incorporation of techniques such as paired comparisons of sound quality and/or perceived intelligibility for selection and/or adjustment of electroacoustic characteristics.

aid(s), we have met the goals selected at the levels of *impairment, activity, participation, HQL,* and *satisfaction.* These data can be used to demonstrate treatment efficacy for individual patients and/or as part of program evaluation. The discussion focuses on measures appropriate for use in the adult, particularly veteran, population. It is important to note that outcome assessment for children requires age-appropriate tests, tasks, and approaches.

MEETING CLINICAL GOALS AT THE LEVEL OF IMPAIRMENT: THE VERIFICATION PROCESS

As discussed, the general goal at the level of impairment is to improve audibility of speech, while maintaining listening comfort. This goal is accomplished through the selection of appropriate electroacoustic parameters and other hearing aid characteristics (i.e., style, arrangement, circuitry). Although 2-cc coupler measurements may be used to ensure that the hearing aid satisfies manufacturer quality control standards and to make initial adjustments on the hearing aid, it is now standard practice to use real-ear measurements (probe microphone measurements of real-ear insertion gain [REIG] and real-ear aided response [REAR], or functional gain for severe to profound losses) to individually adjust the parameters of the hearing aid and verify results. The primary goals of this verification process are to ensure that the measured electroacoustic characteristics are as close as possible to those prescribed for the patient and that the hearing aid provides adequate audibility of the important speech energy without feedback or loudness discomfort.

PITFALL

Assuring audibility at comfortable listening levels does not guarantee an improvement in quality of life.

Root–Mean–Square Difference

Documentation that the impairment-related goals have been met can be accomplished in several ways. For example, one approach would be to specify the root-mean-square (rms) difference between the REIG from the target frequency response. Byrne (1992) has described such a procedure with the following formula:

$$\text{Rms Difference} = \sqrt{\frac{d_1^2 + d_2^2 + d_3^2 + d_4^2}{4}} \qquad (1)$$

Where $d_1^2 \ldots d_4^2$ equals the difference between the target gain and measured gain at 500, 1000, 2000, and 4000 Hz. Byrne discovered that his subjects were able to detect a difference in the sound quality of the hearing aid with an rms difference of as little as 3 dB.

Articulation Index

Another approach to verifying hearing aid selection uses the articulation indices (AI). The AI provides a numerical value between 0.0 and 1.0. Higher AI scores are achieved by placing more of the acoustic speech signal in the audible range. Theoretically, the higher the AI score, the greater the ability to understand speech at comfortable levels. Several methods are available, each with benefits and limitations (e.g., ANSI, 1969; Fletcher, 1953; Pavlovic, 1984, 1991).* The ANSI (1969) and Fletcher (1953) methods require complex calculations and are not appropriate for routine clinical use. The Pavlovic (1984, 1991) methods involve simpler calculations and are easy to use but lack precision. Unfortunately, existing AI approaches that best predict performance are not presently available for clinical implementation (Rankovic, 1997).

PITFALL

Just whose outcomes are you measuring: the patient's or yours? "Hitting the REIG target" is of little value if the patient will not wear the hearing aids because of dissatisfaction with cosmetics or comfort.

Patient Acceptability Factors

In addition to documenting improvements in speech audibility, it is also important to achieve a good physical fit, acceptable cosmetics, adequate volume wheel range, and satisfactory sound quality. The assessment of these important outcomes is typically determined at follow-up visits, through telephone interviews, or by mailed questionnaires.

Acclimatization

After the hearing aid(s) fitting process and a complete orientation to their use and care, patients wear their instruments home for a period of time (at least a few weeks) before obtaining measures that provide validation of the efficacy of hearing aid selection and fitting at a follow-up appointment. During the period between fitting and the follow-up appointment, it is expected that "acclimatization" to amplification may occur at least for some new hearing aid users (Gatehouse, 1992) and that the patient will have experienced a variety of listening environments. Acclimatization may result in improved speech recognition ability over time, particularly for those patients who have more severe losses but also may refer merely to the fact that the patient becomes accustomed to wearing the hearing aids at a higher volume wheel setting or becomes less bothered by such aspects of amplification as the occlusion effect, common background sounds, and the physical presence of the instruments in the ear.

---

*Note that the audioscan® RM500 Real-Ear System/Hearing Aid Analyzer will automatically calculate an AI.

CONTROVERSIAL POINT

Some acclimatization studies suggest that speech recognition outcome measures may change over time. Other investigations failed to demonstrate any significant changes in performance.

MEETING CLINICAL GOALS AT THE ACTIVITY AND PARTICIPATION LEVELS: THE VALIDATION PROCESS

Outcome measures used to validate the efficacy of hearing aid intervention at the activity and participation levels include objective performance measures of speech recognition and self-report measures assessing activity limitations and/or participation restrictions. Each of these categories is discussed.

Objective Performance Measures of Speech Recognition

The use of speech recognition testing as an outcome assessment tool in hearing aid fitting is controversial. Such testing has generally fallen out of favor since the Carhart comparative speech approach to hearing aid fitting (Carhart, 1946) was determined to be too time consuming and the phonetically balanced (PB) word lists were found to be insensitive to small differences among hearing aids (Walden et al, 1983). In addition, it has not been adequately demonstrated that performance on these clinical tests accurately predicts performance in everyday listening environments. Some argue, however, that because the use of phoneme, rather than whole word scoring of PB words, allows for an increase in the reliability of test scores without increasing test time, their use as a hearing aid outcome measure warrants further consideration (Boothroyd, 1998). Furthermore, the application of probability theory to phoneme scores allows for reliable prediction of speech recognition performance for low-predictability sentences (Olsen et al, 1997). However, the use of phoneme scoring does not appear to be gaining widespread acceptance among clinicians.

In recent years new speech in noise testing materials have been developed, ranging from phoneme-level identification tasks to whole-sentence recognition. This topic is discussed in greater detail in *Diagnosis*, Chapter 13. A comprehensive description of speech recognition tests developed for diagnostic and rehabilitative purposes can also be found in Mendel and Danhauer (1997).

Isolated word and syllable tests have recently been supplanted by words in sentence or whole sentence recognition tests, on the assumption that speech that includes contextual cues will have greater predictive validity. Two tests that have seen increasing use both clinically and in hearing aid research are the Speech-In-Noise test (SPIN; Kalikow et al, 1977) and the Hearing-In-Noise test (HINT; Nilson, Soli, & Sullivan, 1994). In the SPIN, a test list consists of 50 male-voice sentences in a background of multitalker babble, one-half of which offer no contextual cues for the final, test word (called

low-predictability [LP] items; scores loosely correlate to monosyllabic word scores), and the other one half of which do have contextual cues for the final word (high-predictability [HP] items). The SPIN is given with fixed speech and noise levels. Percent-correct scores are calculated for the total list and for LP and HP items separately. Scores on the SPIN may be compared for unaided versus aided listening (benefit), but, in addition, comparison of scores for HP versus LP can prove useful in counseling the patient regarding the use of context in word identification.

In the HINT the speech spectrum noise level is fixed at a moderate intensity level. The signal-to-noise ratio (SNR) is varied adaptively to determine the SNR at which a 50% correct sentence performance is obtained. The patient is required to repeat the entire sentence correctly. Two of the benefits of adaptive SNR testing are that for most patients, no ceiling or floor effect exists and the test can be administered quickly. An automated computer format is now available. Caution is advised when using adaptive speech testing procedures to compare performance between hearing aids that have nonlinear signal processing functions, because the input level that yields the target SNR may vary with each hearing aid.

A number of outstanding issues in speech recognition testing remain. Some of the speech materials available do not have normative data, are not available in recorded form, or the recordings are not standardized. One issue that has been noted by some is that the recording or playback process may seriously limit the dynamic range (DR) of the test materials relative to everyday listening environments, which may be an issue in predictive validity, particularly with nonlinear signal processing hearing aids. Finally, questions still exist about what levels the speech and noise should be to represent the "real world," what type of noise should be used, and what loudspeaker array should be used to simulate everyday environments.

PITFALL

Most of the recorded speech materials use a male voice, which may not tap into the perception of important high-frequency phonemes that are so difficult for many patients who have sloping hearing losses.

Subjective Self-Report Measures Examining Activity Limitations and Participation Restrictions

In real-world, rather than clinical or laboratory, conditions the activity of speech understanding and the participation in events that require speech understanding are heavily influenced by contextual factors related to both the environment and the individual. As a result, many questionnaires have been developed to assess the impact of a hearing impairment on the individual in the areas of communication functioning, activity limitation, and participation restrictions. Table 5–2

TABLE 5–2   A comparison of self-report outcome measures

Test Name	Domain	No. Items	Response Mode	Administration Time	Reliability	Scoring
Abbreviated* Profile of Hearing Aid Benefit (APHAB)	Activity/ participation	24 Items 4 subscales with 6 items each AV, EC, RV, BN	Self-report, paper and pencil, computer	10 min or less	.78–.87 by Chronbach's alpha	Equal percentile profiles are determined for unaided, aided, and benefit scores
Client Oriented[†] Scale of Improvement (COSI)	Activity/ participation	5 items	Self-report	N/A	N/A	Patient judges the degree of change attributable to intervention
Communication[‡] Profile Hearing Inventory (CHPI)	Activity/ participation	145 items 25 subscales	Paper and pencil	Phase I: 30–60 min Phase II: 20–40 min Phase III: 20–40 min	.67–.89 as assessed by coefficient X	Results plotted as a profile of scores
Denver Scale of[§] Communication Function	Activity/ participation	25 items	Self-report, paper and pencil	15 min		Plot result as a profile of scores
Hearing[‖] Handicap Inventory - Elderly (HHIE)	Activity/ participation	25 items total 13 items for emotional scale 12 items for social scale	Paper and pencil	10 min	.82 emotional, .93 social, .24 sensitivity section by Chronbach's alpha	% correct 100% max score higher values represent greater perceived handicap
Health[¶] Utilities Index	Activity/ participation	8 attributes with 5–6 levels each	Self-report, paper and pencil	20 min	.767	Uses scoring algorithm to generate both a utility score and a value
Hearing Aid[**] Users Questionnaire (HAUQ)	Activity/ participation	24 items	Self-report, paper and pencil	5–10 min	N/A	Descriptive
Hearing[††] Performance Inventory (HPI)	Activity/ participation	158 items 6 subscales	Paper and pencil	30–45 min	N/A	% of difficulty The lower the score the better performance
MOS SF-36[‡‡] Health Survey	Activity/ participation	36 items 8 subscales	Self-report, paper and pencil	15 min	.78–.9 internal consistency Values for 8 subscales	8 individual subscale scores Physical component scale score and a mental component scale score

* Abbreviated Profile of Hearing Aid Benefit (APHAB)—Cox & Alexander, 1995.
[†] Client Oriented Scale of Improvement (COSI)—Dillon, James, & Ginis, 1997.
[‡] Communication Profile Hearing Inventory (CHPI)—Demorest, & Erdman, 1986.
[§] Denver Scale of Communication Function—Alpiner, Chevrette, Glascoe, Metz, & Olsen,1978.
[‖] Hearing Handicap Inventory Elderly (HHIE)—Ventry & Weinstein, 1982.
[¶] Health Utilities Index—Feeny et al, 1996.
[**] Hearing Aid Users Questionnaire (HAUQ)—Dillon, Birtles, & Lovegrove, 1999.
[††] Hearing Performance Inventory (HPI)—Gioles, Owens, Lamb, & Schubert, 1979.
[‡‡] MOS SF-36 Health Survey—Ware & Sherbourne, 1992.

TABLE 5–2 (continued)   A comparison of self-report outcome measures

Test Name	Domain	No. Items	Response Mode	Administration Time	Reliability	Scoring
Shortened[§§] Hearing Aid Performance Inventory (SHAPI)	Activity/ participation	38 items	Self-report, paper and pencil	N/A	.94 by Chronbach's alpha	% score Higher score represents lower benefit
Sickness[||||] Impact Profile (SIP)	Activity/ participation	136 items 12 subscales	Self-report, paper and pencil	60 min	N/A	Score range from 0–100 with higher indicating poorer health 12 individual category scores, a total score, and physical and psychological dimension scores can be calculated
Satisfaction[¶¶] with Amplification in Daily Life (SADL)	Activity/ participation	19 items	Self-report, paper and pencil	10 min	.59–.88 by Chronbach's Alpha	4 subscales Higher point scores represent higher

[§§] Shortened Hearing Aid Performance Inventory (SHAPI)—Schum, 1993.

[||||] Sickness Impact Profile (SIP)—Bergner et al, 1981.

[¶¶] Satisfaction with Amplification in Daily Life (SADL)—Cox & Alexander, 1997.

provides information about some of the more commonly used self-report outcome measures.

The questionnaires reviewed in detail here meet the following criteria that we consider necessary for clinical use: (1) they are easy to administer in a short period of time; (2) each provides quantifiable preintervention and postintervention scores; (3) test-retest reliability data are available. It should be noted that a plethora of other scales have been developed over the years.* The exclusion here is not intended as a commentary on their psychometric properties or potential use. Rather, we have chosen to focus our discussion on the most commonly used tools that meet our selection criteria for clinical use.

Two well-documented questionnaires warrant special mention although they are not discussed in detail. The first is the Communication Profile for the Hearing-Impaired (CPHI; Demorest & Erdman, 1986), which is an excellent research tool and useful for indepth clinical assessment. With 163 items, however, the CPHI is time-consuming to administer. Another useful instrument is the Hearing Aid Performance Inventory (HAPI, Walden et al, 1984), which at 64 items was quite long. Although shortened versions of the HAPI (SHAPI/SHAPI-E) have been introduced, these inventories provide aided scores only. Because they do not allow for difference scores, their value as an outcome measure is limited.

*See Table 10.1 in Skinner (1988).

PEARL

A clinically practical outcome measure should be easy to administer in a short period of time, provide quantifiable preintervention and postintervention scores, and have established test-retest reliability data.

The HHIE

One of the most commonly used, and studied, outcome measures for audiologic intervention is the Hearing Handicap Inventory for the Elderly (HHIE; Ventry & Weinstein, 1982). The original version, with 25 questions, contains 13 items that are classified as eliciting information from an "emotional" domain and 12 from a "social" domain. The inventory is scored on the basis of the total number of "yes" (4 points), "sometimes" (2 points), and "no" (0 points) responses. The total score (range 0 to 100) provided the clinician with a relative indication of how handicapping the patient perceives the hearing impairment to be. That is, the higher the value, the greater the self-perception of hearing handicap. The questionnaire is repeated after audiological intervention, which may include hearing aids, aural rehabilitation, or both. The change in the HHIE score provides the outcome measure.

When administered in a face-to-face format, a reduction in score of 18.7 points is needed for the clinician to conclude that real benefit has been attained. If a paper-and-pencil format is used, however, test-retest reliability diminishes, and the 95% confidence interval for a true change in score becomes 36 points. An example of an emotional-domain item from the HHIE is "Does a hearing problem cause you to feel embarrassed when meeting new people?" whereas "Does a hearing problem cause you difficulty when listening to radio or TV?" would fall into the "social domain" group of questions.

Variations of the HHIE include the HHIE-S, a 10-item short form version (Ventry & Weinstein (1983); the HHIA, which is a 25-item version including occupationally related questions (and its shortened version, HHIA-S) (Newman et al, 1991); and the HHIE-SP, a 25-item Spanish language version (Gonzalez, 1997). Confidence limits associated with face-to-face and paper-and-pencil administration formats for these measures are presented in Table 5–2. Clinical experience suggests that the HHIE is most effective with inexperienced hearing aid users because experienced users may not accurately recall their "pre-hearing aid" self-perception of hearing handicap after a significant period of hearing aid use.

The APHAB

Another widely used tool for quantifying the changes in activity and participation levels associated with hearing aid use is The Abbreviated Profile of Hearing Aid Benefit (APHAB) developed by Cox and Alexander (1995). This 24-item questionnaire is composed of situational-specific questions that are classified into one of four categories: (1) ease of communication (EC), which examines the communication effort under favorable conditions; (2) reverberation (RV), which examines communication in reverberant environments such as classrooms; (3) background noise (BN), which examines communication in high levels of background noise; and, (4) aversiveness of sound (AV), which examines the unpleasantness of environmental sounds.

Cox (1997) describes the administration and application of APHAB. Patients are asked to indicate the percentage of time they experience problems hearing under these situations. Seven response alternatives range from always to half the time to never. The patient uses these response alternatives to indicate answers to the 24 situational-specific items both "without my hearing aid" and "with my hearing aid." Responses can be recorded in a paper-and-pencil format or keyed directly onto a computer keyboard. A software program available from Cox is used for scoring. The scores generated are displayed graphically and numerically. A subscale score can then be produced for unaided and aided listening. Benefit is defined as the difference between the aided and unaided scores. For individual subscale scores for "EC," "RV," or "BN," a difference of 22 percentage points is needed between aided and unaided scores for the clinician to be reasonably certain that the scores represent a real difference between conditions. When pattern performance across these three subscales is examined, the clinician can be confident that real benefit has been achieved (at least for linear hearing aids) when the aided scores exceed the unaided ones by at least 10 percentage points.

Clinical experience with APHAB suggests several factors to consider in its use. One of these is the administration

format. In one approach the unaided responses are provided before hearing aid fitting, and aided responses are obtained after an appropriate (approximately 30 days) period of hearing aid use. During the second administration, Cox (1997) suggests that reliability and validity are increased if the patients are allowed to see their unaided responses. If they no longer agree with their assessment of their unaided difficulties, they are permitted to change the response. Although this is acceptable, this format differs from the one used when the APHAB was normed, where subjects were asked to provide unaided and aided responses in the same sitting.

Another problem associated with the APHAB is that not all of the situational-specific items are relevant to individual patients. Because patients are discouraged from leaving items blank, they need instruction about how to respond to situations that they do not or are not likely to experience. Finally, some concern exists regarding the reading level associated with the scale. It is recommended that questionnaires and other documents designed for patient use and education (e.g., informed consents, drug information pamphlets) be written at the seventh to eighth grade reading level. The readability level of the APHAB exceeds the eleventh grade level according to the Flesch-Kincaid Grade Level score.

PITFALL

The validity of some self-report questionnaires is limited because they require the patient to respond to situations that the patient does not, and never will, encounter.

The Client-Oriented Scale of Improvement

In contrast to existing scales that list specific questions or situations, the Client-Oriented Scale of Improvement (COSI) (Dillon et al, 1997) requires the patient, with guidance from the clinician, to identify up to five situations that cause the most communication difficulties. At the completion of treatment, the patient assesses the degree to which the identified problems have resolved. Degree of change is ranked on a 5-point scale from worse to slightly better to much better or from hardly ever to occasionally to almost always. A score of 5 corresponds to better/almost always and a score of 1 corresponds to worse/hardly ever. Although this measure promises to have great usefulness, it has not been widely used. One of the concerns about COSI is that its application to program evaluation may be limited because each patient identifies problem situations that are unique to him or her. Dillon et al (1999), however, recently reported their use of COSI and the Hearing Aid Users Questionnaire (HAUQ) as outcome measures for monitoring the National Australian Hearing Services Program. The authors determined that many individual needs identified by the subjects could be classified into 16 categories that can be analyzed for program effectiveness. For example, communication needs associated with hearing or understanding speech in restaurants, parties, or unique social situations can be categorized as "conversation with one or two in noise" or "conversation with group in noise." Approximately 75% of the subjects reported wanting to be able to hear television or radio at normal levels.

The HHIE, APHAB, and other self-report measures assessing activity limitations (i.e., hearing disability) and participation restrictions (i.e., hearing handicap) are useful for documenting hearing aid treatment efficacy according to numerous studies (e.g., Bentler et al, 1993; Cox et al, 1991; Humes et al, 1996; Malinoff & Weinstein, 1989; Mulrow et al, 1990; Newman et al, 1991; Primeau, 1997). Despite the availability and usefulness of these tools, most clinicians reportedly do not use them (Mueller, 1997; Schow et al, 1993). In our own informal survey of VA audiologists, less than 10% of responding clinicians reported routine use of these instruments although most report using some measure of benefit—usually a locally developed instrument. As the need for measurable outcomes increases, however, it is expected that the use of standardized self-assessment measures will become more widespread.

CONTROVERSIAL POINT

Although the COSI may be an effective outcome measure for individual patients, concern exists that it may be inappropriate for analyzing programs. Recent research (Dillon et al, 1999) suggests otherwise.

HEALTH-RELATED QUALITY OF LIFE: AN IMPORTANT OUTCOME MEASURE

Interest is increased in examining the impact of hearing impairment in terms HQL. An assessment of an individual's HQL involves more global considerations than those normally associated with impairment, activity limitations, or participation restrictions, although each of these necessarily have an impact on an individual's perceived HQL. An HQL assessment commonly involves consideration of four separate factors, or domains: (1) *physical* and *occupational* function, (2) *psychological* function, (3) *social* interaction, and (4) *somatic* sensation. HQL assessments are *multifactorial*, that is, they encompass more than one domain of human experience; they are *self-administered*; they are *time-variable*, that is, one's HQL may change from day to day, depending on changes to any one of the four domains; and they are *subjective*. Although specific clinical disciplines such as psychiatry, rehabilitation, cardiology, and oncology use HQL measurements to assess outcome, little is known about how audiological disorders and interventions affect HQL, particularly when compared with other health-related disorders and treatments.

HQL measures can be categorized as *disease-specific* or *generic*. Disease-specific measures are useful for comparing different treatment options for the same health condition. Generic HQL measures, on the other hand, are designed for use across health conditions. For example, a generic HQL measure was recently used to demonstrate the cost-effectiveness of cochlear implantation relative to other health disorders (Wyatt et al, 1995). In choosing a specific or a generic instrument, the benefits and limitations of both approaches should

be considered. Disease-specific instruments are clinically sensible; that is, the questions are similar to those used when talking to a patient anyway. As a result, these instruments tend to be sensitive to the effects of treatments that are directed toward alleviating the specific problems identified. Using disease-specific instruments creates problems, however, when comparing treatment benefits across populations or conditions. Conversely, generic instruments allow comparisons across populations or conditions but may be insensitive to a particular condition and treatment. As a result of these benefits and limitations, the National Institutes of Health consensus statement on HQL (NIH, 1997) currently recommends both types of measures.

PEARL

The National Institutes of Health consensus statement on HQL currently recommends the use of both disease-specific and generic measures when assessing patient outcome.

Disease-Specific Health-Related Quality of Life Measures

The HQL disease-specific instruments were created to measure a specific portion of an individual's health. The questions associated with this type of measure are customized to the HQL burden of a specific disorder and its treatment options. The APHAB, COSI, and other measures summarized in Table 5–2 may be considered as disease-specific HQL measures. For example, Mulrow et al (1990) used the HHIE, a disease-specific measure of hearing aid benefit, in a randomized trial of the effect of hearing aid use on HQL.

Generic Measures

Two styles of generic measures exist: utility measures and health profiles. Utility measures are used to compare medical treatments on a universal scale of 0 to 1. An individual can express positive and negative effects of a health disorder or treatment protocol within one score. One utility measuring device uses a scale, also known as a "feeling thermometer" (Fig. 5–1). A patient may be asked to rank his or her present health state on this thermometer before and after audiological intervention to determine the extent to which our treatment has improved the patient's perceived quality of life.

Standard Gamble

Another utility measure technique is known as the "standard gamble" (Fig. 5–2). In this approach the patient is offered a choice between two alternatives: living with health state "B" with certainty (which is presumably their present health state) or gambling on treatment "A." Treatment "A" can lead to either perfect health or immediate death. The interviewer manipulates the probabilities of perfect health and death in choice "A" until the patient is indifferent between his or her present health state ("B") and choice "A." Obviously, the higher the probability of death the patient is willing to

Utility Measures
Visual Analog Scales

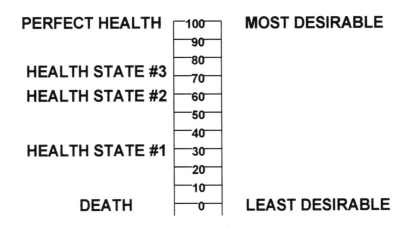

Figure 5–1   An example of a generic, utility measure known as a "feeling thermometer." The patient is asked to rate their overall quality of life on the thermometer before and after treatment. The difference may indicate the degree to which intervention has improved the patient's overall quality of life. (From Feeny et al [1996b], with permission.)

consider, the lower is the health state (or quality of life) inherent in remaining with choice "B."

Although the standard gamble is most commonly used for theoretical purposes to elicit "utility values" associated with serious life-threatening diseases such as cancer and heart disease, this technique may be useful in determining the impact of an individual's hearing impairment on his or her overall perceived quality of life. It might be useful, for example, to apply the standard gamble approach to potential cochlear implant recipients, particularly if candidacy continues to become less stringent. Instead of choosing between "perfect health" and "immediate death," the choice for the cochlear implant candidate might be "normal hearing" and "total deafness." If the patient is reluctant to gamble on a small risk of total deafness, the clinician may assume that the patient perceives his quality of life to be relatively good and not likely to significantly improve with an implant, even if hearing is substantially improved.

Time Trade-Off

An alternate approach to the standard gamble, is time trade-off (Fig. 5–3). In this technique the patient is offered a choice between living a normal life span in his or her present health state or a shortened life span in perfect health. The interviewer reduces the life span spent in perfect health until the

patient is indifferent between the shorter period of perfect health and the longer period in the less desirable state. An individual who is willing to "trade-off" a significant part of his or her life for a shorter life in perfect health is revealing a great deal about his or her perceived quality of life.

Profiles

Health profiles are designed in the form of a questionnaire and provide individual scores for each category of health separate from a general health score. Three generic profiles are referenced in the audiological literature: (1) Sickness Impact Profile (SIP; Bergner et al, 1981); (2) MOS SF-36 Health Survey (SF-36; Ware & Sherbourne, 1992); and (3) Health Utilities Index (Feeny et al, 1996). Information about these measures is included in Table 5–2. The SIP measures sickness-related behavior by either direct report from the individual or from observations by another respondent referring to the individual. The MOS SF-36 measures eight subscales of general health that can be categorized into physical and mental components of health status. Recently, another version of the SF-36, titled the SF-36V, was formulated specifically for use in the VA population. The Health Utilities Index requires individuals to select their level of functioning within each of eight attributes. The scoring algorithm derives a utility score from 0

Utility Measures

• **Standard Gamble Approach:**

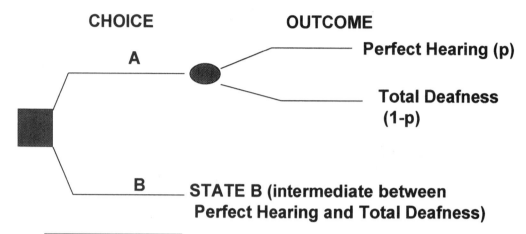

Figure 5–2 Standard gamble technique to determine the degree to which a patient's hearing impairment impacts on their perceivd quality of life. (p) = the probability of perfect hearing; (1-p) = the probability of total deafness. (p) and (1-p) are manipulted until the patient is indifferent between choice A with its associated risk and choice B, their present health state. (Modified from Feeny et al [1996b], with permission.)

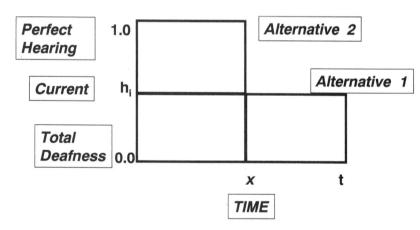

Figure 5–3 Time trade-off technique to determine perceived quality of life associated with hearing loss. h_i = perceived quality of life; t = total years of life remaining; x = total time with perfect hearing. x and t are manipulated until the patient is indifferent between a normal life-span with existing hearing and a shorter life expectancy with "perfect" hearing. (From Feeny et al [1996b], with permission.)

to 1, with "1" representing maximum functioning. The Health Utility Index has not been used in hearing aid research.

The SIP and the SF-36 were designed to measure the impact of illness and disease on an individual's HQL. The SIP is devised of multiple subscales with a grand total of 136 items. It is time consuming and not easy to administer, which limits its clinical usefulness. The SF-36 is much shorter, easy to administer, and is gaining popularity within quality of life research (Spilker, 1996).

One reason that HQL assessment is receiving increased attention throughout healthcare is that the outcomes data obtained can be combined with economic data to examine the cost-effectiveness of particular treatments. In one approach

the relationships among cost, benefit, and time are examined and reported in terms of dollars spent for each quality adjusted life year (QALY) gained. For example, Mulrow et al (1990) by use of the HHIE determined that hearing aids were a very cost-effective treatment for veterans with sensorineural hearing loss, costing only $200 per hearing QALY gained. The concept of QALY and other economic assessments of outcome will be discussed in greater detail later in this chapter.

Satisfaction Outcome Measures

The measurement of *satisfaction* as a clinical outcome presents unique problems. Whereas measures of impairment, activity, participation, and HQL can be referenced to a specific treatment intervention, a patient's perception (judgment) of satisfaction involves a constellation of many factors that are peripheral to the treatment. These may include but are not limited to expectations of success; perceived value; cosmetic appeal; comfort; ease of use; and competent, efficient service delivery.

The concept of value warrants elaboration. For paying patients, the issue is fairly clear—they can return the hearing aid if they do not believe they are getting their money's worth. For our VA patients it is problematic. Individuals might keep the instruments even if they are dissatisfied, because no economic incentive exists to return the aids. However, for these individuals, the concept of value is often related to such non-economic factors as their perception of service-related entitlement. Interestingly, an investigation of the impact of cost on perceived benefit (Newman et al, 1993) revealed that HHIE scores were no different between groups of insured and uninsured hearing aid recipients.

The most common way of documenting satisfaction is through questionnaires. Unlike measures such as the APHAB and HHIE, satisfaction surveys have not been standardized. Numerous surveys are available, however, throughout the healthcare industry. The most extensive instrument is the MarkeTrak series developed by Kochkin (1992, 1997) for the hearing aid industry and allows for the evaluation of satisfaction for device and service delivery. Other questionnaires include the following:

- Hearing Aid Users Questionnaire (HAUQ; Dillon et al., 1997), an 11-item clinical instrument developed and evaluated on an Australian adult population that assesses both device and service delivery satisfaction (Dillon et al, 1997).

- ASHA Consumer Satisfaction Measure that focuses primarily on service delivery.

- Satisfaction with Amplification in Daily Life (SADL; Cox, 1997), a recently developed 15-item instrument that attempts to determine the patient's level of satisfaction among several hearing aid–related dimensions, including

perceived positive and negative effects of amplification, service and cost, and perceived effect on personal image.

Finally, many clinics have developed their own measures to assess patient satisfaction.

PEARL
A comprehensive outcome assessment is best achieved by using a combination of instruments designed to measure the treatment effect on impairment, activity, participation, satisfaction, and health-related quality of life.

THE ECONOMICS OF OUTCOMES

The emphasis on the "bottom line" in healthcare has refocused discussion of outcomes to the costs and the results of treatment. It is no longer sufficient to demonstrate that an intervention has made a difference in the impairment, participation, activity, satisfaction, or quality of life domains. Sufficiency now demands that the outcome has been achieved at "reasonable costs." The definition of "reasonable" is often left up to the entity paying the bills—the insurer, HMO, government agency, or patient. It is becoming increasingly important for audiologists to understand the concepts of healthcare economics to analyze their costs, compare the costs of different treatment options, operate efficient and competitive practices, and determine costs as a function of benefit achieved for audiological intervention. An understanding of healthcare economics is essential for analyzing costs and benefits of present services and for planning future programs. The discussion following is designed to introduce the reader to the basic concepts of healthcare economics. Table 5–3 illustrates the differences among several commonly used health economic measures. For a comprehensive treatment of the subject, the interested reader is referred to Drummond, et al (1997) or Spilker (1996).

TABLE 5–3 A comparison of cost analysis procedures

This Economic Measure	Answers This Question	As Measured By
Cost analysis	How much does it cost me to deliver my service?	Dollars
Cost-benefit analysis	Will the generated revenue or cost avoidance associated with delivering my service, exceed my expenditures?	Dollars vs. dollars
Cost-effectiveness analysis	Which service option, among several, offers the best clinical results for each	Clinical improvement (%, dB, etc.) per dollars spent
Cost-utility analysis	Which service option, among several, offers the largest improvement in quality life, as determined by the patient, for each dollar spent?	Dollars per quality adjusted life years

CONTROVERSIAL POINT

Can the sale of digital hearing aids costing more than twice as much as high-end analog instruments be justified if no significant difference exists in outcome between the two technologies?

Cost Analysis

Cost analysis is the simplest and most straightforward of healthcare economic analyses. It answers the question, "What does it cost to deliver my service?" To answer this question, the clinician needs to identify the resources required to deliver the service. These resources can be separated into direct and indirect costs. Figure 5–4 illustrates how a spreadsheet can be used to calculate the cost of an audiological assessment. Labor costs include not only the time spent by the audiologist with the patient but also the time spent by the receptionist who checks the patient in and schedules the patient for a return appointment and the file clerk who is responsible for locating the file, transporting it to the clinic, and reshelving the records. Fringe benefits must also be included in the calculation of labor costs. These include vacation and sick time, employer-paid health and disability insurance, employer contributions to retirement and social security programs, and workman's compensation. Fringe benefits can add 25% to 30% to the labor costs. Supplies and materials used for the procedure are also considered as direct costs. The indirect costs are primarily associated with equipment and space. If these are leased, the costs can be easily calculated. If the equipment and space (building) are owned, the costs are depreciated over the life expectancy of the equipment and building.

A spreadsheet can be a very powerful tool for cost analysis purposes. The clinician can easily manipulate components of the analysis (salary, equipment, time) to examine various alternatives and the resultant costs. For example, the clinician or manager can answer the following questions: "How will my audiological evaluation costs change if I buy a new audiometer?" "What will happen if I reduce my evaluation time by 10 minutes?" "How will my costs be affected by the 10% increase in the lease for my office space?" Figures 5–5A to 5–5E provide some examples of spreadsheets used to analyze the costs of several audiological procedures.

Although a cost analysis is critical for determining the dollars spent to deliver services, it reveals nothing about the value of those services; that is, what are the benefits achieved for the dollars spent? In economic evaluation of healthcare services the costs of treatment, both direct and indirect, are compared with the measured outcomes resulting from the treatment. Three methods are used to evaluate the relationship between costs and outcomes. *Cost-benefit analyses* measure outcome by assigning monetary values to morbidity and suffering incurred from treatment. *Cost-effectiveness* evaluations measure outcomes as specific increments of clinical effects such as percent correct for word recognition tasks when comparing various hearing aids. Finally, *cost-utility analyses* measure outcomes in terms of quality-of-life produced by the clinical effects. Cost-utility analyses are widely used in the medical field because this type of analysis allows for comparison of the cost-effectiveness between different treatment interventions.

Cost-Benefit

A cost-benefit analysis (CBA) answers the question, "If I apply this intervention strategy, will the dollars earned or saved exceed the dollars spent?" A CBA requires assigning monetary units to both the costs of treatment and the benefits achieved. For example, the costs of a balance rehabilitation program, including evaluation and therapy (as calculated through a cost-analysis process), are compared against the dollars saved by reducing the need for office visits and medication or the dollars gained by allowing the individual to return to work. If the money gained or avoided exceeds the money spent, the service can be considered as "cost-beneficial"—an outcome dearly appreciated by CEOs. However, healthcare is not a manufacturing business where the price of a widget must exceed the cost of manufacturing the widget for the outcome to be considered successful. As a society, we do not treat cancer or kidney disease with the expectation that the monetary benefits associated with treatment will exceed the costs spent on that treatment. An expectation exists that properly delivered healthcare will improve outcomes in domains that are not necessarily economic. Nonetheless, a CBA may be a useful exercise when comparing treatment alternatives that have the potential to reduce personal or societal costs.

Willingness-to-Pay

A special subset of cost-benefit analysis is the willingness-to-pay (WTP) concept. That is, how much is the individual willing to pay for the increased benefits associated with the intervention? Several examples in the audiologic literature have examined this issue. Palmer et al (1995) asked subjects to make sound quality judgments while listening to class A and class D amplifiers. The subjects were then asked how much they would pay for a hearing aid with the associated sound quality. The results indicated that the subjects would be willing to pay up to $200 more for a hearing aid with better sound quality. Newman and Sandridge (1998) compared objective and subjective outcome measures among subjects who were fitted with three levels of hearing aid technology. Although more than 75% of the subjects preferred the fully digital technology, one third of those switched their preference to a lower level of technology after being informed of the cost.

Some problems are associated with WTP assumptions. The same amount of money may be perceived as having inherently greater or lesser *value* depending on one's income. An individual who earns minimum wage is likely to assign a much greater value to hearing aids for which he or she is willing to pay $500.00 than an individual earning a six-figure salary.

Cost-Effectiveness

A cost-effectiveness analysis (CEA) compares the costs of treatment alternatives against a specific outcome measure that is a result of that treatment. For example, we accept the fact that improved intelligibility in noise is a highly desirable outcome of hearing aids. We may want to examine the cost-effectiveness of several hearing aid alternatives—a single microphone, analog instrument; a single microphone, fully digital hearing aid; and a dual microphone, digitally

PROCEDURE: AUDIOLOGICAL ASSESSMENT (AA)

NUMBER OF PROCEDURES:

I. DIRECT COSTS:

A. LABOR COSTS:

POSITION	SALARY/HOUR[1]	PROCEDURE TIME (MIN)	COST/PROCEDURE
Audiologist			$ -
Receptionist			$ -
File Clerk			$ -
			$ -
			$ -

[1] Divide yearly salary by 2080 to determine SALARY/HOUR and multiply this value by .26 (or other %) to account for fringe benefits.

Total Labor Costs Per Procedure $ -

B. SUPPLIES & MATERIALS:

ITEM	COST PER ITEM	NO. PER PROCEDURE	COST/PROCEDURE
Specula			$ -
Boxes			$ -
Glue			$ -
Impression Material			$ -
Earphone Covers			$ -
Impedance Tips			$ -
Insert Phones			$ -
Miscellaneous			$ -

Total Supplies & Materials Costs Per Procedure: $ -

Figure 5–4   An example of a spreadsheet for analyzing costs associated with a comprehensive audiologic assessment. (*Figure continued next page.*)

83

TOTAL DIRECT COSTS PER PROCEDURE: $ -

FIGURE 5–4 (continued)

II. INDIRECT COSTS:
A. EQUIPMENT COSTS:

ITEM	PURCHASE COST	LIFE EXPECTANCY	DEPRECIATED VALUE	COST/ PROCEDURE
Computer				
Audiometer				
Immittance				
Otoscope				
Sound Booth				
Real Ear				
.				

Total Equipment Costs Per Procedure:

B. BUILDING DEPRECIATION

	ACTUAL COST	CONTRACT	TTL M&R
		$ -	

# SQ FT	COST/ SQ FT	AUDIO SQ FT	TOTAL COST	COST/ PROC
			$ -	

BLDG COST/YR

BLDG COST/YR is calculated by dividing the cost of the building by 40 (life expectancy)

Total Building Depreciation Costs Per Procedure: $ -

C. ADMINISTRATIVE SUPPORT:

TTL DIRECT COSTS/PROC   % ADMIN SUPPORT(DEFAULT IS 15%)

$ -   0.15

Total Administrative Support Costs Per Procedure: $ -
TOTAL INDIRECT COSTS PER PROCEDURE: $ -
TOTAL COST PER AUDIOLOGICAL ASSESSMENT: $ -

Figure 5–4   (continued)

PROCEDURE: AUDIOLOGICAL ASSESSMENT (AA)
NUMBER OF PROCEDURES: 1622

I. DIRECT COSTS:

A. LABOR COSTS:

POSITION	SALARY/ HOUR[1]	PROCEDURE TIME (MIN)	COST/ PROCEDURE
Audiologist	$33.35	60	$ 33.35
Receptionist	$13.52	5	$ 1.13
File Clerk	$13.52	3	$ 0.68

[1] Divide yearly salary by 2040 to determine SALARY/HOUR and multiply this value by .25 to account for fringe benefits.

Total Labor Costs Per Procedure $ 35.15

B. SUPPLIES & MATERIALS:

ITEM	COST PER ITEM	NO. PER PROCEDURE	COST/ PROCEDURE
Specula	$ 0.01	1	$ 0.01
Boxes	$ 0.50	1	$ 0.50
Glue	$ 0.10	1	$ 0.10
Impression Material	$ 0.30	2	$ 0.60
Impedance Tips	$ 0.01	1	$ 0.01
Insert Phones	$ 0.20	2	$ 0.40
Miscellaneous	$ 0.10	1	$ 0.10

Total Supplies & Materials Costs Per Procedure: $ 1.72

TOTAL DIRECT COSTS PER PROCEDURE: $ 36.87

Figure 5–5A An example of a spreadsheet for analyzing costs associated with an audiologic assessment. *(Figure continued next page.)*

II. INDIRECT COSTS:

A. EQUIPMENT COSTS:

ITEM	PURCHASE COST	LIFE EXPECTANCY	DEPRECIATED VALUE	COST/PROCEDURE
Computer	$ 2,500.00	10	$ 250.00	$ 0.15
Audiometer	$ 12,500.00	10	$ 1,250.00	$ 0.77
Immittance	$ 6,700.00	13	$ 515.38	$ 0.32
Otoscope	$ 350.00	10	$ 35.00	$ 0.02
Sound Booth	$ 22,500.00	20	$ 1,125.00	$ 0.69
Real Ear			$ -	$ -
			$ -	$ -

	ACTUAL COST	CONTRACT	TTL M&R	COST/ PROC
Maintenance & Repair	$ 458.00	$ 2,500.00	$ 2,958.00	$ 1.82

Total Equipment Costs Per Procedure: $ 3.78

B. BUILDING DEPRECIATION

BLDG COST/YR	# SQ FT	COST/ SQ FT	AUDIO SQ FT	TTL COST	COST/ PROC
$ 3,750,000	850000	$ 4.41	1500	$ 6,618	$ 4.08

BLDG COST/YR is calculated by dividing the cost of the building by 40

Total Building Depreciation Costs Per Procedure: $ 4.08

C. ADMINISTRATIVE SUPPORT:

TTL DIRECT COSTS/PROC	% ADMIN SUPPORT
$ 36.87	0.15

Total Administrative Support Costs Per Procedure: $ 5.53

TOTAL INDIRECT COSTS PER PROCEDURE: $ 13.39

TOTAL COST PER AUDIOLOGICAL ASSESSMENT: $ 50.26

Figure 5–5A (*continued*)

COST ANALYSIS
PROCEDURE: HEARING AID EVALUATION & FITTING

LABOR COSTS:

POSITION	SALARY/ HOUR[1]	PROCEDURE TIME	COST/ PROCEDURE
Audiologist	$33.35	30	$ 16.68
Receptionist	$13.52	2	$ 0.45
File Clerk	$13.52	1	$ 0.23

Total Labor Costs: $ 17.35

SUPPLIES & MATERIALS:

ITEM	COST/PROCEDURE
Real Ear Tubes	$0.05
Hearing Aids (2)	$736.00
Batteries (8)	$1.36
Miscellaneous	$0.05

Total Supplies & Materials Costs: $ 737.46

EQUIPMENT COSTS:

ITEM	DEPRECIATED VALUE[2]	PROCEDURES/ YEAR	COST/ PROCEDURE
Computer	$330.00	1,800	$ 0.18
Otoscope	$67.50	1,800	$ 0.04
Real Ear System	$1,890	1,800	$ 1.05
Maintenance	$228.75	1,800	$ 0.13

Total Equipment Costs: $ 1.40

OTHER COSTS:

ITEM[3]	COST/PROCEDURE
Administration Support (15%)	$ 113.22
Engineering Support (4%)	$ 30.19
Building Mgt Support (2%)	$ 15.10

Total Other Costs:	$ 158.51
TOTAL COST PER HEARING AID EVALUATION (2 INSTRUMENTS):	$ 914.72
(1 INSTRUMENT):	$ 546.72

Notes:

[1] Based on audiology grade of GS-12/5 and clerical grade of GS-4/5, +25% fringe benefits

[2] Straight depreciation plus 5% per year inflation factor

[3] Based on labor and materials costs

Figure 5–5B An example of a spreadsheet for analyzing costs associated with a hearing aid evaluation and fitting.

COST ANALYSIS
PROCEDURE: AURAL REHABILITATION (AR)

LABOR COSTS:

POSITION	SALARY/ HOUR[1]	PROCEDURE TIME	COST/ PROCEDURE
Audiologist	$33.35	90	$ 50.03
Receptionist	$13.52	2	$ 0.45
File Clerk	$13.52	1	$ 0.23
Total Labor Costs:			$ 50.70

SUPPLIES & MATERIALS:

ITEM	COST/PROCEDURE
Pt Education Materials	$ 3.00
Miscellaneous	$ 1.00
Total Supplies & Materials Costs:	$ 4.00

EQUIPMENT COSTS: None

Total Equipment Costs:	$ -

OTHER COSTS:

ITEM[3]	COST/PROCEDURE
Administration Support (15%)	$ 8.21
Engineering Support (4%)	$ 2.19
Building Mgt Support (2%)	$ 1.09
Total Other Costs:	$ 11.49

TOTAL COST PER AURAL REHABILITATION SESSION	$ 66.19

Notes:

[1] Based on audiology grade of GS-12/5 and clerical grade of GS-4/5, +25% fringe benefits

[2] Straight depreciation plus 5% per year inflation factor

[3] Based on labor and materials costs

Figure 5–5C An example of a spreadsheet for analyzing costs associated with aural rehabilitation procedures.

COST ANALYSIS
PROCEDURE: HEARING AID ORIENTATION (HAO)

LABOR COSTS:

POSITION	SALARY/ HOUR[1]	PROCEDURE TIME	COST/ PROCEDURE
Audiologist	$33.35	30	$ 16.68
Total Labor Costs:			$ 16.68

SUPPLIES & MATERIALS:

ITEM	COST/PROCEDURE
Patient Education Materials	$ 1.00
Total Supplies & Materials Costs:	$ 1.00

EQUIPMENT COSTS: None

Total Equipment Costs:	$ -

OTHER COSTS:

ITEM[3]	COST/PROCEDURE
Administration Support (15%)	$ 2.65
Engineering Support (4%)	$ 0.71
Building Mgt Support (2%)	$ 0.35
Total Other Costs:	$ 3.71

TOTAL COST PER HEARING AID ORIENTATION SESSION	$ 21.39

Notes:

[1] Based on audiology grade of GS-12/5 and clerical grade of GS-4/5, +25% fringe benefits

[2] Straight depreciation plus 5% per year inflation factor

[3] Based on labor and materials costs

Figure 5–5D An example of a spreadsheet for analyzing costs associated with hearing aid orientation.

COST ANALYSIS
PROCEDURE: HEARING AID FITTING FOLLOW-UP (F/U)

LABOR COSTS:

POSITION	SALARY/ HOUR[1]	PROCEDURE TIME	COST/ PROCEDURE
Audiologist	$33.35	30	$ 16.68
Receptionist	$13.52	2	$ 0.45
File Clerk	$13.52	1	$ 0.23
Total Labor Costs:			$ 17.35

SUPPLIES & MATERIALS:

ITEM	COST/PROCEDURE
Miscellaneous	$ 0.50
Total Supplies & Materials Costs:	$ 0.50

EQUIPMENT COSTS: None

Total Equipment Costs:	$ -

OTHER COSTS:

ITEM[3]	COST/PROCEDURE
Administration Support (15%)	$ 2.68
Engineering Support (4%)	$ 0.71
Building Mgt Support (2%)	$ 0.36
Total Other Costs:	$ 3.75

TOTAL COST PER HEARING AID FITTING FOLLOW-UP SESSION: $ 21.60

Notes:

[1] Based on audiology grade of GS-12/5 and clerical grade of GS-4/5, +25% fringe benefits

[2] Straight depreciation plus 5% per year inflation factor

[3] Based on labor and materials costs

Figure 5–5E   An example of a spreadsheet for analyzing costs associated with hearing aid fitting follow-up.

TABLE 5–4 An example of a hearing aid cost-effectiveness analysis

Hearing Aid (half-concha)	Cost (retail) ($)	Outcome Score (% improvement on CUNY-NST Test) (%)	Cost per % Increase (cost-effectiveness) ($)
A. Single-channel, single-program, dual-microphone, analog	1104.42	24	46.02
B. Dual-channel, multiple-program, single-microphone, digitally programmable	1357.74	16	84.86
C. Multiple-channel, multiple-program, single-microphone, fully-digital	3472.64	18	192.92

programmable hearing aid—by determining the relative cost per intelligibility point gained (Table 5–4). Until recently, little research has examined the relative cost-effectiveness of hearing aid intervention. Newman and Sandridge (1998), however, conducted a comprehensive benefit, satisfaction, and cost-effectiveness analysis comparing three hearing aids representing different levels of technology: a one-channel linear hearing aid, a two-channel, nonlinear hearing aid, and a multichannel, multiband, digital signal processing (DSP) hearing aid. The investigators found that the subjects scored higher on a speech recognition test with the DSP instrument, but no significant differences were found among the instruments on the self-report measure of benefit or satisfaction survey. The CEA revealed that it cost $49.67 for each percentage point improvement achieved with the single-channel linear hearing aid compared with $51.88 with the two-channel, nonlinear instrument, and $109.76 with the DSP.

An HMO may use the results of the CEA in Table 5–4 to determine which hearing aid technology an insurer will cover or the maximum hearing aid allowance. However, these choices may not coincide with patient satisfaction. The outcome measure used in the CEA may not be the one of primary interest to the patient. The patient may place a premium on cosmetics, the ability to change programs, or simply possessing the latest technology. As discussed earlier in this chapter, a large number of outcome measures exist from which to choose (objective performance measures of speech recognition and self-report measures assessing activity limitations and/or participation restrictions), any one of which may represent a better measure of outcome than percent correct, for example. Another limitation of CEA is that it cannot be used to make comparisons across programs. For example, although we may know that it costs $46.02 for each 1% improvement in intelligibility with hearing aid A, and the same amount of money for each 1-mm reduction in blood pressure with medicine C, we know nothing about the how improved hearing compares to reduced blood pressure in improving that individual's quality of life. Nor are we able

to determine which $46.02 expenditure represents the better use of scarce healthcare dollars. Cost analyses that measure the association between cost and quality of life are best examined using cost-utility analyses (CUA).

CONTROVERSIAL POINT

A cost-effectiveness analysis recently reported in the literature revealed that it cost $49.67 for each percentage point improvement achieved with a single-channel linear hearing aid compared with $109.76 with a fully digital signal-processing instrument.

Cost-Utility Analysis

A CUA focuses on the quality of health outcome achieved by a particular intervention. The analysis typically involves determining: (1) the costs of treatment, both direct and indirect, for each intervention approach; (2) the change in scores as a function of treatment on a HQL instrument; and (3) the estimated quantity of years of life remaining that any treatment effects may influence HQL (usually the life expectancy of the individual as indicated on actuarial tables). These data are then used to calculate the cost of treatment for different diseases or disorders per QALY. QALYs are used in a CUA to put a monetary value on specified treatment protocols. Although CEAs and CUAs are similar from the cost perspective, they differ from the outcome perspective. CEAs examine the cost per unit of some specific outcome achieved; CUAs examine the cost per quality of life year gained.

Table 5–5 illustrates how CUAs may be used to examine the effects of various hearing aid intervention options on costs per HQALYs. Examples 1 and 2 demonstrate that the cost per

TABLE 5–5 Four examples of quality adjusted life year calculations

QALY example #1	QALY example #3
Age of patient – 70 Cost of hearing aids - $2,000/pair Benefit obtained - 25% (APHAB) Life expectancy – 5 years Cost per QALY = $\dfrac{\$2,000}{.25 \times 5}$ = $1,600.00	Age of patient – 5 Cost of implant - $50,000 Benefit obtained – 30% (open set monosyllables) Life expectancy – 70 years Cost per QALY = $\dfrac{\$50,000}{.30 \times 70}$ = $2,380.95
QALY example #2	QALY example #4
Age of patient – 70 Cost of hearing aids - $4,000/pair Benefit obtained - 60% (APHAB) Life expectancy – 5 years Cost per QALY = $\dfrac{\$4,000}{.60 \times 5}$ = $1,333.33	Age of patient – 65 Cost of implant - $50,000 Benefit obtained – 70% (open set monosyllables Life expectancy – 10 years Cost per QALY = $\dfrac{\$50,000}{.70 \times 10}$ = $7,142.86

QALY for more expensive instruments may be *lower* if the improvement in outcome is high enough. On the other hand, examples 3 and 4 illustrate that even a very large difference in outcome cannot overcome the effects of longevity when intervention is begun early enough (assuming the device does not need to be replaced). Such an analysis may be very useful for insurers and healthcare planners when determining what services to offer as part of a comprehensive healthcare plan. Wyatt et al (1995) conducted a CUA on cochlear implants and compared the implant costs with those associated with other common medical interventions. The results of this analysis are summarized in Table 5–6. Cochlear implants compare very favorably with other high-cost medical interventions because of the age at which the patients received their implants and the benefits achieved from using the device. The power of early intervention is nicely illustrated with the neonatal intensive care example. This resource-intensive intervention can cost hundreds of thousands of dollars but may be a "bargain" when the costs and benefits are spread over an individual's lifetime.

TABLE 5–6 Results from Wyatt et al (1995) investigating the cost per quality adjusted life year provided by cochlear implants as compared to other medical devices and services

Technology	Cost/QALY
Neonatal intensive care	$7,968
Cochlear implant	**$9,325**
Coronary artery bypass	$11,255
Coronary angioplasty	$11,485

PEARL

Quality adjusted life year analyses demonstrate that maximum benefit is achieved per dollar spent when intervention is begun as early as possible.

CONCLUSIONS

As the demand for outcome measures increases in healthcare, audiologists need to incorporate measures such as those reviewed in this chapter as part of their standard clinical protocol. It is not enough for patients to simply express satisfaction with the services or devices they receive. Audiologists must be able to document the impact of those services through the use of standardized measures of objective or subjective benefit and satisfaction.

Measuring outcomes is nothing more than applying the scientific method to a clinical application. We develop a hypothesis that a particular hearing aid with specific features (independent variables) will have a certain effect on the activity and participation domains and the quality of life of our patient (dependent variables). We apply the chosen treatment to our patient, measure and analyze the results, and determine whether we have proven our hypothesis. In a sense every clinical intervention is a scientific experiment.

Clinicians are probably familiar with many of the measures presented in this chapter and have likely used the data they provide to adjust hearing aid parameters, counsel patients, or assess satisfaction. Table 5–7 illustrates how some of these measures can be applied to the WHO and audiology domains described earlier in this chapter. The measures selected for this table were chosen for their clinical practicability. They are easy to use, quickly administered and scored,

TABLE 5–7 Clinically useful measures to assess outcomes in the WHO, generic, and audiology domains

WHO Domains	Generic Domains	Audiology Domains	Outcome Measure
Impairment		Verification	2 cc/REM functional gain
Activity/participation		Validation	HINT (objective) SPIN (objective) HHIE (subjective—new users) APHAB (subjective—experienced users) COSI (subjective—new and experienced users)
	Quality of life	Validation	HHIE (disease-specific SF36V (generic)
	Satisfaction	Validation	Selected items from MarketTrack SADL HAUQ

and empirically tested. It is important for us to realize that these and many of the other outcome measures available to us can be used to demonstrate to administrators, insurers, referral sources, other healthcare providers, our patients and their families that hearing aids are an effective and economical treatment for hearing impairment. As audiology continues to compete in the healthcare marketplace, we can demonstrate that our services have a positive impact on activity limitations, participation restrictions, and reduced health-related quality of life associated with hearing loss.

"Research is good. Results are better."—Lyndon Johnson

ACKNOWLEDGMENTS

The members of the VA Audiology Task Force on Outcome Measures who contributed to this chapter include Harvey Abrams, Theresa Hnath-Chisolm, Carol Sammeth, Gerald Schuchman, and Anne Strouse. Other contributors to the task force include Lucille Beck, William Delaune, Kenneth Heard, and Rachel Ridge. The task force was supported, in part, through funds provided by the Rehabilitation Education Program, Department of Veterans Affairs.

REFERENCES

ALPINER, J., CHEVRETTE, W., GLASCOE, G., METZ, M., & OLSEN, B. (1977). The Denver Scale of Communication Function. Unpublished manuscript, University of Denver. In: J. Alpiner (Ed.) (1978): *Handbook of adult rehabilitative audiology* (1st ed.) (pp. 53–56). Baltimore: Williams & Wilkins.

ANSI S3.5. (1969). *American national standards methods for calculation of the articulation index.* New York: American National Standards Institute.

BENTLER, R., NIEBURH, D., GETTA, J., & ANDERSON, C. (1993). Longitudinal study of hearing aid effectiveness I: Objective measures. *Journal of Speech and Hearing Research, 36;*808–819.

BERGNER, M., BOBBITT, R., CARTER, W., & GILSON, B. (1981). The Sickness Impact Profile: Developments and final revision of a health status measure. *Medical Care, 14;*57–67.

BESING, J.M., & KOEHNKE, J. (1995). A test of virtual auditory localizaiton. *Ear and Hearing, 16;*220–229.

BOOTHROYD, A. (1998). Hearing aids outcome evaluation. Paper presented at the *Conference on Outcome Measurement for Hearing Aids,* Los Angeles, CA.

BYRNE, D. (1992). Key issues in hearing aid selection and evaluation. *Journal of the American Academy of Audiology, 3;*67–80.

CARHART, R. (1946). Tests for selection of hearing aids. *Laryngoscope, 56;*780–794.

COX, R. (1997). Administration and application of the APHAB. *Hearing Journal, 50;*32–48.

COX, R., & ALEXANDER, G. (1995). The Abbreviated Profile of Hearing Aid Benefit. *Ear and Hearing, 16;*176–186.

COX, R., & ALEXANDER, G. (1997). *Measurement of Satisfaction with Amplification in Daily Life (SADL).* Paper presented at the American Academy of Audiology Convention, Ft. Lauderdale, FL, April 1997.

COX, R., ALEXANDER, G., & GILMORE, C. (1991). Objective and self-report measures of hearing aid benefit. In: G. Studebaker, F. Bess, & L. Beck (Eds.), *The Vanderbilt Hearing Aid Report II.* Monkton, MD: York Press.

CRANDALL, C. (1998). Hearing aids: Their effects on functional health status. *Hearing Journal, 51;*22–30.

DEMOREST, M., & ERDMAN, S. (1986). Scale composition and item analysis of the Communication Profile for the Hearing-Impaired. *Journal of Speech and Hearing Research, 29;*515–535.

DILLON, H., BIRTLES, G., & LOVEGROVE, R. (1999). Measuring the outcomes of a national rehabilitation program: Normative data for the Client Oriented Scale of Improvement (COSI) and the Hearing Aid Users Questionnaire (HAUQ). *Journal of the American Academy of Audiology, 10;*67–99.

DILLON, H., JAMES, A., & GINIS, J. (1997). Client Oriented Scale of Improvement (COSI) and its relationship to several other measures of benefit and satisfaction provided by hearing aids. *Journal of the American Academy of Audiology, 8;*27–43.

Drummond, M., O'Brien, B., Stoddart, G., & Torrance, G. (1997). *Methods for the economic evaluation of healthcare programmes.* (2nd ed.). New York: Oxford University Press.

Feeney, D., Torrance, G., & Furlong, W. (1996a). Health utilities index. In: B. Spilker (Ed.), *Quality of life and pharacoeconomics in clinical trials.* (2nd ed.) (pp. 239–252). Philadelphia: Lippicott-Raven.

Feeney, D., Torrance, G., & Labelle, R. (1996b). Integrating economic evaluations and quality of life assessments. In: B. Spilker (Ed.), *Quality of life and pharmacoeconomics in clinical trials* (2nd ed.) (pp. 85–95). Philadelphia: Lippicott-Raven.

Fletcher H. (1953). *Speech and hearing in communication.* Krieger: New York.

Gatehouse, S. (1992). The time course and magnitude of perceptual acclimatization to frequency responses. Evidence from monaural fitting of hearing aids. *Journal of the Acoustical Society of America, 92;*1258–1268.

Giolas, T., Owens, E., Lamb, S., & Schubert, E. (1979). Hearing Performance Inventory. *Journal of Speech and Hearing Disorders, 44;*169–195.

Gonzalez, G. (1997). *The hearing handicap inventory for the elderly: Spanish language version.* Unpublished master's thesis. University of South Florida.

Harford, E. (1993). The impact of the hearing aid on the evolution of audiology. *1993 Carhart Memorial Lecture to the Annual Meeting of the American Auditory Society,* Phoenix, AZ, April 15, 1993.

Humes, L., Halling, D., & Coughlin, M. (1996). Reliability and stability of various hearing aid outcome measures in a group of elderly hearing aid wearers. *Journal of Speech and Hearing Research, 39;*923–935.

Jennings, M.B., & Head, B.G. (1994). Development of an ecological audiological rehabilitation program in a home for the aged. *Journal of the Academy of Rehabilitative Audiology, 27;*73–88.

Jerger, J., Chmiel, R., Florin, R., Pirozzolo, F., & Wilson, N. (1996). Comparison of conventional amplification and an assistive listening device in elderly persons. *Ear and Hearing, 17;*490–504.

Kalikow, D., Stevens, K., & Elliot, L. (1977). Development of test of speech intelligibility in noise using sentence materials with controlled word predictability. *Journal of the Acoustical Society of America, 61;*1337–1351.

Kochkin, S. (1992). MarkeTrak III identifies key factors in determining consumer satisfaction. *The Hearing Journal, 45;*39–44.

Kochkin, S. (1997). Subjective measures of satisfaction and benefit: Establishing norms. *Seminars in Hearing, 18;*37–47.

Malinoff, R., & Weinstein, B. (1989). Measurement of hearing aid benefit in the elderly. *Ear and Hearing, 10;*354–356.

Mendel, L.L., & Danhauer, J.K. (1997). *Audiologic evaluation and management, and speech perception assessment.* San Diego: Singular Publishing Group.

Mueller, G. (1997). Outcome measures: The truth about your hearing aid fittings. *Hearing Journal, 50;*21–32.

Mulrow, C., Aguilar, C., Endicott, J., Tuley, M., Velez, R., Charlip, W., Rhodes, M., Hill. J., & DeNino, L. (1990). Quality of life changes and hearing impairment. *Annals of Internal Medicine, 113;*188–194.

National Institutes of Health. (1997). *Quality of life assessment: Practice, problems, and promise.* Proceeding of a Workshop, October 1990. National Institutes of Health, Bethesda, MD.

Newman, C.W., Hug, G.A., Wharton, J.A., & Jacobson, G.P. (1993). The influence of hearing aid cost on perceived benefit in older adults. *Ear and Hearing, 14;*285–289.

Newman, C., & Sandridge, S. (1998). Benefit from, satisfaction with, and cost-effectiveness of three different hearing aid technologies. *American Journal of Audiology, 7;*115–128.

Newman, C.W., Weinstein, B., Jacobson, G.P., & Hug, G.A. (1991). Test-retest reliability of the Hearing Handicap Inventory for Adults. *Ear and Hearing, 12;*355–357.

Nilson, M., Soli, S., Sullivan, J. (1994). Development of the Hearing in Noise Test for the measurement of speech reception thresholds in quiet and in noise. *Journal of the Acoustical Society of America, 95;*1085–99.

Olsen, W., VanTassell, D., & Speaks, C. (1997). Phoneme and word recognition for words in isolation and in sentences. *Ear and Hearing, 18(3);*175–188.

Palmer, C.V., Killion, M.C., Wilber, L.A., & Ballard, W.J. (1995). Comparison of two hearing aid receivers-amplifier combinations using sound quality judgments. *Ear and Hearing, 16;*587–598.

Pavlovic, C.V. (1984). Use of the articulation index for assessing residual auditory function in listeners with sensorineural hearing loss. *Journal of the Acoustical Society of America, 75;*1253–1258.

Pavlovic, C.V. (1991). Speech recognition and five Articulation Indexes. *Hearing Instruments, 42;*20–23.

Pichora-Fuller, M.K., & Robertson, S.R. (1994). Hard of hearing residents in a home for the aged. *Journal of Speech Language Pathology and Audiology, 18;*278–288.

Primeau, R. (1997). Hearing aid benefit in adults and older adults. *Seminars in Hearing, 18;*29–36.

Rankovic, C.V. (1997). Prediction of speech reception for listeners with sensorineural hearing loss. In: W. Jestedt (Ed.), *Modeling sensorineural hearing loss.* Mahwah, NJ: Lawrence Erlbaum.

Schow, R., Balsara, N., Smedley, T., & Whitcomb, C. (1993). Aural rehabilitation by ASHA audiologists: 1980–1990. *American Journal of Audiology, 3;*28–38.

Schum, D. (1993). Test-retest reliability of a shortened version of the Hearing Aid Performance Inventory. *Journal of the American Academy of Audiology, 4;*18–21.

Skinner, M. (1988). *Hearing aid evaluation.* Englewood Cliffs, NJ: Prentice Hall.

Spilker, B. (1996). *Quality of life and pharacoeconomics in clinical trials.* (2nd ed.). Philadelphia:Lippicott-Raven.

Testa, M.A., & Simonson, D.C. (1996). Assessment of quality of life outcomes. *New England Journal of Medicine, 234;*835–840.

Turner, R. (1998). The hearing aid expert: audiologist, dealer, or otolaryngologist? *American Journal of Audiology, 7(2);* 5–19.

Ventry, I., & Weinstein, B. (1982). The hearing handicap inventory for the elderly: A new tool. *Ear and Hearing, 3;*128–134.

Ventry, I., & Weinstein, B. (1983). Identification of elderly people with hearing problems. *ASHA, 25;*37–42.

Walden, B., Demorest, M., & Hepler, E.L. (1984). Self report approach to assessing benefit derived from amplification. *Journal of Speech and Hearing Research, 27;*49–56.

Walden, B., Schwartz, D., Williams, D., Holum-Hardegen, L., & Crowley J. (1983). Test of the assumptions underlying comparative hearing aid evaluations. *Journal of Speech and Hearing Disorders, 48;*264–273.

WARE, J.E., & SHERBOURNE, C.D. (1992). The MOS 36-item short-form health survey (SF-36): I. Conceptual framework and item selection. *Medical Care, 30;*473–481.

WHO. (1980). *International classification of impairments, disabilities and handicaps—A manual of classification relating to the consequences of disease.* Geneva: World Health Organization.

WORLD HEALTH ORGANIZATION. (1997). Towards a common language for functioning and disablement: *ICIDH-2 Beta-draft for Field Trials.* Geneva: World Health Organization.

WYATT, J., NIPARKO, J., ROTHMAN, M., & DELISSOVOY, G. (1995). Cochlear implant cost effectiveness. *The American Journal of Otology, 16;*52–62.

Chapter 6

Human Resources Management in Audiology

David A. Zapala

Whenever individuals unite to work toward a common goal, they can be seen as a human resource that should be organized and managed wisely. This concept applies not only to business concerns but also to professionals and their organizations. The principle message of this chapter is that, as professionals, each of us is a human resource that contributes to the collective health of the discipline and profession of audiology. How we contribute forges our individual and collective future in the service of persons with hearing impairment.

This chapter approaches human resources management from a broad perspective. Specifically, human resource management is discussed from the point of view of the individual professional, the employer, and the profession. Thus the major sections of this chapter are entitled "Self-Management," "Practice Management," and "Ownership of the Profession." No effort is made to be comprehensive in this treatment. Human resources problems, particularly when they involve employer/employee relationships, are complex and best managed by professionals in the area of human resources and law. The approach taken here is to present the principal themes that run throughout one's professional life and to point out potential roadblocks to the advancement of the individual and profession.

SELF-MANAGEMENT

Most audiologists have three professional relationships: with their patient, their profession, and their employer. In this section factors that affect these relationships are presented from the point of view of the individual audiologist.

Relationship with the Patient: Personal and Professional Propriety

Any professional who offers his or her service to the community holds a trust. Professional status implies that, in a given area of enterprise, laypersons cannot reasonably obtain the expertise held by professionals, and may not be able to act in their own best interest without the assistance of one more knowledgeable (Fox & Battin, 1978). Because the consumer must rely on the judgment of the professional, the professional holds a fiduciary responsibility to the consumer. That is, the professional is expected to act in a manner that is in their client's or patient's best interest. It is the professional's expertise and fiduciary relationship that is purchased by the patient, not just a product or service.

From the profession's prospective, audiologists do not treat disease with medication or surgery. We improve people's ability to function or communicate in the face of impaired hearing or balance.* The only way to do this is to change the behavior of those we would help. Audiologist-directed behavior change can only occur when the practitioner is perceived as holding a high standard for personal propriety and professional knowledge. So it stands to reason that these attributes are important assets for all audiologists.

---

*This should not be taken to mean that audiology does not play a significant role in the diagnosis and treatment of ear disease. Over the last several decades, the audiologist's diagnostic tests have improved the physician's ability to diagnosis and treat ear disease. Furthermore, audiologists are well trained to manage cerumen, detect signs and symptoms of ear disease, and refer when necessary. Nevertheless, diagnosis and treatment of ear disease remains the role of the physician. Audiologists diagnose and treat functional deficits in hearing, which may or may not be related to ear disease. Thus at its core the audiologist's intervention improves one's ability to function or communicate in the face of impaired hearing.

Audiology: Practice Management. Edited by Hosford-Dunn, Roeser, and Valente. Thieme Medical Publishers, Inc., New York © 2000

TABLE 6–1 Ethical and personal proprietary standards

SECTION 21. Subject to the due process requirements of the Uniform Administrative Procedures Act, compiled in Title 4, Part 5, any person registered under this part may have his license denied, revoked or suspended for a fixed period to be determined by the council for any of the following causes:

(1) Conviction of an offense involving moral turpitude. The record of such conviction, or certified copy thereof from the clerk of the court where such conviction occurred, or by the judge of such court, is sufficient evidence to warrant revocation or suspension;

(2) Securing a license under this part through fraud or deceit;

(3) Unethical conduct, gross and/or repeated acts of ignorance or insufficiency in the conduct of his practice;

(4) Knowingly practicing while suffering with a contagious or infectious disease;

(5) Use if a false name or alias in the practice of his profession; and

(6) Violating any of the provisions of this part.

From Tennessee Code Annotated; Title 63, Chapter 17, Part 2, Section 21.

In general, professionals are held to a higher standard of conduct than others in the work force, primarily because of their fiduciary responsibilities. As professionals, audiologists are not exempt from these standards. Most licensure statutes have sections detailing standards for personal propriety and ethical behavior. An example of such a section is shown in Table 6–1.

These statues are designed to protect the public from professionals who have poor character and are thus unworthy of the public trust. They are based on the assumption that the individual who is worthy of professional status will stand a test of good citizenship. For example, most statutes specifically require that the professional be free of felony conviction, have no evidence of fraudulent activities, be in general good moral standing as judged by peers, and require the applicant to follow a professional code of ethics (typically modeled after the American Speech-Language-Hearing Code of Ethics or the American Academy of Audiology Code of Ethics, which are reprinted in Appendix I in this volume).

Employers and other accrediting agencies might require higher minimum standards of good citizenship. For example, many agencies receive government funds and must provide evidence of a drug-free environment (Whiting, 1994). In passive enforcement a drug-related arrest may be enough for disciplinary action. In active enforcement random tests may be required. Other requirements might include standards to ensure against sexual harassment, and gender or cultural or racial discrimination, or set minimum requirements for employee health status or creditworthiness (Paulson & Layton, 1995; Whiting, 1994).

Professional propriety refers to actions involved in professional practice. The American Speech-Language-Hearing Association's Certification of Clinical Competence and the American Academy of Audiology's Board Certification Program require that the professional maintain minimum standards in the areas of professional propriety, experience, and knowledge. These are embodied in both organizations' codes of ethics.

Standards imposed by employers and other agencies are not the only standards to which the professional must subscribe. They are a minimum. What might a patient expect from an audiologist in terms of personal propriety and ethical behavior? What would fellow colleagues expect? In general, patients expect at least three things beyond the audiologist's knowledge and fiduciary responsibility. They are empathetic care, integrity, and preservation of personal autonomy.

PEARL

"Patients don't much care what you know until they know that you care."

Anonymous

Empathetic care means the ability to understand the patient's circumstance as if it were your own (empathy) and have compassion for the patient. Integrity means the ability to be truthful and to act consistent with a moral and ethical code. Preservation of personal autonomy means including patients as active participants in their own care. To include patients as participants in the treatment process, they must be informed of treatment options, participate in the selection their treatment, hold some responsibility for compliance with the treatment plan, and participate in the assessment of treatment outcomes (Beuf, 1979; Inlander et al, 1988).

Delivering empathetic care with integrity while preserving personal autonomy is harder than it seems. In fact, it is a lifelong process that starts with a commitment to basic values, self-evaluation, and a desire to improve. Issues of integrity become more complex as one ventures further into the field of audiology. For example, are professionals showing integrity when they accept gifts from manufacturers for using products? Are audiologists ever tempted to recommend the hearing aid with the highest profit margin over a less profitable alternative? Am I always "on time" and "focused" when I see patients? The wise professional is always vigilant for signs of self-delusion, substandard care, and potential conflicts of interest. This is necessary to maintain his or her fiduciary responsibility to patients. (For further discussion, see Chapters 3 and 9, in this volume.)

This is not a chapter about ethics. However, a profession is made up of individual practitioners. We are defined as much by the actions of our peers as our own actions or those of our professional societies. In the long term an individual's personal and professional propriety is recognizable in the marketplace and contributes to the perception of the profession as a whole.

Relationship with the Profession: Personal Growth

Most audiologists selected their profession out of a strong desire to help others. Audiology is a young, dynamic, growing field. A way to learn more or improve outcomes always exists. Often the same desire to help that attracted the student into the field propels the accomplished practitioner to innovate or master a new area. Thus it is not surprising that audiologists feel a need and an obligation for continuing education and self-development.

The process of planning for continued growth begins soon after the audiologist leaves graduate school. Few audiologists are perfectly prepared for professional life immediately after graduating. At some point during the fellowship year, the new audiologist begins a process of self-evaluation. In several areas the fellow's clinical skill will fall short of the demands of independent clinical practice. Although this can leave the new audiologist feeling inadequately trained and frustrated, it really heralds the beginning of the next stage in self-development. It is only through honest self-evaluation that the audiologist can prioritize deficit areas. Once deficit areas are prioritized, a plan for further education and skill development can be made. Later, when the audiologist has developed clinical acumen, this same process of self-assessment will spark efforts to broaden and diversify areas of expertise. The process continues throughout one's professional life—always with the goal of improving one's ability to contribute to the health and well-being of the community.

Audiologists have several tools with which to develop their knowledge base and clinical skills. Professional journals are available in audiology, medicine, and the basic sciences. Textbooks and formal continuing education course work can improve the didactic knowledge of the audiologist. The habit of reading professional literature and completing course work starts in graduate school and continues throughout one's professional life. No better way to develop the knowledge base of the practitioner exists.

Developing clinical skills often takes more than didactic instruction. For example, one can be well read yet have difficulty determining the appropriate course of action when confronted with an incomplete clinical picture. Furthermore, because audiologists are in the business of behavior change, the clinician's interpersonal skills play as important a role as professional knowledge. Two powerful methods are available to help improve clinical skills. They are structured formal case presentations and mentorship.

Structured formal case presentations are situations in which a difficult or interesting case is presented to a group of peers (Zapala, 1996). The role of the presenter in these "case staffings" is to present the case information in as efficient method as possible, with the factors that influenced the clinician's decision making clearly evident. The role of the peer group is to respectfully listen and offer insight into how the case could have been managed better. This is not an adversarial situation. The presenter must be willing to take some criticism as a price of improved clinical decision making. The listener must be tactful

enough to offer suggestions in a helpful manner, remembering that his or her turn will come in time. For staffing to work, a bond of trust must exist between a group of colleagues dedicated to improving clinical efficacy. When care is taken to maintain this bond of trust, routine staffing can be the best way to sharpen clinical judgment. An example of a staffing presentation is shown in Table 6–2.

Mentorship is vital to the life of any discipline or profession. (See Minghetti et al [1993] for an interesting treatment of this topic.) This is a personal relationship in which a clinician with knowledge in a given area helps an audiologist/student acquire that knowledge. Mentoring relationships are particularly important in the early years of one's professional life. During this period, a combination of encouragement and "hands-on" instruction by a senior clinician can spark a lifetime of learning and service.

Mentoring relationships continue to be helpful throughout the course of one's professional life. Audiology offers a multitude of opportunities to serve and reap reward. One of the best ways to determine whether a new area of interest is worthy of the time and effort required for mastery is to identify potential mentors in the area. Mentors can be faculty members in university or research settings, other experienced practitioners, or individuals in other professions with special knowledge or experience. They help the audiologist by offering guidance in the development of new skills, provide personal feedback about the audiologist's progress, and provide a glimpse of the lifestyle that might be enjoyed once a new area is mastered. One plays the role of student or mentor many times in the course of personal growth. In many ways it is this collegial sharing that keeps the profession vital.

> ### PITFALL
>
> **On occasion an audiologist graduates with the misunderstanding that it is not necessary to continue the path of self-learning taught in graduate school. Nothing could be further from the truth. Self-learning must continue throughout one's professional life just to maintain minimal standards.**

In discussing self-development within the professional arena, it is easy to end with issues of continuing education and skill development. However, audiology is not practiced in a vacuum. Political and legislative initiatives often promote or threaten our ability to practice independently. As members of a profession, we have a responsibility to be informed and act proactively to protect and strengthen our right to practice. More on this topic will be offered in the third section of this chapter.

Relationship with an Employer: Being Managed

Accepting a job offer requires a commitment and investment for both the employee and the employer. From the employer's point of view, the audiologist will "cost" a significant amount of time and money for training, orientation, and continuing education. Furthermore, he or she will cost their salary plus 30% to 75% in indirect costs (Whiting, 1994). So the employer

TABLE 6–2   Example structure case staffing

1. Who (demographics) has what chief complaints (when possible, note onset and progression of symptoms; separate medical from auditory/communicative)

   EXAMPLE: A 7-week-old infant was seen in follow-up after failing an otoacoustic emission hearing screen before discharge and again 4 weeks after discharge. Test results obtained at 4 weeks suggest a strong chance of sensorineural hearing loss. This is the first birth in a young family (mother and father are 19 and 21 years, respectively). Good extended family support is present. However, the mother's parents are not supportive of the parent's efforts to follow-up with the audiological evaluations to date. No risk factors were associated with the birth, specifically, no history of hearing loss was present in any of the known family members. The family was sent to our clinic to confirm or refute the results of the referring hospital and, if necessary, to develop a management plan for the family.

2. Background and related information

   EXAMPLE: (continued): At the 4-week visit, OAEs were absent to 80-dB pSPL clicks (TEOAEs, ILO88, quick screen differential mode). An ABR, obtained at the 4-week visit, demonstrated click-evoked responses down to 40-dB nHL in the right ear, and 55-dB nHL in the left ear. High-frequency tympanometry yielded patterns consistent with the Van Hues model at 220 Hz and 1000 Hz (Y, G, B) in both ears. In addition, an ipsilateral acoustic reflex was measured in the left ear at 95 dB.

3. Subjective and objective assessment

   EXAMPLE: (continued): Parents present with sleeping child. No physical sign of cranial facial malformation is present. TEOAEs were absent in the left ear, and a possible emission was detected in the 700-Hz region (SNR 4 dB, absolute level was -10-dB SPL) distortion product emissions (DPOAEs) were absent between 1000-Hz and 8000 Hz (L1-L2: 65 to 55 dB, F1/F: 1.2, 4 points/octave) bilaterally. DPOAEs were present between 1000 and 1500 Hz using 70-70 (L1-L2) primaries in the right ear. They were absent in the left ear. ABR was identical to prior study, except I obtained a threshold of 35 dB on the right side (latency prolonged). Otologic evaluation: no middle ear effusion, normal infant head and neck examination, R/O congenital hearing loss.

4. Impressions (information that is dictating your management)

   EXAMPLE: (continued)
   1. Suspect at least mild sensorineural hearing loss bilaterally, greater in the left ear.
   2. Communicatively significant?
   3. At risk for progressive hearing loss.
   4. Parent anxiety, with family members that may impede further compliance.

5. Management actions and outcome

   EXAMPLE: (continued): I told the parents that I was reasonably sure that a hearing loss was present. However, I am not sure that it is great enough to warrant the use of hearing aids at the present. I told them I would present this in staffing and call them with our conclusions. I am not sure they will return.

6. Problems (best to list in order of importance; your colleagues may modify the list)
   1. I am not sure whether this is communicatively significant. Should I initiate an early intervention program or just monitor hearing?
   2. Do I have enough information?
   3. Parents are now less sure of the diagnosis and may not remain compliant.

What would you do?

---

is gambling that the ultimate contribution the audiologist makes to the business will exceed the hiring costs. It is easy to see where the employer might expect a commitment from the audiologist to constantly improve performance.

From the audiologist's point of view, employment offers a venue for practicing audiology and contributing to the health and well-being of the community. It is also a chance to exchange clinical service for financial reward and an opportunity for professional growth and career advancement. When audiologists become employees, they take on a set of responsibilities and allegiances to the employer. These allegiances

must be held along with fiduciary responsibilities to the patient. In most cases employer allegiances are not in conflict with the audiologist's fiduciary responsibilities or their obligations to their profession. However, incongruent allegiances can occur. It is always best to discover these before accepting employment. The only way to accomplish this is for the applicant to know his or her own obligations and allegiances beforehand and be able to explore the mission, goals, and methods of the organization with which employment is sought.

Allegiance to an employer is dictated in part by the nature of the employment relationship. Audiologists may be hired as independent contractors, technical service providers, part-time employees, or full-time employees. When audiologists are hired as independent contractors, they have a more distant relationship to the employers. They may be paid more than a full-time employee. However, they are essentially self-employed and are responsible for self-employment tax. The employer has no obligation to the contractor, does not contribute to the contractor's income tax responsibilities, and provides no benefits. The allegiance to the employer in this case is driven solely by the audiologist's prerogatives. Independent contractors will be discussed in greater detail in following sections.

Technical service providers are employed by an agency, which in turn contracts with a client service provider. For example, an audiology group may hire an audiologist and send him or her to several otolaryngologist's offices to cover their clinics. The audiologist is hired by the audiology group. So they hold an allegiance to that agency. Holding the interests of the agency in mind, the audiologist would also consider the needs of the agency's client, but only to the extent that this is in the interest of the agency.

Part-time and full-time employees might share more of a stake in the success of the employer than other types of employees. Full-time employees in particular may enjoy greater career advancement opportunities and may thus feel greater allegiance to their employer.

How important are these allegiances and how do they make an impact on one's behavior? Two factors bear on this question. First is the issue of personal propriety. If one agrees to work in a certain situation, it is best to show integrity and perform the job to the best of one's abilities. The second factor is the legal doctrine called "employment at will." This doctrine, which is incorporated into the laws of most states, gives the employer the right to fire an employee without cause unless the employee's civil rights have been violated (Hosford-Dunn et al, 1995; Whiting, 1994). By design, this gives the employer the upper hand when dealing with the performance of an employee.

Ideally, both the employer and the employee share the same mission. Both then share in the successive achievements of the practice. However, even when good alignment exists between the mission, goals, and methods of the employing agency and the audiologist, conflicts in perceived obligations may occur. No perfect rule exists for settling these disagreements. In general, a professional's first obligation is his or her fiduciary responsibility to the patient. The next obligation is to stay within the bounds of legal and ethical professional practice. The final obligation is to the employer.

What should an employer expect when hiring an audiologist? A good starting place is found in Dr. Michael Chial's 25 points for developing professionalism (see Table 6–3). Students at the University of Wisconsin–Madison are presented with this list at the start of their clinical experiences. It lays a good foundation for future professional development.

HUMAN RESOURCE ISSUES IN PRACTICE MANAGEMENT

The career paths of many audiologists eventually lead to management positions. Every audiologist/manager wants to

create an innovative, high-quality audiology service. It does not take long for new managers to realize that their ability to accomplish this will depend less on their personal clinical acumen than on their ability to attract, develop, and keep a skilled, motivated, energetic group of workers (audiologists and others) who are aligned with the goals of the organization.* This working definition is the "heart" of human resources (HR) management. Many texts on HR management focus on the bewildering array of the laws, standards, and tasks that must be addressed by large corporations. To be sure, the HR management complexities increase with the size of the employing agency. However the "heart" of the task remains the same.

PEARL

The heart of HR management is the ability to attract, develop, and keep a skilled, motivated, energetic group of workers who are aligned with the goals of the organization.

Attracting, developing, and keeping a skilled workforce is a basic human resource function for any company. Staff turnover increases training costs and makes it more difficult to maintain consistent, high-quality service. One estimate places the cost of replacing an employee at 500 times their hourly rate (Whiting, 1994). In audiological practices turnover is even more costly. Successful audiologists are highly trained, having mastered the science and technology of modern hearing care. They also establish close trusting relationships with their patients. When an audiologist leaves an organization, their technical expertise and those personal relationships are lost. So from a patient care perspective, it is important to maintain a stable, skilled workforce.

The other part of the "heart" of HR management is maintaining a motivated group of workers who are aligned with the goals of the organization (Labovitz & Rosansky, 1997). This is a leadership function. An often-quoted adage is "you manage supplies and equipment, you lead people." To do this, an organization's leadership must communicate its mission and goals in a way that inspires understanding and commitment in its membership (Bick, 1997; Levine & Crom, 1995). Communication is also important to ensure that the right people focus on the right tasks at the right time (Larwood, 1984; Schlesinger et al, 1992). Therefore good HR management includes the communication of information that motivates and directs the activities of the workforce.

So how does one attract and develop a skilled, motivated group of audiologists and keep them aligned with the goals of the organization? This discussion will focus on three critical areas: organization and staff planning, attracting and hiring staff members, and developing and retaining a competent staff.

Organization and Staff Planning

The organizational plan defines each position in an organization by the key processes and tasks performed and how

---

*This definition was derived by the author from essays by Hosford-Dunn et al (1995), Kishel and Kishel (1993), and the book *The Power of Alignment* by Labovitz and Rosansky (1997).

TABLE 6–3 Professionalism

Audiology is a professional discipline. Professions require certain behaviors of their practitioners. Professional behaviors (which may or may not directly involve other people) have to do with professional tasks and responsibilities, with the individuals served by the profession and with relations with other professions. Included among professional tasks are education and training. The following conveys expectations about the behaviors of those who seek to join this profession.

1. You show up.
2. You show up on time.
3. You show up prepared.
4. You show up in a frame of mind appropriate to the professional task.
5. You show up properly attired.
6. You accept the idea that "on time," "prepared," "appropriate," and "properly" are defined by the situations, by the nature of the task, or by another person.
7. You accept that your first duty is to the ultimate welfare of the persons served by your profession and that "ultimate welfare" is a complex mix of desires, wants, needs, abilities, and capacities.
8. You recognize that professional duties and situations are about completing tasks and about solving problems in ways that benefit others, either immediately or in the long term. They are not about you. When you are called on to behave as a professional, you are not the patient, the customer, the star, or the victim.
9. You place the importance of professional duties, tasks, and problem solving above your own convenience.
10. You strive to work effectively with others for the benefit of the person served. This means you pursue professional duties, tasks, and problem solving in ways that make it easier (not harder) for others to accomplish their work.
11. You properly credit others for their work.
12. You sign your work.
13. You take responsibility for your actions, your reactions, and your inaction. This means you do not avoid responsibility by offering excuses, by blaming others, by emotional displays, or by helplessness.
14. You do not accept professional duties or tasks for which you are personally or professionally unprepared.
15. You do what you say you will do, by the time you said you would do it, and to the degree of quality you said you would do it.
16. You take active responsibility for expanding the limits of your own knowledge, understanding, and skill.
17. You vigorously seek and tell the truth, including those truths that may be less than flattering to you.
18. You accept direction (including correction) from those who are more knowledgeable or more experienced. You provide direction (including correction) to those who are less knowledgeable or less experienced.
19. You value the resources required to perform duties, tasks, and problem solving, including your time and that of others.
20. You accord respect to the values, interests, and opinions of others that may differ from your own, as long as they are not objectively harmful to the persons served.
21. You accept the fact that others may establish objectives for you. Although you may not always agree with those goals or may not fully understand them, you will pursue them as long as they are not objectively harmful to the persons served.
22. When you attempt a task for the second time, you seek to do it better than you did the first time. You revise the ways you approach professional duties, tasks, and problem solving in consideration of peer judgments of best practices.
23. You accept the imperfections of the world in ways that do not compromise the interests of those you serve.
24. You base your opinions, actions, and relations with others on sound empirical evidence and on examined personal values consistent with the above.
25. You expect all the above from other professionals.

Adapted from Chial (1998), with permission.

those relate to the mission of the organization (Carnegie, 1995; Larwood, 1984). The staff plan describes how people will be managed within the organization. The two are related but not identical (Hosford-Dunn et al, 1995). For example, a receptionist position may be in the organizational plan. However, the staff plan may be to fill the position when the business can support hiring a new employee. This will become more evident as the discussion proceeds. This section will focus on two aspects of organizational and staff planning.

First, attention will be directed at defining the organizational structure and the job positions within the structure. Then some regulatory considerations for the employer-employee relationship will be discussed.

Organizational Structure and Job Descriptions

Before anyone can be hired, the potential employer must define who is needed to perform what tasks. This process starts by examining the organizational model that is defined in the business plan. The organizational model answers the "form follows function" edict. That is, one first defines the functions that must be achieved by the organization. Then one designs an organizational model that can achieve those functions efficiently and effectively (Larwood, 1984; Schlesinger et al, 1992).

Typically, the organizational model identifies two different types of associates. First, an inevitable set of outside consultants provide needed skills to the organization. These typically include an accountant, attorney, banker, financial planner, insurance agent, and perhaps a bookkeeper, collection agency, and computer consultant. Because of the unique set of skills each professional brings to the enterprise, they are typically identified as management consultants within the business plan of the organization (Hosford-Dunn et al, 1995; Paulson & Layton, 1995). The business plan may or may not identify the management consultants by name. Their importance rests in what skills they bring to the enterprise (although individuals with a good reputation can make the organization look more attractive to potential investors).

The same philosophy holds true for the organization's staff membership. The clinic's staff should be organized around the skills required to accomplish the organization's mission. This is accomplished by developing an organizational model. According to Schlesinger et al (1992), the model defines the following form/function issues:

- The key tasks and processes that must be accomplished to provide targeted services
- The positions within the organization and the skills required for each position to ensure completion of assigned tasks
- An organizational structure that (a) allocates responsibilities, activities, and authority to individuals, and (b) coordinates these individuals with others in the organization
- A performance-appraisal system to provide feedback to each person about their efforts to achieve the tasks and processes of their position
- A reward system, including pay, benefits, and intangibles such as status, career development opportunities, and the chance to contribute to an important objective
- A selection and development system for attracting and training employees

In a solo audiology practice the organizational model is very simple: all jobs fall within the job description of the owner, who is self-motivated and intrinsically aligned with the goals of the organization. As practices grow, audiologists, support personnel, and other professionals may be hired. In these small organizations one manager can use face-to-face communication to direct, monitor, and coordinate the activities of others.

Informal communications systems break down as the organization grows. A single manager can no longer deal with everyone on a one-on-one basis. In these cases decisions may be made without important information, tools, or controls. More fatally, charismatic workers may informally take on leadership functions and make decisions that may not be compatible with the mission and goals of the organization. For these reasons, it is wise to develop an organizational model and staff plan that addresses the preceding six aspects regardless of the size of the organization.

The first four aspects of the organizational model just defined delineate the job responsibilities, skill requirements, and performance measurements for each position. In addition, they establish a chain of command between job positions to define the flow of information and decision-making prerogatives. This information can be communicated formally through an organizational diagram and specific job descriptions. The job description is a tool that documents the role, responsibilities, performance expectations, and location in the chain of command for each position within an organization (Hosford-Dunn et al, 1995). Typical items for a job description include the following:

- Job title: One or two identifying words such as audiologist or business manager.
- Job statement: A sentence or two that defines how a person in this position contributes to the goals of the organization.
- Major/minor duties: The major aspects of the job that relate the skills of the individual with performance standards and expectations for the position. An example for a receptionist might be: "Greets patients cheerfully."
- Relationships: This delineates the organizational structure and chain of command. For example, a supervisor may oversee the performance of several individuals and report to a director.
- Qualifications: This specifies the minimum educational and licensure requirements, experience level, physical abilities, travel demands, and other perquisites to qualify for the position.

An example organizational diagram and job description are presented in Figure 6–1 and Appendix A at the end of this chapter, respectively. Hosford-Dunn et al (1995) and Welch and Fowler (1994) also offer example job descriptions for independent practices and large clinics, respectively.

An entire organization can be structured using this approach. When implemented successfully, each employee understands his or her responsibilities and performance expectations, understands how decisions are made and by whom, and understands how information should flow through the organization. From clearly defined job descriptions, the manager should be able to define and measure the important aspects of an individual's job performance. This is critical for providing accurate feedback on performance (Carnegie, 1993; Schlesinger et al, 1992). It is also helpful for determining whether poor performance is due to an employee motivation problem, a skill deficit, or an overall problem with the process (Levine & Crom, 1995). Finally, having a rigorously defined job description and performance appraisal system helps protect the employer from litigation when an employee is discharged for inadequate job performance (Whiting, 1994).

Regulatory Considerations in Employer-Employee Relationships

Several legal doctrines and federal mandates define the employer-employee relationship. This section will review several of the more commonly applied rules of employment. However, this review is not comprehensive, nor is it meant to replace legal or professional counsel. The reader is cautioned

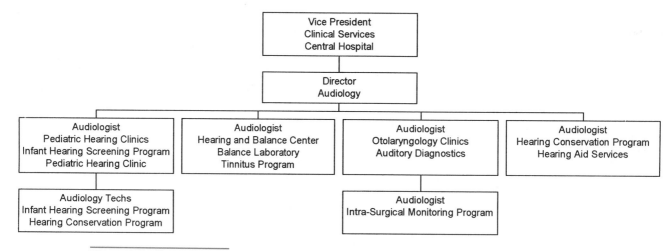

Figure 6–1   Example organizational chart of a hospital-based audiology department.

to seek the services of a competent HR professional before employing individuals in a private practice.

Employment-At-Will Doctrine

"Employment-at-will" refers to the common law doctrine that holds that either an employer or employee can terminate an employment relationship at any time, and for any reason, or for no reason at all (Hosford-Dunn, 1995). Although this is generally true, Whiting (1994) identifies several exceptions to the employment-at-will doctrine.

- Written or implied contracts may stipulate that termination can only occur for "good cause" or "just cause." This is a common policy in large organizations or in some union contracts. An audiologist may or may not be offered an employment contract, depending on the organizations' staffing plan. If neither a written or implied contract is in force, employment is "at will."

- Violations of public policy may limit employment-at-will prerogatives. For example, discharging an employee would be illegal if the discharge was based on the employee's race, gender, age, national origin, religion, physical handicap, mental disability, marital status, or union activity.

- An employer may inadvertently lose the "employment-at-will" prerogative when discipline is inconsistently applied and results in the perception that discrimination has taken place. For example, if other employees perceive that one employee is able to arrive late for work without reprimand, they may feel discriminated against on the basis of race, gender, age, and the like, when they are reprimanded or discharged for a similar behavior. The result can be litigation and loss of the employer's employment-at-will prerogative with other employees if the court sides with the discharged employee. Therefore it is important to develop, communicate (verbally and in writing), and enforce policies and procedures consistently.

- Another way an employer may inadvertently lose the "employment-at-will" prerogative is by implying permanent employment. For example, statements such as "during your probationary period you may be discharged for

any reason" may be taken to mean that a higher standard than employment-at-will is in place after the probationary period. Similarly, offering a "yearly salary" may be interpreted that employment is for a year period. Such misunderstandings imply a promise for continuing employment. The result can be litigation when an employee is discharged and loss of the employer's employment-at-will prerogative with other employees if the court sides with the employee.

Because of these potential problems, it is wise to provide written notification that employment is "at will" and "may be terminated by either the employee or employer at any time, for any reason or no reason at all, without cause or notice." (Whiting, 1994). This is best accomplished within the context of an employment agreement (following).

Employment Agreements

It may be that an audiologist enters into a formal contract when he or she accepts a position. These are sometimes called employment agreements or service contracts (Desmond, 1994; Hosford-Dunn et al, 1995). These contracts define whether the employee is "at will" and describe the compensation package, termination provisions, restrictive provisions, time to be devoted to the business, vacation and sick days, and any fringe benefits that will be provided. Restrictive provisions are designed to protect the employer. Typical restrictive provisions include (1) noncompete/nonsolicitation clauses, (2) patient and practice confidentiality clauses, and (3) antiprivacy clauses. Noncompete/nonsolicitation clauses ensure that while the employee works for the business and for some time after termination, the employee will not interfere with the practice's patients or contracts (Hosford-Dunn et al, 1995).

Patient and practice confidentiality clauses protect patient information and trade secrets such as pricing, contractual and vendor relationships, business strategies, and methods of business. Antiprivacy clauses protect against the theft of intellectual property such as computer programs, forms, correspondence, and the like (Hosford-Dunn et al, 1995).

Two factors should be considered when developing protective provisions. First, they must be specific and fair.

Noncompete and nonsolicitation clauses need to have a limited scope. They must apply to a reasonable geographical region and must restrict competition for a reasonable time period. "Reasonable" is typically defined in regional court cases and may vary from state to state. Consequently, it is important to have these clauses and all aspects of the employment agreement reviewed by an attorney who is familiar with local standards (Whiting, 1994).

The second consideration is that enforcement of restrictive provisions is not automatic. Rather, violations must be adjudicated through civil litigation. If the restrictive provisions are considered unfair to the employee, they may be unenforceable by legal decree. Hosford-Dunn et al (1995) recommend that a "comprehensive severability clause" be incorporated into employment agreements. This clause protects the remaining scope of a set of restrictive provisions if one part of the agreement is disallowed by legal decree.

Other Laws and Regulations that Impact the Employer-Employee Relationship

Sexual Harassment

Employers have the responsibility to maintain a workplace that is free from sexual harassment, discrimination, or intimidation of any form (Whiting, 1994). Larger organizations are required to have a written policy banning sexual harassment. However, as a preventive measure, all organizations should have these policies in writing (Paulson & Layton, 1995). Furthermore, employers may be held vicariously liable for the actions of subordinates in the organization if written policies are not enforced (Jandt, 1990). Because this area is evolving and the stakes can be so great, it is imperative that sexual harassment policies be in written form and reviewed by the organization's attorney (Hosford-Dunn et al, 1995; Paulson & Layton, 1995; Whiting, 1994).

Other Regulations

Several other laws and regulations commonly impact the employer/employee relationship. These are summarized in Table 6–4, which was adapted from the Employer's Resource Group (1993) and Whiting (1994). Review of these laws and regulations is beyond the scope of this text. Moreover, some only impact organizations that employ more than a certain minimum number of employees. Consultation with HR and legal professionals is strongly encouraged to understand how these regulations might impact an individual practice situation.

Other Regulations that Impact the Right to Practice

Several other regulations may impact the staff and organizational plan. First, most states have licensure requirements for an individual to practice as an audiologist. State licensure agencies are listed in Appendix B at the end of this chapter. Associated with licensure are the rules and regulations for the legal practice of audiology. Verification of license status is certainly an important requirement when employing a potential staff member. Furthermore, the rules and regulations for legal practice of audiology must be understood and followed. In addition, providers of Medicaid services are required to have a Certificate of Clinical Competence in Audiology (CCC-A) or equivalent to receive payment for audiology services. Consequently, current ASHA standards of practice and code of ethics will influence the practice of audiology within an organization (see Battle [1994]). Finally, depending on the venue, voluntary standards may apply. For example, The Commission on Accreditation of Rehabilitation Facilities (CARF) accredits rehabilitation agencies, The Joint Committee on Accreditation of Healthcare Organizations accredits hospital and other healthcare organizations, and the ASHA Professional Services Board (PSB) accredits agencies that provide speech-language or hearing services. Compliance with the standards of these agencies is often required by third-party payers.

Common Law Causes of Action: Wrongful Discharge

Several common law doctrines may also lead to litigation on the basis of "wrongful discharge." According to Whiting (1994), wrongful discharge occurs when the implied covenant to act in "good faith and fair dealing" is breached by the employer, and by doing so the employee is damaged. Five common causes of this type of common law "tort" are as follows:

- Breach of implied contract
- Workers' compensation retaliation
- Invasion of privacy
- Fraudulent misrepresentation
- Defamation

Breach of implied contract was discussed in the section describing "employment at will" and will not be reviewed here. *Workers compensation retaliation* may occur when an employee is injured on the job and starts collecting workers' compensation. The company then discharges the individual to avoid making the compensation payments. In this situation the injured worker can claim workers compensation retaliation and sue for lost wages and other damages. *Invasion of privacy* occurs when an employee's name, likeness, "private" information, or information that places the employee in a false light is released to the public without consent.

The remaining two causes of tort action require special attention because they may be more commonly encountered in organizations similar to audiology practices. *Fraudulent misrepresentation* occurs when an employer makes representations that are known to be false, to induce an employee to take certain action, and the employee acts on these representations to their detriment. For example, if a potential employer attempts to induce an applicant to accept a job offer by promising the potential for a long-term career with the organization when the true aim is to simply hire the applicant for a short-term purpose, the employer is guilty of fraudulent misrepresentation. For this reason and for the purpose of protecting employment-at-will prerogatives, it is wise to honestly and explicitly describe the expected employment arrangement in the form of an employment agreement.

Defamation occurs when publishing or providing information about someone that is false and injures that person's reputation. Two types of defamation are libel and slander. Libel refers to written defamatory statements and slander denotes spoken defamation. Defamation may occur when making statements about an individual's performance, character, or

TABLE 6–4 Summary of major laws and regulations affecting human resource management*

Law or Regulation	Brief Summary
Wages, Hours, and Conditions of Employment	
Fair Labor Standards Act (FLSA)	Sets minimum wage standards, overtime pay rules, record-keeping requirements, and child labor restrictions.
Walsh-Healey Public Contracts Act	Employers w/certain government supply contracts must pay time and a half to employees working more than 40 hours/wk.
McNamara-O'Hara Service Contract Act (MOSCA)	Employers w/certain government service contracts must pay specified minimum hourly rates and fringe benefits.
Davis-Bacon Act	Employers w/certain government public works contracts must pay specified minimum hourly rates and fringe benefits.
Family and Medical Leave Act (FMLA)	Employers with more than 50 employees must offer employees up to 12 wk unpaid, job-protected leave annually for certain family and medical reasons.
Employment Practices	
Title VII of the Civil Rights Act of 1964	Prohibits discrimination because of race, color, national origin, religion, sex, pregnancy (including childbirth or related condition).
Title I of the Americans with Disabilities Act of 1990	Prohibits discrimination in terms, conditions, and privileges of employment against individuals with disabilities who, with or without reasonable accommodation, can perform essential functions of job.
Section 1981, Title 42 U.S.C. (Civil Rights Act of 1966)	Prohibits racial and ethnic bias in employment.
Executive Order 11246	For government contractors, requires antidiscrimination clause in contract plus written affirmative action plan for single contract of $50,000+ and 50+ employees.
Age Discrimination in Employment Act (ADEA), including Older Workers Benefit Protection Act (OWBPA)	Prohibits age discrimination in employment, including benefits, for employees 40 or older.
Equal Pay Act of 1963 (EPA)	Prohibits pay differentials on basis of sex in substantially equal work requiring skill, effort, and responsibility under similar working conditions. No exemption for executive, administrative, professional, and outside sales employees.
Rehabilitation Act of 1973, Section 503	Requires affirmative action and nondiscrimination in employment of handicapped persons.
Rehabilitation Act of 1973, Section 504	No discrimination against, denying benefits to, or exclusion from participation including employment, by any qualified handicapped individual.
Employee Polygraph Protection Act of 1988 (EPPA)	Generally prohibits the use of "lie detectors" and lie detector results in private employment. Limited exemptions apply for certain internal investigations.
Federal Military Selective Service Act	Gives employee returning from U.S. military service the same wages, benefits, and rights as the employee would have received had he or she not left. Discrimination against reservists barred.
Jury System Improvement Act	Provides that an employer cannot discharge, or threaten to discharge, an employee for serving on a federal jury.
Vietnam Era Veteran Readjustment Assistance Act	Requires affirmative action regarding Vietnam-era veterans and disabled veterans.
Immigration Reform and Control Act of 1995 (IRCA)	Prohibits hiring of illegal aliens. Requires verification and record keeping of work authorization documents.
Drug-Free Workplace Act of 1988	Establishes drug-free awareness program and makes good faith effort to carry out; requires penalties or rehabilitation for employees convicted of workplace drug offenses.

TABLE 6–4 (continued)   Summary of major laws and regulations affecting human resource management*

Law or Regulation	Brief Summary
Employment Practices (continued)	
Department of Transportation Drug Testing Regulations	Requires employers to conduct drug tests of certain employees in compliance with strict regulations; provide education and minimal Employee Assistance Programs (EAPs).
Worker Adjustment and Retaining Notification Act (WARN)	With some exceptions, requires 60-day notice to employees and state and local governments before layoffs of 50 or more employees.
Taxes, Insurance, and Employee Benefits	
Social Security Act (FICA)	As of 1992, employer and employee each must contribute 7.65% of wages up to $55,500 and 1.45% on excess up to $130,200. Withholding required. Wage base subject to annual adjustment.
Federal Unemployment Tax Act (FUTA)	Must contribute 0.8% (varies with credits for participation in state unemployment programs) up to $7000 of each employee's wages.
Employee Retirement Income Security Act of 1974 (ERISA)	Requires extensive pension and welfare plan reporting, plus disclosure to plan participants and beneficiaries; minimum participation vesting and funding standards for pension plans, including profit-sharing plans; plan termination insurance for pension plans.
Consolidated Omnibus Budget Reconciliation Act of 1985 (COBRA)	Requires provision of continuation coverage under employer's group health plan to employees, spouses, and/or dependent children on the occurrence of specified events, including termination of employment or reduction in hours.
Labor Relations	
Health Maintenance Organization Act (HMO)	Specific employers must offer membership in a qualified HMO if available where employees live.
National Labor Relations Act (NLRA)	Covers employee rights to engage in protected concerted activity and organize or decertify union.
Railway Labor Act	Regulations co-union elections/mandatory dispute-resolution processes.
Occupational Safety and Health Act (OSHA)	Employer must furnish safe employment according to designated workplace standards; record keeping; no retaliation against employees for exercising rights.
Consumer Credit Protection Act, Title III (Federal Wage Garnishment Law)	Restricts garnishment w/holding to 25% or less of disposable income. Allows larger deductions for support or alimony garnishment. No discharge for one or more garnishments of one debt.
Fair Credit Reporting Act	Discloses to applicants/employees intent to use investigative consumer report and, on request, nature/scope of investigation. Must inform applicant/employee if credit report is related to adverse action and disclose credit agency.
State Laws and Regulations	
State Labor Regulations	Provides for Workers' Compensation benefits after a work-related injury.
State Licensure Acts	Provides the definition of the profession and the legal right to practice.

*NOTE: Listing is not complete and not all listed laws may apply to a specific organization. Seek professional advice before acting on this information.

ethics, as might occur during a performance review, discharge interview, or reference check. In general, the following must occur for a prima facie case defamation:

1. A false or derogatory statement made about a person.

2. The statement was "published" to a third person.

3. The statement caused actual damage or the statement falls into a "defamation per se" category, which presumes harm and permits the award of damages without proof of actual injury.

In professional circles it is common to receive requests for employment or character references. It is important to carefully choose the information given out for these references. Any negative statement may lead to the loss of a significant and potentially profitable career goal. Such a loss can be considered "actual damage" and result in litigation. In general the truth is a defense against defamation. However, one must go to court to prove the truth, which is costly and time consuming. Furthermore, although the truth is the best defense against a defamation suite, it is always difficult to prove an opinion. If a reference is to be given, stick to *facts* that are documented unambiguously in the employee's record. Alternately, many organizations have chosen a policy of providing limited information for employment references (Desmond, 1994; Whiting, 1994). Many provide only a simple verification of employment statement.

PITFALL

Example of defamation: "She was a good employee. However, she liked to party too much and frequently arrived late to work."

Analysis: "Party too much" is an opinion about the cause of a behavior about which the employer may have no direct knowledge. Better to note that the employee was counseled about being late for work after checking the employees record and finding a signed, written tardiness warning.

Protections Against Legal Action—Seek Professional Help

Obviously, several pitfalls can be encountered when entering into an employer-employee relationship. Several actions can protect the employer from the deleterious effects of litigation. It is important to clearly communicate (preferably in writing) the nature of the employment arrangement, performance expectations, and applicable rules and regulations to avoid misunderstandings (Hosford-Dunn et al, 1995; Paulson & Layton, 1995). Consistency and fairness in enforcing rules and regulations is also important (Whiting, 1994). HR professionals insist on a policy and procedure manual to formalize the employer-employee relationship (Jandt, 1990; Paulson & Layton, 1995). Given the cost of legal action, it is always advisable

to have HR and legal professionals review the organizational plan before it is in place and when conflicts arise.

Attracting and Hiring Staff Members

Once the organizational structure and job descriptions are in place, a great deal of detail is known about the type of person best suited for each position in the organization. Assuming that the organization has a need and can financially support adding a new employee into a position, the next task is finding that best person for each position. How a candidate is selected depends on the position to be filled, the current job market, and the current needs of the business.

Hiring or Contracting

One of the first decisions that needs to be made when filling a position is whether the position should be full time and permanent. Full-time, permanent employment requires a great deal of commitment on the part of the employer. Employees receive pay and benefits regardless of changes in the organization's profitability (Paulson & Layton, 1995). This level of commitment may not be reasonable, particularly in the case of small or start-up organizations and particularly when the position is not one involved in direct patient care. Creative and fair alternatives to full-time positions exist.

Secretarial and support staffs are not directly involved with patient care. Furthermore, their skills are commonly available in the job market. Consequently, secretarial and support staff might be better "outsourced" to an employment agency (Hosford-Dunn et al, 1995; Paulson & Layton, 1995). The agency hires the person, pays all employment taxes and benefits, and then contracts that person to the business as a temporary employee. The cost per hour may be greater than if the support person were a full-time employee. However, no commitment exists on the part of the clinic to keep the contract employee. Furthermore, the level of commitment made by the contract employee may be greater than a full-time associate. This is because the contract employees continued employment is directly related to the employer's day-to-day satisfaction with their job performance (Paulson & Layton, 1995).

In some circumstances audiologists can be engaged as contractors. This model is more common in larger cities where more than one practice may have a need for audiology services on an "as-needed" basis. If the audiologist is holding himself or herself out as an independent contractor, great care must be taken to ensure that IRS regulations are not broken (Desmond, 1994). If a contract is written that defines the audiologist as an independent contractor and the IRS finds that the person did not meet the requirements of independent contractor status, the organization may be responsible for back taxes and penalties (Paulson & Layton, 1995). Consultation with the organization attorney and accountant is necessary before entering into this type of relationship. Further information can be obtained from IRS publication 937.

SPECIAL CONSIDERATION

Independent contractor status is appealing to many audiologists who wish to develop an independent practice. In contracting audiology services to physicians, these audiologists are able to develop a stable income stream while developing other referral sources. However, care must be exercised to ensure that the contracting audiology services qualify under IRS rules for independent contractor status. Do audiologists schedule or otherwise direct their activities with sufficient independence to meet minimum IRS requirements for independent contractor status? Review of IRS publication 937 with a knowledgeable tax consultant is recommended before entering into these relationships.

Hiring Employees

In general hiring an employee involves six steps: (1) determining what is needed, (2) employee recruiting, (3) prescreening and reference checking, (4) interviewing and testing, (5) selecting the applicant, and (6) orientation.

Determining Exactly What Is Needed

By having up-to-date organizational and staff plans, the job description and requisite skills have been defined. These help define a "candidate profile" or the minimum requirements for a position (Whiting, 1994). Other factors may also influence this profile. For example, each organization has a culture or personality. This captures the behavioral patterns, values, and attitudes that members use to guide organizational life (Larwood, 1884; Schlesinger et al, 1992). Candidates who share these attitudes may appear more attractive to the hiring organization.

PITFALLS

- Looking for an ideal candidate
- Using the last person in the position as a guide
- Having an inflexible organizational/staff plan

Employee Recruiting

Hosford-Dunn et al (1995) identify four methods of recruiting staff members. They are networking, advertising, using employment agencies, and using walk-ins. Networking involves keeping active relationships with other professionals.

Communicating the availability of a job position to individuals likely to encounter qualified applicants increases the success of the search. Professional colleagues, local educational institutions, the alma maters of current staff members, Internet list servers and professional sites, and industry contacts (hearing aid manufacturers, equipment and service representatives) are productive contacts. Siropolis (1990) suggests that a combination of advertising and networking is often the most successful and quickest means of filling a position. Moreover, the search is accomplished with limited expense to the organization.

Advertising positions available is sometimes an effective tool. The strategy for advertising depends on the relative scarcity of the qualified candidates in the local job market. In general, advertisements should be designed to appeal to candidates with the personality and job skills that are being sought. When advertising for support staff, the response is sometimes overwhelming. Consequently, the ad needs to state job specifications clearly to discourage unqualified respondents. They should not violate equal employment opportunity (EEO) guidelines. Specifically, they should not specify gender, race, age, religious affiliation, physical or mental health as a condition for employment (Whiting, 1994). Although the EEO Commission is a federal agency, each state has its own Human Rights Commission. Specific EEO guidelines may vary on a state-by-state basis. Because of this, the services of an HR expert are helpful in questionable cases.

Placing help wanted ads in local or regional newspapers can be an effective means of filling support positions. It is less successful for finding audiologists unless a large population of audiologists is in the area. In these situations the advantage of advertising in the mass media must be weighed against the disadvantage of giving competitors information about the organization's staffing situation. Blind advertisements do not identify the practice and use the publication's address or a post office box to receive correspondence. The value of placing a blind ad is that the practice does not reveal its intentions to potential competitors (Hosford-Dunn et al, 1995).

When advertising for audiologists, it is often more productive to look for qualified candidates through national publications and trade journals (*Advance Magazine, Hearing Instruments, The Hearing Journal*). Again the Internet has a number of sites that post job positions. The ASHA, (www.asha.org), AAA (www.audiology.org), and Audiologyinfo.com (www.audiologyinfo.com) Web sites have vehicles for this purpose. National and state conventions are also good places to look for potential applicants. Clinical fellowship positions are best promoted by posting position available announcements at regional universities and are most productive in the late spring and summer.

Filling audiology positions can be a lengthy process. Publication lead times can be as long as 90 days. Once someone responds to a national ad, travel time will be required for interviewing. If the job offer is accepted, time for relocating is needed. Consequently, unless someone local is interested in the position, finding an experienced audiologist can take many months (Hosford-Dunn et al, 1995). Moreover, the more technical the position or the more experience required, the longer it takes to fill the position.

State and federal employment agencies often maintain lists of unemployed workers in the area according to job category

(Paulson & Layton, 1995). This can be a rich source of applications for nonprofessional positions. In some cases tax benefits and other inducements may be available if a long-term unemployed worker is hired off of one of these lists. However, care must be taken to ensure that the potential employee has the skills necessary to fulfill the job requirements.

There are also private agencies that will search and do the initial screening of candidates. They are most effective in filling jobs requiring special or professional skills. Private employment agencies are appealing because if they do not have the right person to fill the position, they will go out and find such people. However, they can be expensive, usually 10 to 30 % of the first years' salary (Tway, 1992).

Occasionally a resume will appear serendipitously when a position is available. Although this can save an incredible amount of time when the applicant is well qualified, this is obviously not a good staffing strategy to use. Practice building requires a more active commitment on the part of the manager to ensure the right person is hired for the job. Nevertheless when an unsolicited resume is sent to an organization, it is good form to respond to it in writing. If a position is available, this can be pointed out and the applicant can enter the prescreening process. If no positions are available, a letter should still be written, if for no other reasons than to acknowledge the job seeker as a colleague, wish them well, guide them to other job openings, and incorporate them into the practice's network (Hosford-Dunn et al, 1995).

Prescreening and Reference Checking

Before time is spent interviewing, a system for prescreening applicants should be undertaken. Several prescreening tools are available. The simplest prescreening tool is a resume review with transcripts and letters of recommendation (Desmond, 1994). For nonprofessional positions, resumes may not be all that informative, and the employer may feel overwhelmed with the number of seemingly qualified candidates. In such cases it is helpful to use a telephone prescreening interview before an application is accepted. During the telephone interview, the following questions should be asked:

- Where does the applicant work currently?
- If not now employed, where did the applicant work last?
- How long did the applicant work there?
- Why did the applicant leave?
- What did the applicant do?
- What was the applicant's rate of pay?

This line of questioning is repeated until it is established that the applicant does or does not have the perquisite qualifications for the job. Very little information about the job requirements should be provided during the prescreening interview. This limits the applicant's ability to tell the interviewer that he or she had a specific skill, solely on the basis that the interviewer stated that was a skill that was desirable. If the applicant is not qualified for the position, the conversation should be terminated by explaining that "we are looking for someone else whose background and qualifications more closely meet our requirements." The advantage of the strategy is that nonqualified applicants are not given an opportunity to set the stage for litigation if that is their objective (Whiting, 1994).

Prescreening is also necessary when filling professional positions. As mentioned before, resumes, personal and professional references, employment histories, and license status are helpful tools in assessing minimum qualifications. Because of the threat of lawsuits, written references seldom contained negative information (see "Defamation" section). However, carefully thought out telephone interviews with reference sources can yield information that might not have been put in writing (Desmond, 1994). One question that may elicit good information is "would you hire this person back?" Sometimes, a failure to respond to this question is as meaningful as a response.

At this stage of prescreening, another advantage to blind advertisements becomes apparent. Applicants can be screened on the basis of resume information and references before learning the potential employer's identity. This strategy may also decrease the organization's exposure to litigation (Whiting, 1994).

Interviewing and Testing

The purpose of the initial preemployment interview is to discover information about the applicant that is not on his or her resume or application. The purpose is not necessarily to tell the applicant about the job or the organization. Several books are available that provide a good overview of interviewing techniques, objectives, and pitfalls (see for example Yate [1994]). This section will review the major steps in the interview process. The first step is to prepare well for the interview. Review the job description for accuracy. Prepare your questions in advance, and ensure that the process and questions are applied consistently across all candidates (see Table 6–5 for examples of open-ended questions). The Equal Opportunity statutes and Americans with Disabilities Act limit or eliminate questions that could be construed as discriminatory. The law prohibits questions about race, age, religion, marital status, child-care arrangements, transportation, or handicap status (Paulson & Layton, 1995; Whiting, 1994). Table 6–6 presents some examples of legal and problematic questions.

It is advisable to have more than one person interview viable candidates. Part of the interview process is to determine how well the applicant's personality matches the culture of the organization. Furthermore, interviews for professional positions can be quite intense. It helps to break the interview up into smaller segments to decrease the stress level of candidates and give them time to loosen up. Finally, the time commitment shown by the organization is a sign of respect to the applicant.

It is also important to prepare applicants for the interview. Let them know before they arrive what the interview schedule will be like. This is particularly important when interviewing for professional positions. Start the interview with courteous and friendly small talk to relax candidates. Explain the hiring process early in the interview. Specifically explain

TABLE 6–5 Selected examples of open-ended questions

Area	Example Questions
Communication skills	Tell me about a time when you had to use speaking skills to make a point that was important to you.
	Give me an example of a time when you built motivation among subordinates and what rewards you got out of that experience.
Problem-solving skills	Give me an example of when you had to make a quick decision.
	Describe a situation when several coworkers were angry about a company policy. What did they do? What did you do? Why?
Organizational skills	How did you set priorities for your staff in previous jobs? How did you update them?
	Let's suppose you could devise a procedure that would get your work done in an hour less a day. How would you spend that extra time?
Customer service	Give me an example of when you had to be flexible and creative to meet new customer requirements?
	What are some of the behaviors and attitudes you want your staff to practice to ensure excellent customer service?
Leadership skills	In past supervisor roles, how many did you supervise? In what areas?
	How did you deal with employee conflict?
	What type of employee behavior makes you angry?
	What's your philosophy in dealing with low morale of staff?
Audiology specific	Why did you chose to become an audiologist?
	What is the most difficult clinical case you have experienced?
	What is the most rewarding thing you have done as an audiologist?
	What aspect or job in audiology really gets you excited? What do you like to do?

when they can expect to hear if the position is offered and set a deadline beyond which they can conclude someone else has been selected. From then on, the goal is for the applicant to do all of the talking. Following the "80-20 rule," the interviewer should talk 20% of the time and listen 80% of the time (Whiting, 1994; Yate, 1994).

The interviewer will want to determine candidates' knowledge bases; ability to think on their feet; their level of maturity and self-awareness; their motivations, values, and attitudes; their ability to handle stress; and their overall ability to contribute to the organization. Remembering the 80-20 rule, preselect open-ended questions that relate directly to written job requirements. When more than one person is involved as an interviewer, it is helpful to assign specific areas of assessment to each interview. For example, one audiologist might probe the candidate's knowledge base in auditory diagnostics and pediatric patient care. Another might look for computer skills and the ability to fit programmable hearing aids. Again, each area of inquiry should relate directly to the written job description.

When interviewing for support positions, it may be helpful to formally test the candidate's ability to perform specific tasks. Typing, math, filing tests, or observation of computer use can access specific clerical skills. Professional skills can be observed by having the audiologist work with a patient (Desmond, 1994).

Under certain highly restricted conditions, applicants may be asked to take sample health examinations.* These examinations are obtained to ensure that the applicant has no communicative diseases. The results cannot be used as grounds for not hiring. Rather, reasonable accommodations must be

---

*Title 1 of the Americans with Disabilities Act places severe restrictions on the use of health examinations in the screening and hiring process. Preoffer examinations are prohibited. ADA does not prohibit voluntary tests. An offer may be contingent on satisfactory results of a medical examination. However the results cannot be used to withdraw the offer unless they show that the potential employee is unable to perform tasks required of the job. ADA includes people with AIDS, HIV, and rehabilitated drug abusers in its definition of "disabled." The ADA does not require, however, that employers hire persons who are known drug users or who have contagious diseases (Jenkins, 1993; cited in Hosford-Dunn et al, 1995).

TABLE 6–6 Selected examples of legal and potential problem questions

Category	Legal Questions	Ill-Advised Questions
1. Citizenship or national origin	Can you show proof of your eligibility to work in the United States? Are you fluent in any language other than English?* *Ask this only if it applies to the job being sought.	Are you a U.S. citizen? Were you born here?
2. Religion or political beliefs	Will the working hours, as described, pose any problem for you?* *You may inquire about weekend availability only if it is required for the job being sought.	What is your religion? Which church do you attend? What are your religious holidays?
3. Race	None	
4. Military status	Have you ever served in the Armed Forces? Did you receive any experience/training relating to this position?	In what branch of the military did you serve? What type of discharge did you receive?
5. Sexual identification	Have you worked or attended school under another name?	Are you male or female? Have you ever been married?
6. Family status	Do you have any responsibilities that conflict with job attendance or travel requirements? (If you ask this, you must ask it of all applicants.)	Are you married? What is your spouse's name? What is your maiden name? Do you have any children? Are you pregnant? What are your child-care arrangements?

made. Applicants may also take a urine test to determine substance use or abuse. Audiological practices often operate in proximity to other healthcare providers. It is detrimental to the practice's reputation if an employee or associate is suspected or caught abusing substances illegally in the medical environment (Hosford-Dunn et al, 1995).

If formal testing is used, it is a good strategy to test with the least expensive tests first. If an applicant fails one of the less expensive tests, the evaluation process can stop before unnecessary expenses are incurred (Paulson & Layton, 1995; Whiting, 1994).

When the interview is completed, the interviewee should be given a chance to ask questions. These are often just as informative as their formal responses. One difficult question to answer involves salary. Early in the search process, it may be more productive to ask: "How much money are you looking for?" At the conclusion of the interview, you may want to provide serious candidates with a ballpark salary range. Always thank the applicant and document the highlights of the interview (Whiting, 1994).

It is not uncommon for applicants who have not been offered a position to call back just to confirm the decision. In these cases, it is important to tell them that somebody else was selected "whose background and qualifications more closely matched our requirements." Telling them why they were not hired or answering questions about what they could have done differently or better may expose the organization

to litigation if the applicant perceives discrimination (Paulson & Layton, 1995; Whiting, 1994).

Selecting the Candidate

When the top candidates have been selected, the most promising prospect is generally brought in for a final interview. This is the final opportunity to make sure that the candidate is the right person for the position. Whiting (1994) suggests that this is the time to fully describe the job to the applicant. This "job preview" presents the applicant with a realistic description of the job situation, including any positive and negative aspects. The applicant should have a good understanding of the positive attributes of the organization and its mission, the importance of the job to the organization, and how their background and qualifications qualify them for the position. They also need to know to whom they will be reporting, their advancement opportunities, and any fringe benefits. In this way the potential employee understands the terms and benefits of employment.

A tentative salary and benefit package may be presented. However, the position might not be formally offered until a few days after the interview. The final interview is designed to provide just enough information to ensure that the candidate can make an informed judgment about the position's desirability. Making that judgment should take some time. Moreover, the organization has a psychological advantage if they are seen as having other selection options (Hosford-Dunn et al, 1995). Making an offer at the final interview may show desperation and decrease the perceived value of the offer. Tway (1992) suggests making the offer 24 hours after the final interview if all goes well.

SPECIAL CONSIDERATION

Firing an employee is traumatic for both the organization and the employee. Keeping an employee who is not producing is demoralizing to employees who are dedicated and work hard. No manager who has gone through firing an employee is capricious in how he or she chooses new employees. Hire well.

Compensation levels vary from one community to another and also according to current market conditions. The practice must determine the current market conditions and make an appropriate offer. Additional negotiations are not uncommon before the practice and the candidate agree to a final package (Hosford-Dunn et al, 1995).

Once the applicant accepts the offer of employment, the employer is required under federal law to check for alien status (Hosford-Dunn et al, 1995; Whiting, 1994). The new employee must complete a form I-9 (employment eligibility verification.) Depending on the employee's citizenship status, the new employee must either demonstrate proof of U.S. citizenship, or provide one or more of the following: (1) a certification of naturalization, (2) an alien registration card, or (3) a current Immigration and Naturalization Service (INS) employment authorization with proper passport identification, depending on immigration status. A list of acceptable documents for establishing identity and/or employment eligibility is shown in Table 6–7. In addition, the employer must establish the employee's tax status. For federal and state income taxes, this is determined from the employee's responses on the IRS W-4 form. The organization will also need to determine Social Security, Medicare, Federal Unemployment, and State Unemployment withholding. The organization's accountant will help set up the employee's tax and benefit withholding.

Orientation Period

In many organizations the first few months of employment are described as a "probationary period." The implication is that the employee is being evaluated during this period and may be discharged if performance is unsatisfactory. Many human resource specialists advocate against this term because it implies that employment-at-will status will change after the employee finishes the probationary period (Whiting, 1994). Rather than placing an employee on "probation," they suggest providing an "Orientation Period." The orientation period focuses on developing the new employee, without implying a promise of "permanent" employment after the period has passed.

The goal of the orientation period is to familiarize the new employee to the organization with the responsibilities of their position. This starts with an explanation of the values and mission statement of the organization (Whiting, 1994). Every other aspect of the organization should be presented in terms of how each relates to the mission of the organization. Under-

standing the values and mission of the organization will help new members approach their job tasks in a way that is congruent with the current objectives of the organization.

The orientation process starts on the first day. A number of administrative topics must be covered early in the process. These include an orientation to payroll practices, company policies and procedures, the daily routine, employee relation's policies, and employee benefits (Whiting, 1994). In healthcare settings, additional information may be disseminated. These include infection control procedures, OSHA safety programs, and procedures for dealing with medical emergencies if medically frail patients are to be seen (Hofkosh, 1975; Lubinski, 1994; Zapala, 1996). No employee can assimilate all this information at once, and some will not ask many questions. This information should be in written form so that the employee can refer to specific areas as needed (Paulson & Layton, 1995).

Orientation procedures must also clearly define the vital processes and outcomes for which the employee is responsible and any quality indicators that may be used to measure job performance. Examples may include audiologist's ratings on patient satisfaction surveys, length of time per evaluation, or number of hearing aid returns per number sold. Careful orientation procedures help maintain employee's confidence, communicate and reinforce practice policies and procedures, and address positive and negative behavior. Employee confidence and satisfaction will increase as the knowledge of the job expectations is communicated and reinforced (Hosford-Dunn et al, 1995; Welch & Fowler, 1994.)

Many organizations provide a mentor to the new employee early in the orientation process. The mentor's role is to help the new employee in his or her new surroundings and answer simple questions in the absence of the supervisor. Mentors also help demonstrate the performance expectations of the organization. For example, new audiologists may need help formatting reports and correspondence or determining when clinical policy may call for a specific evaluation or referral. Most of these issues should be addressed in a protocol manual to ensure uniformity of quality service across practitioners (see next section on staff training). Nevertheless such manuals cannot address all the contingencies that might be encountered in clinical practice. In these cases the judgment of an experienced clinician can go a long way in promoting clinical skill and audiologist confidence.

Occasionally, it becomes apparent that the new employee is not well suited to the tasks of his or her position. In these cases it is better to let the employee go early in the orientation process (Hosford-Dunn et al, 1995; Whiting, 1994). Discharging a marginal employee well past the orientation period is more stressful because he or she has acclimatized to the job.

Developing and Retaining a Competent Staff

An audiologist can practice from several different venues. Moreover, one of the attractions of a career in audiology is the fact that it is dynamic and growing. Consequently, an audiologist's skills and the venues from which one may practice are in constant evolution and development. Continued training and education, both self and organization directed, is vital to developing and maintaining a competent audiology

TABLE 6–7   List of acceptable documents for establishing identity and/or employment eligibility

LIST A Documents that Establish Both Identity and Employment Eligibility	LIST B Documents that Establish Identity	LIST C Documents that Establish Employment Eligibility
1. U.S. passport (unexpired or expired) 2. Certificate of U.S. citizenship (INS Form N-560 or N-561) 3. Certificate of naturalization (INS Form N-550 or N-570) 4. Unexpired foreign passport, with 1-551 stamp or attached INS Form 1-94 indicating unexpired employment authorization 5. Alien registration receipt card with photograph 6. Unexpired temporary resident card (INS Form 1-688) 7. Unexpired employment authorization card (INS Form I-68BA) 8. Unexpired reentry permit (INS Form 1-327) 9. Unexpired refugee travel document (INS Form 1-571) 10. Unexpired employment authorization document issued by the INS that contains a photograph (INS Form 1-6888)	1. Driver's license or ID card issued by a state or outlying possession of the United States provided it contains a photograph or information such as name, date of birth, sex, height, eye color, and address 2. ID card issued by federal, state, or local government agencies or entities provided it contains a photograph or information such as name, date of birth, sex, height, eye color, and address 3. School ID card with a photograph 4. Voter's registration card 5. U.S. military card or draft record 6. Military dependent's ID card 7. U.S. Coast Guard Merchant Mariner Card 8. Native American tribal document 9. Driver's license issued by a Canadian government authority For persons less than age 18 who are unable to present a document listed above: 10. School record or report card 11. Clinic, doctor, or hospital record 12. Day-care or nursery school record	1. U.S. social security card issued by the Social Security Administration (other than a card stating it is not valid for employment) 2. Certification of birth abroad issued by the Department of State (Form FS-545 or Form os-1350) 3. Original or certified copy of a birth certificate issued by a state, county, municipal authority, or outlying possession of the United States bearing an official seal 4. Native American tribal document 5. U.S. citizen ID card (INS Form 1-197) 6. ID card for use of resident citizen in the United States (INS Form I-179) 7. Unexpired employment authorizsation document issued by the INS (other than those listed under List A)

Employee must show item from list A or any combination from list B and C. (Taken from INS, Form I–9 [rev. 11-21-91].)

staff. The obligation of the audiologist to maintain a regimen for self-development was addressed earlier in this chapter. This section will focus on the organization's interest in the development of a competent staff.

From a service organization's point of view, survival depends on the ability to consistently deliver high-quality services as cost-effectively as possible (Hosford-Dunn et al, 1995; Jandt, 1990). Audiological services are delivered within the context of an audiologist/patient relationship. Consequently, consistently delivering a high-quality service requires that individual audiologists within the organization hold to a common standard of quality for each service delivered.

Moreover, as professionals, most audiologists recognize the obligation to contribute to the mission of the organization by seeking to enhance the quality and efficiency of the services they provide through the organization. Thus the organization must have some system to coordinate and train new audiologists to meet existing quality standards and to foster innovations that improve quality or efficiency. (For full discussion of this topic, see Chapter 4 in this volume.)

Training to Meet Existing Requirements

The first step in developing a competent audiological staff occurs when the organization hires the best applicants. Once hired, the new audiologist learns the administrative aspects of the position as described previously. Orientation to the technical and clinical aspects of a practice may require more time. Audiology is very equipment dependent. Larger clinics may have several different pieces of equipment that accomplish the same task (for example, there may be more than one type of auditory-evoked potential system). Clinical information management systems have increased in both complexity and power with the integration of newer computer systems (Jacobson, 1994). Thus the orientation process must result in proficiency in the use of clinical equipment, clinical test techniques, assessment protocols for various patient types (basic comprehensive examinations, tinnitus and balance assessments, infant and pediatric assessments, etc.), and the information management system for audiological services (documentation of clinical encounters, test forms, reports and letters to referral sources, outcome assessment results, billing, scheduling, etc.).

In large clinics the orientation to the technical and clinical aspects of practice is formalized (Zapala, 1996). First, most facilities have protocols established for each test or test battery used by the clinic. In most cases each test protocol documents the applicable patient selection criteria, the data collection method, reporting procedure, and expected cross checks. An example protocol is shown in Table 6–8. The formal process of assessing competency begins with an initial skills assessment. Here the new audiologist demonstrates that he or she has the skill to perform each test by either performing the test under supervision or showing that he or she performed the test in the past at an appropriate level of competence. An example form for cataloging clinical skills is shown in Appendix C at the end of the chapter.

Once clinical skills are cataloged, a personal plan for development is established. It identifies deficits in the audiologist's clinical armamentarium and prioritizes which skills should be developed first. This process need not be restricted to new audiologists. Many clinics have established these systems as part of a yearly performance appraisal and some accreditation agencies such as the Joint Commission for the Accreditation of Healthcare Organizations require yearly competency evaluations. The value of the yearly evaluation goes beyond satisfying external requirements. A yearly evaluation helps focus the audiologist and the organization on the long-term development of the individual, the organization, and the profession. Further recognition of formal mastery helps bolster the sense of accomplishment of the individual and identifies potential mentors for other less experienced staff members. Finally, if a career ladder is to be developed (e.g., recognition of a senior audiologist with mastery of a wide range of skills), formal assessment of competency is invaluable.

Clinical Case Staffing

The ability to perform a test does not necessarily imply good patient care. Audiological patient care involves the diagnosis and management of auditory-based functional deficits, patient education, and the art of directing patients to act in their own best interests. Within this context, accurate test performance comprises a small part of clinical practice. How does one evaluate or, more importantly, enhance patient care abilities? One tool is the practice of case staffing. Case staffing is a peer review process in which an audiologist formally presents a case and seeks advice from colleagues (see Table 6–2). Assessment choices, treatment plans, and outcomes are discussed. If necessary, literature reviews and outside mentors are consulted to improve the breadth of the learning experience. The peers award the presenting audiologist a score for the quality of the patient care provided. Each audiologist maintains a casebook documenting every case presented and the peer-awarded score. At the end of the year, this information is also used to establish the audiologist's competency. The expectation is that every year the casebook will document how the audiologist is managing cases of increasing complexity with improving outcomes.

Three advantages exist to staffing cases formally.

1. Accomplishment in some of the aspects of patient care is documented for accreditation purposes. This is a necessary task in some practice environments but is not an adequate justification for the practice.

2. Second benefit is seen in critical self-examination and accountability that naturally follows from holding oneself accountable for clinical outcomes.

3. Finally, all the participants learn to think in terms of quality care and patient outcomes and come to consensus about what constitutes quality patient care. In this sense, staffing can be a real team-building activity.

Staffing is difficult to do when interpersonal relationships are not open and honest in the office. Ideally, one chooses to staff those cases that were problematic. Lack of trust or respect among staff members can lead to personal attacks during staffings. This must be strongly discouraged. The ethic should be that case presentations are a professional exercise. Personal differences should be left at the door. Thus to use this important tool, a professional culture conducive to this activity must prevail within the organization. The concept of the professional culture will be discussed in the following section.

Performance Appraisal

Performance appraisal can refer to two separate processes. In the first an individual's performance is monitored and constructive feedback is given with the goal of improving performance. This is the leadership function that optimally

TABLE 6–8 Example clinical protocol

Department of Audiology				
			THIS	REPLACES
☐ Administrative		INDEX:	Tech27765	
✗ Technical			DPOAE	
☐ Office Procedure		DATE:	01/30/96	
		PAGE:	1 of 2	

ORIGINATOR	Chief of Audiology
SUBJECT	Procedure 27765 DPOAE Infant Hearing Screen
PURPOSE	To detect hearing impairments greater than 40 dB HL in newborns that may significantly impede natural speech, language, and cognitive development.
PATIENT SELECTION	Newborns and infants less than 6 months of age who are at low risk for central forms of hearing hearing loss and are able to rest quietly for the screening procedure.
PROTOCOL	1. Instrument: GSI 60 DPOAE system.
	2. Data: Distortion product otoacoustic emissions are obtained from primaries at 1500, 2000, 3000, and 4000 Hz (geometric mean frequency.) L1-L2 = 65- to 55-dB SPL in the earcanal, F_1/F_2 ratio = 1.2. Maximum permissible earcanal level in the region of the expected primary is 15 dB peak SPL. A minimum of 60 frames must be averaged. A DP is present when the SNR is + 13 dB.
	3. Method: The earcanal is inspected and a probe inserted such that no acoustic leak from the earcanal and no evidence of an occluded probe port are present. Either a sequential or simultaneous presentation mode is acceptable.
	4. Validation: Either by cross check or retest.
REPORTING	"Pass" = Three of four expected DPs detected with amplitudes > −5 dB SPL in at least one ear. "Refer" = Any nonpass test.
EXPECTED CROSS CHECKS	None as a screening procedure.
ADDITIONAL CROSS CHECKS	TEOAEs, ABR, tympanometry if middle ear effusion suspected.

Alterations in protocol or reporting must be documented on screening form with explanation of how procedures varied and why alteration was neccessary.

instructs, motivates, and directs the activities of employees. Optimal ongoing performance appraisals correct deficit performance while leaving employees feeling that they have self-direction, they are competent, and they are contributing to a worthy goal (Byham & Cox, 1988). More often than not, it is these feelings that lead to employee commitment and longevity (Labovitz & Rosansky, 1997).

PEARL

Correct errors in private with prior warning and reward in public with prior announcement.

The second type of performance appraisal is more problematic. In larger organizations a yearly performance appraisal process is often tied to merit-based pay increases (Hofkosh, 1975). Giving merit raises on the basis of performance may make intuitive sense. However, some see problems with this type of reward system. W. E. Demming, a leader in the total quality movement, believes such appraisals are devastating to organization performance and individual achievement (Walton, 1986). The problem, in Demming's view, is that in most organizations most of the factors that affect individual performance are beyond the control of the individual. Rather, they reflect problems in the process or systems that underpin performance. This is not to say that individuals do not make choices and are sometimes not productive. Rather, the focus should be on ensuring that employees are properly trained and are in an environment that promotes quality before too much focus is placed on individual ability.

It is not always obvious how to improve systems or processes, particularly when the processes have not changed in several years. One method of determining whether a process can be improved is by "benchmarking for best practices." The concept behind benchmarking is simple. An organization, in this case an audiology department, compares its productivity against other departments with similar circumstance. If areas exist in which the audiology department's performance does not compare favorably, a process or system may need to be improved. Benchmarking is a way of identifying what is possible for an organization. However, it should not be used to define what individuals can do unless all process issues have been solved. For further discussion of benchmarking, see Chapter 4 in this volume.

Individual performance appraisals are a fact of life for many audiologists. Those that are performed well help the audiologist see personal growth opportunities and new development challenges. Constant feedback about growth and performance on a daily basis are key to ensuring that performance appraisals are a positive experience. If a surprise deficit area is seen on an annual performance review, the supervisory and leadership process has failed (Delbecq, 1985; Walton, 1986). Barring unforeseen surprises, the evaluation should review the employee's abilities and performance (which should be readily apparent from their case book); adherence to the value system of the organization; growth over the year; and areas of weakness or areas where new skills can be obtained.

When Performance Flounders

Discipline is the process used to train, correct, and mold behavior. It is the basis for giving continued feedback to employees about their performance. Whiting (1994) identifies two types of discipline. Negative discipline emphasizes punishment for breaking rules. Positive discipline assumes that employees are adults who have self-respect and a desire do what is expected of them. As long as a rule has been communicated to such employees and that rule is perceived to be reasonable, employees will generally obey the rule (Jandt, 1990).

When performance flounders, the supervisor should first assess whether a problem exists with a procedure or the knowledge base of the employee (Byham & Cox, 1988; Jandt, 1990). If this is the case, retraining or redesigning the work process should solve the problem. If this is not the case and the employee repeatedly demonstrates that he or she will not change inappropriate work behaviors, formal corrective action is required.

For corrective action to be effective, employees must first know what is expected of them and why. Policies, procedures, rules, and regulations must be communicated to employees, preferably in writing. Furthermore, employees must believe that the expectations of the organization are reasonable. Consequently, it is important that employees understand why the policies and procedures are in place (Jandt, 1990; Whiting, 1994).

Traditionally, corrective action has been based on the concept of progressive discipline (Delbecq, 1985; Jandt, 1990; Whiting, 1994). Typically four levels of progressive discipline exist: verbal warnings, written warnings, suspension, and discharge. In general, the first time an employee commits a minor rule violation, a friendly reminder or warning is all that is necessary. A written warning is given to an employee who commits a more serious violation or who fails to improve after repeated verbal warnings. Written warnings should contain the following information:

- The reason for the disciplinary action
- Date of the disciplinary action
- Action to be taken
- Description of the incident causing the disciplinary action
- What will happen if the employee violates the rule again
- What the employee agrees to do to correct his or her behavior
- A place for the employee to sign and date the form
- A place for the supervisor to sign and date the form

Written warnings should be placed in the employee's personnel file.

Suspension, with or without pay, is usually reserved for employees who commit very serious violations of the rules or have committed repeated violations with written warnings. Whiting (1994) recommends that it is wise to have more than one manager in the meeting where the suspension is given, and it is desirable to suspend with pay. Suspending without pay seldom results in improved performance. The employee should be charged with deciding whether he or she wants to return to work the following day. The employee should understand that everyone must follow the rules and no exception will be given. If the employee decides to stay after this type of ultimatum, it is more likely that he or she will attempt to be compliant.

The final step in progressive discipline is discharge. A constructive discharge occurs when management creates a situation in which the employee is not able to exercise free choice when deciding whether to resign. In some cases a constructive discharge leaves the employee eligible for benefits that he or she may not obtain if fired (Whiting, 1994).

Before offering a constructive discharge or terminating an employee, the following questions should be addressed:

- Was there a written rule regulation covering the type of activity for which the employee is being discharged?
- Was the employee informed about these rules and regulations, either through written or verbal communications?
- Have these rules been administered in a fair and consistent manner?
- Is there adequate written documentation in the form of written disciplinary actions to support the discharge?
- Has there been a fair investigation of the facts surrounding the case to ensure that you were aware of all of a possible circumstances?
- Has the employee been presented with an opportunity to present his or her side of the story?
- Have the employee's past record and time of service been considered?
- Is it fair to the organization and the employee to terminate employment?
- Would it seem fair to a judge?

If all nine questions can be answered yes, the employee should probably be discharged. Whenever possible, it is best to review each case with the personnel department or a consulting HR specialist to ensure that no legal exposure to the termination is present. Employees should be paid for all of hours worked up until the time they are terminated. They also have a right to continue their group insurance under Consolidated Omnibus Budget Reconciliation Act of 1986 (COBRA) as long as they are not discharged for gross misconduct (e.g., theft, fraud, embezzlement, physical assault, etc.).

If it is determined that an employee should be discharged, the supervisor should conduct a discharge interview. Whiting (1994) recommends that at least two managers or, in small practices, the owner and an unbiased witness be present for the interview. The interview should last no more than 2 or 3 minutes. The supervisor should explain that it is necessary to terminate the employee and briefly give the reason why. The procedure for obtaining the final paycheck should be explained. The employee should be escorted to his or her work area to clean up the desk and then escorted to the door. It is good form to wish them well in the future. Most discharged employees are not bad people. They were simply hired for the wrong job. Nevertheless, firing an employee is traumatic for both the organization and the employee. No manager who has gone through this process is capricious in how he or she chooses new employees.

OWNERSHIP OF THE PROFESSION

A saying exists that "all ships rise at high tide." The meaning is simple: When times are good, everyone prospers, so all have an obligation to work for good times. The same principle applies to Audiology. Audiology is both a discipline and a profession. Both require good stewardship. All audiologists and hearing scientists have an obligation to support the development of the discipline and the profession for the sake of the hearing impaired and the future of the profession. The following sections suggest ways in which the practitioner can support both the profession and the discipline.

Minding the Discipline

The profession of audiology is founded on the bedrock of basic and applied science. A healthy scientific discipline provides the theories that underpin new understandings of clinical problems and new treatments (Minghetti, 1994). Audiologists are well trained in the scientific underpinnings of the profession in graduate school. In practice, a strong background in clinical research is essential to the evaluation of new technologies and clinical methods that inevitably evolve. Without this knowledge, clinicians might become overly influenced by manufacturer's claims and profit margins rather than the best clinical evidence and optimum clinical outcomes. So the first obligation to the profession is to keep current in the scientific discipline that underpins the profession.

A second way to help maintain a healthy scientific discipline is to support those individuals and institutions that contribute to the discipline. This may include lobbying for increased funding from the National Institutes of Health or simply helping to enroll subjects in a graduate student's research project. Collaborations between clinicians and researchers are vital for both groups. Clinicians benefit from the repeated exposure to basic science practices. Researchers benefit from exposure to common clinical problems that can be better managed with new data, information, or theory.

Ultimately, no gulf should exist between researcher and clinician. In fact, many have argued for a clinician/researcher as one person, whereas others are just as adamant that the two cannot be joined. (See Minghetti et al [1993] for a recent treatment of this old issue.) This issue is too broad to address in detail here. However, the important consideration from an HR perspective is our own expectation. Few would disagree that more research may result in systematic improvements in the quality of service delivered by clinicians (Goldberg, 1991). A clear need exists for continued research, strong theory development, and improved clinical methods. What does this mean for our expectations of ourselves as academicians or as practitioners? If the need is so great, perhaps we should look toward different, more efficient collaborative models between researchers and practitioners to meet the need. As the profession moves toward a formal professional doctorate, more will be expected of practitioners in the way of clinical research. But we should not wait for this to happen. All of us as owners of the profession share the responsibility to our patients to promote the art and science of audiology. We should always look for ways to innovate, collaborate, and share our knowledge with others.

Developing the Profession

Unlike a discipline, which can be understood from a completely scholarly viewpoint, a profession is defined within the context of the marketplace. From this perspective, the profession is the translation of the knowledge base of the discipline into goods or services that are valued by the market. Following the definition in *The American Heritage Dictionary of the English Language* (1996), two attributes are commonly ascribed to a "profession." First, the market perceives that part of the value of an individual practitioner's goods or services is a by-product of considerable training and specialized study. Second, the market perceives that all practitioners of the profession have a common identity, share a common level of training and study, and offer a high minimum level of quality in the goods or services offered.

Professional status offers several advantages to its members. First, individual practitioners share the market's value of their services without each individual first developing a reputation. Second, professions are more able to capture markets because they can promote the relationship between their group identity and the value of their goods or services. Third, following the saying that: "all ships rise at high tide," the group affiliation that is part of professional status allows members to work as a group to promote common interests. As such, they truly become a human resource.

The value of professional status is determined by market perceptions. Consequently, professionals invest in efforts that enhance value of their services in the market and promote the association between high value and professional affiliation. These activities are often accomplished through professional organizations.

Professional organizations perform at least one of three core functions. These core functions are as follows.

1. Facilitate the development and dissemination of new knowledge to their membership
2. Self-police by establishing guidelines for entry into the profession and determination of what is and what is not acceptable professional practice
3. Protect the interests and enhance the position of the profession within the marketplace

Facilitating the development and dissemination of new knowledge to their membership helps the profession develop more efficient and effective goods and services. Self-policing helps maintain the quality of goods and services provided by the profession. Both these functions enhance the perceived value of the profession within the market. Protecting the interests and position of the profession within the marketplace involves ensuring that the market has optimum exposure and access to the profession. All three functions are often accomplished within the same organization. So, for example, members of professional audiology organizations (e.g. ASHA, AAA, ADA) may be grappling with the acceptance of a new clinical technique, lobbying for a new licensure law, establishing practice guidelines, promoting the profession to third-party payers, and disciplining a member for an ethics violation.

Except in very restrictive circumstances (such as the Bar Association), membership in a professional organization is voluntary. Achieving the objectives of the organization (and, hopefully, the goals of the profession) requires an investment of financial support, time, effort, and involvement on the part of the membership. Many believe this is a professional obligation (Williams, 1994); particularly in view of the benefits afforded to the practitioner if the organization enhances the perception of the profession of audiology within the marketplace.

Acculturation

Many professions develop a sense of responsibility for participation in the profession through a process of acculturation. In this use of the term acculturation means maintaining a culture among professionals that promotes the health of the profession. For example, most professional schools (medical, legal, and military schools in particular) maintain close relationships with practitioners in the profession. It is not uncommon for practitioners to sponsor social activities with students for the sole purpose of helping new members in training to network. These social activities help the students identify clinical mentors and establish professional bonds that build group cohesion. Later, these relationships promote diplomacy in solving internal controversies, and promote united action when there is an external threat to the profession.

Audiology also has several vehicles for professional acculturation. Both the ASHA and AAA have affiliated student organizations. Most state organizations promote student participation through reduced membership fees and special clinical forums. Individual practitioners support the process by taking students in clinical externship and offering clinical fellowship positions. All of these activities acculturate new members into the profession.

The value of acculturation extends beyond initial entry into the profession. Audiologists often compete with each

---

PEARL

Acculturation promotes diplomacy in solving internal controversies and united action when an external threat to the profession is present. Because these are vital to the survival of the profession, each member is responsible for developing collegial interpersonal relationships with other members of the profession.

---

other in professional practice. Competition can be a positive influence in that the search for a competitive advantage can lead to improvements in service delivery. Competition can also have a negative effect when the importance of maintaining a healthy profession gives way to issues of commerce. When competitive pressures break down professional relationships, the parties are trading the future of the profession for short-term gain. This is never a good trade.

By working to build positive relationships and sharing innovations with colleagues, the overall knowledge base of the profession grows. Furthermore, when outside forces threaten the professional prerogatives of audiology, members are more likely to become involved for the common good. One approach to promote this type of collegiality is taken by the American College of Surgeons. Fellowship in

---

TABLE 6–9 American College of Surgeons Fellowship Pledge

Fellowship Pledge

Recognizing that the American College of Surgeons seeks to exemplify and develop the highest traditions of our ancient profession, I hereby pledge myself, as a condition of Fellowship in the College, to live in strict accordance with its principles and regulations.

I pledge myself to pursue the practice of surgery with honesty and to place the welfare and the rights of my patient above all else. I promise to deal with each patient as I would wish to be dealt with if I were in the patient's position, and I will set my fees commensurate with the services rendered. I will take no part in any arrangement, such as fee splitting or itinerant surgery, which induces referral or treatment for reason other than the patient's best welfare.

Upon my honor, I declare that I will advance my knowledge and skills, will respect my colleagues, and will seek their counsel when in doubt about my own abilities. In turn, I will willingly help my colleagues when requested.

Finally, I solemnly pledge myself to cooperate in advancing and extending the art and science of surgery by my Fellowship in the American College of Surgeons.

Fellowship Pledge, American College of Surgeons. No Date. Reproduced with permission.

this prestigious organization requires that the potential members subscribe to the Fellowship Pledge, which is shown in Table 6–9.

By subscribing to this oath, the American College of Surgeons promotes an ethic of placing the patient and the profession ahead of commerce. This ethic creates a heritage or standard that ensures the health of the profession. Perhaps audiology should develop a similar pledge.

The vehicle for most professional relationships within audiology is our professional organizations. These groups serve as coordinators of our human resources. They help organize and act in ways that are in our own professional interest. However, it is not the organization's responsibility to meet the needs of the profession. Rather, it is the membership—the professionals who make up the profession—who have the ultimate responsibility. Yet, participation in these organizations is less than optimal, particularly at the state and local levels. Many reasons for this exist, and a full treatment of the topic is beyond the scope of this chapter. However, a very real cost is present with low participation levels. Most state level organizations, the very organizations that address licensure and other right-to-practice legislation, have meager membership rosters. This means a small group of dedicated audiologists are expected to do the work of the profession. The need to participate in state level organizations simply to develop and protect audiology's expanding scope of practice continues. No one else will protect our interests in our absence.

CONCLUSIONS

This chapter has dealt with HR issues from a very broad prospective. On the microlevel, audiology is a high-technology endeavor. Successful practice requires that the individual master complex assessment and management tools. However, we are about human perception and communication.

CONTROVERSIAL POINT

Most issues involving the right to practice, such as licensure, scope of practice, minimum qualifications to practice, and, increasingly, provider reimbursment issues, are decided on the state level. Yet membership in state professional organizations is low relative to national organizations. It may be wiser to invest more in state organizations to promote changes at the state level than to expect national organizations to influence decisions that are decided at the state level.

Our contribution is not our machinery. Rather, the difference between a good audiology practice and a great practice is the "high touch" or "human factor." Wise stewardship is necessary to capitalize on the human potential of our profession. As professionals, we are responsible for our own development and the promotion of our discipline and profession. Without this, we cannot maintain our fiduciary responsibilities to our patients. It is hoped that this chapter has presented some principles that will aid in this endeavor.

On a macro level, audiology is a young, growing profession. As we mature, we will face many issues and threats, both internal and external, that will impact our long-term future. It will become increasingly important for us to develop and maintain a cohesive group culture. This starts with an ethic that promotes the development of the profession and discipline, places the patient and the profession before commerce, reinforces respect for colleagues, and promotes coordinated action to advance the initiatives of the profession and those it would serve.

Appendix A
Example Audiologist
Job Description

JOB TITLE: Audiologist
DEPARTMENT: Audiology-Hearing and Balance Center
SUPERVISOR: Director of Audiology

JOB SUMMARY: The audiologist is responsible for evaluating, treating, and counseling with the pediatric, adult, or geriatric patient with hearing disorders in accordance with professional and corporate quality standards. Models appropriate behavior as exemplified in corporate value system and the operating mission, which reflects commitment to total quality improvement.

JOB FUNCTIONS (major and minor duties)

1. *Conducts* hearing and balance evaluations for inpatients and outpatients, including neonates, pediatric patients, adolescents, adults, and geriatric patients, and *assesses* the history, medical diagnosis, social, and communicative condition of the patient through testing and interview to establish a basis for patient treatment (type I services).

   A. Through history, interview, and formal diagnostic testing, characterizes the perceptual abilities and physiological state of the auditory system in neonatal, pediatric, adult, and geriatric patients.

   B. Understands otologic and neurological diagnostic processes well enough to obtain audiological information that will help the physician distinguish between competing etiological entities in a given patient.

   C. Generates written communications for treating physicians that are timely, clear, and succinct.

   D. Understands the theory behind established clinical protocols and can modify diagnostic procedures to meet the needs of the patient/customer without sacrificing test reliability or validity.

   E. Has expertise in at least two of the following areas and provides inservice and professional training in same: Infant and pediatric audiology, diagnostic audiology, forensic and occupational audiology, amplification and aural rehabilitation, balance and spatial orientation.

   F. Provides all services with a caring, empathetic manner, holding to the highest professional, ethical, and legal standards.

2. *Determines* patient's perceptual and communicative needs and *formulates, implements, and measures* the efficacy of an audiological rehabilitation treatment plan (type II service).

   A. Interprets the results of hearing evaluation data within the context of the patient's perceptual, social, and communicative needs, identifies deficit areas; and communicates this information clearly to the patient as the first step in rehabilitation

   B. Together with the patient and significant others develops a rational treatment and monitoring plan, including the use of amplification, assistive listening devices, aural rehabilitation, and counseling as indicated.

   C. Demonstrates knowledge of current amplification technologies, fitting practices, and validation procedures

   D. Monitors treatment effectiveness and modifies treatment plans when necessary for optimal treatment outcomes.

   E. Develops and assesses impact of family-based education to facilitate carryover of new skills into everyday environments.

3. Together with other audiology staff members, *develops* methods to identify hearing-impaired patients in the hospital and community and *facilitates* community awareness of hearing impairment and its management (type III service).

   A. Uses basic and advanced diagnostic technologies to screen the hearing of at-risk populations.

   B. Develops and maintains data management systems to facilitate efficient follow-up of at risk patients.

   C. Presents information within the community to promote awareness of hearing impairment and its management.

   D. Participates in studies designed to assess the effectiveness of hearing screening programs.

   E. Develops new methods and systems to promote hearing healthcare within the hospital and community.

4. *Promotes* professional practice of all members of the departmental care team.

   A. Supports the team concept among all staff; participates in mutual problem solving to achieve positive outcomes and improve quality of services; documents incidents of critical nature; participates in departmental meetings.

   B. Demonstrates initiative in identifying opportunities for self-development and enhancement of professional competency through self-study, on-the-job training, and attending professional meetings.

C. Demonstrates effective customer relations skills, promotes a positive work environment, and contributes to the overall team effort.

D. Participates in quality monitoring and evaluation activities and implements measures to ensure hospital, JCAHO, and other quality standards are met.

E. Works together with audiology, other department staff, and administration in sharing and giving information and support as needed in a manner of dignity, respect, and helpfulness as exemplified in the corporate value system, total quality improvement process (TQI), and the organization mission statement.

5. *Performs* other job functions as needed.

6. *Acts* in a manner consistent with the following value system.

A. Demonstrates dedication to *quality*.
- Makes effort to do each job function correctly.
- Keeps persons informed who should and need to be informed.
- Takes responsibility for problems, questions, or issues and makes effort to solve or get someone who can, rather than passing on the problem.
- Identifies barriers to efficiency and effectiveness in own job, department, or other areas and suggests ways to improve.

B. Demonstrates dedication to fairness.
- Treats others with dignity and respect.
- Promotes cooperation and teamwork among co-workers.
- Works and behaves in a manner that does not create problems or provoke negative reactions from others.
- Demonstrates support of corporate and department policies to ensure consistency of impact on others.

C. Demonstrates dedication to customer service (internal or external).
- Provides quick service.
- Is polite in interactions, which includes body language and tone of voice.
- Demonstrates a concerned and caring attitude.
- Communicates needed information to those who need to know.
- Provides clean environment that gives appearance of professionalism.
- Provides a quiet atmosphere by low-key interactions demonstrating a professional demeanor in the work unit and in any affiliated facility.
- Takes initiative to offer assistance when needed.
- Takes initiative to coach fellow associates to appreciate and demonstrate customer-focused behaviors.
- Goes beyond the specific demands of his or her job to serve the customer better.
- Stays focused on the customer as long as needed.

D. Demonstrates dedication to integrity.
- Is honest in all interactions.
- Demonstrates a work ethic that is exemplified by reporting to work on time; not taking excessive breaks; working until end of shift; and not wasting time.
- Is honest in timecard and time off reporting.
- Reports own errors to correct problems and develop trust.
- Demonstrates behavior that is consistent with the ASHA and AAA Code of Ethics.

PERSONAL CONTACTS

Internal: The audiologist has daily contact with associates, supervisors, and managers in audiology, in other areas of rehabilitation services, and in other hospital departments, such as nursing floors.

External: The audiologist has daily contact with physicians, patients, patients' family members.

Supervision given: Lead responsibilities are to direct and to monitor performance of audiometric technicians as assigned by director.

Physical demands/conditions: Exposure to patient body fluids; ability to react quickly to emergency situations; ability to read and write to communicate both orally and in writing with other individuals; normal vision, including peripheral vision; occasional travel within the region; some lifting of equipment weighing up to 35 lb.

MINIMUM QUALIFICATIONS

1. A. Possession of a current license to practice in the state of Tennessee as an audiologist (master's degree required for licensure).

   B. Possession of current certificate of clinical competence in audiology from the American Speech-Language-Hearing Association, or current Board Certification from the American Academy of Audiology or equivalent.

2. Knowledge of audiology methods and techniques in two or more of the following areas (2 years' experience desirable): industrial audiology; pediatric audiology, including hearing aid fitting, aural rehabilitation, and community-based programming; infant hearing assessment, including otoacoustic emissions and evoked potentials; educational audiology, including assessment and management of auditory language/learning disabled (CAP) children; advanced differential diagnostic testing of otologic and neurological patients; assessment of spatial orientation, including ENG, rotational tests, posturography, and behavioral assessment.

3. Ability to understand and prepare moderately complex written materials, such as patient records.

4. Prepared by education, training, or experience to work with the adult, geriatric, pediatric, or neonatal patient.

5. Ability to communicate verbally with Associates, physicians, and other outside professionals.

6. Ability to work without close supervision and to exercise independent judgment.

7. Ability to organize multiple tasks and projects and maintain control of work flow.

Appendix B
State Speech-Language Pathology and Audiology Regulatory Agencies and State Regulatory Agencies for Hearing Aid Dispensing

B1. The following is a listing of the agencies that regulate speech-language pathologists and audiologists through state licensure, certification, or registration. In some states, different boards regulate the dispensing of hearing aids. Please see Appendix B2: State Regulatory Agencies for Hearing Aid Dispensing for all information regarding state regulation of hearing aid dispensing.

Alaska
Division of Occupational Licensing
(applies only to audiologists)
P.O. Box 110806
Juneau, AK 99811-0806
(907) 465-2695
(907) 465-2974 (Fax)

Alabama
Alabama Board of Examiners for Speech Pathology
and audiology
400 S. Union Street
Montgomery, AL 36104
(334) 269-1434
(334) 409-0680 (Fax)

Arkansas
Arkansas Board of Examiners in Speech Pathology
and Audiology
101 East Capitol, Suite 211
Little Rock, AR 72201
(501) 682-9180
(501) 682-9181 (Fax)

Arizona
Audiologists and Speech-Language Pathologists
Licensing Program
1647 East Morten Avenue, Suite 160
Phoenix, AZ 85020
(602) 255-1177 ext. 4307
(602) 255-1109

California
Speech Pathology and Audiology Examining Committee
1434 Howe Avenue, Suite 86
Sacramento, CA 95825-3240
(916) 263-2666
(916) 263- 2668 (Fax)

Colorado (applies only to audiologists)
Audiologists and Hearing Aid Dealers Registration
1560 Broadway, Suite 680
Denver, CO 80202
(303) 894-2464
(303) 894-2821 (Fax)

Connecticut
SLP and Audiology Licensure
Department of Health
P.O. Box 340308
Hartford, CT 06134-0308
(860) 509-7560

Delaware
Board of Audiology, SLPs and HAD
P.O. Box 1401, Cannon Building, Suite 203
Dover, DE 19903
(302) 739-4522, ext. 215
(302) 739-2711 (Fax)

Florida
Board of SLP and Audiology
Department of Health
1940 North Monroe
Tallahassee, FL 32399-0778
(904) 488-0595
(904) 921-5389 (Fax)

Georgia
Georgia Board of Examiners for SLP and Audiology
166 Pryor Street, S.W.
Atlanta, GA 30303-3465
(404) 656-3933
(404) 651-9532 (Fax)

Hawaii
Board of Speech Pathology and Audiology
P.O. Box 3469
Honolulu, HI 96801
(808) 586-2693
(808) 586-2689

Illinois
Illinois Department of Professional Regulations
320 West Washington Street
Springfield, IL 62786
(217) 782-8556
(217) 782-7645 (Fax)

Indiana
Indiana Speech-Language Pathology and Audiology Board
402 West Washington Street, Room 041
Indianapolis, IN 46204
(317) 232-2960 (Applications)
(317) 233-4407 (Director)
(317) 233-4236 (Fax)

Iowa
State Board of SLP and Audiology Examiners
Bureau of Professional Licensure
Lucas State Office Building
4th Floor
Des Moines, IA 50319-0075
(515) 281-4408
(515) 281-3121 (Fax)

Kansas
Speech-Language Pathology/Audiology Advisory Board
109 S.W. 9th Street
Topeka, KS 66612-2218
(913) 296-0056
(913) 296-7025 (Fax)

Kentucky
Board of Examiners of SLP and Audiology
P.O. Box 456
Frankfort, KY 40602
(502) 564-3296 ext. 223
(502) 564-4818 (Fax)

Louisiana
Louisiana Board of Examiners for SLP and Audiology
11930 Perkins Road, Suite B
Baton Rouge, LA 71108
(504) 763-5480
(504) 673-3085 (Fax)

Massachusetts
Board of Registration for Speech-Language Pathology and Audiology
100 Cambridge Street, Room 1513
Boston, MA 02202
(617) 727-1747

Maryland
Maryland Board of Examiners for Audiology, HADs and SLPs
4201 Patterson Avenue
Baltimore, MD 21215
(410) 764-4725
(410) 764-5987 (Fax)

Maine
Board of Examiners on Speech Pathology and Audiology
35 State House Station
Augusta, ME 04333
(207) 624-8603 x48609
(207) 624-8637 (Fax)

Minnesota
Minnesota Department of Health
121 East Seventh Place
P.O. Box 64975
St. Paul, MN 55164-0975
(612) 282-5629
(612) 282-3839 (Fax)

Missouri
Missouri Board of Registration for the Healing Arts
3605 Missouri Boulevard
Jefferson City, MO 65102
(573) 751-0098
(314) 751-3166 (Fax)

Mississippi
Mississippi State Department of Health
Professional Licensure
P.O. Box 1700
Jackson, MS 39215-1700
(601) 987-4153
(601) 987-3784 (Fax)

Montana
Board of SLPs and Audiology
Bureau of Professional Licensing
111 North Jackson Street
Helena, MT 59620
(406) 444-3091
(406) 444-1667 (Fax)

North Carolina
North Carolina Board of Examiners for SLP and Audiology
P.O. Box 16885
Greensboro, NC 27416-0885
(910) 272-1828
(910) 272-4353 (Fax)

North Dakota
Board of Examiners on Audiology and SLP
Bureau of Educational Services and Applied Research
P.O. Box 7189
Grand Forks, ND 58202-7189
(701) 777-4421
(701) 777-4365 (Fax)

Nebraska
Board of Examiners in Audiology and SLP
Department of Health
301 Centennial Mall Street
Lincoln, NE 68509
(402) 471-0547
(402) 471-3577 (Fax)

New Hampshire
Board of Speech Language Pathologists
(only for speech-language pathologists)
2 Industrial Park Drive, Suite 8
Concord, NH 03301-8520
(603) 271-1203
(603) 271-6702 (Fax)

New Hampshire Board of Hearing Care Providers
(includes Audiologists)
Office of Health Planning and Review
6 Hazen Drive
Concord, NH 03301
(603) 271-4604
(603) 271-4141 (Fax)

New Jersey
Audiology and SLP Advisory Committee
New Jersey Division of Consumer Affairs
124 Halsey Street, 6th Floor
Newark, NJ 07102
(201) 504-6390
(201) 648-3355 (Fax)

New Mexico
SLP, Audiology and AUD Practices Board
Regulation and Licensing Department
P.O. Box 25101
Santa Fe, NM 87504
(505) 827-7554, ext. 24
(505) 827-7548 (Fax)

Nevada
Nevada State Board of Examiners for Audiology and Speech
Pathology
P.O. Box 70550
Reno, NV 89570-0550
(702) 857-3500
(702) 857-2121 (Fax)

New York
State Board for SLP and Audiology
Room 3013 CEC
Empire State Plaza
Albany, NY 12230
(518) 473-0221
(518) 473-6995 (Fax)
Web: http://www.nysed.gov/prof/profhome.htm

Ohio
Board of SLP and Audiology
77 South High Street, 16th Floor
Columbus, OH 43266
(614) 466-3145
(614) 644-8112 (Fax)

Oklahoma
State Board Examiners for SLP and Audiology
P.O. Box 53592
Oklahoma City, OK 73152
(405) 840-2774
(405) 840-2774 (Fax)

Oregon
Board of Examiners for SLP and Audiology
800 NE Oregon Street, #21
Portland, OR 97232
(503) 731-4050
(503) 731-4207 (Fax)

Pennsylvania
Board of Examiners in Speech, Language and Hearing
P.O. Box 2649
Harrisburg, PA 17105-2649
(717) 783-1389
(717) 787-7769

Rhode Island
Board of Examiners in SLP and Audiology
Rhode Island Department of Health
3 Capitol Hill, Room 104
Providence, RI 02908-5097
(401) 277-2827
(401) 277-1272 (Fax)

South Carolina
South Carolina Board of Examiners in Speech Pathology
and Audiology
P.O. Box 11329, Suite 101
Columbia, SC 29211
(803) 734-4253
(803) 734-4284 (Fax)

Tennessee
State Board of Communication Disorders and Sciences
Speech Pathology and Audiology
426 5th Avenue N Floor 1
Nashville, TN 37214-1010
(615) 532-5160
(615) 532-5164 (Fax)

Texas
State Board of Examiners for SLP and Audiology
1100 West 49th Street
Austin, TX 78756-3183
(512) 834-6627
(512) 834-6677 (Fax)
Web: http://www.tdh.state.tx.us/hcqs/plc/speech.htm

Utah
Division of Occupational and Professional Licensing
P.O. Box 146741
160 East 300 South
Salt Lake City, UT 84114-6741
(801) 530-6632
(801) 530-6511 (Fax)
Web: http://www.commerce.state.ut.us/web/commerce/dopl/dopl1.htm

Virginia
State Board of Audiology and Speech Pathology
6606 West Broad Street, 4th Floor
Richmond, VA 23230-1717
(804) 662-7390
(804) 662-9943 (Fax)

Washington
Board of Audiology, Speech and Hearing Instrument Fitters
Department of Health
Health Service Unit Two
1300 SE Quince Street
Olympia, WA 98504-7869
(360) 586-0205
(360) 586-7774 (Fax)

Wisconsin
Council on SLP and Audiology
Department of Regulation and Licensing
P.O. Box 8935
Madison, WI 53708-8935
(608) 266-1396
(608) 267-0644 (Fax)

West Virginia
West Virginia Board of Examiners for SLP and Audiology
P.O. Box 854
Dunbar, WV 25064
(304) 766-1096

Wyoming
State Board of Examiners in SLP and Audiology
2020 Carrey Avenue
Suite 201
Cheyenne, WY 82002
(307) 777-7780
(307) 777-3508 (Fax)

B2. This is a listing of state agencies that regulate the dispensing of hearing aids. In some states, hearing aid dispensing by audiologists and nonaudiologists is regulated by the same board. In other states, hearing aid dispensing by these groups is regulated by different boards. This listing is for hearing aid dispensing only. Please see Appendix B1 (State Speech-Language Pathology and Audiology Regulatory Agencies) for state agencies responsible for regulating audiologists and speech-language pathologists.

Alabama
Licensed Audiologists Speech Pathology and Audiology
P.O. Box 20833
Montgomery, AL 36120-0833
(334) 269-1434
(334) 269-1434 (Fax)

Nonaudiologists:
Board of Examiners for Hearing Aid Dealers' Board
Bureau of Healthcare Standards
434 Monroe Street
Montgomery, AL 36130-3017
(334) 269-1434

Alaska
Licensed Audiologists and Nonaudiologists
Division of Occupational Licensing
Hearing Aid Dealers' Section
P.O. Box 110806
Juneau, AK 99811-0806
(907) 465-3811
(907) 465-2974 (Fax)

Arizona
Licensed Audiologists and Nonaudiologists
Audiologists' and Speech-Language-Pathologists'
Licensing Program
1647 East Morten Avenue, Suite 160
Phoenix, AZ 85020
(602) 255-1144

Arkansas
Licensed Audiologists
Board of Examiners in Speech Pathology and Audiology
101 East Capitol, Suite 103
Little Rock, AR 72201
(501) 682-9180
Betty Bass, Office Manager

Nonaudiologists
Board of Hearing Aid Dispensers
305 N. Monroe
Little Rock, AR 72205
(501) 663-5869

California
Licensed Audiologists and Nonaudiologists
Hearing Aid Dealers' Examining Committee
1420 Howe Avenue, Suite 12
Sacramento, CA 95825-3230
(916) 263-2288
(916) 920-6377

Colorado
Licensed Audiologists and Nonaudiologists
Audiologists' and Hearing Aid Dealers' Registration
1560 Broadway, Suite 670
Denver, CO 80202
(303) 894-2464

Connecticut
Licensed Audiologists
SLP and Audiology Licensure
Department of Health
P.O. Box 340308
Hartford, CT 06134-0308
(203) 509-7560

Nonaudiologists
Department of Health Licensure Applications,
Examinations and Licensure
150 Washington Street
Hartford, CT 06106
(203) 566-4068

Delaware
Licensed Audiologists and Nonaudiologists
Audiology, SLP and Hearing Aid Dispensing Board
Division of Professional Regulation
Cannon Building, Suite 2303
Dover, DE 19903
(302) 739-4522, ext. 215
(302) 739-2711

District of Columbia
Licensed Audiologists and Nonaudiologists
Department of Consumer and Regulatory Affairs
Division of Pharmaceutical, Radiological
and Medical Devices Control
614 H Street, N.W., Room 1016
Washington, DC 20051
(202) 727-7218

Florida
Licensed Audiologists
Board of SLP and Audiology
Department of Professional Regulation
1940 North Monroe
Tallahassee, FL 32399-0778
(904) 487-3041
(904) 921-5389 (Fax)
Lucy Gee, Executive Director

Nonaudiologists
Department of Professional Regulation
1940 North Monroe Street
Tallahassee, FL 32399-0797
(904) 487-3041
(904) 921-5389 (Fax)

Georgia
Licensed Audiologists
Georgia Board of Examiners for SLP and Audiology
166 Pryor Street, S.W.
Atlanta, GA 30303-3465
(404) 656-6719
(404) 651-9532 (Fax)

Nonaudiologists
Examining Boards Division
166 Pryor Street, S.W., Suite 401
Atlanta, GA 30303
(404) 656-3912

Hawaii
Licensed Audiologists and Nonaudiologists
Licensure Branch of HADs and Fitters
Professional and Vocational Licensing Division
P.O. Box 3469
Honolulu, HI 96801
(808) 586-3000

Idaho
Licensed Audiologists and Nonaudiologists
Hearing Aid Dealers' and Fitters' Bureau
1109 Main Street, Owyhee Plaza, Suite 220
Boise, ID 83702
(208) 334-3233

Illinois
Licensed Audiologists and Nonaudiologists
Board for Hearing Aid Dispensers
Consumer Protection Program
Department of Public Health
Division of Health Assessment and Screening, 2nd floor
535 West Jefferson Street
Springfield, IL 62761
(217) 782-4733

Indiana
Licensed Audiologists
Speech-Language Pathology and Audiology Board
402 West Washington Street
Indianapolis, IN 46204
(317) 233-4407
(317) 233-4236 (Fax)

Nonaudiologists
HADs' Committee
402 West Washington Street, Suite #41
Indianapolis, IN 46204-2739
(317) 233-4407
(317) 233-4236 (Fax)

Iowa
Licensed Audiologists and Nonaudiologists
Board of Examiners for Hearing Aid Dealers
Department of Public Health
Lucas State Office Building, 4th Floor
Des Moines, IA 50319-0075
(515) 281-4401

Kansas
Licensed Audiologists and Nonaudiologists
Board of Hearing Aid Examiners
600 North St. Francis
P.O. Box 252
Wichita, KS 67201
(316) 264-8870

Kentucky
Licensed Audiologists and Nonaudiologists
Licensure Board for Specialists in Hearing Instruments
P.O. Box 456
Division of Occupations and Professions
Frankfort, KY 40602-0456
(502) 564-3296
(502) 564-4818

Louisiana
Licensed Audiologists
Board of Examiners for SLP and Audiology
11930 Perkins Road, Suite B
Baton Rouge, LA 71108
(504) 763-5480
(504) 673-3085 (Fax)

Nonaudiologists
Board of Hearing Aid Dealers
2205 Liberty Street
Monroe, LA 71211-6016
318-362-3014

Maine
Licensed Audiologists and Nonaudiologists
Board of Hearing Instrument Dealers and Fitters
Office of Licensing and Regulation
35 State House Station
Augusta, ME 04333
(207) 624-8603
(207) 624-8637

Maryland
Licensed Audiologists and Nonaudiologists
Board of Examiners for Audiology, HADs and SLPs
Department of Health and Mental Hygiene
4201 Patterson Avenue
Baltimore, MD 21215-2299
(410) 764-4725
(410) 764-5987

Massachusetts
Licensed Audiologists
Board of Registration for Speech-Language Pathology and Audiology
100 Cambridge Street, Room 1513
Boston, MA 02202
(617) 727-1747

Nonaudiologists
No HAD Regulation

Michigan
Licensed Audiologists and Nonaudiologists
Department of Consumer and Industry Services
BOPR—Office of Commercial Service Licensing Division
P.O. Box 30243
Lansing, MI 48909
(517) 335-4403
(517) 373-2795

Minnesota
Licensed Audiologists and Nonaudiologists
Health Occupations Programs
Board of Examiners for Hearing Aid Dealers
717 S.E. Delaware Street
Minneapolis, MN 55440-5620
(612) 282-5620

Mississippi
Licensed Audiologists and Nonaudiologists
Professional Licensure / Hearing Aid Specialists
P.O. Box 1700
Jackson, MS 39215-1700
(601) 987-4153
(601) 987-3784 (Fax)

Missouri
Licensed Audiologists and Nonaudiologists
Board of Hearing Instrument Specialists
P.O. Box 471
Jefferson City, MO 65102
(573) 751-0240
(573) 526-3481

Montana
Licensed Audiologists and Nonaudiologists
Board of Hearing Aid Dispensers
Professional and Occupational Licensing Division
111 North Jackson Avenue
Helena, MT 59620-0513
(406) 444-5433

Nebraska
Licensed Audiologists and Nonaudiologists
Board of Hearing Aid Instrument Dispensers and Fitters
Division of Professional and Occupational Licensure
P.O. Box 94986
Lincoln, NE 68509-5007
(402) 471-2299
(402) 471-3577

Nevada
Licensed Audiologists and Nonaudiologists
Board of Hearing Aid Specialists
3172 North Rainbow, Suite 141
Las Vegas, NV 89108
(702) 226-5716

New Hampshire
Licensed Audiologists and Nonaudiologists
Board of Hearing Aid Dispensers
Office of Health Planning and Review
6 Hazen Drive
Concord, NH 03301
(603) 271-4604
(603) 271-4141 (Fax)

New Jersey
Licensed Audiologists and Nonaudiologists
Hearing Aid Dispensers Examining Committee
124 Halsey Street, 6th Floor
Newark, NJ 07102
(201) 504-6331

New Mexico
Licensed Audiologists and Nonaudiologists
SLP, AUD and HAD Practices Board
Regulation and Licensing Department
P.O. Box 25101
Santa Fe, NM 87504
(505) 827-7554, ext. 24
(505) 827-7095 (Fax)

New York
Licensed Audiologists
State Board for SLP and Audiology
Room 3013 CEC
Empire State Plaza
Albany, NY 12230
(518) 473-0221
(518) 473-6995 (Fax)

Nonaudiologists
Licensing Hearing Aid Dealers
Department of State Division of Licensing Services
84 Holland Avenue
Albany, NY 12208-3490
(518) 474-4429

North Carolina
Licensed Audiologists and Nonaudiologists
Hearing Aid Dealers and Fitters Board
401 Overlin Road, Suite 111
Raleigh, NC 27605
(919) 834-0430
(919) 833-9954

North Dakota
Licensed Audiologists and Nonaudiologists
Board of Hearing Instrument Fitters and Dispensers
825 25th Street
Fargo, ND 58103
(701) 237-9977

Ohio
Licensed Audiologists
Board of SLP and Audiology
77 South High Street, 16th Floor
Columbus, OH 43266
(614) 466-3145
Nonaudiologists
Hearing Aid Dealers and Fitters Licensing Board
P.O. Box 118
Columbus, OH 43266-0118
(614) 466-5215

Nonaudiologists
Hearing Aid Dealers and Fitters Licensing Board
P.O. Box 118
Columbus, OH 43266-0118
(614) 466-5215

Oklahoma
Licensed Audiologists
State Board Examiners for SLP and Audiology
P.O. Box 53592
Oklahoma City, OK 73152
(405) 840-2774
(405) 840-2774 (Fax)

Nonaudiologists
Hearing Aid Division
Occupational Licensing Service—0203
Oklahoma State Health Department
1000 N.E. 10th Street
Oklahoma City, OK 73117-1299
(405) 271-5217

Oregon
Licensed Audiologists and Nonaudiologists
Hearing Aid Dealers Board
Health Division Licensing Programs
700 Summer Street, NE, Suite 100
Salem, OR 97310
(503) 378-8667 ext. 4306
(503) 585-9114 (Fax)

Pennsylvania
Licensed Audiologists and Nonaudiologists
Hearing Aid Dealers and Fitters
Department of Health
Bureau of Quality Assurance
Room 930
Health and Welfare Building
Harrisburg, PA 17120
(717) 787-8015

Rhode Island
Licensed Audiologists
Rhode Island Department of Health
3 Capitol Hill, Room 104
Providence, RI 02908-5097
(401) 277-2827
(401) 277-1272 (Fax)

Nonaudiologists
Board of Hearing Aid Dealers and Fitters
3 Capitol Hill, Room 104
Providence, RI 02908-5097
(401) 277-2827
(401) 277-1272 (Fax)

South Carolina
Licensed Audiologists
South Carolina Board of Examiners in Speech Pathology
and Audiology
PO Box 11329, Suite 101
Columbia, SC 29211
(803) 734-4253
(803) 734-4284 (Fax)

Nonaudiologists
Commission for Hearing Aid Specialists
Department of Health and Environmental Control
Division of Health Licensing
2600 Bull Street
Columbia, SC 29201
(803) 737-7202
(803) 737-2202

South Dakota
Licensed Audiologists and Nonaudiologists
Board of Hearing Aid Dispensers
P.O. Box 654
Spearfish, SD 57783-0654
(605) 642-1600
(605) 642-1756

Tennessee
Licensed Audiologists
Board of Communication Disorders and Sciences
287 Plus Park Boulevard
Nashville, TN 37247-1010
(615) 367-6223
(615) 367-6210 (Fax)

Nonaudiologists
Hearing Aid Dealers Counsel
Board of Communication Disorders and Sciences
287 Plus Park Boulevard
Nashville, TN 37247-1010
(615) 367-6223
(615) 367-6210 (Fax)

Texas
Licensed Audiologists
Board of Examiners for SLP and Audiology
1100 West 49th Street
Austin, TX 78756-3183
(512) 834-6627
(512) 834-6677 (Fax)

Nonaudiologists
Board of Examiners in the Fitting and Dispensing
of Hearing Instruments
1100 West 49th Street
Austin, TX 78756-3183
(512) 834-6784
(512) 834-6677

Utah
Licensed Audiologists
Bureau Manager Health Prof. Lic.
P.O. Box 45805
160 East 300 South
Salt Lake City, UT 84145-0805
(801) 530-6628
(801) 530-6511 (Fax)

Nonaudiologists
Hearing Instrument Specialists
Division of Occupational and Professional Licensing
160 E. 300 South Street
Salt Lake City, UT 84144-6741
(801) 530-6511

Vermont
Licensed Audiologists and Nonaudiologists
Office of Professional Regulation
Hearing Aid Dispensers Advisors
109 State Street
Montpelier, VT 05609-1101
(802) 828-2191

Washington
Licensed Audiologists and Nonaudiologists
Board of Audiology, Speech-Language-Pathology
and Hearing Instrument Fitters
Department of Health
Health Service Unit Two
PO Box 47869
Olympia, WA 98504-7869
(360) 753-1817
(360) 586-7774

West Virginia
Licensed Audiologists
West Virginia Board of Examiners for SLP and Audiology
P.O. Box 2136
Weirton, WV 26062
(304) 797-5108
(304) 797-4112 (Fax)

Nonaudiologists
Board of Examiners for Hearing Aid Dispensers
701 Jefferson Road
South Charleston, WV 25309
(304) 558-7886

Wisconsin
Licensed Audiologists and Nonaudiologists
Hearing and Speech Examining Board
Council on SLP and Audiology
Department of Regulation and Licensing
P.O. Box 8935
Madison, WI 53708-8935
(608) 266-1396
(608) 267-0644 (Fax)

Wyoming
Licensed Audiologists and Nonaudiologists
Board of Hearing Aid Specialists
2020 Carey Avenue, Suite 201
Cheyenne, WY 82001
(307) 777-7788

Modified from a listing on the ASHA Web Page
(www.asha.org), November 10th, 1998.
Used with permission.

Appendix C
Example Record of Competency

RECORD OF COMPETENCY EVALUATION

DEPARTMENT OF AUDIOLOGY

		Key:
Name:		P = Reviewed Policy
		0 = No Knowledge of Procedure—Optional skill
Job Title:		1 = Didactic knowledge of procedure
		2 = Performs procedure w/ supervision
Supervisor:		3 = Basic Competence; performs procedure w/o supervision
		4 = Master/Mentor: teaches and assess competency
Date:		Modifiers: NI—Needs Improvement
S.S. #:		R—Retraining Required
		N/A—Not Applicable
		O—Optional skill

Scores awarded on the basis of case staffing performance (5 cases, successfully completed procedures by vote of peers) or oversight of Audiologist rated as a master in the area assessed. For new hires, transfers, and promotions: This record will be administered at the beginning of departmental orientation and will be filed in the departmental file. Those items highlighted (*) must be completed prior to the end of departmental orientation. (Complete and update at least annually for **all staff** and keep in the Associate's departmental file.)

Competencies	Date	Code	Initial
Technical Competencies:			
I. Basic Comprehensive Examination			
a. Case History			
b. Pure tone Audiometry			
c. Speech Recognition Testing			
d. Tympanometry			
e. Acoustic Reflex Testing			
f. Clear Statement of Clinical Impressions			
g. Statement of Recommendations			
II. Cochlear-Retro cochlear Differential			
a. PI-PB Testing			
b. SSI-PI Testing			
c. Acoustic Reflex Decay Testing			
d. UCL			
e. Electrocochleography			
f. ABR-AEPs			
g. MLR-AEPs			
h. Transient Otoacoustic Emissions			
i. Distortion Product Otoacoustic Emissions			
III. Brain stem-Cerebral Differential			
a. Masking Level Differences			
b. SSI-ICM			
c. SSI-CCM			
d. Temporal Patterns and Tonal Patterns			
e. SSW			
f. Late and Endogenous AEPs			
IV. Spatial Orientation Assessments			
a. ENG—Visual Tracking (gaze, saccadic & smooth pursuit)			
b. ENG—Optokinetic induced eye movements			
c. Spontaneous, Positional & Positioning Nystagmus Assessment			
d. Bi-thermal Caloric Testing			
e. Vertical and single eye recording techniques			
f. Assessment of eye movements through Frenze Lenses			
g. Detection of Toulio and Hennabart signs			
h. Postural Sway Foam and Dome assessments			
i. Bedside evaluation of VOR, VVOR, OPN, pursuit, Saccadic eye movements, posture and head/neck orientation			
j. Development of Functional Treatment Plan			
k. Performs canalith repositioning and monitors effectiveness			

Competencies	Date	Code	Initial
l. Orchestrates multi-disciplinary balance rehab. treatment programs			
V. Tinnitus Assessment and Rehabilitation			
a. Tinnitus Matching			
b. Assessment of Residual Inhibition			
c. Prescription of Maskers			
d. Multi-disciplinary management Strategies & counseling			
VI. Special Populations			
a. Non-organic loss: Stenger Tests			
b. Non-organic loss: Lombard Tests			
c. Nonorganic loss: LOT tests			
d. Childhood central auditory abilities (CAA)—Figure Ground assessment			
e. Childhood central auditory abilities (CAA) sequential memory assessment			
f. Childhood central auditory abilities (CAA) short-term memory assessment			
g. Childhood central auditory abilities (CAA) auditory maturity assessment			
h. Childhood educational audiology—academic achievement assessment			
i. Childhood educational audiology—IEP and least restrictive environment			
j. Childhood educational audiology—monitoring IEP implementation			
k. Pediatric audiology: visual reinforcement audiometry			
l. Pediatric audiology: COR play audiometry			
m. Adult audiology: hearing handicap communication assessments			
n. Aural rehabilitation—ASL interpreting			
o. Adult audiology: aural rehabilitation—ALD Rx and dispensing			
p. Aural rehabilitation—hearing aid selection and fitting			
q. Aural rehabilitation—environment adaptation strategies			
r. Electroacoustic assessment and modification of hearing aids			
s. In situ probe measurements			
VII. Infant hearing assessment			
a. High-frequency tympanometry			
b. Otoacoustic emission screening			
c. Family contact protocols			
d. Auditory-evoked potential assessment of the infant			
VIII. Hearing conservation programming			
a. Plan and implement yearly monitoring service			
b. Consult re: management of STS cases			
c. Consultant re: selection and verification of hearing protective devices			
d. Plan, implement, and evaluate employee education program			
e. Consultant re: ADA and hearing impairment			
IX. Student/resident instruction			
X. Basic computer literacy			

REFERENCES

The American Heritage Dictionary of the English Language. (Ed. 3). (1996). Houghton Mifflin Company. Electronic version licensed from INSO Corporation.

BATTLE, D. (1994). Certification and licensure. In: R. Lubinski & C. Frattali (Eds.). *Professional issues in speech-language pathology and audiology.* (pp. 38–51). San Diego, CA: Singular Press.

BEUF, A.H. (1979). *Biting off the bracelet: A study of children in hospitals.* Philadelphia: University of Pennsylvania Press.

BICK, J. (1997). *All I really need to know in business I learned at Microsoft.* New York: Simon & Schuster/Pocket Books.

BYHAM, W.C., & COX, J. (1988). *Zapp: The lightning of empowerment.* New York: Fawcett Columbine.

CARNEGIE, D. (1995). *Leadership training for managers: Team building skills for today's quality-conscious organizations.* Garden City, NY: Dale Carnegie and Associates.

CHIAL, M. (1998). Viewpoint: Conveying expectations about professional behavior. *Audiology Today, 10*(4),25.

DELBECQ, A. (1985). Influence of professional behavior: The management of norms and discipline. In: R. Schenke (Ed.), *The physician in management* (pp. 179–192). Forrestville, MD: Artisan Printing.

DESMOND, A. (1994). Personnel management. In: *Development and management of audiology practices.* Report by the American Speech-Language-Hearing Association (ASHA) Ad Hoc Committee on Practice Management in Audiology (pp. 67–70). Rockville, MD: ASHA.

Employer's Resource Group. (1993). *Jack Katz's nightmare.* Rockville, MD: BNA Communications.

FOX, D., & BATTIN, R. (1978). *Private practice in audiology and speech pathology.* New York: Grune & Stratton.

GOLDBERG, B. (1991). Digging for truth. *ASHA, 33*(1); 37–48.

HOFKOSH, J.M. (1975). Personnel management. In: R.J. Hickok (Ed.). *Physical therapy administration and management* (pp. 50–90). Baltimore: Williams & Wilkins.

HOSFORD-DUNN, H., DUNN, D.R., & HARFORD, E. (1995) *Audiology business and practice management.* San Diego, CA: Singular Publishing Inc.

INLANDER, C., LEVIN, L., & WEINER, E. (1988). *Medicine on trial.* Englewood Cliffs, NJ: Prentice Hall.

JACOBSON, G. (1994). Office automation. In: *Development and management of audiology practices.* Report by the American Speech-Language-Hearing Association (ASHA) Ad Hoc Committee on Practice Management in Audiology (pp. 25–30). Rockville, MD: ASHA.

JANDT, F.E. (1990). *The manager's problem solver.* Glenview, IL: Scott Foresman and Company.

JENKINS, M.D. (1993). *Starting and operating a business in Arizona.* Grants Pass, OR: Oasis Press.

KISHEL, G.F., & KISHEL, P.G. (1993). *How to start, run, and stay in business.* New York: John Wiley & Sons, Inc.

LABOVITZ, G., & ROSANSKY, V. (1997). *The power of alignment.* New York: John Wiley & Sons, Inc.

LARWOOD, L. (1984). *Organizational behavior and management.* Boston, MA: Kent Publishing.

LEVINE, S.R., & CROM, M.A. (1995). *The leader in you: How to win friends, influence people and succeed in a changing world.* New York: Simon & Schuster / Dale Carnegie and Associates.

LUBINSKI, R. (1994). Infection control. In: R. Lubinski & C. Frattali (Eds.), *Professional issues in speech-language pathology and audiology* (pp. 269–281). San Diego, CA: Singular Press.

MINGHETTI, N.J., COOPER, J.A., GOLDSTEIN, H., OLSWANG, L.B., & WARREN, S.F. (EDS.), (1993). *Research mentorship and training in communication sciences and disorders: Proceeding of a national conference.* Rockville, MD: American Speech-Language-Hearing Foundation.

PAULSON, E., & LAYTON, M. (1995). *The complete idiot's guide to starting your own business.* New York: Simon & Schuster/ Alpha Books.

SCHLESINGER, P.E., SATH, V., SCHLESINGER, L.A., & KOTTER, J.P. (1992). *Organization: Text, cases, and readings of the management of organizational design and change* (3rd ed.). Homewood, IL: Irwin.

SIROPOLIS, N. (1990). *Small business management.* Boston: Houghton Mifflin.

TWAY, P. (1992). *People, common sense and the small business.* Crozet, VA: Betterway.

WALTON, M. (1986). *The Deming management method.* New York: Perigee Book.

WELCH, C., & FOWLER, K. (1994) Human resource management. In: S.R. Rizzo, & M.D. Trudeau (Eds.), *Clinical administration in audiology and speech-language pathology* (pp. 93–132). San Diego, CA: Singular Publishing Group.

WHITING, R. (1994). *Hiring and firing within the law.* Carrollton, TX: Whiting and Associates.

WILLIAMS, P. (1994). Professional organizations. In: R. Lubinski, & C. Frattali (Eds.), *Professional issues in speech-language pathology and audiology* (pp. 14–25). San Diego, CA: Singular Press.

YATE, M. (1994). *Hiring the best: A manager's guide to effective interviewing* (4th ed.). Holbrook, MA: B. Adams.

ZAPALA, D. (1996). Professional issues in hospital practice. *Seminars in Hearing, 17*(3);261–274.

Chapter 7

Marketing Principles

Wayne J. Staab

Outline

PITFALL

Too much of today's "marketing," unfortunately, is based on the reliance of a hearing aid product or hearing aid technology with the assumption that if it can be made a little better, success will inevitably follow. However, without a program to make oneself unique in the patients' minds, technological superiority alone no longer guarantees success or even a position in the race.

Because the practice of audiology exists and is defined through its involvement with hearing aids primarily, this chapter emphasizes marketing principles that address issues related to hearing aids rather than diagnostic or other rehabilitative procedures. Transitional applications to diagnostics and/or other rehabilitative procedures can be made by changing the terminology.

The complexities and volatility of the hearing healthcare marketplace dictate that marketing must be an ongoing or daily activity. The market is dynamic and ever changing. Too much of today's "marketing," unfortunately, is based on the reliance of a hearing aid product or hearing aid technology; assuming that if it can be made a little better, success will inevitably follow. However, without a program to make oneself unique in the patients' minds, technological superiority alone no longer guarantees success or even a position in the race. Even good products will not sell themselves. In the long run, hearing aid patient needs and desires define the products. As they change, so must the product because evolving patients demand evolving products. Just as product complexities make it easier to make products different, they also make it difficult for the patient to understand the differences that do exist. If the differences do not exist in the patient's mind, they do not exist in the marketplace.

The ever-changing marketplace presents several challenges that include the following: (1) survival in the marketplace as the hearing healthcare system changes, (2) the perception of the product/service delivered as a commodity for which price is the only distinguishing feature, (3) the inability to define sufficient "benefit" with amplification to patients having a hearing impairment, and (4) the management of a successful business with the understanding that it involves more than being a skilled audiologist (see Chapter 8 in this volume for related information).

With projections suggesting hearing healthcare as a growth industry, competition and consumerism are shifting much of the emphasis of the marketplace away from the system as we know it today, resulting in alternative and nontraditional sites and purveyors. Added to this, and contributing to challenges, are changes in the state of the economy, changes in tax laws and government regulations, FDA investigations in the United States into hearing aid dispensing practices and pricing, negative media publicity, perceptions on the part of the consumer that the only real difference between dispensers is their name, and health care reform proposals that have and are expected to continue to affect the stability and growth of the hearing healthcare industry. A reality check of the significance of good hearing to the patient complicates matters further. For example, those of us who provide services to people having hearing impairment are often adamant in our belief that hearing is very important. The unfortunate reality is that to many people with hearing impairment, loss of hearing is not that big a deal. This discrepancy between audiological perception of the "problem" and consumer reality mandates in large part the necessity for a chapter on marketing principles.

137

Do these incursions and perceptions suggest that only negatives exist and not opportunities? On the contrary, opportunities do exist. As a prime example, the aging of America will contribute to the growth of the population with hearing impairment. Mature Americans who accounted for 8.1% of the population in 1950 are expected to grow to 20.4% of the population by 2050, according to the U.S. Census Bureau (USA Today, 1996). In addition, new computer-based programming technologies, hearing and hearing aid test equipment, hearing aids, and office automation systems have the potential of contributing to diagnosis, productivity, quality assurance, hearing aid performance, and patient satisfaction. A significant hurdle will be the acceptance of and motivation for a person to act relative to their loss of hearing.

How is the hearing healthcare professional to meet these challenges and take advantage of opportunity in both the short run and long run? This question has no single answer. However, a rational, market-based response can be made by preparing goals and strategies and then using the basic precepts embodied in good business planning: know your market; know your market's needs; present appropriate products and services; price according to market conditions; and merchandise, advertise, and sell.

The purpose of this chapter is to explain marketing principles that can be used to bridge the transitions in meeting the challenges identified and to help narrow the discrepancy between perception and reality in the marketplace. The contents relate more specifically to marketing than to sales principles, explain key marketing concepts, suggest methods to foster practical marketing skills, and provide step-by-step descriptions and analyses of the tools needed to design and implement a complete marketing plan.

HEARING AID DISPENSING AS A BUSINESS

Despite the "audiology as a profession" rhetoric, it is significant to recognize that an audiological practice is a business foremost. Being just a professional does not generate business, but business and its subsequent demand can and does create a profession. (A Glossary of marketing terms is available in Appendix A.)

Failure to understand and accept these realities is almost a certain roadmap to failure—failure both professionally and financially. What does your road map look like as you make plans in your practice? In their article on "The Marketing Challenge," Jelonek and Staab (1994) suggest that you ask yourself the following questions: What do you anticipate in dollars or unit sales? How will you compete against similar competitors, much less with "managed care" and large retail operations? How will your office be different from other dispensing practices in your marketing area? Will you be able to increase your net income 15% or so per year so that funds can be set aside for your retirement and your childrens' educations? More specifically, will you be able to survive another 5 years? Will you be financially successful, just comfortable, or out of business? What are the amounts of savings and investments your business must provide for you on the day you retire to do this comfortably? Table 7–1 can be used to assist you in obtaining an estimate to the last question, which may in turn drive business decisions to provide you with answers to the other questions. Another ballpark estimate of your retirement needs can be obtained from the American Savings Education Council internet site: http://www.asec.org/bpk-comp.htm.

With business as a focus, what business concerns are most frequently addressed by today's dispensing audiologists? Over a 2-year period during which 18 intensive marketing programs were offered to those dispensing hearing aids, the following list of issues (unranked) was cited most frequently as requiring attention by attendees (Staab & Jelonek, 1994b, 1995b):

TABLE 7–1   How much you'll need in retirement

(General estimate of how much money is needed in savings and investments to retire comfortably. The formula gives a rough idea of how much you will need on the day you retire. Modify as desired.)
- Determine what you need for annual income in retirement. Use $50,000 a year as an example.
- Estimate what you expect for an average rate of return on your investments. Planners say 8% is a good figure.
- Estimate inflation. About 4% a year is reasonable.
- Subtract the inflation rate from your rate of return. That leaves 4%, which is what your investments will earn after inflation.
- Divide your desired income by the after-inflation return: $50,000 divided by 4% equals $1.25 million. That is your goal if you expect all your retirement income to come from your investments. If you will get a company pension, have income from other investments and Social Security, you will need less.

(USA Today Retirement Planning Hot Line, 1998)

- Building revenue
- Generating new patients—expanding markets served
- Generating referrals
- Competing with a referral source
- Competing with price discounters

- Meeting personal financial needs (added as being very important, but only after the suggestion was made)
- Working with HMOs, PPOs, and the like
- Marketing on a limited budget

Hearing aid dispensing is considered a small business activity. Small businesses constitute 99.7% of the businesses in the United States (21.3 million), provide 54% of the work force, 52% of all sales, and generate 50% of the private sector product (White House Conference on Small Business Issue Handbook, 1994). They also have the greatest risk. Statistics indicate that 25% fail before the end of the second year (*White House Conference on Small Business Issue Handbook,* 1994). This is somewhat consistent with data stating that 50% of small businesses failed within the first 5 years of operation in 1980 (Bank of America, 1988) but more difficult to resolve with data stating that as many as 80% survive at least 4 years (Inc., 1995). Regardless, risk is associated with small business and emphasizes the necessity of a marketing plan to ensure that your practice not only has a start but also survives and grows.

The amount of personal financial investment risk, and hence reward, varies with the management structure of the practice you are in. Audiologists working for an Ear, Nose, and Throat practice, public-funded agency, a hospital or other clinic that has patients referred from internal sources for hearing aids and services have considerably less risk (this is not to minimize the risk of job or income loss). Understandably, the rewards are not as great either because of the reduced financial investment risk involved. Audiologists who put their finances and reputations on the line as free-standing diagnostic and dispensing audiology practices have much greater risk and investment and rightly expect to reap the financial benefits of that risk. Capital equipment purchases, leases, utilities, taxes, time, salaries, and the hearing aids themselves represent substantial financial and personal commitment. Daily concerns center around running the business, the patient base, and cash flow.

MARKETING VERSUS SALES

Marketing is the understanding of, and delivering or responding to, *consumer needs;* whereas sales is providing for our financial needs as businesspersons—in other words, looking out for *our needs.* This distinction is not always as clear in actual practice, but the differentiation must be understood if we are to succeed in business. Table 7–2 "Why customers are lost," although generic to business, suggests strongly the need for being aware of patient needs.

TABLE 7–2 Why customers are lost

- 1% die
- 4% move
- 11% competitive inroads
- 16% product dissatisfaction
- 68% quit because of an ATTITUDE of indifference by someone who works in your office

Marketing Skill Priorities

The development of marketing skills should be as much a priority as hearing evaluation and hearing aid dispensing skills. The dispensing audiologist must understand the fundamental principles of marketing and have basic marketing skills. Skills that are essential include (Staab & Jelonek, 1994a, 1994b, 1995b) the following:

- How to set reasonable, achievable marketing and financial goals.
- How to analyze competitors and patients and develop competitive marketing offerings and programs that meet patient needs and wants.
- How to identify, or develop, and then use competitive advantages.
- How to develop a profitable line of products and services that meet patient needs while ensuring the audiologist's ability to learn, control, and knowledgeably apply technology.
- How to competitively and profitably price products and services.
- How to sell, that is, *personally market*, products, technologies, and services.
- How to design a market communications program for current patients, prospective patients, and referral sources.
- How to market without advertising. How to market more effectively.
- How to develop and successfully implement marketing programs.

MARKETING ACTION PLAN

Management by crisis is how much of the marketing in audiology practices occurs today. However, crisis management, alone, cannot and should not dictate the development of sales or promotional programs. Market planning should not be a one-time event initiated with the start-up of a business or the need for a bank loan. Communications and sales programs must reflect the unique demographic character and lifestyle of local populations. It must be recognized that mature populations are not a homogeneous group having uniform needs and purchasing behaviors. To that end, a marketing action plan is needed. Unfortunately, only 38% of audiologists report having a preplanned marketing program (Skafte, 1998).

The successful professional must have a marketing action plan that can readily adapt to competitive events or changing patient behavior; it must be dynamic in that it is modified constantly to changing market needs. A marketing action plan is a marketing and financial road map of how you are going to get from your current position to your desired destination. It describes how you will allocate scarce resources (time, finances, personnel) to reach that destination. It outlines strategies and programs that will enable you to traverse a highly competitive landscape. It should include also a method to measure how well the plan's goals were met. Figure 7–1 illustrates the basic flow of the overall marketing action plan.

Marketing Process

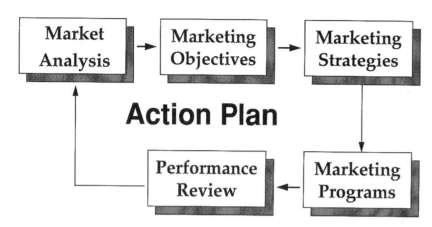

Figure 7–1 Action plan for the marketing process, indicating the flow of events.

As you continue planning, assess the viability of your internalized or written market plan using the following nine point questionnaire modified from Jelonek and Staab (1994):

1. *Do I have specific quantified goals for the coming year?* Are these sales units, billable revenue, patients, growth, productivity?

2. *Who are my current and prospective patients?* What are their demographics, lifestyles, and what will motivate them to purchase hearing aids?

3. *Who are my key competitors?* What marketing actions are they likely to take in the coming year? What are their relative marketing strengths and weaknesses?

4. *What is my competitive advantage?* How am I going to advance or succeed competitively?

5. *How am I going to use technology, products, service and office equipment to achieve my marketing and financial goals?* Do I have marketing programs organized to take advantage of these features? Do I have procedures and protocols in place that will ensure product performance and patient satisfaction?

6. *Do my pricing and sales strategies reflect competitive actions and positions?* Have I changed these strategies from last year? Am I just copying the actions of my competitors? Do my strategies support the achievement of my goals?

7. *What is my market communications program?* How am I going to communicate with my current patients, prospective patients, referral sources? What message am I going to give them?

8. *What resources do I have and how will I allocate them to achieve my goals?* How will I use my money, time, personnel?

9. *What are the potential barriers to achieving my goals?* Is it the economy, competitors, personal knowledge or skill, finances? What can I do to eliminate or minimize these barriers?

Having a marketing action plan is essential to your professional survival and continued success. A plan does not have a magical starting date. It can begin January 1 or March 13. The date does not determine its success. The actual development of the plan can be self-directed, guided by outlines or texts, or accomplished by means of a group seminar. It should, however, be written because the very act of writing goals, strategies, and tactics is a commitment to their completion.

Market Analysis Action Plan

*Where Is Your Business and
What Is Your Market Potential?*

The hearing aid marketplace is an ever-changing entity, and the audiologist must be able to rapidly adjust the practice to accommodate the recognized changes. Markets are driven by the relationships and interactions of its players, with no member of the market isolated from the other. This means that what affects one segment of the market is likely to affect your practice as well. This requires an ongoing market analysis (a snapshot of the marketplace at a point in time), which is essential to find new ways to compete and grow an existing practice.

This analysis should provide you with specific answers about what the served market is, as well as about the entire market. Such a review of the general market that you function in and also of your own business should be performed routinely. This can be as sophisticated as you would like, taking as little as a few hours to several days, but should include monitoring your market in terms of its conditions or trends, growth, stagnation, or decline. Market analysis is used to assist in planning successful marketing strategies and programs and to evaluate the performance of the general market plan.

Market Analysis (Situational Analysis)

The purpose of market analysis is to determine the status of your practice and where it is going. It is here that an assessment of the market is determined from the market structure (definition, size, growth), market conditions (economic, social, environmental, governmental), demographics (age and income), and competition. The simple worksheet at the end of this chapter can be used to gather such information, but this can be made much more elaborate if you choose to do so.

These data are then used to focus on a *segment* of the total hearing aid market by offering products and/or services for this segment. It is unrealistic to believe that you will serve the entire market. A market analysis should be done at least annually, or more frequently if market conditions change. Market analysis should be regarded as an annual checkup of the local market that assesses the market environment, the market profile, an analysis of the patient, and a competitive analysis.

Before initiation of a market analysis, the following informational resources should be obtained, limiting the gathering of data to an area approximating 80% from where your patients are expected to come:

- Geographical and population information: This should consist of such information as Zip codes, census data, psychographics, maps covering your market area (to plot competitors, referral sources, etc.), income, age demographics, geographical mix, home or business breakdowns by area, or any other information that allows you to analyze the population within your area.

- Economic information: This is often found in local newspapers, from the Chamber of Commerce, banks, or local business publications if the area is sufficiently large.

- Competitive information and/or referral sources: Yellow pages, professional directories, sales representatives, the competition themselves, advertising/promotion, news stories, state membership, registration or licensing lists, local newspapers, and meetings/conventions are sources of this information.

- Industry information: Each year the hearing aid trade publications provide information about State sales (trends, volume, sources of revenue, expenditures), sources of competition, pricing, and so forth.

- Public and commercial resources: Many of these resource data sources can be obtained from the public library, Internet, Chamber of Commerce, government offices, commercial sources, and so forth.

Market Definition (Area, Scope of the Market)

Simple ways to identify your market may be to limit it to: (a) the geographical area where your current patient base lives or works (general demographics are available from the public library or from the Internet), or (b) define it by the geographical area from which you are drawing large clusters of new patients (take this from your office visit statistics). When viewed in these ways, your market can be identified by a list of Zip codes, cities, or counties (Action Plan, Market Definition, Appendix B).

Market Size (Numbers)

How is your market size determined? It is determined generally by summing the population statistics from the market definition (Action Plan, Market Size, Appendix B). The actual number of persons with hearing impairment can be calculated as 9.4% of the market size. If based on a percentage of the population statistics, is it a percentage of the overall population in your marketing area or a percentage of your served market (defined later).

An alternate method to market size estimation is to base it on the total number of hearing aids sold within the geographical served area. One method is to guesstimate the monthly unit new sales of hearing aids in competitors' offices on the basis of the number of persons a given office employs (Action Plan, Market Size, Appendix B) or on the basis of industry sales per average office. Or you can estimate competitor office unit sales from your unit sales on a per person employed basis. Soliciting comments from manufacturers' representatives can also provide you with "ballpark" figures. Hearing aid sales by competitive offices could provide insight into the total population served. Realize, however, that approximately 60% of the sales are binaural, thus reducing the market penetration somewhat.

Does a market size exist that is required in which your practice can exist and grow? I am not aware of any data from the hearing aid industry to this effect. Jelonek (1992a) estimates that the dispenser-to-population ratio in the United States is 1:26,267, and the dispenser-to-older-than 65 population is estimated at 1:3,245. She suggests that a population of approximately 30,000 is sufficient per dispenser, that less than 20,000 is very competitive, and that with 18,000 it is difficult to survive. Despite these suggestions, what is perhaps more critical are the (a) age and income of the population, (b) the incidence of hearing impairment in the population considered, and (c) the type of marketing program(s) provided, even when faced with a greater number of competitors than the market would seem to support. For example, when comparing city populations of 35,000, a 48% statistic of individuals 65 years of age and older in Sun City, Arizona, is likely to support more dispensing operations than a 14% 65 plus age group in another city of the same size. Keep in mind also that although the hearing aid sales market potential is anywhere from 40 to 80% of the hearing-impaired market, industry statistics indicate that the actual market penetration is only about 20%.

How many hearing aids sold in your market area should be sufficient for your practice? The answer lies in the determination of whether enough new units are sold within your marketing area to sustain you and your competitors with the total number of projected units per month (year).

Market Growth—Measurement

Just as important as the market size is the expected growth of the market in question. Is it growing, stable, or shrinking, and by what percent? What are the long-term growth prospects for your market? Is population growth city or county related, is it due to low- or no-growth policies of local governments, are you growing more or less than the market? If less, you are losing market share. If more, you are gaining market share. No advantage exists in investing in a market that is shrinking in total population or total hearing aid sales volume (Action Plan, Market Growth, Appendix B). Some of the issues that influence population trends include the economic health of a community, taxes, the quality of life, rates of employment, business openings or closings, social conditions, crime, education, and pollution.

Market Conditions

What market conditions currently affect your business or are likely to affect your business within the next 3 to 5 years? Are these positive or negative influences? These may be somewhat difficult to quantify, but an attempt should be made to identify at least the economic, social, environmental, and governmental influences on your practice. If recognized, planning can be performed to minimize or take advantage of these as they occur. For example, plant closings often signal a reduction and distribution change in a population. The chamber of commerce in a community can provide information about employment opportunities and industries that draw certain groups of individuals. With the information age, do not forget data available from the Internet. Market data resources are available also from the public library and often include incomes, demographics, growth, age comparisons, trends, and environmental conditions. Action Plan, Market Conditions, Appendix B provides a check-off list of issues that are worthy of consideration.

Do market conditions have an impact on hearing aid sales? It is reasonable to expect they do, depending on the type and populations affected. For example, high employment might signal sales opportunities to populations who do not normally have large discretionary funds. Interest rates can have serious implications to retirees whose living standard is tied explicitly to savings. Higher interest rates (resulting in higher CD returns, money market funds, bonds, etc.) signal increased discretionary income and greater opportunities for hearing aid purchase. A bull stock market and low national rates of inflation generally provide income increases not required for the necessities of life.

Industry trends and conditions can influence your market as well. New technologies supported in part by manufacturers can stimulate consumer interest and hearing aid sales purchases. Pricing policies, discount schedules, warranty plans, and return policies all affect the way dispensers operate their businesses (Jelonek, 1992b).

Consumer Analysis: Age and Income Demographics for Your Market

This is the title listed on the simple Action Plan, Market Analysis Part 5, Appendix B, but is often more extensive than an analysis of age and income only. It ordinarily includes both demographic and behavioral profiles. Demographic variables often list age, gender, income, occupation, race, marital status, housing, education, family size, and so forth. Behavioral profiles include psychographics, purchase tendencies, risk concerns, interests, and driving forces.

Consumer analysis is an attempt to more specifically target your market. It is from much of these data that actual marketing programs will be developed. Collectively, consumer analysis data can be used to determine the age, retirement populations, disposable income, activity level, how geographically concentrated the market is, and potential purchasing levels of the population in question. Purchasing decisions are influenced heavily, especially by seniors, on the basis of interest rates, certificates of deposit, and other investment incomes. They are more likely to purchase when investment income is high.

In the action plan example (Action Plan, Market Analysis Part 5, Appendix B), comparisons of age and income are made to national statistics but could be made to city, state, or county data, whichever is available or of interest. The data that follow, in Tables 7–3 through 7–8, Figures 7–2 through 7–4 and Appendix B are intended to provide summary data for simple comparisons.

Tables 7–3 and 7–4 provide examples of the type of age and income data that are useful when comparing markets (Staab & Jelonek, 1995b). Both provide information relative to the United States, for five states, and for select Zip codes

within four of the five states. Table 7–3 provides age statistics, and Table 7–4 provides household income statistics. This kind of information is available from various sources. (These specific data were purchased from CACI Marketing Systems, 1995, http://www.demographics.caci.com.)

Keep in mind when using such statistics to direct marketing efforts toward the elderly population that the older individual is either well aware of loss of hearing function sufficient to create problems in understanding the speech of others or may be unaware of information-bearing signals in his or her acoustic environment. Regardless, marketing practices that stress the loss of hearing as a function of aging serve only to remind the person of the inevitable changes in life that reduce one's participation in it. The elderly seem not to be as intimidated by the loss of sensory function as they are by the changes in interpersonal relations and the ability to actively participate in social activities—that should be the message (Sandlin, 1992).

Information of Use When Comparing Markets

Served Market

When estimating the size of your market from population statistics, understand that an overall hearing impaired market and a served market exist. Seldom, if ever, are they the same. What is the difference? The hearing-impaired market consists of the total number (percentage based on estimates) of individuals in the population considered to have a measurable hearing loss, regardless of how that marketing area is defined. The served market is a realistic expectation of those individuals within your marketing area that are accessible to hearing aid sales from your office.

Many audiologists use misguided information about their served market, using instead, the entire hearing-impaired population within their area. However, allowances must be made for those populations not being served by your office and may exclude numbers associated with veterans, the deaf, the institutionalized, children, health maintenance organizations, age, income and demographic populations within your area, insurance or industrial companies that have plans in which you or your patients do not participate, those having mild hearing impairments who do not believe that their hearing is severe enough to require hearing aids, and other exclusionary market segments. In reality, elimination of these members could reduce the served market to much less than the 9.4% noninstitutionalized, national average. On the other hand, concentration of efforts within retirement communities could lead to a much higher percentage.

Whatever the served market, it should reflect the exceptions identified in the previous paragraph. This will require estimates on your part because every marketing area is expected to be different from all others. For example, you may have a geographical population of 35,000 people. A general hearing-impaired population of 9.4% would suggest 3290 persons with hearing impairment. However, when adjustments are made for age, type of employment, and so on, the number could be significantly different.

The Hearing-Impaired Population by Age, Degree of Loss, and Life Expectancy

The total population in the United States for 1995 was estimated at 261,000,000 individuals (Census Bureau, not dated).

TABLE 7–3 The use of age demographics in the market analysis. Comparisons can be made to the United States in general, to the state, city, or Zip code, and by different age groupings.

ZIP CODE OR COUNTY	POPULATION MEDIAN AGE 1995	POPULATION AGE DISTRIBUTION					POPULATION AGE DISTRIBUTION			
		<18	45-64	65-84	85+	65+	45-64	65-84	85+	65+
USA	34.00	26.10	18.30	9.60	1.10	10.70	48,130,143	25,248,600	2,893,069	28,141,668
CALIFORNIA	32.60	27.10	19.50	11.40	1.40	12.80	6,192,089	3,619,991	444,560	4,064,551
FLORIDA	37.40	29.90	20.00	16.90	2.00	18.90	2,838,079	2,398,177	283,808	2,681,985
ILLINOIS	34.00	26.20	19.50	11.30	1.40	12.70	2,305,055	1,335,750	165,491	1,501,241
INDIANA	34.10	26.20	19.90	11.50	1.40	12.90	1,154,102	666,944	81,193	748,137
NEW YORK	35.00	24.20	20.50	12.00	1.50	13.50	3,731,333	2,184,195	273,024	2,457,219
NEW YORK										
10021 New York	42.40	10.20	27.50	15.10	2.70	17.80	29,700	16,308	2,916	19,224
10022 New York	47.60	7.80	32.10	19.60	2.80	22.40	10,223	6,242	892	7,134
10028 New York	40.60	11.70	27.60	11.90	2.00	13.90	11,873	5,119	860	5,979
INDIANA										
46342 Hobart	35.20	22.40	30.70	20.80	11.70	32.50	9,862	6,682	3,759	10,440
46368 Portage	33.90	27.80	22.60	12.00	1.00	13.00	10,051	5,337	445	5,782
46410 Gary	37.20	23.20	21.80	14.80	1.50	16.30	6,928	4,703	477	5,180
ILLINOIS										
60120 Elgin	30.40	32.00	15.00	6.80	0.90	7.70	7,107	3,222	426	3,648
60123 Elgin	33.00	28.50	18.20	9.70	1.40	11.10	8,926	4,757	687	5,444
60178 Sycamore	34.50	28.00	20.60	10.80	1.10	11.90	3,188	1,671	170	1,841
CALIORNIA										
92025 Escondido	30.80	30.00	16.50	8.10	1.60	9.70	6,836	3,356	663	4,019
92056 Oceanside	28.00	22.70	12.30	8.60	0.80	9.40	6,204	4,337	403	4,741
92128 San Diego	43.10	12.90	19.70	24.70	3.00	27.70	7,253	9,094	1,105	10,199
95825 Sacramento	34.00	84.10	17.80	12.60	1.80	14.40	4,948	3,503	500	4,003
95608 Carmichael	37.30	76.70	23.00	13.70	1.60	15.30	13,291	7,917	925	8,841
95661 Roseville	35.30	72.10	22.70	9.20	1.70	10.90	5,354	2,170	401	2,571
94588 Pleasanton	33.40	26.10	23.30	4.10	0.20	4.30	4,913	864	42	907
94550 Livermore	32.00	27.90	20.80	6.90	0.70	7.60	13,605	4,513	458	4,971
94583 San Ramon	34.30	25.90	23.90	4.60	0.30	4.90	9,214	1,773	116	1,889
96002 Redding	33.10	29.10	20.00	11.60	1.40	13.00	6,273	3,639	439	4,078
96003 Redding	35.20	26.10	20.70	14.00	1.30	15.30	7,365	4,981	463	5,444
96007 Anderson	35.10	29.80	20.30	13.30	1.30	14.60	4,452	2,917	285	3,202
96067 Mt. Shasta	39.70	24.50	25.40	13.70	1.40	15.10	1,724	930	95	1,025
96080 Red Bluff	36.20	27.70	20.60	15.20	1.80	17.00	5,419	3,999	474	4,472
96097 Yreka	39.70	25.30	23.40	16.00	2.40	18.40	2,139	1,463	219	1,682

From Staab and Jelonek (1995b), with permission.

TABLE 7–4 The use of income demographics in the market analysis. United States, state, city, and Zip codes can be compared in terms of median incomes, rank order, and by income ranges. Age and income could be identified as well (not from this table, however).

ZIP CODE OR COUNTY	HOUSEHOLD INCOME MEDIAN 1995	NAT'L RANK	STATE RANK	MEDIAN 2000	HOUSEHOLD INCOME DISTRIBUTION					AVG
					Less than $15,000	$15,000-24,999	$25,000-49,999	$50,000-99,000	$100,000-149,999	$150,000-or More
USA	$33,610	-	-	$32,972	20.50	20.50	33.80	23.70	4.20	2.00
CALIFORNIA	$38,099	15	-	$37,122	16.90	14.10	32.50	27.80	5.60	3.00
FLORIDA	$31,524	27	-	$31,216	20.00	18.00	34.90	21.40	3.60	2.00
ILLINOIS	$35,865	19	-	$35,492	18.90	14.70	34.30	25.50	4.40	2.20
INDIANA	$36,137	18	-	$36,848	16.50	15.30	36.90	26.00	3.90	1.40
NEW YORK	$33,826	23	-	$32,749	22.20	14.80	31.60	24.10	4.60	2.07
NEW YORK										
10021 New York	$57,762	96	93	$54,148	10.10	8.20	25.00	26.80	11.10	18.80
10022 New York	$61,114	97	95	$57,535	10.00	7.50	23.70	26.30	12.50	19.90
10028 New York	$58,319	96	94	$54,761	9.40	7.70	26.40	26.30	12.00	18.20
INDIANA										
46342 Hobart	$40,731	84	79	$40,611	11.60	13.60	36.30	32.10	4.20	2.20
46368 Portage	$41,353	84	81	$42,968	12.60	12.70	37.60	31.80	4.10	1.30
46410 Gary	$41,645	85	82	$41,078	11.20	11.30	38.30	32.90	5.30	0.90
ILLINOIS										
60120 Elgin	$40,252	83	82	$40,599	12.00	13.30	38.40	31.30	4.10	0.90
60123 Elgin	$44,355	88	87	$45,951	11.70	10.80	34.80	33.90	6.70	2.10
60178 Sycamore	$40,303	83	82	$42,825	12.30	12.30	38.20	31.50	4.10	1.50
CALIORNIA										
92025 Escondido	$33,107	66	45	$32,411	17.50	18.50	35.10	21.90	4.60	2.30
92056 Oceanside	$35,112	71	49	$34,022	11.70	18.50	41.30	24.80	4.60	0.80
92128 San Diego	$51,702	94	86	$50,551	8.50	8.60	30.60	37.60	2.90	4.80
95825 Sacramento	$29,514	56	34	$27,852	19.40	20.20	38.90	17.00	9.90	1.90
95608 Carmichael	$37,867	79	58	$35,786	14.50	13.90	34.40	27.80	2.70	3.90
95661 Roseville	$49,677	92	83	$47,454	12.00	11.00	27.30	38.90	5.50	3.00
94588 Pleasanton	$61,756	97	94	$60,648	2.50	5.20	27.00	49.40	7.80	3.50
94550 Livermore	$53,061	94	87	$51,984	8.60	7.80	28.80	44.20	12.40	2.10
94583 San Ramon	$65,701	98	96	$62,821	3.90	4.60	22.70	49.30	8.50	4.40
96002 Redding	$27,819	49	28	$25,927	22.60	21.30	34.90	18.40	15.20	0.80
96003 Redding	$26,534	43	24	$24,550	27.40	19.50	33.90	16.80	1.90	1.00
96007 Anderson	$23,508	28	15	$21,002	31.70	20.40	35.00	11.40	1.40	0.30
96067 Mt. Shasta	$25,775	39	21	$23,407	28.00	20.40	29.80	19.00	1.20	1.00
96080 Red Bluff	$25,389	36	20	$24,956	27.40	21.60	33.60	14.80	1.70	0.60
96097 Yreka	$21,645	22	10	$19,760	31.10	24.90	29.60	12.00	1.90	0.60

From Staab and Jelonek (1995b), with permission.

The total, civilian, noninstitutionalized hearing-impaired population is estimated at 9.4%, and of the total U.S. population at 11.2%. The incidence of hearing loss ranges from 4.4 to 27.8% and reflects variations in defining hearing loss, measurement procedures, intended use of the data, and so on. The percentage used in this chapter to describe the total hearing-impaired population is 9.4% because it appears to be based on the best and most extensive data analysis (Fig. 7–2). This calculation provides hearing-impaired totals as shown in Figure 7–3 in the United States of approximately 25 million. Mild hearing losses account for 47.3% (11.6 million) of the hearing-impaired total, moderate losses at 29.0% (7.1 million), severe losses at 16.6% (4.1 million), and the profound deaf category at 7.1% (1.7 million). World population percentages are expected to be similar; however, most other countries report much lower percentages, reflecting the lack of methods to adequately evaluate hearing on the total population and also reflecting the lower significance of the role of hearing in their cultures. Data for Figures 7–2 through 7–4 and Table 7–5 are derived from: Gentile (1975); Glorig and Nixon (1960); Goldstein (1984); HIA (Hearing Industries Association) (1984); Jatho (1969); Moscicki, et al (1985); NCHS (1981); NCHS: Rowland (1980); NHIS (1977); NHIS: Adams & Hardy, (1989); Ries (1982); Roberts (1968); U.S. Department of Health and Human Services (1988); Wilder (1975); and Williams (1984).

Population projections show that a continuing and increasing incidence exists, especially in the older than 65 category for hearing impairment (Fig. 7–4). Projections for the total population from 1995 through 2050 are 261,000,000; 276,000,000; 300,000,000; 350,000,000; and 392,000,000. Life expectancy is projected to change from 76.3 years of age in 1995 to 82.6 years of age in the year 2050. The percentage of individuals older than 65 is expected to move from about 13% today to a little more

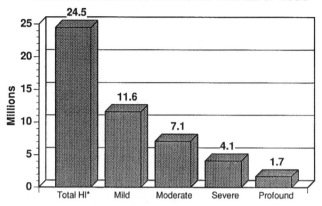

HEARING IMPAIRED IN THE U.S. BY DEGREE OF LOSS

(In Millions: Based on best available statistics)
***9.4% of the total population)**

Figure 7–3 "Best estimate" of people with hearing impairment in the United States by degree of loss by Staab (1991). Projected from the following data: Gentile (1975); Glorig and Nixon (1960); Goldstein (1984); HIA (Hearing Industries Association) (1984); Jatho (1969); Moscicki et al (1985); NCHS (1981); NCHS: Rowland (1980); NHIS (1977); NHIS: Adams & Hardy (1989); Ries (1982); Roberts (1968); U.S. Department of Health and Human Services (1988); Wilder (1975); and Williams (1984).

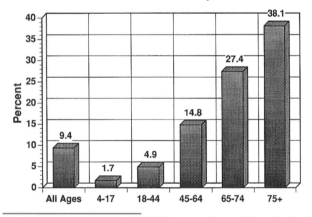

Prevalence of Hearing Impairment in the Civilian, Non-institutionalized Population

Figure 7–2 "Best estimate" of the prevalence of hearing impairment in the civilian, noninstitutionalized population by Staab (1991). Projected from the following data: Gentile (1975); Glorig and Nixon (1960); Goldstein (1984); HIA (Hearing Industries Association) (1984); Jatho (1969); Moscicki et al, (1985); NCHS (1981); NCHS: Rowland (1980); NHIS, (1977); NHIS: Adams & Hardy (1989); Ries (1982); Roberts (1968); U.S. Department of Health and Human Services (1988); Wilder (1975); and Williams (1984).

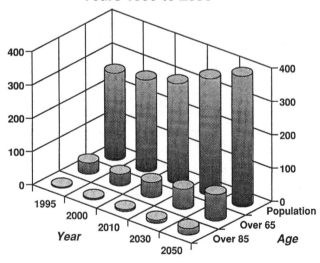

Projected Total Populations in Millions Years 1995 to 2050

	1995	2000	2010	2030	2050
Total Population	261	276	300	350	392
Over 65	33.9	35	45	60	78.4
Over 85	3	4.2	5.7	9	19

All numbers are in millions

Figure 7–4 Projected total population in millions, with the >65 and the >85 age groups identified. Years 1995 to 2050, U.S. Census Bureau.

than 20% in the year 2050 (USA Today, 1996). Individuals older than 85 comprised about 3 million in 1995 and are expected to increase to about 19 million (1 in 20) in the year 2050.

Trends in U.S. population demographics are reflected in Tables 7–4 to 7–7 and show a population older than 65 increasing from 11.3% in 1980 to 23.5% in the year 2080. This reflects an increasing life expectancy from about 47 years of age in 1900 to approximately 78 years of age today, and an expectation of extending further. This age group is of particular importance to audiology because it reflects the age group that is most likely to seek hearing services, especially hearing aids. It is roughly estimated that currently approximately 65% of all hearing aids are sold to individuals 65 years of age and older.

Some interesting statistics emerge from the U.S. Census Bureau in a study financed by the National Institute on Aging (USA Today, 1996) on the status of the elderly, considered to be those 65 years of age and older:

- The 65 and older population will grow from one in eight today to one in six by 2020 and one in five by 2050.
- By 2020, the nation's elderly population will total 53.3 million—a 63% increase over the current elderly population of 33 million.
- By 2020 nine other states will look a lot like Florida today (the largest proportion of elderly) at 2.5 million or 18.6% of the total population.
- In eight states, the number of people age 65 and older will more than double by 2020.
- The elderly population increased 11-fold from 1900 to 1994. The population younger than 65 increased just threefold.
- Of 80 million elderly projected for 2050, 8.4 million will be African American, 6.7 million will be of races other

than white or African American, and 12.5 million will be Hispanic.

- The percentage of elderly living in poverty declined from 24.6% in 1970 to 12.9% in 1992.
- The ratio of elderly people to working-age people (age 20 to 64) will nearly double between 1990 and 2050.
- In 2020, 25% of Floridians will be elderly. Arizona will have the largest percentage of seniors after Florida: 19.6%.
- The number of elderly will at least double in eight states between 1993 and 2020. The fastest growth will be in Nevada, where the older than 65 group will surge 116%.

Other age group statistics and information that are of interest are as follows:

- The number of centenarians – 100 years and older – more than doubled since 1980 to nearly 50,000. Four in five were women.
- Five states with the highest proportions of people age 85 and older in 1993 were in the Midwest: Iowa, North Dakota, South Dakota, Nebraska, and Kansas.
- From now until 2014, someone will turn 50 every 7.5 seconds.
- The old of 2020 will be healthier than their parents of 1920.
- Seniors 85 and older are the fastest-growing age group. They are expected to more than double to 7 million in 2020.

Lifestyle Demographics

Lifestyle demographics provide information about the types of goods and services that are important to people and that help drive their activities and purchases. Table 7–8 is a sampling of issues that were investigated for the cities and Zip codes identified and listed as a percentage of households that

DEMOGRAPHICS - 100 YEARS

		General Population							Hrg. Impaired Population		
Year	Total Pop. (Thous.)	Population by Age Group (Thous.)					% 65+	% Total Pop. Hrg. Imp.*	Total Hrg. Imp (Thous.)	Total 65+** (Thous.)
		18-24	25-34	35-44	45-64	65+				
1980	227,704	30,347	37,593	25,881	44,493	25,714	11.3	8.1	18,444	11,804
1985	238,631	28,739	41,788	32,004	44,652	28,608	12.0	8.6	20,522	13,134
1990	249,657	25,794	43,529	37,847	46,453	31,697	12.7	9.1	22,719	14,540
2000	267,955	24,601	36,415	43,743	60,886	34,921	13.0	10.1	27,063	17,320
2030	304,807	26,226	37,158	40,168	70,810	64,580	21.2	11.8	35,967	23,019
2080	310,762	25,296	37,237	38,222	73,748	73,090	23.5	13.0	40,399	25,855

Population Statistics Source: Census Bureau: Projections of the U.S. by Age, Sex, and Race: 1983-2080, Series P-25, No. 952.

Hearing Impaired Population Data was derived from data presented by Gentile, (1975); Glorig and Nixon, (1960); Goldstein, (1984); HIA (Hearing Industries Association), (1984); Jatho, (1969); Moscicki, Elkins, Baum, and McNamara, (1985); NCHS, (1981); NCHS, (1980); NHIS, (1977); NHIS, (1989); Ries, (1982); Roberts, (1968); U.S. Department of Health and Human Services, (1988); Wilder, (1975); and Williams, (1984).

* This % takes into consideration that the total percentage of the population with hearing impairment will increase as the population ages.

** This is based on 64.0% of those over 65 having a hearing impairment.

TABLE 7–5 Demographics—100 years. This projects the general and hearing-impaired populations from 1980 through 2080 for various age groups, both in numbers and in percent.

TABLE 7–6   Probability a 65-year-old will live until age:

Age	Percentage
70	95.5
80	78.0
90	43.9
100	9.6

Conclusion:

The older you get, the older you'll probably get!

TIAA-CREF magazine, 1998

TABLE 7–7   What will life expectancies be thirty years from now?

Life-expectancy prognostications are as varied as weather forecasts, depending on which forces the demographer believes exert the strongest influence. The two basic schools of thought are that (1) aging is controlled by a biological clock, so that life expectancy will not increase after it hits the built-in lifespan, or that (2) medical breakthroughs and healthier lifestyles will override any biological clock.

Researchers at Duke University, examining mortality trends, have concluded that the human life span's limit is currently 130. Other demographers estimate the practical limit to life expectancy at about 85 years; still others estimate "the average child born today may survive to age 95 or 100, with no inherent limit to human longevity in sight." (*Science* magazine, July 5, 1996).

With all this in mind, working people should heed the words of the composer Eubie Blake: "If I had known I was going to live this long, I would have taken better care of myself." Blake lived to be 100.

TIAA-CREF magazine, 1998

participate in that particular activity (Staab & Jelonek, 1995b). These can be compared with each other and also to the average in the United States (top line). Other areas of interest that were represented in this comparison (but not shown) include real estate, investments in stocks and bonds, wines, electronics, home video games, personal computers, photography, science fiction and new technology, stereos and tape recorders, VCRs, cable TV, bicycling, boating, bowling, golf, physical fitness, jogging, snow skiing, tennis, walking, watching TV, camping and hiking, fishing, hunting and shooting, motorcycles, recreational vehicles, wildlife and the environment, automotive work, reading, church, gambling, coins and stamp collecting, crafts, dieting, crossword puzzles, current affairs and politics, sweepstakes, gardening, grandchildren, health foods, home workshop, household pets, needlework, self-improvement, sewing, and veterans programs. The identification of populations that have higher-than-normal or lower-than-normal interests in certain areas provides significant information about how to market to that audience and

with what kind of message. For example, Zip code 10010, under dining out, suggests a population that may be more affluent (35.70% participating) as opposed to Zip code 15636 (13.90% participating). It also suggests that hearing instruments that allow for speech understanding in noise might offer a better message to those who dine out often. Lifestyle demographic information can tell you much about the population in your served market, and this should be taken into consideration when developing your marketing action plans. As an example, using messages that suggest hearing aids associated with grandparenting to a group that does not list grandparenting high on their list (Californians) is not a good use of your marketing efforts and expenditures. This group might be more responsive to materials that illustrate travel in the message. Lifestyle demographic interest differences often make it difficult to use a manufacturer's mass-produced advertising and promotional literature by everyone throughout the country. It can certainly explain why the same piece of literature pulls better in some places than in others. (These data were obtained from services purchased from CACI Marketing Systems, http://www.demographics.caci.com. CACI is one of a number of companies that provides information on updated and projection demographics and consumer data and trends, including lifestyle demographics.)

Market Analysis—Competition

Your business does not function in a vacuum. You have competition, and that competition is able to influence the success of your practice. It is, therefore, important to not only analyze the market potential and your own business but that of the competition as well. This is key to the identification of market opportunities and the development of marketing strategies and promotions.

Profile and Evaluate the Distribution Structure of the Local Market

Competition is anyone who, in the eyes of the consumer, provides substitute products or services to yours, who promotes in your market, or who shares referral sources. Table 7–9 provides a checklist of competitive analysis variables. If the competition is superior, their products and services will be chosen over yours. If they are inferior, they are vulnerable and represent a marketing opportunity for you.

Analyze the competition from the perspective of your patients. Who are your competitors? Why have patients chosen their services? Analyze their strengths and weaknesses (personally, educationally, and professionally). What would you say they do best? What do your patients and referral sources say about them? What is their facility, market share, growth rate and potential, equipment, accessibility, ambiance, length of time in business, image, and marketing message? How many offices and service centers do they have, what kind of staff (type and number)? For what are they known? This analysis should be performed to determine whether your competition has a marketing advantage that will make it difficult for your plans to succeed. This information can be obtained by reviewing the yellow pages, reading competitive advertising, a drive-by of their facility, or by asking potential patients what they think about a given practice. Businesses that have a competitive advantage are rewarded in that they

City	Zip Code	1990 Population	CUL Good Life Cultural/Arts Events — % Households Participating	CAR Good Life Career-Oriented Activities — % Households Participating	FLY Good Life Frequent Flyer — % Households Participating	FAS Good Life Fashion Clothing — % Households Participating	ART Good Life Fine Arts/ Antiques — % Households Participating	FOR Good Life Foreign Travel — % Households Participating	GOU Good Life Dining Out — % Households Participating	HFD Good Life Hshld Furn Decorating — % Households Participating	MON Good Life Money Making Opportunities — % Households Participating
UNITED STATES			15.10%	11.90%	11.50%	12.70%	10.30%	13.10%	20.20%	19.10%	9.20%
STRATFORD	06497	49,495	16.70%	11.70%	17.30%	14.40%	9.70%	16.90%	24.60%	19.90%	9.40%
BRIDGEPORT	06606	41,861	14.60%	12.00%	11.50%	19.90%	8.40%	17.10%	25.30%	19.60%	11.00%
TRUMBULL	06611	32,236	18.00%	12.90%	27.40%	15.50%	11.50%	21.10%	25.90%	21.80%	9.00%
DARIEN	06820	13,449	24.70%	13.10%	40.20%	16.10%	19.30%	34.50%	35.30%	25.90%	8.20%
NORWALK	06850	14,019	19.20%	16.10%	28.00%	18.20%	12.40%	23.40%	31.10%	19.90%	10.20%
WESTPORT	06880	21,737	32.00%	18.30%	45.20%	17.20%	21.20%	37.50%	35.20%	25.10%	10.20%
HACKENSACK	07601	36,932	19.40%	15.80%	22.30%	21.30%	11.20%	24.50%	27.80%	19.10%	12.00%
BOGOTA	07603	7,824	13.00%	15.10%	11.70%	12.60%	10.80%	17.50%	24.40%	17.50%	10.70%
HASBROUCK HTS	07604	11,489	12.40%	13.70%	17.30%	17.60%	8.40%	16.40%	25.60%	24.50%	7.60%
BERGENFIELD	07621	24,580	14.00%	8.70%	18.40%	15.50%	8.40%	20.10%	24.40%	18.10%	5.80%
PARAMUS	07652	25,059	17.00%	13.20%	24.40%	18.30%	10.00%	25.70%	26.60%	19.00%	12.90%
TEANECK	07666	37,815	27.60%	19.00%	24.80%	16.50%	13.00%	28.50%	25.40%	19.20%	10.50%
DENVILLE	07834	14,554	18.40%	15.80%	28.20%	13.90%	12.80%	21.60%	28.30%	24.70%	11.60%
MORRISTOWN	07960	38,515	27.10%	18.70%	38.00%	17.10%	16.50%	30.50%	29.80%	21.10%	8.90%
NEW YORK	10003	49,308	47.20%	25.10%	34.60%	24.10%	26.40%	43.90%	34.40%	18.30%	7.20%
NEW YORK	10010	24,606	43.00%	23.90%	33.80%	24.80%	21.70%	44.70%	35.70%	20.50%	9.00%
NEW YORK	10016	45,192	41.00%	25.90%	36.00%	30.30%	22.80%	44.30%	33.90%	21.20%	9.70%
NEW YORK	10021	93,571	42.60%	22.60%	40.30%	27.80%	25.90%	47.10%	34.60%	21.40%	9.30%
NEW YORK	10028	41,373	25.40%	21.20%	26.50%	21.60%	17.70%	56.00%	27.50%	23.80%	10.90%
NEW YORK	10128	48,417	41.80%	24.30%	40.30%	25.20%	22.30%	43.90%	34.50%	21.00%	8.40%
BRONX	10461	37,530	13.50%	12.10%	10.30%	19.00%	8.00%	18.50%	26.20%	19.00%	10.80%
BRONX	10465	27,638	11.00%	9.50%	10.70%	18.70%	7.20%	16.90%	26.80%	22.60%	11.60%
BRONX	10467	64,302	16.10%	13.90%	8.90%	21.50%	7.80%	19.60%	22.10%	19.20%	13.70%
MIDDLETOWN	10940	37,232	14.50%	13.00%	10.20%	15.20%	9.00%	14.00%	22.60%	18.20%	11.30%
BROOKLYN	11203	59,995	20.80%	17.30%	10.00%	25.50%	7.10%	28.60%	22.90%	20.10%	16.10%
BROOKLYN	11204	50,923	11.40%	9.90%	9.60%	20.70%	8.20%	19.80%	26.20%	17.00%	12.50%
BROOKLYN	11214	58,783	12.60%	10.40%	9.90%	19.60%	8.70%	19.00%	28.60%	18.30%	11.50%
BROOKLYN	11223	53,105	12.20%	9.10%	10.60%	21.60%	8.50%	20.00%	25.70%	20.00%	11.30%
BROOKLYN	11225	48,321	22.10%	15.60%	10.90%	27.60%	9.00%	28.30%	25.40%	20.10%	14.50%
BROOKLYN	11226	76,678	20.90%	17.50%	8.00%	28.40%	8.80%	26.90%	25.50%	20.30%	18.90%
NEWBURG	12550	34,816	13.20%	12.50%	11.10%	14.80%	9.00%	14.60%	24.80%	18.50%	10.90%
NEWBURG	12553		13.80%	13.30%	14.20%	15.60%	9.10%	15.40%	23.60%	24.50%	9.80%
GREENSBURG	15601	43,164	14.20%	9.80%	11.50%	44.10%	8.90%	8.00%	18.10%	20.90%	8.90%
HARRISON CITY	15636	3,313	7.70%	7.50%	9.70%	9.60%	7.60%	5.70%	13.90%	26.80%	10.80%
MURRYSVILLE	15668	8,860	19.70%	16.00%	29.60%	12.30%	11.10%	16.80%	19.50%	22.70%	7.50%
COATESVILLE	19320	29,226	10.70%	10.00%	9.50%	15.40%	10.70%	10.80%	21.60%	19.30%	7.70%
DOWNINGTOWN	19335	24,438	13.70%	14.30%	24.00%	13.30%	11.10%	15.40%	24.50%	23.30%	8.40%

TABLE 7–8 Lifestyle demographic sample data. The percentages indicate the population within the Zip codes identified that are likely to engage in the activity listed. This is a sampling only of the categories of lifestyle interests that can be evaluated and that are useful in directing marketing efforts. (From Staab & Jelonek [1995b], with permission).

COMPETITOR ANALYSIS CONSIDERATIONS
(Much information can be obtained from just thinking)

Defensive Position:
- Is the competition satisfied with his/her current position? If so, good.
- What likely future moves or shifts will they make and how dangerous are they to you?

Offensive Position:
- Where are they vulnerable?
- What might you do to cause them to respond vigorously (good or bad)?

A **Competitor Profile** is the way that an analysis can be approached. Think of competitors as those who make your business life more miserable.

1. What are the competitors' strengths and weaknesses?
2. What are the competitors' strategies?
3. Competitors' have long memories and will hang onto something that has worked for them in the past.

☐ Facility
    ☐ Location
    ☐ Ownership
    ☐ Decor
    ☐ Type of facility
☐ Financial
    ☐ Profitability
    ☐ Cash flow
    ☐ Cash reserves
    ☐ Prices
    ☐ Discounts
    ☐ Staying power
☐ Product/Services
    ☐ Product or services mix
    ☐ Product brand
    ☐ Test equipment

☐ Market share
    ☐ Customer base
    ☐ Sales volume
    ☐ Distribution area
    ☐ Referral sources
☐ People
    ☐ Credentials
    ☐ Sales style
    ☐ Knowledge
    ☐ Communication skills
    ☐ Staff size
☐ Advertising/Promotion
    ☐ Media used
    ☐ Amount used
    ☐ Types used

TABLE 7–9   Variables to consider when conducting a competitive analysis. (From Staab & Jelonek [1995b], with permission.)

have performance that consistently is better than others, have continuous referrals, enjoy generous walk-in business, have a high incidence of word-of-mouth referrals, have a market share that is stable or growing, show close rates on advertising and promotion leads that are high, and which have high name recognition among hearing aid users and referral sources.

Competition can be analyzed from either a defensive or offensive position. If defensive, attempt to determine whether he or she seems satisfied with the current position. If so, this can prove advantageous to you. If they are likely to move or shift position, what will these shifts be and how dangerous are they to your practice? If analyzed from an offensive position, look to where the competition is vulnerable. What might you do to cause them to respond vigorously to your program(s), and how might you expect them to respond?

After you have finished analyzing your competition, analyze your practice in the same way. Determine whether you have a competitive advantage and, if not, how will you motivate people to frequent your practice (objectives, strategies, and tactics)? It is *key* that you identify and develop your competitive advantage. Unfortunately, most people do not perform such an analysis. However, without a competitive advantage, a dispensing operation will not achieve and sustain superior market performance.

When do you have a competitive advantage? This occurs when you have a product or service that is as follows (Jelonek, 1992a):

- *Unique.* The product or service is not available from others.
- *Has value.* Patients believe that for their dollar, they are receiving an exceptional value or deal. This value might be evidenced by the image of your practice, by your specialization, by the superiority of the product itself, differentiation, or through exclusivity.
- *Is defendable.* Your offering is difficult to copy or might include provisions that exclude others from providing something similar.
- *Is sustainable.* It has a momentum that can continue for a reasonable period of time without encroachment.

PEARL

You have a competitive advantage when your product or service is unique, has value, is defendable, and is sustainable (Jelonek, 1992a).

What are some ways or issues involved in the development of a competitive advantage? The following approaches are suggested (Staab & Jelonek, 1994b, 1995b):

Cost

Cost can be a competitive advantage only if everything associated with this offering can be obtained and provided at a lower cost than by the competition. This includes the entire management of the business as well. If a cost advantage exists, the focus should be on the cost, not on the price of the product. Selling a product or offering service at a low cost alone, or for a short period of time, does not provide a cost advantage. In reality, few practices are able to offer cost as a competitive advantage. Selling at a low price without a cost advantage is a certain route to failure.

> ## PITFALL
>
> **Selling a product or offering service at a low cost alone, or for a short period of time, does not provide a cost advantage. In reality, few practices are able to offer cost as a competitive advantage. Selling at a low price without a cost advantage is a certain route to failure.**

Focus

Specializing in a certain type of service or product or on a specific segment of the market might give you a competitive advantage. Examples of this could include home service, cochlear implants, working with children, concentration on celebrities, service centers, the latest technology, private label products, and so on. The specialty cannot be in name only. You must have associated with you all the skills, knowledge, and equipment to keep you ahead of the competition.

Timing

This assumes that you can quickly and easily offer new products or services to the market. Or, it might mean that you are able to offer the products and services that others offer, but more quickly, with greater accessibility, and with greater quality.

Differentiation

What do you do or have that is unique to the marketplace? Are you able to offer a value that others cannot and present it in a distinctive manner? Do you have credentials that others do not have, hospital or academic training program privileges, knowledge, quality, skills, offerings, a delivery system, managed care, cerumen management, equipment? In what you do, is it the distinguishing characteristic or competitive strength of your practice?

However you differentiate your practice from others, make certain that you present your offering with added value, realizing that value is determined by the patient, not by you. Patients often consider cost, time, accessibility, and outcome as factors that determine value. It is this feature that the consumer will often refer to when asked about your business. If what you are offering is not perceived by the patient as having added value, it is considered a commodity, for which price is the only distinguishing competitive feature.

> ## PITFALL
>
> **If what you are offering is not perceived by the patient as having added value, it is considered a commodity, for which price is the only distinguishing competitive feature.**

In a series of marketing seminars on hearing aids comanaged by me, attendees were asked to identify what they thought their competitive advantage was. Almost without exception, each suggested that they were very caring and understanding of their patients, that they related to them extremely well, and that they considered them as people rather than as patients. They believed that their interaction with the patients was their primary competitive advantage. They considered this interaction with their patients to be very special, and perhaps it was. However, this relationship does not provide the basis for a competitive advantage because literally everyone in the room expressed the same "competitive advantage." How does this meet the requirements of uniqueness, value, defendable, and sustainable? In other words, rather than being a competitive advantage, what they were expressing was a measure of "standards of performance." This was *expected* of them to manage a business successfully.

Appendix C at the end of this chapter provides an action plan outline for determining your competitive advantage. It is important to have one so that you can be differentiated from the competition. It gives your office a focus, drives your marketing strategies and programs, gives you an identity, and positions you relative to competition in the minds of your patients. Analysis of competition is a tool in establishing uniqueness of your office. Your resourcefulness in using this information is the key to a successful practice.

> ## CONTROVERSIAL POINT
>
> **The special care, understanding, and attention you give to your patients is not considered a competitive advantage—it should be considered a "standard of performance."**

How to Use Market Analysis Data

Market data are used to help determine market sales potential, to assess the competitive intensity of the market, to develop market programs, to facilitate strategic planning, to determine service offerings and pricing levels, to target direct mail programs, to identify office locations and design, to determine what types of services and products should be offered, to develop promotional programs, and to select and direct market communications. The market potential is determined by a number of factors, including population size and growth rate, population mix, income and occupations, community economic health, and dispenser/population ratios.

Marketing Objectives

Goals or objectives?—Goals are fine, but objectives may be better. Both are important. The difference between them is that one is qualitative and the other is quantitative. The convention is that goals are qualitative and objectives are quantitative, but if you reverse these that is fine also, as long as you quantify your *thinking*.

Goals should be considered for both personal and business reasons. Personal goals might consist of achieving income, preparing for retirement, or enjoying a particular lifestyle, among others. Business goals might consist of increasing unit sales, increasing gross sales, increasing net income, improving productivity, expanding market position, increasing profitability, decreasing debt, repositioning the practice, expanding of the practice with a new office, developing new patients, developing new markets or referral sources, increasing cash flow, lowering the return rate, decreasing the resale time period, increasing the lifetime value of current patients, increasing response rates to prospect mailings, decreasing patient attrition, providing better patient service, and so on. These are all examples of worthwhile goals frequently listed with proposals on which marketing strategies are built.

It follows, naturally, that if goals are quantified, resulting objectives—if achieved—will provide a basis for measuring the value of the goal. For example, selected goals just defined could be restated into the following list of objectives:

- *Increase unit sales* by 10% from 20 units per month to 22 units per month without a decrease in gross profit margin.
- *Decrease debt* by 40% without absorbing more than a 10% loss from gross profits.
- *Increase the lifetime value of current patients* by 15% from an average of $8000 to $9200.
- *Increase response rates to prospect mailings* by 10% from 2 to 2.2%, while keeping the number of pieces mailed constant.
- *Decrease patient attrition by 20%* from 10 to 8%, without increasing marketing costs by more than $50 per first-time purchaser.

- *Reduce the average inbound call wait time* from 30 to 20 seconds, without increasing total inbound telemarketing costs by more than 8%.

Regardless of how goals or objectives are stated, they should be (a) put to writing, (b) quantified, (c) realistic, and (d) limited in number.

In the hierarchy of events, goals or objectives are at the tip of a triangle, strategies are below this and should support the goals, and the bottom level consists of the tactics, which are the day-to-day programs to allow the practice to reach its objectives (Fig. 7–5).

Marketing Strategies

Marketing strategies are developed as general directions used to achieve the goals or objectives. They are the "how to" but not the detailed activity. The detailed activities are the tactics (specifics) and are presented later in the marketing action plan under "Promotion."

Positioning is central to all marketing strategies. It is difficult to provide services and products if they are not proper for the market, if they are priced incorrectly, if the practice is not known to the market, or if the practice lacks a credible image (Hosford-Dunn et al, 1995a). Positioning is accomplished through strategies implementing the "marketing mix" categories of product, price, promotion, place, and people. How you position yourself relative to these categories defines the image of your practice. Such categorization is not necessary normally when detailing strategies, however, because seldom do so many exist as to call for such a categorization. In fact, for small businesses, the number of objectives, strategies, and tactics should be kept to a manageable number—which generally translates to "relatively few."

Still, to assist in understanding what these categories refer to, and how they help to build the image of the practice, the following brief explanations are provided.

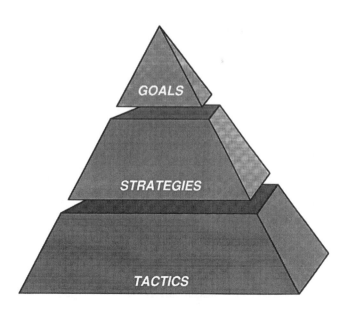

Figure 7–5   The arrangement of marketing features. Goals (objectives) define the overall direction of the business. Strategies are developed as general directions used to achieve the goals or objectives. The programs (tactics) consist of the day-to-day, detailed activities (specifics) that allow the practice to survive and grow.

Product

Product refers to the overall nature of the goods and services one provides to one's patients. Product strategies involve the selection of products, the number of and brands managed (including also product skills, knowledge, and expertise), hearing analyses, outcome measurements, services, warranties, and return policies. Which products to use are often decided by the image, profit margins, investment, technology, reliability, and by what the supplier is able to help the audiologist with professionally and personally. This decision appears to be made on the basis of both product performance and business realities. For example, most dispensing audiologists have come to grips with the initial euphoria of the Americans With Disabilities Act and recognize that persons with hearing impairment are not beating a path to their door to purchase assistive listening devices. Most find that their practices are sufficiently inventoried if they have alerting devices (especially for the doorbell or phone), something for television use, a telephone amplifier, and a hard-wired remote microphone-to-earphone communication device.

Suggestions for deciding how to position a product in the marketplace (modified from McKenna, 1986) follow.

Understand Market Trends

If new technology is critical to your market, position your practice as the technology leader through your product offerings. For example, offer digital hearing aids; not just a single brand, but all digital brands to support that image.

Focus on Intangible Positioning Factors
Having to do with Quality

A constant emphasis on new products (tangible items), while ignoring unrelated services, can have immediate adverse effects when the new product becomes obsolete. Obsolescence can occur rather quickly with some new products or technologies.

Focus on a Specific Audience
and Serve it Better than Anyone Else

You might choose to concentrate on home care service with the aged who have difficulty transporting to your office, or with children.

Experiment and Pay Attention to Market Reaction

You may have preconceived ideas about products and services for a particular market, but they may not be consistent with consumer performance. For example, at one time many thought that in-the-canal and completely-in-the-canal hearing aids were not for the elderly because they might have difficulty managing the controls. The reality is that many elderly can manage and prefer the smaller instruments. Failure to test this with elderly patients results in many being treated at a facility other than yours.

Price

Price defines your pricing strategy and methods and is integral to your marketing plan. Price strategies relate to pricing options, increased value, added services, multiple-tiered services, and products. Pricing must be consistent with the perceived value of your offerings and still allow your practice to survive, grow, and meet the overall financial goals as stated in your business plan. Because price plays such an important role in establishing the success and image of your practice, it is discussed separately.

Promotion

Promotion includes media advertising, publicity, brochures and literature, personal selling, sales promotion, direct marketing (including mail and telemarketing), patient education, and sales incentives. Although advertising is a part of promotion in the marketing mix, it is not the only way to promote. Advertising is a subset of promotion and is discussed later in this chapter; it is not just another word for marketing.

Place

Place refers to where your practice is located and by whom and when your offerings are made. It defines also your target geographical trade area: city, county, state, region, and so on. Place strategies include office location and design, relocation, the tracking of clientele, increasing outside service calls, remodeling/enlarging, the integration of new technologies, additional financing (long or short term), and functional uses of facilities. Suggestions for practice location are made in Chapters 8 and 13 in this volume.

People

People defines your staffing needs and division of labor relative to marketing and sales. People strategies are often patient based. These can involve existing patients, potential patients, or referral sources (from patients, the medical community, third party, or managed care). They often involve a knowledge of the lifestyle demographics and psychographics of the population in question. This category is not always identified separately in the "P's" of the marketing mix as is done here but is listed under the "place" category.

Having discussed in general the role of strategies in the market program, the following examples of strategies that support a goal (nonqualified marketing objective) are presented. The specific strategies used would depend on how the objective was quantified.

Objective: To increase profitability
Strategies:

1. Eliminate unprofitable activities
2. Increase prices
3. Sell premium priced products
4. Emphasize cost reductions
5. Sell more products or services
6. Add point-of-purchase products
7. Decrease spending
8. Improve effectiveness of patient service
9. Cross-train personnel

As can be identified in this example, even though the objective is price related, the strategies cover a range of product mix elements: product, price, promotion, and people. Place was not a marketing strategy in this example. The critical element in strategic planning is to ensure that the strategies proposed help achieve the overall objective with which they are associated. At least one or more strategies should be present for each objective.

Price As a Marketing Strategy

> ### SPECIAL CONSIDERATION
>
> The pricing decision must reflect management's objectives, satisfy customers, and ensure competitive status in the marketplace.

Pricing is often considered the cornerstone of the marketing plan. It helps determine not only current sales and earnings but, much more fundamentally, who your patients and competitors will be in the future. Whatever the price, it must reflect the business objectives, satisfy patients, and ensure a competitive status in the marketplace. The basic plan is to determine the pricing objective, to target the market, and then to provide appropriate pricing strategies. (NOTE: An excellent overview of pricing, with detailed examples to audiological practice, is presented by Hosford-Dunn et al, [1995b]. Readers who are interested in more specific details are encouraged to read Chapter 14 of this source.)

The price you charge for your products and service can determine the success or failure of your overall business. Some practices set prices on simple criteria such as recovery of costs, percentage markup over cost, competitors' prices, or the market price leader. The problem with such approaches is that they fail to take into account numerous other factors that affect the pricing decision. For example, would it not seem prudent to consider such issues as the patient base and mix, consumer demands, competitive forces, economic conditions, availability of money, and changes in interest rates? It is because of these issues, and others, that each practice should develop independently its own pricing policies and objectives. *These decisions are essential because changing price levels affect cash flow and margins more rapidly than any other marketing decision.*

Pricing Objectives

What are your pricing objectives? Do they include profit, return on investment, improved cash flow, liquidation of aging inventory, or increased sales volume or market share? In establishing pricing objectives, the *ultimate sales and profit* objectives must first be determined. To accomplish this, at least the following issues must be resolved first:

- Disagreements must be ironed out over objectives within your own organization.
- The fundamental conflict between buyer and seller must be considered.
- Sellers view price as (a) expected revenue, (b) an accumulation of costs, and (c) a marketing feature (high prices indicate product quality—low prices provide a marketing advantage).
- The buyer views the purchasing decision on the basis of the perceived value of the product and on its price compared with the competition.

What approach should be used when establishing sales and profit objectives? Three general pricing objective categories have been identified : (1) profit oriented, (2) sales

oriented, and (3) the status quo (Hosford-Dunn et al, 1995b). These authors also review the target measures and pricing methods for each of these categories. The explanations of approaches that follows is intended to serve as guidelines for determining your general pricing objectives.

> ### PEARL
>
> General pricing objectives include increasing profitability, increasing sales, gaining market share, eliminating competition, promoting an image of quality or service, discouraging any new competitors from entering your market, being accepted as a price leader in the market by competitors, restoring order to a disorderly market.

Price for Profit

Price for profit is the most logical pricing objective and most practices use the "cost plus" approach to obtain it. However, to achieve a predetermined profit, specific goals must be established, a specific percentage of sales as a rate of return on investment (ROI) or as a rate of return on assets managed (ROAM).

Maximize Profit

When used as a short-term objective, maximizing profit may be incompatible with the almost certain long-term goal of profit maximization. For example, for some who have chosen to dispense primarily premium priced hearing aids or charge high prices in an introductory product stage, high gross revenues may be realized, but the use of this approach may also prevent the practice from gaining its ultimate market share because of the practice's increased dependence on a smaller number of consumers. In addition, high gross revenues do not necessarily translate into high profits.

Achieve a Certain Return on Investment

Prices are set to generate the level of profit necessary to achieve a targeted ROI (predetermined) desired. This is a pricing approach based on net profit goals for an *average* sales volume, rather than on *actual* volume. A danger is that achieving this volume may take precedence over realizing adjustments that might allow an immediate high rate of cash return.

EXAMPLE: Hearing aid sales of 8 per month = 96/y
Fixed cost of product per year = $1000/aid or $96,000/y*
Variable cost of product per year = $800/aid or $76,800/y
Desired profit margin = 20% ROI (but, select your own)

---

*With nontangible items no cost is associated with the product alone (for example, a hearing test), but variable costs are associated with giving the test. Tangible items, such as hearing aids, have both fixed and variable costs (fixed cost of $1000/unit and a variable cost of $800/unit to dispense and maintain the instrument in this example). The average cost per unit of products or services sold would be the sum of total fixed and variable costs, divided by the number of services or products sold. Using the information above:

$$\text{Selling price} = \frac{\text{Net profit}}{\text{Sales}}$$

Selling price =

$$\frac{[(100 + \%\text{ROI})/100] \times (\text{Expenses} + \text{Cost of goods sold})}{\text{Sales (Number of products sold)}}$$

$$\text{Selling Price} = \frac{1.2 \times \$96,000 + \$76,000}{96 \text{ units/y}}$$

$$= \$2,150/\text{hearing aid}$$

A very simple method to determine how large the ROI must be to ensure an acceptable return after taxes and inflation is:

$$\text{Break-even point} = \frac{\text{Rate of inflation (\%)}}{100 - \text{Rate of tax on gain}}$$

As a general point of information and as an example, with inflation at 6%, a business in the 40% tax bracket must have net returns of more than 10% to come out ahead.

Price for Cash Flow

At times you may have to adopt policies that conflict with profit objectives. For example, if you have committed large sums of money for a particular direct mail program on programmable hearing instruments, a pricing policy may have to be set in place, temporarily, which returns the maximum cash within a specific period.

Price to Increase Sales

Pricing, either up or down, can have an impact on sales volume faster than any other marketing technique. However, similar results can be achieved by improving product quality, service, or delivery. One must fully understand the implications of price reductions on gross profit margins (and the increase in product or service unit sales required) before instituting such programs (Table 7–10). For example, if a decision is made to offer a price discount (such as 30%) and an attempt is made to maintain the same gross profit (i.e., 50% which is the sales minus the cost of goods sold), an increase in sales dollar volume of 42.86% would be required. This would amount to an increase in unit sales from 20 to 28.57 units. These figures would change if different scenarios were sought (Staab, 1986). To determine the impact of a price increase, review the break-even analysis in Figure 7–8 (see p. 158 in Section on Break-Even Analysis).

IMPACT OF DISCOUNTS ON GROSS PROFIT
(50% gross profit margin used in this hearing aid sale example)

Sales Dollars and Unit Increase Required to Maintain a 50% Gross Profit if Discounts are Offered. Modify numbers as required.

Selling Price	= $1000 – changes with discount offered, column (b)
Costs	= $500 (assumes this is constant to offset volume purchasing lost)
Average Sold	= 20 units/month
Sales Volume	= $20,000/mo (based on selling price of $1000)

(a) % Discount	(b) Selling Price/Aid	(c) Sales $ – Discount	(d) New Sales Volume With No Unit Increase	(e) Profit Margin (%)	(f) Sales Volume Increase Needed to Get Back to 50% Gross Margin	(g) Unit Increase Needed to Get Back to 50% Gross Margin
0%	$1000	$20,000 – $0	$20,000	50.00%	0%	0
5%	$950	$20,000 – $1000	$19,000	47.37%	5.26%	1.05
10%	$900	$20,000 – $2000	$18,000	44.44%	11.11%	2.22
15%	$850	$20,000 – $3000	$17,000	41.18%	17.65%	3.53
20%	$800	$20,000 – $4000	$16,000	37.50%	25.00%	5.00
25%	$750	$20,000 – $5000	$15,000	33.33%	33.35%	6.67
30%	$700	$20,000 – $6000	$14,000	28.57%	42.86%	8.57

(a)	Percent discount per aid
(b)	Selling price of aid minus the discount ($1000 X discount % in (a))
(c)	Monthly sales volume with discount shown ($20,000 minus monthly discount)
(d)	Discounted monthly sales volume
(e)	Profit Margin (Selling price minus costs)/Selling price X 100
(f)	Sales volume increase required to get back to 50% gross margin (% increase of 20,000 over (d))
(g)	$20,000 divided by discounted selling price (b). Subtract 20 monthly average from the calculated figure.

TABLE 7–10 The impact of price discounts on gross profit margins. The greater the discount the greater the increase in units of product or service that are required to stay at the same profit margin. Shown also are the dollar volume increases required to continue to achieve the same profit margin (50% in this example), and the number of additional instruments that must be sold at each discount level. The figures change with different scenarios. See text for explanation.

Price to Maintain or Increase Market Share

Pricing to maintain or increase market share is a fairly common practice but is often misunderstood. The theory is that market share increase (new unit sales or patients) is a more meaningful measure of success than growth in sales dollars because expanding market share may permit a business to accomplish its long-term objectives more easily as a result of the broader patient base. For this reason prices are sometimes set to ensure high sales volume, even at the expense of short-term profits.

Price to Stabilize Market Prices and Margins

Pricing to stabilize market prices and margins is often done as a reaction to competition, especially during times of rising prices (but can be done when prices are falling as well). This should be used with caution because adjusting prices to competitors often triggers price wars.

Price to Follow the Law of Supply and Demand

Pricing to follow the law of supply and demand tailors the pricing strategy to selling less for a higher price, or more for a lower price.

• • •

A couple of pricing approaches that may not be directly related to increased profits or sales volume include (1) Pricing to maintain image, in which a high price implies quality, value, or prestige; and (2) Limiting the degree of price hikes, an example is if a 10% price increase is projected for next year, the increase can be tempered by initiating two 5% increases—one now or in another 6 months and the other a year from now.

From Objectives to Strategies

It is not possible to anticipate every variable affecting the market but one should be aware of the following general rules:

• With few exceptions, an increase in the price of a product will lead to a fall in the demand for that product. Conversely, a reduction in the product price will lead to an increase in demand for that item.

• No practice will be a product leader over its entire product line. In a competitive marketplace, even the strongest company will have weaknesses in some areas.

• Any pricing policy must be flexible enough to allow for minor price adjustments on the basis of prevailing market conditions. To allow this flexibility, the pricing policy should have a basic reference point price. The price is then modified to take into account variations within a product line, market structure, geographical location, competition, terms, and quantity.

Pricing Strategy

Not until all conflicts related to objectives are resolved can strategies be put into effect. To facilitate decisions regarding pricing strategies, the following must be done:

• Have a pricing policy that sets the basic philosophy for the entire marketing plan; price above, equal to, or less than that of the competition. When setting this basic philosophy, remember that smaller practices may not be able to offer some products or services that are priced well above or well below the competition.

• Consider the relationship between pricing and the product's life cycle (see Fig. 7–13). The price in the growth stage is usually different (higher) than when in the mature stage.

• Establish and define your pricing objective.

Specific Pricing Strategies

For price-influencing factors, see Figure 7–6.

"Cost Plus" Pricing

Cost plus pricing is the simplest approach, but often the least rewarding. The reasoning is that operating expenses at least must be recovered. *Total operating expenses are calculated, and a percentage markup is added for profit.* What goes into total operating expenses? These generally include costs of all material, labor, and overhead. It fails to consider what the consumer is willing to pay and differences in the product mix. This approach is best used for determining the *minimum* price to charge.

Markup Pricing (Standard Markup Pricing)

Markup pricing also has the advantage of simplicity. This adds a percent value to the *cost* of the products or services, including overhead. It is often a constant percentage added to each product or service (a doubling or tripling of the cost). The markup is *usually a percentage of the selling price that is added to the cost and not the actual earnings.* For example, a hearing aid that has a wholesale cost of $1000 and is sold for $2000 has a 50% markup, not a 100% markup. This is also sometimes referred to as the gross profit, gross margin, or markup.

$$\text{Markup} = \frac{\text{Selling price} - \text{Cost of product}}{\text{Selling price}} \times 100$$

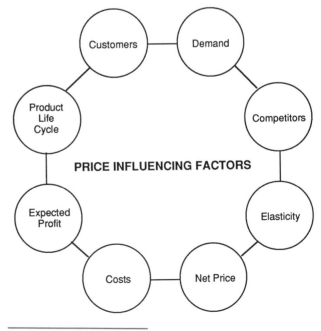

Figure 7–6 Price-influencing factors.

$$\text{Markup} = \frac{\$2000 - \$1000}{\$2000} \times 100 = 50\%$$

$$\text{Selling Price} = \frac{\text{Cost of product}}{100 - \text{Markup}} \times 100$$

$$\text{Selling Price} = \frac{\$1000}{100 - 50\%} \times 100 = \$2000$$

This approach does not attempt to determine what the product is actually worth to the patient. Be aware, however, that using a percentage markup can lead to underpriced labor-intensive products and overpriced material-intensive products. Its efficiency is undermined by the failure to reap the maximum profits (when patients are willing to pay a higher price for the product or service).

Consumer Pricing

Consumer pricing determines that price must be based on the *consumer-perceived values* and not on one's costs. This is often used by businesses that offer specialized products and services where each can be priced individually on the basis of costs, expenses, and profit margins. Pricing strategies based on ROI often fall in this category. This type pricing often takes a multitiered approach where products and prices are offered at more than one level, and the consumer selects on the basis of what he or she is willing to pay.

Inflation Pricing

Inflation pricing complicates pricing strategies because it drives costs up, whereas the experience curve tends to go down (especially in the case of new products). If set too low, prices may not be able to keep up with inflation, or if too high, may not generate the volume needed for one to stay in business. This is not ordinarily used in audiology. Instead, other approaches are modified to compensate for inflation.

Competitive Pricing (Follow the Leader)

Competitive pricing is one of the simplest pricing approaches. Basically, fees are set at or less than those of competitors, without regard to profitability. Because dispensing audiologists often use the same products or services (which can substitute for each other), price is certainly a factor, and this is the approach used by many. In some highly competitive markets this may be the most reasonable approach. Competitive pricing necessarily affects the price you can charge and what the competition can charge relative to your practice. But, what should you do if your competitor raises or lowers prices? Before changing your price relative to theirs for the same or similar products (i.e., hearing aids), consider the following:

- What are the competitor's reasons for his or her prices? Do you have the same cost pressures? Are they attempting to seek immediate cash, a liquidation of stock, or are they an aggressive competitor seeking market share?
- Consider responding with a nonprice-related strategy, such as higher quality, better distribution, or an extended warranty.
- If the competitor offered a lower price, consider offering a lower-priced product to compete with the offering.

- If the competitor offered a higher price, consider both your own costs and possible consumer reaction to the higher cost.

Many audiologists mimic the market leaders when it comes to pricing. Unfortunately, this assumes that the leaders know what they are doing.

CONTROVERSIAL POINT

Many audiologists mimic the market leaders when it comes to pricing. However, this assumes that the leaders know what they are doing.

Price Skimming

Price skimming deliberately sets a high price on products to maximize short-term contributions. This is often used with new products. A potential bonus is that the product or service may develop prestige, because high prices usually denote high quality. However, one must make certain that the service and quality are commensurate with the price or consumer resentment and loss of sales will develop.

Low-Ball Pricing

Low-ball pricing is often used by extremely aggressive companies or those struggling to gain market share. In some cases the products are sold at a loss. This is an attempt to buy market share in the short term, with an expectation that they will be able to attain profits in the long term.

Penetration Pricing

Penetration pricing revolves around the "experience curve" theory. The philosophy states that when prices are set deliberately low, a large market share can be captured quickly, resulting in economies of scale such that unit costs are low. The success or failure of this approach depends on the speed with which economies of scale can be achieved (and depends on the size of purchase discounts, low competition, no returns, and efficient use of overhead). This is often a high-risk strategy. This pricing approach is used also at times with low-cost, high-volume products such as hearing aid batteries.

Opportunistic Pricing

Opportunistic pricing can occur during severe supply shortages when patients are willing to pay more for products they value. This is seldom used in dispensing practices because substitute products seem to be readily available.

Price Bundling (or Unbundling)

Price bundling (or unbundling) occurs when different products are sold together at a single price. This is very common with hearing aids, especially behind-the-ear instruments where the ear mold is sold as a part of the hearing aid. It occurs as well with the hearing aid evaluation cost being a part of the hearing aid sale. Or a service contract is sold as part of the instrument sale but not broken out with a separate fee. Unbundling occurs when each component of a product package or service is identified with a separate price. Audiologists are split almost equally on bundling or unbundling costs (Skafte, 1998).

Loss Leader Pricing

Loss leader pricing is sometimes used to offer a full line of products and services or to attract new patients. The intent is to attract patients to company products that are profitable (free hearing aid batteries with the hope that the patient will later purchase new hearing aids or free hearing testing to sell hearing aids) by offering something else at below or no cost.

Defensive Pricing

Defensive pricing occurs when a loss of market share is anticipated. It is more common with established businesses as an attempt to discourage competitors to enter or to remain in the market. The discounted pricing is strategically timed to affect the competitor when he or she is most vulnerable.

Price Milking

Price milking is sometimes used by mature companies who wish to leave the market or when a product life cycle has entered the mature stage. Maximum profits are sought by setting prices at levels higher than the market would normally justify. A certain percentage of patients who are loyal to a particular product will pay the higher price even though marketing costs may have been significantly reduced.

Demand-Oriented Pricing (Market-Oriented)

Demand-oriented pricing is modified pricing according to the demand. Prices are raised when demand is high and lowered when demand is low. One type of demand-oriented pricing is

margin analysis. Margin analysis is a method that searches for the best price and also identifies a range of profitability on the basis of demand (Hosford-Dunn et al, 1995b). These authors provide excellent examples of this to the audiological discipline. It does lend itself well to computer spreadsheets once a few basics are understood. Readers are encouraged to read the referenced material for details.

Thoughts on Setting the Price: Average, Over, or Underpricing?

This section will provide a philosophical explanation of the consequences when the price is not set appropriately. According to Miles (1986), one of the key steps to avoid in pricing is that of "average pricing." Pricing should reflect the true competitive value of what is being provided even as conditions change. When this is achieved, no money is left on the table unnecessarily on the one hand, and no opportunities are opened for competitors through inadvertent overpricing on the other hand. As a representative of the Boston Consulting Group, he states that average pricing is a major cause of gains and losses of market position. Figure 7–7 is a simplified diagram to facilitate this statement.

No average cost to an average patient exists. As a result, some are overcharged (overpriced) and others are undercharged (underpriced). In *overpricing* "low-service" patients are forced to subsidize the "high-service" segments. This is likely to result in a loss of those patients being overcharged, but a gain in

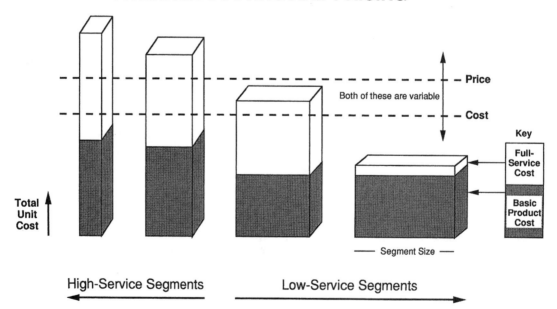

Figure 7–7 Simplified diagram of the dangers of average costing and pricing. The shaded portion of each box represents the basic product cost of the product for the segment size identified. The unshaded portion of each box indicates the total full-service cost of the product (everything other than the basic cost that goes into the delivery). The dotted "cost" line represents the average cost of the sale, including the full-service cost and the basic product cost. Using this average cost for setting price, if you charge too high a price (overpricing: dotted "price" line), the "low-service" patient segment is being forced to subsidize the "high-service" segment. If the price is set too low (underpricing), there is a failure to charge up to the full value of what is being delivered to less price-sensitive patients. (Adapted from Miles [1986], with permission.)

market share among those being undercharged. The result may be a business that is apparently growing but has mysteriously decreasing profit margins. Or worse, a focused competitor could capture this business and still have ample margins. Progressive expansion by competitors could occur with them moving to the next most overcharged segment. This would leave you with high-service segments at the "average" price.

In *underpricing* a failure to charge up to the full value of what is being delivered to less price-sensitive patients exists (although focusing on this much smaller group can be quite rewarding financially). Underpricing overlooks the fact that price is frequently a key indicator of quality. More often, though, underpricing is the result of the seller's lack of understanding of consumers' needs, business economics, options available, and criteria for selection to gauge their price sensitivity. If sufficient margins do not exist, your practice will cut back on what differentiates you from the others. Design, features, quality, innovations, and service will suffer. In addition, opportunities will open for the insightful competitor.

A somewhat related issue to underpricing is the lower selling price on hearing aids and other services demanded by most managed health care programs as one of the conditions for dispenser participation. In many of these programs the selling price of a hearing aid may fall below the established full-service cost (Fig. 7–7). The price to nonmanaged care patients will have to be adjusted upward to subsidize the low gross profit business, or the audiological practice may find itself in a financially losing situation. Awarded discounts for volume purchases should not be passed on to these programs because this practice further exacerbates the problem.

What is needed to help set the price appropriately?

1. An understanding of the full costs of serving specific customer segments. Use a periodic in-depth review and analysis to obtain this information. Average costs often come from pooled data allocated such that they disguise the true cost of doing business with different service level patients.

2. Up-to-date assessment of competitors' costs to serve the same segments. Try to find these out in detail.

3. Thorough understanding, from patients' perspectives, of their needs, decision criteria, and available alternatives.

4. An assessment of patients' likely responses, including price sensitivity, to potential offerings that promise to provide new value.

Interestingly, three of the five deadly business sins identified by Drucker have to do with pricing. These are (1) the worship of high profit margins and of "premium pricing," (2) mispricing a new product by charging "what the market will bear," and (3) cost-driven pricing (reported in Hosford-Dunn et al, 1995b).

When all is said and done, what are the basic marketing steps related to pricing?

1. Determine the minimum price you can offer your product for (cost-plus) and still remain in business.

2. Select the market segment you desire to satisfy with that pricing structure (target market).

3. Determine an image for the product/service that will satisfy that target market. Attach the price that is compatible with this image.

4. Test the price.

Test the Price

Although a number of approaches could be used to test the price, multiple uses of the break-even point can provide you with much of the information you are seeking. It allows you to perform "what if" analyses rather quickly.

Break-Even Analysis

Perhaps a good approach to use when making pricing decisions is that of break even-analysis. It basically states that certain fixed costs must be covered to break even. This technique considers the fixed versus variable costs and the total costs of doing business to determine the break-even point (in units and dollars). Once this point is exceeded, profits increase in direct proportion to the level achieved beyond this point. This method works best when products are rather homogeneous.

To Figure a Break-Even Point:

Assumes:	*Total fixed costs* (costs unaffected by volume: lease, taxes, administration, insurance, etc.)	$96,000/y
	Variable costs (costs that vary with volume: direct labor, telephone, power, hearing aids, supplies, commissions, etc.)	$500/unit
	Average selling price	$1200/unit
	Available for fixed costs	$700/unit

Calculation of Break-Even Point Volume in Unit Sales:

$$BEP = F/(S-V)$$

BEP = break-even point; F = total fixed costs; S = selling price; V = variable cost/unit

$$BEP = \frac{\$96,000}{\$1,200 - \$500} = 137.14 \text{ units/y or } 11.43/\text{mo}$$

To recover the $96,000 in fixed costs, 137.14 units would have to be sold in 1 year or an average of 11.43 units/mo at $1200/unit.

Another way to show this is illustrated in Figure 7-8 and is set up as a chart in this example on a *monthly* basis ($8000/mo fixed costs). The remaining assumptions are the same as in the previous example. This shows that 11.43 units and $13,716/mo is required to break even. The profit increases substantially once the break-even point has been exceeded. The break-even chart provides a method to visually monitor the impact of sales on profit, cost, and volume.

Break-even point to figure the effect of a price change:
Using the same break-even formula, if the selling price of the product goes down to $1000/unit and all other costs remain constant, the break-even volume will now be 192 units/y or 16 units/mo. Figure 7–8 shows only the break-even point at a sales price of $1200/unit. Other prices can be drawn on the chart—or overlaid.

Projecting the prices and necessary unit sales necessary to achieve target ROIs before taxes:
The break-even point can be used to determine prices and necessary unit sales to achieve target ROIs before taxes. For example, if you wished to make $150,000 before taxes, had fixed overhead of $50,000, and variable costs per unit of $500, how many units would have to be sold at a price

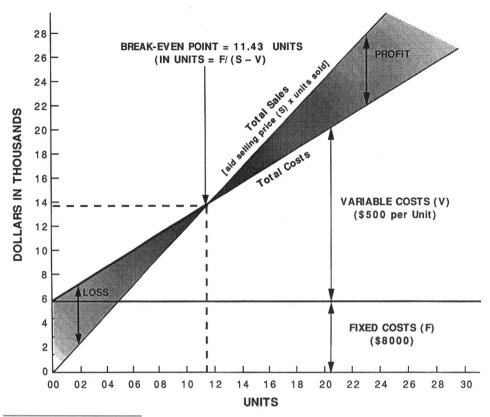

Figure 7–8 Break-even analysis chart based on a 1-month projection (although this could be displayed yearly as well). Fixed and variable costs are compared with projected units and revenues. In this example from the text, fixed costs, regardless of how many units are sold, are $8000. The variable cost per unit is $500. At a selling price of $1200, the sale of 11.43 units will yield $13,715 revenue, and costs and revenue will equal each other. (Or, another way to explain this is that when 11.43 units are sold, total cost is 11.43 times $500, or $5715, plus $8000, or $13,715.) At the same price, the sale of each unit above 11.43 yields profit.

of $1200? The contribution margin in this case is $700 (suggested unit selling price minus the variable unit costs). Seven hundred divided into $150,000 is 214.29 units that would have to be sold at $1200/unit. Scenarios can be projected by changing the number of units and selling price, assuming all other factors remain the same.

Legal and Ethical Issues Related to Pricing and Consumer Contacts

Activities that inform, persuade, or communicate in some way with the market attract attention of regulatory agencies. As a result, regulations have been promulgated that are intended to protect the consumer.

The list of regulations that follows is not meant to be all inclusive (adapted from Lear Siegler, Inc. Antitrust Laws Policy Guide, 1988) and a comprehensive discussion is not within the scope of this chapter. Each audiologist is encouraged to check with the laws and regulations in his or her own state. The actions discussed are unlawful only if they are taken by joint agreement with one or more competitors. However, it is a mistake to think that such an agreement must be either formal or conspiratorial. The government's position is that ordinarily no legitimate reason exists for competitors to be

discussing such subject and to do so risks investigation and possible indictment by the Justice Department.

Antitrust Regulations

Antitrust regulations govern the acts of business. The basic purposes of these laws are to promote vigorous, free, and open competition in the marketplace. They are based on the belief that such competition provides the best guarantee that the American consumer will obtain the best product at the lowest price. The salient features of these regulations require stating because many dispensing audiologists are unaware of them and the potential consequences of seemingly innocent conversations with others about their business practices.

Price fixing is illegal. Section 1 of the Sherman Antitrust Act of 1980 prohibits "every contract, combination... or conspiracy in restraint of trade of interstate commerce." Probably the clearest and most widely publicized violation of the act is price fixing between competitors—agreements between competitors to set prices, to establish minimum or maximum prices, to establish a common pricing system, or to otherwise affect competitive pricing in the industry. Several Supreme Court cases have dealt with a mere exchange of information among competitors concerning recent and specific price quotations to identified patients. Even when no express commitment was made by these competitors to adhere to any price schedule and the prices charged by them were not uniform, the court found that the exchange of price information constituted sufficient "concerted action" with the expectation that reciprocal information would be given on request, with the effect that prices were kept within a specified range.

For this reason it is important to avoid the exchange of sensitive business information with competitors. For example, even a seemingly innocuous activity such as the exchange of current price lists could conceivably constitute a violation of Section 1 of the Sherman Act because of its natural tendency to produce uniform prices, even in the absence of any agreement to fix prices. It is expected, of course, that as a vigorous competitor the dispensing audiologist will obtain as much information as possible about the competition and the market for products, prices, or services. However, the point to remember is that such information should not be discussed openly with competitors to set prices or discounts, terms or conditions of sale, the creditworthiness of patients, profit margins or costs, or bids or intent to bid, and so on.

Interestingly, the proscription against price fixing does not apply only to the price but to all terms and conditions of sale. Thus agreements as to credit charges, discounts, service charges, delivery terms, and the like are all per se illegal.

Pricing of products and services should be made on the basis of all relevant factors and not exclusively on prices charged by competitors.

The Formation of Monopolies is Illegal

The Clayton Act of 1914 was passed to strengthen Section 2 of the Sherman Antitrust Act by preventing the formation of monopolies.

Unfair Competition is Illegal

This was established with the Federal Trade Commission Act of 1914. This was passed to deal with unfair methods of competition not covered by the Clayton Act. The Federal Trade Commission (FTC) is empowered to take action against any business practices that are deemed harmful either to competing firms or to consumers.

Price Discrimination

Price discrimination can be illegal (Robinson-Patman Act of 1936) if the same product is sold to different patients at different prices, unless it is performed as a justified approach to meet competition or is based on the costs of servicing the customers. This supplemented Section 2 of the Clayton Act.

Regulation of Promotional Activities
(Tax Reform Act of 1986—Federal Trade Commission)

These make an impact on the use of coupons and in-package promotions and other offers, including warranties. Unfair trade practice laws sometimes make it unlawful for retailers to sell products below cost.

Phony Price Lists are Illegal

Wheeler Lea Amendment in 1938 to the FTC.

Advertising and Sales Promotion Claims Documentation

Be certain documented evidence is in the files for claims made in advertising and sales literature. In general, statements made in advertising, sales literature, or orally will be held to violate Section 5 of the Federal Trade Commission Act if they have the capacity or tendency to deceive, considered in light of the entire advertisement, the entire sales brochure, or the entire sales presentation. The test for determining deception is the effect of the statement on the ordinary or average person. Failure to qualify affirmative representations that are too broad also may constitute deception. In other words, a half truth may be just as false as a whole lie. The FTC, for example, holds that any claim that the average person would relate to safety of a product is a factual claim. Furthermore, absence of knowledge that a claim is false will not defeat an FTC proceeding.

Risk Reduction

This topic most often elicits two types of thinking attributed to consumers: "Will I get my money's worth?" And, "Will the hearing aids or products/services purchased live up to my expectations?" In reality, hearing aid purchasers face at least five types of risk when making their buying decision. These are monetary, functional, social, psychological, and physical (Settle & Alreck, 1989: Staab & Jelonek, 1995a). The magnitude of each depends on the characteristics of the buyer and on the type of hearing aids or services being considered.

- *Monetary risk* is the fear that the purchased product/service will provide less value than the price leads the buyer to expect.
- *Functional (performance) risk* occurs when buyers have alternative brands, styles, services, and so on to choose from.
- *Social (occupational) risk* relates to the affiliation or social status associated with the purchase of a good, (i.e., "...hearing aids are for old people").
- *Psychological risk*: "Did I do the wrong thing by buying these hearing aids?"
- *Physical risk*: "Will they hurt? Will I feel them? Will they be uncomfortable?"

Buyers risk can be reduced by a number of methods. Figure 7–9, adapted from Settle and Alreck (1989), identifies 24 of these (some more significant than others). The oval shadings indicate the expected success of methods that seem to function best to reduce risk for each of the risk categories identified.

Targeting promotions to fairly small, sharply defined audience segments means much more than just using highly selective media. It demands tailoring message content to the preferences and buyer risk profiles of each segment. What is required, as much as anything, is matching the hearing products and their promotional message (the language, social situation, and psychological state) to the social and internal realities of the target market segment. "The best approach to reducing consumers' sense of risk is to provide successful performance and service with their current hearing aids. Nothing has more effect on hearing aid sales (either positive or negative) than previous experience" (Staab & Jelonek, 1995a). Figure 7–10 identifies the type of risk and the hearing aid purchasers who are most sensitive to each of the categories.

Buyer Risk Types & Reduction Modes

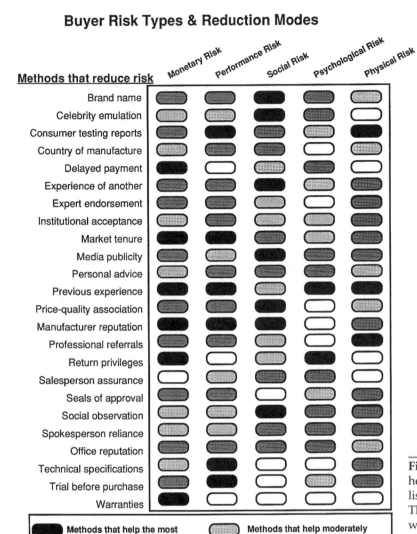

Figure 7–9 Overview of the types of risk a hearing aid purchaser may face, and a partial listing of methods used to help reduce that risk. The shading of the oval indicates the extent to which the methods used actually help reduce the risk involved. (Modified from Settle & Alreck [1989], with permission.)

MARKETING PROGRAMS (TACTICS)

Marketing programs are the day-to-day sales promotional activities or tactics that generate the business to finance the practice. Programs direct how you interact with your patients. They emphasize the harsh realities of managing a business (set prices, policies, shape patient perceptions) and require detailed planning (objectives, strategies, programs, deadlines, schedules, budgets, itemization). Marketing program efforts generally receive cursory rather than the specific attention they require. Often the programs offered consist of reactive marketing efforts to competitive programs. In this sense much of what we do is similar to the reactions of sheep—follow what someone else is doing.

A successful hearing aid marketing program requires targeting the market with the right blend of activities. If no marketing plan and programs support it, the practice may not reach the proper market or, even worse, may lose its existing market. To identify how marketing programs fit into the overall marketing plan, recall that the market analysis targets market segments, identifies marketing opportunities, and establishes the competitive advantage. Goals and objectives direct the marketing strategies, which in turn outline how the goals and objectives are to be obtained. Marketing programs (tactics) are developed to address a specific problem or take advantage of an immediate market opportunity. To this end a number of marketing programs are generally required. These can be developed as individual programs or as part of a series of complementary synergistic programs serving different marketing strategies. The extent to which they are developed depends on the limited resources available (funds, labor, time, personnel). Figure 7–11 identifies changes in dispenser uses of marketing media over the past several years, which in turn, suggest changes in the kinds of marketing tactics used.

Many audiologists believe that if they do what the competition does (average = consistent with the competition) they are doing as much as is required. However, the average is just as close to the bottom as it is to the top. To be successful, rather than average, programs must result from the end product of detailed, systematic planning. This planning can be done using the same flowchart provided for the overall marketing program (Fig. 7–1). The discussion that follows identifies related issues to successful marketing programs.

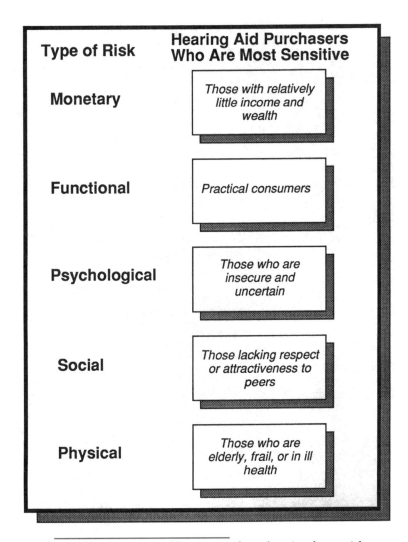

Figure 7–10   Forms of hearing products/services buyer risk.

Main Promotional Activities

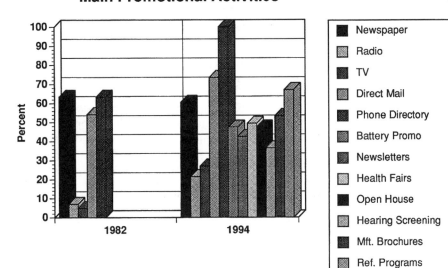

Figure 7–11   Dispenser trends of the promotional mix over the past few years. An increasing number of advertising and promotional activities exists and with a higher percentage of use. (From Cranmer [1983], pp. 9–12; and Skafte [1995], pp. 16, 18, 20, 24–27, 53, 60, 61.)

The Promotional Mix

The tactics for presenting a promotional mix consist of a combination of personal selling (oral and face-to-face), advertising (paid presentation), public relations (your image with a public interest), and sales promotions. The offer might focus on just one element of the marketing mix (product, price, promotion, or place) or on linking multiple marketing elements.

When developing market plans, the dispensing office or clinic is rarely included as part of the marketing mix. This is unfortunate because in hearing aid dispensing the office should be considered as a dynamic marketing tool that can support sales, attract new patients, and help generate referrals (Jelonek & Staab, 1994). The authors suggest the use of a checklist as in Table 7–11 to evaluate your office. Is it patient-oriented? Does it contribute to, or undermine, your marketing efforts?

Programs Should Be Highly Focused on the Target Market

To whom should the message be directed? Decide whether it should be for existing patients, prospective patients, referral

TABLE 7–11   Checklist to evaluate your office when considering its use as a marketing tool

Office Checklist

How does your office check-out? Is it consumer-friendly?
Does it support sales, service efforts, and consumer expectations?

Neighborhood
- ❏ Accessible by car
- ❏ Nearby parking
- ❏ Accessible by public transportation
- ❏ Safe (crime rate) during daylight hours
- ❏ Neighborhood ambiance: retail
- ❏ Neighborhood ambiance: professional
- ❏ Neighborhood ambiance: medical
- ❏ Neighborhood ambiance: residential

Office building
- ❏ Visible, easy-to-read signage: (Business or building name, street address)
- ❏ Easy to find office location: (On or near well know streets, locations)
- ❏ Accessible office suite: (Stairs, elevators, ramps, hallway length, directions within bldg.)
- ❏ Building ambiance: retail
- ❏ Building ambiance: professional
- ❏ Building ambiance: medical
- ❏ Building ambiance: residential
- ❏ Building condition: (Cleanliness, decor, smell, temperature, safety)

Office
- ❏ Decor: positive, professional or retail image
- ❏ Decor: consistency
- ❏ Lighting: easy-to-see, easy-to-read
- ❏ Furniture: easy-to-sit in and stand-up from
- ❏ Furniture: stable, secure
- ❏ Easy access and movement for clients with limited mobility, poor eyesight, using assistive devices (canes, walkers, wheel chairs, oxygen tanks)
- ❏ Test equipment looks professional, high tech, up-to-date
- ❏ Test equipment is visible
- ❏ Client can see computer screens and participate in the fitting or testing process: (Hearing aid fitting systems, hearing aid analyzers, real ear equipment)
- ❏ Offices: clean, uncluttered
- ❏ Dedicated offices for audiometric testing, fitting, service
- ❏ Accessibility of real ear test systems, hearing aid analyzers, hearing aid programming devices, computers
- ❏ Well-organized literature stands and tasteful POP displays
- ❏ Magazines, books, etc. related to hearing

Evaluation
Rate each of the above areas according to the following:
1. Excellent
2. Above average
3. Average
4. Below average
5. Poor
If you rated any of the categories average or below, immediate action should be taken to improve your office as a marketing tool

sources, third-party payers, or some other group. Is the message to be targeted to a certain age group, sex, income, lifestyle, or purchase-decision style or group? Proper focus allows resources to be concentrated and increases the probability that the program will be successful.

Where to Present the Messages

Is this done better in the print media (yellow pages, newspapers, direct mail, printed materials, etc.), audio/visual media (television/cable, radio, television, or the Internet), outdoor media, personal contacts, advertising specialties, or through private label? Regardless, use a story (headlines and content) and visuals to get attention, to direct the message, and to motivate potential purchasers to action.

Promotional Tasks

Promotional tasks for all the above are either to inform, persuade, or remind consumers about the products or services offered. Do you intend to provide awareness, value, life enhancement, education, a call to action, or to position your practice competitively? If product related, the approach is closely tied to the stage of the product's life cycle. Regardless, the "offer" is important.

Promotional Tips in Message Presentation

Promotional tips should include a strategy of explaining the benefits, adding value, target as specifically as possible, cross-promote if a program does well, use a theme identified to your office, focus your message, and always ask the question the consumer will ask, "what's in it for me?"

Limited Life Span

A limited life span is characteristic of marketing programs. They are generally short-term programs lasting from a few days to perhaps a few weeks. Seasonal programs have their own built-in life span (Christmas, summer maintenance, May is Better Hearing Month, year-end offering, Cheyenne Frontier Days). It is possible that some programs will take on a life of their own after being initiated. Loss or damage, programmable hearing aids, or "essentially invisible" hearing aids are examples.

Advertising and Promotion
Advertising

Advertising consists generally of media marketing (television, radio, newspapers, consumer/business publications, print media, etc.). It is purchased as a commodity with the content controlled by the advertiser. It tends to use a shotgun approach in that it scatters its message of a broad objective toward the product or service. Immediate action is not expected. It should, however, eventually contribute to sales through its attempts to disseminate information, persuade purchasers, and to influence attitudes. Advertising is used because products and services do not normally sell themselves. Therefore advertising is used as a predominant message as to how consumers form opinions about the products they buy, about the services they seek, and about the businesses they patronize. Its role is, purely and simply, to communicate, to a specified market, information and develop a frame of mind that stimulates action. If advertising is not intended to contribute to immediate sales, some have questioned its importance, . . . but not advertising is like winking in the dark; you know what you're doing, but nobody else does. According to a survey by the American Association of Advertising Agencies, the average person is exposed to more than 16,000 different advertising messages every day. Of these, the average person remembers about six – meaning that something else may be required to complete the sale (Staab, 1992).

PEARL

Not advertising is like winking in the dark; you know what you are doing, but nobody else does.

Advertising creates awareness, including long-term recognition. It helps to build your identity, to position yourself relative to the competition, and to build and sustain momentum. The message should always be clear, it tells the real "story." A famous example of a story gone wrong, albeit through translation, was John F. Kennedy's announcement to the people of Berlin . . . "Ich bin ein Berliner!" JFK thought he said, "I am a citizen of Berlin!" To some, what he 'really' said was, "I am a jelly doughnut!" ("Berliner" is a German type of "jelly doughnut.")

Public Relations (Publicity)

This marketing function relates the image of your practice with the public interest. According to Stevens (1984), public relations is an effective marketing technique intended to (a) make your personal expertise known to the public, (b) promote respect for your services, and (c) provide a useful public service by imparting reliable information to a knowledge-hungry society. It is not always easy to get the attention of the press, but if you do, use it as follows:

- Identify the appropriate person to whom information should be sent.
- Try to send information on a periodic basis.
- Articles or interviews are perceived by the public as more objective than advertisements.
- Free publicity is generally better than paid-for advertising.
- The message should be informative and educational, rather than promotional.
- Use public relations to help create your image.

Advertising objectives and strategies must be developed within the context of the marketing plan. They are generally divided into three basic categories: to inform, to persuade, or to remind (Fig. 7–12).

Basic Approaches to Advertising

How to Establish an Advertising Budget

The following list of approaches has been identified (Berkowitz, 1992):

- What you can afford (what is left over after managing all other expenses).
- Competitive parity (based on what the competition does without regard to goal differences).
- Fixed percentage of sales. This does not allow for experimentation, countercyclical promotions, and opportunities. It is good to maintain a close relationship between expenses and sales per business cycle.
- Percentage on future sales projections. This avoids using last year's figures for this year's budgeting.
- Unit of sales/fixed dollar amount
- Task/objective approach based on the media selected, frequency, reach, continuity, repetition, ad size, length of commercial requirements, and so on.
- Co-op advertising with manufacturers to increase advertising budget. (Yellow pages ads under brand name listings and also for direct mail inserts, newspaper ads, etc.).

The Message

The message should emphasize awareness, interest, desire, credibility, or action. An acronym that can be used for this is "SIMPLE:" (stop the reader, interest the reader in finding out more, motivate the reader to want the product, persuade the reader that the product is right for him or her, logical reason for purchase, and ease the path to purchase) (Berkowitz, 1992).

Benefits, not features, should be sold. This approach determines the way patients perceive your business. A systematic approach to layout design (Ogilvy, 1983) follows the "KISS" principle (keep it simple, stupid):

PEARL

Keep it "SIMPLE:" stop the reader, interest the reader in finding out more, motivate the reader to want the product, persuade the reader that the product is right for him or her, logical reason for purchase, ease the path to purchase.
(Berkowitz, 1992)

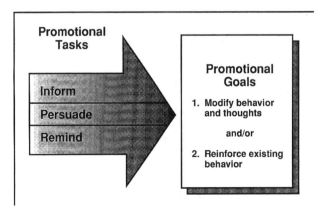

Figure 7–12 Promotional tasks are either to inform, persuade, or remind consumers about products and/or services. The choice of which to use depends largely on the product life cycle.

- Use familiar serif type face.
- Use upper and lower case print.
- Reading (or scanning is from top to bottom, and if the layout is proper, can increase readership by 10%).
- Illustration on top (a picture is worth a thousand words).
- Headline under illustration. Headlines have five times the readership as body copy.
- Copy under headline should emphasize the benefits. As few as 5% may actually read the body copy, so use short sentences, short paragraphs, and the language of everyday conversation.
- Add a tracer so that the source of the ad can be determined when the patient sets an appointment.

Advertising Media

Newspapers provide good local coverage and depth penetration. Having a wide range of appeal and a broad acceptance, their highest readership percentage is in the 45- to 64-year age group. They allow for good timing and space flexibility and are an ideal medium for ads with clipout inquire forms. Limitations are their relatively short life (1 day), strong competition from all kinds of other ads, and the fact that the reader spends, on average, 34 minutes reading the paper, with only 18% of this (6 minutes) reading ads (Braun, 1981). The frequency with which ads should be placed varies. Berkowitz (1992), in reporting data from Gensch (1970), suggests that 13 exposures over 52 weeks is preferred over 13 in 13 weeks. The first three to four get lost in the masking of other ads, the fifth and sixth exposures are the ones that register with readers, and the seventh and eighth are those that register with the individual. Exposures from 7 to 10 are important for their repetition and reminder value.

Newspaper media kits (available from other media as well) allow for the determination of the following:

- Which papers will reach the maximum number of your target audience?
- Daily circulation figures to determine days with highest readership (for scheduling).
- Advertising rates (usually cost per thousand).
- Section in which to place the ad.

Weekly papers and *shopping papers* are alternate approaches used to reach a localized circulation and keep costs low.

Television is often economically beyond the reach of small business. However, in small market areas, cable TV, public access channels, and paid programming have become more accessible and affordable.

The advantages of television is that it combines sight, sound, color, motion, and drama. It commands high attention and high exposure, along with the opportunity to project an image and deliver a message to people in their own homes with significant power and persuasiveness.

Weaknesses include its high absolute cost, the amount of clutter in fighting for the viewer's attention, brief exposure (30 seconds generally), and less audience selectivity. It takes several exposures before a reaction is obtained and involves a higher cost, which is determined by the audience size, time of day, and commercial length.

As with newspapers, use the station representatives as a source of target market information. The message often involves slice of life, testimonials, offers for demonstrations, and problem solving. Name identification and repetition are very important for recall. The use of an attention grabber in the first frame can be used for visual surprise, along with closeups, sound effects, reinforcement of the offer by having it appear in print, and showing the product in use. The use of videotape has reduced the cost of commercials and has speeded up the production process. TV can be used more frequently than radio because it offers both visual and auditory stimulation and therefore does not have same fatigue factor (Berkowitz, 1992).

Radio offers an advertising medium that is highly selective and that is also very fragmented (all news, talk shows, music, ethnic programs, etc.). Commercial units are of 10, 30, and 60 seconds, with time grids (morning and evening drive times: 5 to 10 AM and 3 to 7 PM; daytime, evening overnight; and weekend). Radio offers a variety of packages (including combinations of day and evening, etc.). Radio benefits include mass use, high geographical and demographical selectivity, and low cost. Advantages are that the listener tunes to stations, not programs, compared with TV (where one watches programs and not channels). Limitations of radio are that it is presented in audio only and therefore requires numerous repetitions because it is ancillary to other activities in which the listener is involved. As such, it attracts a lower attention level than TV. Rate structures are not standardized. The task is to get people to listen. To accomplish this, the following elements are used: surprise, arousal of curiosity, repeated promise of the benefit, and repeat identity. Radio account executives will be able to help you determine which radio stations are appropriate for you. They will provide you current market research to allow you to make an informed decision and match your prospects to the correct ratio station. Know also that the radio station will assist you in writing and producing the commercial. Except for rare conditions, there should be no additional cost for development of the advertisement (as opposed to TV).

Outdoor advertising is more limited in scope and is used much less frequently by audiologists than any of the other media approaches. This consists of the use of billboards, benches, bus signs, taxi advertising, and so on. These offer little flexibility because their size, and often their content, is highly standardized, regulated, and disciplined. The message view time is extremely short (2- to 3-second message read time). It is considered supplementary to support other major media.

Promotion

Promotion is often associated with all activities other than personal selling, advertising, or public relations. Compared with advertising, promotional activities use more of a rifle approach. Promotions have specific objectives and are intended to stimulate immediate action. They are more precise than advertising. The goals of promotional programs are to modify behavior and thoughts and/or to reinforce existing behavior. Promotional activities are relatively short term, usually no longer than 2 weeks. They should be directed toward the consumer and should stimulate a specific action. Originally this was referred to as sales promotion and was used largely as a defensive or retaliatory price weapon. Today this activity is used to build long-term business and to convert consumers to full-fledged patients. As such, it is considered a strategic tool and not just an opportunistic tactic. Sales promotion is used to (a) combat the intensification of competition because of increasing numbers of audiologists without comparable increases in hearing aid sales or profits, (b) satisfy patient wants rather than needs, (c) promote sales during economic decline with the purpose of retrenching and surviving, (d) increase market share during good business times, (e) create new patients, (f) build a list of qualified prospects, and (g) build the dispensing practice image (Staab, 1992).

Sales promotion should continue in times of heavy demand because the market is dynamic and patient loyalty is a "sometime thing." Heavy demand also draws more competition, requiring promotional activities to maintain market share. In the face of a declining demand for products or services, promotional activities may discourage competitors from entering the marketplace.

Salient Characteristics of the Promotional Mix

The Purpose of Sales Promotion
The purpose of sales promotion is to change the image and shape of the demand curve for the products and services offered.

The Primary Objectives
The primary objectives are generally short-term activities above and beyond the normal advertising or routine selling activities.

What Sales Promotion Is
- A short-term activity
- Directed toward the consumer
- Intended to stimulate some specific action by means of (a) informing, (b) persuading, or (c) reminding. Audiologists must find new ways to attract first-time patients and to maintain their existing patients.

Factors That Influence the Promotional Mix

The Amount of Funds Available for the Promotion
The amount of funds available for promotion is the true determinant of what the promotional mix will be.

The Nature of the Market
The influence of the nature of the market is felt in at least three ways: (a) geographical scope of the market, (b) market concentration, and (c) type of patients.

The Nature of the Product
Are hearing aids considered a shopping, specialty, or unsought good (Staab, 1990)? The promotional approach will be different, depending on the consumer's perception. Equally important is whether the audiologist is using a "push" or "pull" strategy. Pushing strategies are more likely to use advertising, point-of-purchase, or personal selling to convince the consumer to purchase products being "pushed" in the promotion. If the consumer demands certain products, this is indicative of a "pull" strategy.

The Stages of the Product's Life Cycle
Advertising and promotional strategies relate closely to the market situation and should vary depending on the life cycle stage of the product (Fig. 7–13). If not product related, strategies can be used to correct misinformation (all hearing aids are the same), to reduce consumer risk and/or fears, to create an image, to suggest new uses of a product, and so on.

In the *introductory stage* of a product the market situation is that the patient does not realize that the product or service is wanted or even how it will help. Personalized attention is required and the interest is in features and functions. Early innovators and early adopters are likely to be involved. The promotional strategies are to inform and educate, to let them know of the existence of the product, what it is, its satisfying benefits, and how it is to be used.

The *growth stage* involves a market situation in which patients are now aware of the benefits of the product or service, it has good acceptance, and requires much less personal selling. Consumers are interested in the *use* of a particular product (primary demand) in contrast to the *demand* for a particular product (selective demand). The promotional strategies here are to stimulate selective demand—to show why this model or test is desirable. Promotion and advertising should be increased.

The *maturity-saturation stage* is entered into by the late adopters. Competition has intensified and sales have leveled off. Late adopter buyers are somewhat immune to promotion, depending primarily on word-of-mouth referrals. The strategy used at this stage is to use promotions and advertising techniques to get them to purchase *your* products (persuasion). Promotions at this stage are costly and often contribute to profit *decline*.

In the *sales decline stage* sales and profits are declining. New and better products are being produced. The strategy is to cut back on all promotional efforts unless something has occurred that can revitalize the offering. This occurred with behind-the-ear (BTE) hearing aids when programmability became a new feature and existed initially with BTE instruments only.

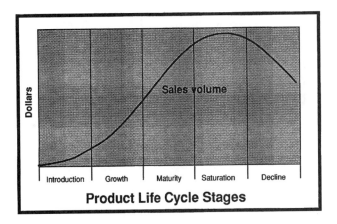

Figure 7–13 Stages of a product life cycle. The needs of the patient varies with each stage and should be reflected in the marketing strategies, programs, and funds expended. See the text for an explanation.

How to Present the Promotional Program

As has been mentioned previously, the presentation of the promotion program (Fig. 7–14) mirrors the general marketing program (Fig. 7–1). The primary difference is that the activities of the promotion program are related to specific activities rather than to the major marketing program. Basic elements in the promotional presentation (adapted from Staab, 1992) follow. It is important to remember that each of these steps should be *brief.* This is no place to establish yourself as a researcher or writer.

Identify Market Opportunity or Threat (Situation Analysis)

Although the overall marketing objectives set the stage in establishing the promotional objectives, this phase should not repeat those same objectives but should add new dimensions.

This phase describes the opportunity or competitive threat. The market and market conditions are then analyzed to determine whether the opportunities or threats are worth pursuing in your served market. Use market data from the overall market analysis data earlier in this chapter. Identify possible courses of action.

Marketing programs are often set for smaller market segments where the message can be directed very specifically. This often results in less complicated programs, making them more personal and easier to develop and evaluate. How you choose to segment the market depends on what your program is intended to do. In general, the closer your program offering meets the needs of the target, the better the results are expected to be.

Examples of opportunities include unserved or poorly served patient needs, products or services not being provided, competitor financial or management problems, discontinued or resold offices, competitor inactivity, changes in personnel, encourage new uses of hearing aids, basic industry marketing changes, or population adjustments. Threats exist when new technology is introduced in a timely fashion by competitors, additional offices are added in your marketing area, negative FDA or consumer announcements, highly financed and visible competition, the stock market drops dramatically, the economy changes for the worse, heavy advertising and promotions to your market segment are made by others, exclusivity of a product or service takes business from you, and the introduction of a price discount offering that could have an immediate impact on your sales. All situations that lead to potential opportunities or threats cause patients to re-evaluate purchasing decisions.

Some situations do not lend themselves well to sales promotion. It is not recommended when the product is inadequate or overpriced, when overnight success is expected, when the cost of the promotion is so costly that the investment might be better spent on improving service, when used with an established product with declining market share (i.e., BTE hearing aids), or when the sales promotion is used alone. A sales promotion requires support from other marketing areas.

Set Strategies That Will Provide Means To Resolve the Market Opportunity or Threat

Think of strategies at this level that are extensions of the general marketing strategy. These could be achieved using the strategies (partial listing) that follow:

- Sample consumers' interests in a given hearing aid or related services.
- Convert patients from other dispensers, rather than merely borrowing patients.
- Deplete inventories of existing hearing aids, batteries, or other supplies that have become excessive to make room for new products.
- Encourage the sales force (if one exists) to focus on a particular product or service.
- Induce the trial of hearing aids, a specific test, or some other service available.

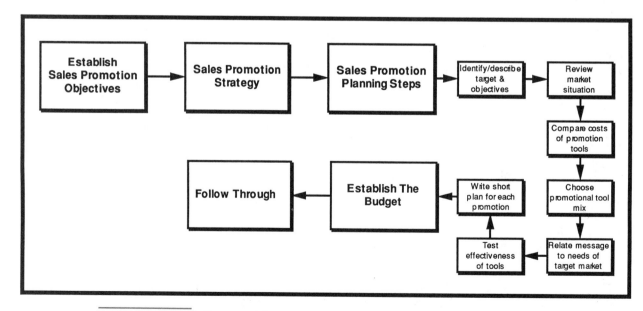

Figure 7–14 Block diagram of the marketing programs (promotional; tactical) phase of the overall marketing process action plan. Detailed steps of the sales promotion plan are included.

- Create excitement about a product or call attention to use of products or services in new and unusual ways.
- Increase consumer demands for hearing aids or some other service or product supplied by your practice.

Sales Promotion Planning Steps

Define who and where the target group(s) are

This is perhaps the most important ingredient to the success of the promotion. According to the Direct Mail Marketing Association (DMMA), the success of the marketing campaign is attributed as follows: 15% on the copy, 25% on the offer, and 60% on how well the target market is defined (The Competitive Advantage, 1986). Include information about the targets' habits, characteristics, wants, and needs. What appeals to this market segment?

SPECIAL CONSIDERATION

The success of the marketing campaign is attributed as follows: 15% on the copy, 25% on the offer, 60% on how well the target market is defined. (The Competitive Advantage, 1986).

Review the market situation (product, sales history, stage of life cycle, competitive strategies)

These factors, along with the sales trends, pricing, and budget constraints, determine the optimum promotion mix.

Know the capabilities of different promotional approaches and comparative costs

Keep files on the competition as reference material.

Choose the promotional tool(s) that are best suited to reach the target with maximum results

You will not usually know what these are before the promotion. However, measure performance so that future promotions can use information on the basis of: (1) your past experience, (2) results of other promotional programs that have been run, and (3) the product's place in its own life cycle.

Relate the theme and message of the promotion to the real or imagined needs of the target market

The market offering is the heart of the marketing program. To motivate the target audience it should have a premium or added value that will encourage them to purchase the offering *now*, not later. As a tangible item, it could be a product, service, or saving. It can also be intangible, such as enhanced performance, self-image enhancement, or patient support. The offer can be price, product, promotion, delivery (place), or people driven, or a combination of these.

- *Price*-driven examples could include battery club programs, a backup set of hearing instruments at a reduced price, a percent off on cleaning.
- *Product*-driven examples could be digital technology, completely-in-the-canal aids, noise cancellation, array microphone systems.

- *Promotions* often are evidenced as direct mail, newsletters, consultations, and advertising.
- *Delivery* often promotes rapid turnaround, expanded office hours, service centers, and on-site repairs.
- A *people* example could be the use of specific individuals within the office to manage particular patients.

Is there a cost or savings associated with the offer (direct or indirect), and what will its effect be on the marketing program? Does it add value and demand a premium price, or is it an offering of a savings? What will the result be to the final line?

A competitive advantage suggests that the program has value to the potential patient; what's in it for them? Also, can the program manage in the face of competition?

Time limitations specify the start and end of a program. By definition, marketing programs are short but can be repeated if they are cyclical or seasonal. Materials that are media promoted or mailed to the consumer have relatively short response interest. How will you manage inquiries after the termination date of the program?

Test the effectiveness of the promotional tools used

This is very desirable but seldom performed. A simple way to check this is to use a return on promotion (ROP) approach. You will have to decide whether the ROP is acceptable or not.

$$ROP = \frac{Sales - Cost\ of\ sale}{Cost\ of\ sale}$$

Assume: Sales for 1 month = $9000

Cost of sale   = $2000

Sale can be for either days, weeks, months, or cycles)

$$ROP = \frac{\$9000 - \$2000}{\$2000} = \$3500$$

Write a short plan for each promotion

This should be short and include the following:

- Statement of objectives
- Target market(s)
- Message and marketing tools to be used and why
- The time line for the promotion (when it will occur, with dates for start and end)
- How to measure the promotion's effectiveness

Establish the Budget

This includes all resource requirements (the investment in time, labor, funds, personnel, and equipment required to make the program function). Have these been allocated properly? What is the mechanism for financing the program (budgeted funds, existing funds, debt)? Create a budget that itemizes all costs, direct and indirect, and set up a schedule. Calculate a break-even point and project a ROI. Compare the cost and returns of alternate programs. Develop the schedule to allocate personnel, time, duration of the program, and expected results. Consider contingency plans if the program does not progress as expected. The plan should be in written form to prevent omissions and errors.

How much should you budget? Some marketing texts place this figure between 2 and 35% of the total marketing/advertising budget. According to Skafte (1998), the average dispensing audiologist indicated that for 1997, 10% of the budget was used for marketing, down from 13.5% the previous year.

Funds should ideally be allocated to specific sales promotions on the basis of market potentials or past history. Unfortunately, this approach may be difficult to calculate, leading to alternate approaches to establish budgets for these activities:

- *Relation to income.* This is based on a percentage of past or anticipated sales. It is sometimes based on a per *unit* basis. The procedure is simple to calculate. The problem is that if based on past experiences, this makes the program a *result* of sales, when in fact it should *cause* sales.
- *Task or objective.* Determine what the promotion is intended to accomplish and then determine what the cost of the promotional activity must be (or what is acceptable). This is a fairly sound approach that is not too complicated.
- *All funds available.* This requires deep pockets and puts all the eggs into one basket.
- *Follow the competition.* This assumes that what the competition is doing is right. However, their program may not have the same goals, targets, and so forth that you have.

Program Execution and Follow Through

This requires that the schedule and plans that have been set are followed. Results should be monitored to track the progress and success (or failure) of the program. Use some unit of measure that is easy to quantify (new unit sales, new patients, resales, leads generated, inquiries) and be prepared to modify the program to increase its effectiveness or to terminate the program if it becomes a drain on your practice. Results can be used to direct additional marketing programs.

PROMOTIONAL TACTICS (PROGRAMS)

Some Tips for Promotional Programs

(Staab, 1992)

- Try to add value, rather than discounting products.
- Put your imprint on the promotions. Make them exclusive and identifiable to your office.
- Focus on the future. Look for repeat business, not just new business.
- Give your promotions a theme to help reinforce your other promotional efforts.
- Target your promotions as specifically as you can and make the results measurable.
- Try to find ways to reward your best patients, the life blood of your business.
- If the promotion does well, look for cross-promotional opportunities.
- Find ways to make your patient feel good about you and your office.
- Promotions should be presented in a quality manner but within your affordability range.
- If you have a sales staff involved, the promotion should be exciting and rewarding for them to participate in, or it will not perform as well.

- Make the promotions fun and easy to execute.
- Keep testing different promotions, even if specific promotions are working well.
- Design the promotion asking the question, "what do hearing aid consumers want us to do for them," or rephrased, the consumer should be able to ask "what's in it for me?"

A myriad of sales promotional activities exist, but only general categories and examples will be identified and/or discussed here. More complete descriptions can be found in Staab (1992) or in observing what the competition offers. Keep in mind that sales promotion activities are supplementary to advertising. Sales promotions work better on products where advertising has *already* generated recognition and acceptance. Advertising creates value, promotion induces trial, and the product provides the satisfaction. The type and number offered is limited only by your imagination and budget. Promotions that have been successful in the past continue to be reintroduced and modified, reinforcing the belief by many that no promotion device is actually new.

Although most promotional approaches are directed primarily at attracting new patients, few will pay for themselves on this basis alone. They are just as important in retaining existing patients, creating excitement about you and your products, stimulating the sales force (even if it is only you), and combating competitive promotions.

Promotional Programs (Tactics)

Word of Mouth

Experience indicates that word of mouth is the best referral and promotional program available. The opinion (and hence, the message conveyed by patients to others—word of mouth) of a company is generally formed by the products and service provided. The difficult part is how to develop this into a specific plan. What is most important is the message to spread and how it can be done. To illustrate the significance of word of mouth, consider the following statistics from surveys conducted by the Technical Assistance Research Programs Institute in Washington, D.C. and reported by Boyett and Conn in 1991 (Hosford-Dunn et al, 1995a).

Poor Word of Mouth Messages

- Consumers were five times more likely to stop doing business with a company for poor service than for poor product quality or high cost.
- Ninety-six percent of a company's dissatisfied patients never complained to the company, but 90% quit doing business.
- The average dissatisfied patient complains about the company to nine other people. Thirteen percent complain to at least 20 people.
- The cost of losing a patient is five times the annual value of the patient's account.

Good Word of Mouth Messages

- An undifferentiated product accompanied by outstanding service may command up to a 10% price premium.
- A patient who is pleased with a company will tell five other people about the company. Many of these people become patients of the company.

- Almost all patients (95%) with a complaint will stay with a company if their complaint is resolved quickly.
- Improving quality of service is much more cost-effective than other promotional efforts: it costs five times as much to obtain a patient than to keep one.

In-Office or In-Home Demonstrations

Economy is better in the office, but the home offers an environment freer from obligation (it is less threatening and in some cases essential because of limited mobility on the part of the patient).

Special Offers

Special offers are essentially price discounts in that a reduction in price occurs as a result of the offering (two for one, free batteries, a percent off on cleaning, new aids, etc.). Care should be exercised with such promotions because although they may help short-term sales, they can erode profits and dilute the image of your practice. In reality, they are often used as an easy-out solution, to resolve a panic situation, or to generate a database. Their use to reduce a nonworking inventory, however, can work to your advantage. Cash with order or senior citizen discounts fall under this category as well.

Premiums/Incentives

A combination order in which the patient purchases one pack of batteries and receives another free or at a reduced price is an example of a premium. Buy a hearing aid and receive a 1-year supply of free batteries; receive coupons with the purchase of a certain dollar amount, quantity, or during a certain time that can be redeemed for cash or product; mail-in offers of free books or similar literature; direct premiums as gifts to the first 50 individuals who attend an opening; patient-get-patient "finder's" fees, and battery clubs are additional examples of premiums/incentives.

Coupons

The use of coupons may be considered controlled price reduction programs. They are less expensive than other promotional forms, have low up-front costs, and have no cost until they are redeemed. The use of coupons is to encourage trial of the product or service in that the discount reduces the patient's risk. A potential negative must be considered with coupons, however, in that often a feeling is present that the price was too high to begin with. Regardless, coupons have been used to suggest a backup set of hearing aids; the second of a binaural; to clean, recheck, adjust, test, or repair instruments; as an in-pack insert to battery club members for the purchase of additional products; a $ off the next purchase to competitive product users; as a Welcome Wagon introduction to new members of a community; to generate additional purchases by current users, and so on. Physical layout suggestions for coupons suggest a photo rather than a sketch of the product, a person showing the product's use, the use of the words "save" or "savings" as a prominent feature, a touting of the benefits and features, best when printed on one side only, single-product coupons as being best, and a definite expiration date that is not too distant.

Direct Mail

Direct mail has become the largest marketing media in America, commanding 26% of total advertising dollars (Kramer, 1992). This approach allows promotion to be directed to specific markets with greater control than any other media and is the easiest way to reach large numbers of selected prospects. The message comes to the prospect without competition from other advertising or editorial matter and does not have a limitation on space or the format involved. It permits great flexibility in materials, production, is statistically projectable, cost-effective, can be produced and distributed quickly, and can also use professionally prepared materials supplied by manufacturers, but personalized. Its prospects come from lists (compiled, response, or consumer) that can be purchased or self-developed.

Direct mail does not come without its detractors, however. Rising postage and production costs can limit its usefulness, an error in conception or execution can make the marketing effort worthless, mailing lists deteriorate, and some recipients are prejudiced against all direct mail. Objectives of direct mail may be to arouse or renew interest in an office, its products, or its services; to familiarize prospects with products and services available at the office; to encourage continued patronage by current patients and to resell old patients; and to favorably predispose prospects to a personal demonstration of the product or service. Giving proper justice to direct mail is not within the scope of this chapter. An in-depth approach to direct mail by hearing aid-dispensing practices is provided by Kramer (1992).

Point of Purchase

Point of purchase (POP) programs are promotions that relate to products on the counters of your office or in other areas of your practice. Their value is that the product is placed close to or at the point of sale, the only time and place where all the elements of the sale come together (patient, money, and product). POP is intended to capitalize on the impulsive nature of the buyer. The POP becomes a last-minute inducement to purchase a product, and once a consumer picks up a product, the probability of a purchase increases. Additional advantages of POP include low cost, a distinct consumer focus (readily seen), precise target marketing, the communication of new ideas or performance, keep the patient in the office longer resulting in an increased selling opportunity, help to make shopping entertaining, reinforce brand awareness and help deliver a message, enhance the delivery package and benefits, encourage return visits and remind them of you, help sell even when no salesperson is present by allowing patients to "help themselves," and provide a promotion that is easily evaluated. If sold, the POP is working. Some POP promotions that are familiar include hearing aid battery displays, ear wax removal kits, hearing aid listening demonstration comparisons, hearing aid user's guide books, dry and store units to manage cerumen and moisture problems, assistive listening devices, and so on. These are additional sources of revenue that require little involvement by the audiologist but that can be considered for each patient who visits the office.

Posters/Displays

Posters and displays help to hold a person's interest and educate them about the issues and products involved. In addition to posters of hearing aids and pamphlets about their specific uses, testimonial letters on a bulletin board, old hearing aid collections, and waiting room displays that call attention to certain issues at different times of the year are valuable.

House Organs (Newsletters)

Newsletters help develop personal rapport with patients. Quick and easy to read, newsletters present information directly and personally and at relatively little expense. It might be suggested that these are the "softest" hard-sell materials that can be placed in the consumer's hands. It is in newsletters that you are able to fulfill one of your primary responsibilities to consumers, that of offering solution options to their problems and concerns. They select from the options that you have presented the ones that meet their needs. Newsletters can provide patient education, promote new products and services, offer special battery sales, familiarize readers with staff members, provide announcements of changes in office hours, duplicate media content from trade and the consumer press, explain why a given hearing aid might be best for a given population, offer suggestions, tell of audiologist education efforts, summarize articles of consumer interest, present legislative matters, provide maintenance reminders, tell of your community involvement, and present testimonials from satisfied users. These provide an opportunity for you to use your imagination. Newsletters can be distributed at no charge to existing and potential patients, and to referral sources. Publication should be at least two, but better at four, times a year.

Telemarketing

The use of the telephone to promote products or services is construed by most audiologists as something anathema. Ironically, it is used essentially by every practice, at least to a certain extent. Although it is often considered an inbound activity, its outbound functions are not only desirable but also essential to the success of a practice. Some use telemarketing as a follow-up to a direct mail promotion, recognizing that a 35% chance exists that the mailing was discarded without having been read. The call provides a second opportunity to introduce the hearing aid or service and provide a detailed promotional message. It is often used also to qualify or activate a potential patient or to follow up on leads. Without question, telemarketing should be used to set and confirm appointments, provide postorder or postdelivery support, follow-up on service contracts (cleaning, evaluation, accessories, batteries), and confirm that the instruments are working well and answer questions.

SPECIAL CONSIDERATION

Telemarketing should be used to set and confirm appointments, provide postorder or postdelivery support, follow-up on service contracts (cleaning, evaluation, accessories, batteries), and confirm that the instruments are working well and to answer questions.

Yellow Pages Directory

Yellow page promotions are almost a necessity for a business. Whether you believe they are effective or not, when a consumer has opened the yellow pages to a particular section, the decision has already been made to purchase. The only question that remains is, from whom? It is your responsibility to develop a yellow pages listing such that the consumer will consider your practice. Yellow pages salespeople suggest that you use multiple listings, advertise prominently, make your listing stand out (box ad, color, or something else), and that you list in directories of nearby communities and other private directories. All of these are good but expensive if they do not produce results. Issues that you should look to relate to listing all the major brands or services you offer, highlight special features, possibly include a map or description of your location if it is difficult to find, recognize that the size of the ad implies reliability and success, that the length of time you have been in business implies trustworthiness, and that a photo of your building implies a solid status. For many young audiologists trying to attract elderly purchasers, a photograph of your building might be more influential than your photograph.

Open House (Consultation)

Open house programs have met with mixed reviews. The general purpose is to provide for high traffic flow and sales in a short time (3 to 5 days). An outside consultant is often employed to provide technical information about the product in question, to review one's hearing loss and fit them with appropriate instruments, to set appointments, or to set the stage for the audiologist. A combined media approach is used to contact potential attendees, with the mailing list coming from the audiologist or from a purchased mailing list that targets the market. The open house has a theme, generally centering around a factory representative, a new product, solutions to special problems, instrument cleaning, a research study, demonstrations, free hearing testing, a new or remodeled office, or some special event. Discount coupons are often included to help entice attendees. Open house programs can generate substantial cash flow in a short time (but may also require substantial up-front investment if the program is to function properly). A potential drawback of these programs is the possibility of a substantial drop-off in sales after the event, unless some other promotional activity is planned to continue patient participation. Another potential drawback is that the "consultant" may be more interested in generating sales that are less likely to be successful, leaving the practice with unanticipated problems a few weeks after the conclusion of the open house.

Public Relations

Public relations involves the generation of positive publicity for your practice, generally for little or no cost. Publicity can be generated by staging an event at your facility with an invitation to the press to attend. Variations of this can be generated for school field trips, special recognition, hosted seminars, individual office tours for reporters, and so forth. Keep a single-page "media handout" that provides information about you, your qualifications, what your practice does, and your staff. Press releases to all the media can often provide hundreds of dollars in free advertising (remember that the best advertising is often that which you do not pay for). It is important to ensure that the information released is newsworthy. Human interest stories are good (hearing aid donations, special fittings).

Special Event

Some marketing programs are intended to improve recognition of your practice by mass exposure during a short period of time. They seem to work well for products or services that are difficult to differentiate from the competition (think of automobiles). Although not used often by audiologists, they can be good on a local level and seem to provide the greatest impact when the dispensing practice is the sole sponsor of a small event.

Tie-In Promotions

These are not practiced frequently by audiologists. They consist of joint, cooperative, or umbrella promotions that allow different businesses to share a promotion (cost, mailing lists, etc.) and reap the benefits from the members of each of the participants. They function best when the businesses are noncompetitive (hearing aids and eyeglasses, hearing aids and wheelchairs), and generally play on themes, seasons, or synergy. The advantages include enhanced product image, shared media costs, a widened market penetration, expanded product use, and added visibility in nontraditional hearing aid locations. Some of the promotions are cross-branded, meaning that products are joined from the same business environment (hearing aid and batteries in a derived-demand relationship), as common-thread products (hearing aids and ear wax remover), or as complementary use relationships (hearing aids and assistive listening devices). Some tie-in promotions are event-oriented in which they are associated with some major event or celebration that is either community wide or national (Prescott Frontier Days Celebration, Fourth of July, etc.). Many are identified with lifestyle (hearing aids and elderly in nursing homes), seasonal connections (holidays and hearing grandchildren), or with special events (May is Better Hearing Month). Whenever possible, attempt to align and stay with one special event in the community per year. Tie-in promotions are not without their problems, especially when associated with another business or group. Difficulties arise in partner selection, longer lead times for coordination, creative and promotional decisions, and logistical and legal difficulties.

Printed Material

Printed material promotions take many forms. As the name implies, they include almost everything that is printed. This includes brochures, booklets, bulletins, circulars, pricing schedules, business cards, letterheads, manuals, correspondence, and other promotional materials. The important issue is that most elderly (approximately 60% of your patients) have a measured reading level of the eighth grade or less and diminishing vision. This makes it important to use relatively short words and sentences (less than 20-word sentence average) and to use large type print (12 point or larger).

Hearing Screening Programs

Conducted with audiometers or by telephone screening machines, hearing screening programs should be performed practically, ethically, and tastefully. Aside from telephones, they are often performed in pharmacies, clinics, retirement homes, senior centers, or fairs. If done by telephone, they have a much greater impact if not provided on a daily basis, but during limited time periods (about 2 weeks) at select times of the year, not too closely related.

Community Events

Certain events within the community provide important opportunities for your name to come before the people. You can use these to your advantage as a member of any of the committees, as a sponsor of the event, or the fact that you consistently participate in one way or another.

Personal Contacts

"Networking" with other useful and/or important individuals is a term of the 1990s, although the practice has always existed. This is often accomplished through service or professional groups (the Lion's Club, Rotary, Kiwanis, Chamber of Commerce, the country club, churches, etc.).

Advertising Specialties

Advertising specialties provide your message on useful, giveaway items (pens, rulers, fly swatters, caps, key rings, calendars, mugs, etc.). These items should have a fairly long use life, offer repeated exposure to your name, and be practical. If cheap or not useful, they reflect on your practice.

Alternative Print Media

Not used often by audiologists, these consist of package inserts (the message is carried with another's purchased item as often seen in the computer industry), ride-along/co-ops (your message with a number of other advertisers using nonstandard formats), as statement stuffers (including a mailing piece in another's or your own statements), as card decks (along with a number of other unrelated advertisers with the message on similar 3 x 5 inch cards), or as free-standing inserts (most often recognized as loose inserts in newspapers).

Information Lunches

Information lunches bring groups of potential patients together for the purpose of presenting useful information with the intent that it will influence attendees to consider your practice as knowledgeable and a purchase location if and when the product is desired.

Personal Selling

Personal selling is a promotion activity that falls outside the scope of this chapter but is the primary method by which marketing promotion occurs.

CONCLUSIONS

The marketplace of the future will foreshadow a period of change: new products and technologies, quality assurance programs, new competitors, and growing, diverse consumer populations. The way in which we do business, deliver products and services, and compete may change, but that change is not without opportunities for professional growth and financial success.

The hearing healthcare world is changing dramatically, and those who change to meet its needs will succeed. As we move ahead, the ability to target specific markets, monitor costs, and market changes will be critical to maximizing profits. Successful audiologists will be those who are flexible, who rethink their products and services, their marketing strategies, and who adjust to changing market needs.

What marketing challenges will you accept in your next marketing plan? What marketing mountains will you climb? The year ahead is filled with opportunity, and those years that follow, even more so. What is required on your part is a destination, a marketing action plan, basic marketing skills, and a willingness to succeed and persevere.

Appendix A
Glossary

advertising Any paid form of nonpersonal sales or promotional effort made on behalf of goods, services, or ideas by an identified sponsor.

advertising agency A firm that specializes in providing promotional services to other businesses for a fee. Services offered include development of advertising copy, selection of advertising media, and placement of the advertisement.

advertising copy The communication that a prospective buyer actually sees or hears.

advertising media The broadcast or print vehicles through which an advertisement is communicated, such as radio, television, magazines, newspapers, and billboards.

assets The resources that a business uses in attempting to earn a profit.

average markup A single percentage used to determine the selling price of each item in a given product line.

brand A name, term, symbol, or design (or a combination of them) used by a business firm to identify its goods or services and to distinguish them from those of competitors.

budget A planning statement that shows the projected revenues and expenses of an organization.

business Any privately owned and operated organization primarily devoted to securing profits or other benefits desired by its owners or managers.

capital A factor of production, including machines, tools, and buildings used to produce goods and services.

cash An asset that includes currency, checking and savings deposits in commercial banks, cashier checks, bank and postal money orders, and bank drafts.

cash discounts Discount prices offered in return for prompt payment for goods or services.

channels of distribution The various ways that goods flow from manufacturers to industrial customers or ultimate consumers.

compensation The total wages, salaries, and fringe benefits received by employees.

competition The process of determining the price, quality, and available quantity of an item through the impersonal interactions of numerous firms.

consumer behavior How people make buying decisions.

consumer market Individuals or households that purchase goods and services for personal use.

cooperative advertising An arrangement whereby national advertisers and local merchants share the cost of local advertising.

cost of goods sold The direct material costs incurred by a firm in producing its products.

couponing A technique for spurring sales by offering a discount through redeemable coupons.

demand The ability and willingness of consumers to buy specific quantities of a good in a given time period.

direct mail A method of promotion in which the business uses mailing lists to reach its most likely customers.

discount A reduction in the price offered to a customer for prompt payment or for buying in large quantities.

entrepreneur Person who starts a business and takes the financial and personal risks involved in keeping it going.

expense A cost of doing business.

gross profit The difference between a firm's net sales and its cost of goods sold. Also called *gross margin.*

gross sales The total dollar amount of goods sold.

inflation An increase in price levels, often measured by the annual change in consumer or wholesale prices.

interest A sum paid or charged for the use of money or for borrowing money.

inventories In retailing, goods available for sale to the consumer.

inventory control The processes whereby managers determine the right quantity of various items to have on hand and keep track of these items' movement and use within the organization.

labor A factor of production, consisting of the human resources used to produce goods and services.

management The process of coordinating resources to meet an objective.

markdown A reduction in the original retail selling price of an item.

market A group of people who have needs to satisfy, money to spend, and the ability to buy.

market research Research that attempts to find out what products or services the consumer wants; what forms, colors, packaging, price ranges, and retail outlets the consumer prefers; and what types of advertising, public relations, and selling practices are most likely to appeal to the consumer.

market segmentation An approach to marketing in which the marketer splits the total market into smaller, more homogeneous groups, and aims production and selling strategies at these target markets.

market value The price of a good, service, or security as determined by demand and supply.

marketing That area of business that directs the flow of goods and services from producer to consumer to satisfy buyers and to achieve company objectives.

marketing concept The principle that stresses shaping products to meet consumer needs rather than attempting to mold those needs to the products.

marketing mix The blend of the five basic marketing activities (product, place, promotion, people, and price) that a firm uses to reach its target market effectively.

markup The difference between the cost of an item and its selling price.

markup percentage The difference between an item's cost and its selling price, expressed as a percentage.

media All the different means, including broadcasting, publications, and other means, by which information and advertising reaches its audience.

money Anything that is generally accepted as a means of paying for goods and services.

net income The actual profit or loss of a company, obtained by subtracting expenses from revenues.

net operating income Gross profit *less* operating expenses.

net sales The figure obtained after discounts to customers are deducted from gross sales.

objectives Broad, long-term goals that provide direction for an organization.

operating expenses All the costs of business operations that are not included in costs of goods sold.

operating income The income left for a business after operating expenses are deducted from gross income.

organization A group of people who have a common objective.

outdoor advertising Any public information about a company's products or services placed out of doors, including sky-writing and neon signs but consisting mainly of billboards and posters.

penetration pricing An approach to pricing in which the manufacturer introduces the product at a low price, planning to get back the initial investment through big sales.

personal income Total income from wages, salaries, business, professional, receipts, dividends, rent, interest, and government payments to individuals.

personal selling Any personal communication between seller and buyer that is performed by salespeople operating inside or outside the firm.

place The element of the marketing mix that involves finding appropriate channels of distribution, including retailing and wholesaling institutions, to get the product to the target market at the right time and in the right place.

planning Establishing objectives for an organization and determining the best way to accomplish these objectives.

plans The means by which an organization's objectives are achieved.

point-of-purchase display (POP) A device by which a product is displayed in such a way as to stimulate immediate sales.

policy A guideline established by management for a specific type of activity in an organization.

price The element of the marketing mix that involves establishing a monetary value for the product that gives value to the customer and adequate revenue to the producer; also

the money and goods exchanged for the ownership or use of some assortment of goods and services.

price discrimination The practice of charging customers different prices for products of like grade and quality.

price fixing An arrangement among competitors to set prices at designated levels.

price leader The producer who tends to set prices in an industry.

price stability An economic pattern in which prices change very little, on the average, overall.

pricing above the market An approach to pricing in which the marketer charges prices that are higher than those of competitors.

pricing below the market An approach to pricing in which the marketer charges prices that are less than those of competitors.

pricing with the market An approach to pricing in which the marketer charges prices that match those of competitors.

product The element of the marketing mix that involves developing the right good (or service) for the target market; also a physical item or service that satisfies certain customer needs.

product life cycle The stages of growth and decline in sales and earnings through which most products go after they have been introduced in the marketplace.

product line The array of products offered for sale by a business.

product mix The list of all products offered by a seller.

profit The money left over from all sums a business has received from sales after expenses have been deducted.

promotion Persuasive communication designed to sell products, services, or ideas to potential customers.

promotional mix A combination of advertising, personal selling, publicity, and sales promotion designed to communicate persuasively with the target market.

psychographics The study of the behavior or consumers of an individual level.

publicity Any information relating to a business, product, or services that appears in any medium on a nonpaid basis.

receivables Money owed to a business.

recession A decline in the real GNP for two consecutive quarters.

retail selling Direct, face-to-face selling that takes place mostly in department and specialty stores.

retailer An establishment that purchases only consumer goods from manufacturers or wholesalers and sells them to ultimate consumers.

return on investment The total return, or profit, obtained from a project *divided* by the amount of money invested in it.

revenue The financial receipts of a business.

risk management The process of reducing the threat of loss as a result of uncontrollable events.

rules Procedures covering a specific situation.

salary A method of compensation based on the amount of time the employee works, where the unit of time is a week, a month, or a year instead of merely an hour.

sales promotion Those marketing activities other than personal selling, advertising, and publicity that stimulate consumer purchasing and dealer effectiveness.

selling expenses The expenses a firm incurs through marketing and distribution of the products it buys or makes for sale.

skimming A pricing method in which a manufacturer charges a high price during the introductory stage of a product and later reduces it when the product is no longer a novelty.

small business One that is independently owned and operated and is not dominant in its field.

target market The specific group or groups of customers to whom a company wishes to sell its products or services.

theory of supply and demand The theory that the supply of a product will rise when demand is great and fall when demand is low and that prices will be higher when supply is low and lower when supply is great.

trading area The geographical region from which a business draws most of its customers and obtains most of its sales and revenues.

Appendix B
Action Plan

MARKET ANALYSIS

1. MARKET DEFINITION

Define the geographical market you serve
Use zip codes, cities, counties, or multiple counties if in a sparsely-populated area.
Include only those places that account for at least 5–10% of your current client base or
those places from which you draw at least 10% of your new clients.

	ZIP Code	City	County	Multiple Counties
Example 1.	85351			
Example 2.		Fountain Hills		
Example 3.			Yavapi	
Example 4.				Cochise/Havasu
5.				
6.				
7.				
8.				

2. MARKET SIZE

What is the size of your market?

a. Population:

Use zip code, city, or county(ies) (samples)	Sample	Population
Example 1.	85351	31,737
Example 2.	Fountain Hills	11,999
3.		
4.		
5.		
6.		
7.		
8.		

Example | **TOTAL** __43,736__

2. MARKET SIZE

What is the size of your market?

b. Hearing Aid Sales

List all competitors in your geographical market market. Guesstimate their <u>average monthly unit sales</u> of hearing aids. Total these averages to estimate monthly unit sales. **Multiply this number by 12, to estimate total annual <u>unit</u> sales.**

	Your Office		Trad. Disp.	Disp. Aud.	Medical Facil	Other
Example	20	a	15	20	12	10
Example		b	25			
		b				
		d				
		e				
		f				
		g				
Example Totals	240		480	240	144	120

This process can be repeated to determine the total market volume for audiological procedures, surgeries, etc., if this information is important to your practice and planning.

TOTAL 1224

Example

3. MARKET GROWTH

a. Is your market's <u>population</u>:

Growing? ☐   Shrinking? ☐   By what %?_____

Why? _____

_____

What are the long-term growth prospects for your market? _____

_____

b. Is your market's <u>total hearing aid sales volume</u>:

Growing? ☐   Shrinking? ☐   By what %?_____

Why? _____

_____

What are the long-term growth prospects for your market? _____

_____

4. MARKET CONDITIONS

a. What market conditions are **currently affecting your business**? (Population, economic cycles, socio-economic conditions).
(Check off those that apply).

■ **ECONOMIC**
- ❏ Unemployment
- ❏ Plant openings, closings
- ❏ Cost of living
- ❏ Interest rates
- ❏ Inflation

■ **SOCIAL**
- ❏ Crime
- ❏ Senior services
- ❏ Health care services: availability, accessibility
- ❏ Transportation
- ❏ Accessibility of cultural, social sport activities

■ **ENVIRONMENTAL**
- ❏ Pollution
- ❏ Weather extremes
- ❏ Natural disasters
- ❏ Prob. of future natural disasters
- ❏ Traffic congestion
- ❏ Environmental ambience
- ❏ Proximity of parks, open space, vacation sites

■ **GOVERNMENT**
- ❏ Senior services
- ❏ Taxation
- ❏ Licensing laws

b. What market conditions are **likely to affect your business** during the next 3-5 years? (Population, economic cycles, socio-economic conditions).
(Check off those that apply).

■ **ECONOMIC**
- ❏ Unemployment
- ❏ Plant openings, closings
- ❏ Cost of living
- ❏ Interest rates
- ❏ Inflation

■ **SOCIAL**
- ❏ Crime
- ❏ Senior services
- ❏ Health care services: availability, accessibility
- ❏ Transportation
- ❏ Accessibility of cultural, social sport activities

■ **ENVIRONMENTAL**
- ❏ Pollution
- ❏ Weather extremes
- ❏ Natural disasters
- ❏ Prob. of future natural disasters
- ❏ Traffic congestion
- ❏ Environmental ambience
- ❏ Proximity of parks, open space, vacation sites

■ **GOVERNMENT**
- ❏ Senior services
- ❏ Taxation
- ❏ Licensing laws

c. What can you do to minimize the ill-effects of negative events or conditions? How can you take advantage of positive events or conditions?

5. AGE AND INCOME DEMOGRAPHICS FOR YOUR MARKET

What are the age and income demographics for your market? (From demographics data).

Zip Code, City, or County	Age 45–64	65–84	45+	65+	85+	Median Age	Median Income	Nat'l / State Centile
USA	19.30%	11.40%	32.00%	12.70%	1.30%	33.70%	$33,900	
Arizona	18.00%	12.20%	31.40%	13.40%	1.20%	32.90%	$29,833	
Example								
85351	11.00%	68.00%	68.00%	83.00%	15.00%	76.10%	$27,151	45 / 51
Fountain Hills	24.20%	17.70%	17.70%	18.20%	0.50%	40.20%	$44,946	89 / 91
Yavapi	23.50%	25.00%	25.00%	27.00%	2.00%	45.40%	$21,493	18 / 9
Cochise/Havasu	20.20%	22.40%	22.40%	83.00%	2.30%	41.10%	$20,725	15 / 26

Appendix C
Action Plan

Towards 2000™ Marketing Workshop
"8-Point Competitive Analysis"
Used to Determine Your Competitive Advantage

1. COMPETITIVE PROFILE

a. List all competitors in your market (within a certain distance, area, or market profile) .

b. Place an asterisk next to the names of your key competitors (those who are a substitute for you in your served market).

c. Note the ownership, type of business, and professional credentials of your key competitors (**Ownership** = sole proprietor, MD, investor, corporation, hospital,multi-site chain, major company, government, etc. **Type of business** = MD, clinic, HMO, hospital, private practice, hearing aid dispensary, franchise, retail store. **Professional credentials** = audiologist, hearing aid specialist, MD, etc.).

	Name	Location	Ownership/Type	Credentials
Example 1. *	Audiology Associates	5 miles	Private Practice	Audiologist
2.				
3.				
4.				
5.				
6.				
7.				
8.				

2. COMPETITIVE INTENSITY

Total numbers of Competitors _____

Market Size (Population) _____

Population per Office _____

Example:	
Total # of Competitors	= 8
Market size	= 250,000
Population per office	= 31,250

3. COMPETITIVE PERFORMANCE ANALYSIS

<u>Estimate</u> **all** competitors' unit sales per month, market share, growth (compared to overall market), client base. Add revenue if you are able to estimate it.

	Name	Unit Sales HAs	Market Share %	Growth + or -	Client Base Active Users
Example 1.	Audiology Associates	30	25%	Greater	1000
2.					
3.					
4.					
5.					
6.					
7.					
8.					
9.					
10.					
11.					
12.					
13.					
TOTALS					
	# Competitors	Aids Per/Mo	100%	+ or -	# Customers

4. MARKET POTENTIAL

Market Size (Population) _____

Hard-of-Hearing Population (9.4% of Total) _____

40% of HOH Population ===================

60% of HOH Population ===================

Example	Market size	= 250,000
	9.4% = HOH	= 23,500
	What potential of this 23,500 do you believe are potential purchasers?	
	20%	= 4,700
	40%	= 9,400
	50%	= 11,750
	60%	= 14,100

5. MARKET PENETRATION

Cumulative total of client bases ————————

Market Size (Population) ————————

Hard-of-Hearing Population (9.4% of Total) ————————

Population per Office ════════════

Example:	
Client Base	= Total customers from #2
Market size	= 250,000
9.4% HOH	= 23,500
Pop. per office	= 31,250

6. COMPETITIVE STRENGTHS & WEAKNESSES

Assess **key** competitors' strengths and weaknesses. Use a + for strength and − for weakness.

Competitor A

- ❑ Client Base
  - ❑ Size
  - ❑ Location
  - ❑ Income
- ❑ Finances
  - ❑ Assets
  - ❑ Credit Worthiness
  - ❑ Cash
- ❑ Technology
  - ❑ Test Equipment
  - ❑ Programmable Hearing Aids
  - ❑ Computerized Office
- ❑ Knowledge, Skills
  - ❑ Hearing Aids
  - ❑ Audiology
  - ❑ Counseling
  - ❑ Sales
  - ❑ Service
- ❑ Communication Skills
- ❑ Credentials
- ❑ Reputation
- ❑ Visibility, Name Recognition
- ❑ Marketing Communications
- ❑ Office
  - ❑ Location
  - ❑ Decor

COMPETITIVE ADVANTAGE
- ❑ Cost Structure
- ❑ Timing
- ❑ Focus
- ❑ Differentiation   Ⓐ

Competitor B

- ❑ Client Base
  - ❑ Size
  - ❑ Location
  - ❑ Income
- ❑ Finances
  - ❑ Assets
  - ❑ Credit Worthiness
  - ❑ Cash
- ❑ Technology
  - ❑ Test Equipment
  - ❑ Programmable Hearing Aids
  - ❑ Computerized Office
- ❑ Knowledge, Skills
  - ❑ Hearing Aids
  - ❑ Audiology
  - ❑ Counseling
  - ❑ Sales
  - ❑ Service
- ❑ Communication Skills
- ❑ Credentials
- ❑ Reputation
- ❑ Visibility, Name Recognition
- ❑ Marketing Communications
- ❑ Office
  - ❑ Location
  - ❑ Decor

COMPETITIVE ADVANTAGE
- ❑ Cost Structure
- ❑ Timing
- ❑ Focus
- ❑ Differentiation   Ⓑ

Competitor C

- ❑ Client Base
  - ❑ Size
  - ❑ Location
  - ❑ Income
- ❑ Finances
  - ❑ Assets
  - ❑ Credit Worthiness
  - ❑ Cash
- ❑ Technology
  - ❑ Test Equipment
  - ❑ Programmable Hearing Aids
  - ❑ Computerized Office
- ❑ Knowledge, Skills
  - ❑ Hearing Aids
  - ❑ Audiology
  - ❑ Counseling
  - ❑ Sales
  - ❑ Service
- ❑ Communication Skills
- ❑ Credentials
- ❑ Reputation
- ❑ Visibility, Name Recognition
- ❑ Marketing Communications
- ❑ Office
  - ❑ Location
  - ❑ Decor

COMPETITIVE ADVANTAGE
- ❑ Cost Structure
- ❑ Timing
- ❑ Focus
- ❑ Differentiation   Ⓒ

7. YOUR STRENGTHS & WEAKNESSES

Business Assessment. Assess your strengths and weaknesses. Use a **+** for strength and **−** for weakness.

+	−	
___	___	❏ Client Base
___	___	❏ Size
___	___	❏ Location
___	___	❏ Income
___	___	❏ Finances
___	___	❏ Assets
___	___	❏ Credit Worthiness
___	___	❏ Cash
___	___	❏ Technology
___	___	❏ Test Equipment
___	___	❏ Programmable Hearing Aids
___	___	❏ Computerized Office
___	___	❏ Knowledge, Skills
___	___	❏ Hearing Aids
___	___	❏ Audiology
___	___	❏ Counseling
___	___	❏ Sales
___	___	❏ Service
___	___	❏ Communication Skills
___	___	❏ Credentials
___	___	❏ Reputation
___	___	❏ Visibility, Name Recognition
___	___	❏ Marketing Communications
___	___	❏ Office
___	___	❏ Location
___	___	❏ Decor

+	−	
___	___	**COMPETITIVE ADVANTAGE**
___	___	❏ Cost Structure
___	___	❏ Timing
___	___	❏ Focus
___	___	❏ Differentiation

TOTAL ___ ___

How do you rank your competitive situation? Are you positive or negative on these? Add these up to obtain your totals.

8. COMPETITIVE ADVANTAGE

Describe <u>your</u> current and planned Competitive Advantage on the following categories.

❑ Cost
❑ Focus
❑ Timing
❑ Differentiation

Based on these, how is your Competitive Advantage relative to:

Value? _____

_____

_____

Unique? _____

_____

_____

Sustainable? _____

_____

_____

Defendable? _____

_____

_____

COMPETITIVE ANALYSIS

	Competitor	Competitor	Competitor	Competitor	Competitor	Competitor
COMPETITIVE ENVIRONMENT						
(a) Estimated Unit Sales						
(b) Estimated % Custom-Molded						
(c) Estimated % Non Custom						
(d) Market Share Trends						
SUCCESS FACTORS						
(a) Product Quality						
(b) Product Reliability						
(c) Product Price						
(d) Product Recognition						
(e) Company Image						
(f) Product Breadth of Line						
(g) Market Coverage Sales						
(h) Effectiveness						
(i) Location						
(j) Buyer-Seller Relationship						
(k)						
(l)						
(m)						
MAJOR STRENGTH						
MAJOR WEAKNESS						
STRATEGY						

MARKETING STRATEGIES OF COMPETITORS

1. Describe the current **product strategies** employed by primary competitors.
   Competitor A _____
   _____
   Competitor B _____
   _____
   Competitor C _____
   _____

2. Describe the current **pricing strategies** employed by primary competitors.
   Competitor A _____
   _____
   Competitor B _____
   _____
   Competitor C _____
   _____

3. Describe the current **distribution strategies** employed by primary competitors.
   Competitor A _____
   _____
   Competitor B _____
   _____
   Competitor C _____
   _____

4. Describe the current **advertising strategies** employed by primary competitors.
   Competitor A _____
   _____
   Competitor B _____
   _____
   Competitor C _____
   _____

5. Describe the current **sales promotion strategies** employed by primary competitors.
   Competitor A _____
   _____
   Competitor B _____
   _____
   Competitor C _____
   _____

REFERENCES

ANTITRUST LAWS POLICY GUIDE. (1988). Santa Monica, CA: Lear Siegler, Inc.

BANK OF AMERICA. (1988). Steps to starting a business. San Francisco: *Small Business Reporter.* 20 pp.

BERKOWITZ, A. (1992). Advertising to fulfill the marketing plan. In: W. Staab (Ed.), *Applied hearing instrument marketing* (pp. 165–185). Livonia: National Institute for Hearing Instruments Studies.

BRAUN, I. (1981). Building a successful professional practice with advertising. *American Marketing Association Communications.*

CACI MARKETING SYSTEMS. (1995). Internet address: http://www.demographics.caci.com.

CENSUS BUREAU (not dated). *Projections of the United States by age, sex, and race: 1983–2080.* Series P-25. No. 952.

CRANMER, K. (1983). Hearing aid dispensing—1983. *Hearing Instruments,* 34(5);9–12.

GENSCH, D. (1970). Media factors: A review article. *Journal of Marketing Research,* 7(5);216–225.

GENTILE, A. (1975). Persons with impaired hearing United States – 1971. Vital and Health Statistics, Series 10, No. 101, DHEW Publication No. (HRA) 76-1528. Washington, DC: U.S. Government Printing Office.

GLORIG, A., & NIXON, J. (1960). Distribution of hearing loss in various populations. *Annals of Otology,* 69;497–516.

GOLDSTEIN, D. (1984). Hearing impairment, hearing aids, and audiology. *ASHA,* 27;24–31,34–35,38.

HIA (HEARING INDUSTRIES ASSOCIATION) (1984). *A market research study of the U.S. hearing-impaired population.* Washington, DC: The Association.

HOSFORD-DUNN, H., DUNN, D.R., & HARFORD, E.R. (1995a). Marketing. *Audiology business and practice management* (pp. 295–319). San Diego: Singular Publishing Group, Inc.

HOSFORD-DUNN, H., DUNN, D.R., & HARFORD, E.R. (1995b). Pricing. *Audiology business and practice management* (pp. 295–319). San Diego: Singular Publishing Group, Inc.

INC. MAGAZINE. (1995). December. © 1996 Goldhirsh Group, Inc., 38 Commercial Wharf, Boston, MA 02110.

JATHO, K. (1969). Population surveys and norms. *International Audiology,* 8;231–239.

JELONEK, S. (1992a). Conducting a market analysis. In: W. Staab (Ed.), *Applied hearing instrument marketing* (pp. 35–58). Livonia: National Institute for Hearing Instruments Studies.

JELONEK, S. (1992b). The importance of good marketing programs. In: W. Staab (Ed.), *Applied hearing instrument marketing* (pp. 59–88). Livonia: National Institute for Hearing Instruments Studies.

JELONEK, S., & STAAB, W.J. (1994). The hearing aid office as a marketing tool. *Hearing Instruments,* 45(4);27–28,30.

KRAMER, A. (1992). Direct mail. In: W. Staab (Ed.), *Applied hearing instrument marketing* (pp. 187–200). Livonia: National Institute for Hearing Instruments Studies.

MCKENNA, R. (1986). *The regis touch. New marketing strategies for uncertain times* (pp. 7–15). New York: Addison-Wesley.

MILES, A.W. (1986). V. *Pricing. Perspectives marketing series* (pp. 1–5). Boston: The Boston Consulting Group, Inc.

MOSCICKI, E., ELKINS, E., BAUM, H., & MCNAMARA, P. (1985). Hearing loss in the elderly: An epidemiologic study of the Framingham Heart Study Cohort. *Ear and Hearing,* 6;184–190.

NCHS. (1981). Prevalence of selected impairments, United States—1977. DHEW Pub. No. (PHS) 82–1562.

NCHS: ROWLAND, M. (1980). Basic data on hearing levels of adults 25–74 years, United States, 1971–1975. *Vital and health statistics,* Series 11, No. 215, DHEW Publications No. (PHS) 80–1663.

NHIS. *(1977). Hearing ability of persons by sociodemographic and health characteristics: United States.* Vital and health statistics, Hyattsville, MD: National Center for Health Statistics.

NHIS: ADAMS, P., & HARDY, A. (1989). Current estimates from the National Health Interview Survey: United States. *Vital statistics,* 10(173). Hyattsville, MD: National Center for Health Statistics.

OGILVY, D. (1983). *Ogilvy on advertising.* New York: Crown Publishers.

RIES, P. (1982). Hearing ability of persons by sociodemographic and health statistics. *Vital and health statistics,* Series 10, No. 140, DHHS Pub. No. (PHS) 82–1568, Washington, DC: U.S. Government Printing Office.

ROBERTS, J. (1968). Hearing status in examination findings among adults, United States—1960–1962. *Vital and Health Statistics,* Series 11, No. 99, DHEW Publication No. 1000, Washington, DC: U.S. Government Printing Office.

SANDLIN, R.E. (1992). The problem/the market. In: W. Staab (Ed.), *Applied hearing instrument marketing,* (pp. 1–33). Livonia: National Institute for Hearing Instruments Studies.

SCIENCE MAGAZINE. (1996). July 5.

SETTLE, R.B., & ALRECK, P.L. (1989). Reducing buyers' sense of risk. *Marketing communications, January;* 34–39.

SKAFTE, M.D. (1995). A review of the 1994 hearing instrument market. *The Hearing Review,* 1(3);16,18,20,24–27,53,60–61.

SKAFTE, M.D. (1998). The 1997 hearing instrument market – the dispensers' perspective. *Hearing Review,* 5(6);6,8,10,12, 16,18,20,24,26,28,30,32.

STAAB, W.J. (1986). Hearing aid dispensing. In: W. Hodgson (Ed.), *Hearing aid assessment and use in audiologic habilitation.* (3rd ed.). (pp. 266-300). Baltimore: Williams & Wilkins.

STAAB, W.J. (1990). Marketing hearing aids—An overview. In: C. Killingsworth (Ed.), *Directions in marketing audiology: Turning up the volume.* Academy of Dispensing Audiologists.

STAAB, W.J. (1991). *Hearing aids: A user's guide* (p. 39). Phoenix, AZ: Wayne J. Staab Publisher.

STAAB, W.J. (1992). Sales promotion for office traffic control. In: W. Staab (Ed.), *Applied hearing instrument marketing* (pp. 201–254). Livonia: National Institute for Hearing Instruments Studies.

STAAB, W.J., & JELONEK, S. (1994a). Are you finding your competitive advantage? *Hearing Instruments,* 45(7);20–21.

STAAB, W.J., & JELONEK, S. (1994b). *Towards 2000: Hearing aid marketing workshop.* Building Professional Marketing Skills. Phoenix, AZ.

STAAB, W.J., & JELONEK, S. (1995a). Reducing hearing aid purchasers' sense of risk. *Audecibel, January/February/March;* Boston: 19–25.

STAAB, W.J., & JELONEK, S. (1995b). *Towards 2000: Hearing aid marketing workshop.* Building Professional Marketing Skills. Phoenix, AZ.

STEVENS, A. (1984). Public relations: A powerful hearing health-care marketing tool. *The Hearing Journal, October;* 25–28.

TIAA-CREF MAGAZINE. (1998). How long will I live? The view from 100. 12–13.

U.S. DEPARTMENT OF HEALTH AND HUMAN SERVICES. (1988). Aging America: Trends and projections, 1987–88 edition. Washington, DC: U.S. Government Printing Office.

USA TODAY. (1996). Study: 2020 begins age of the elderly. Tuesday, May 21, 4A.

USA TODAY. (1998). Retirement planning hot line.

WHITE HOUSE CONFERENCE ON SMALL BUSINESS ISSUE HANDBOOK: A FOUNDATION FOR A NEW CENTURY. (1994). Prepared by the Office of Advocacy, U.S. Small Business Administration, 1800 G Street, NW, Suite 1233, Washington, DC.

WILDER, C. (1975). Prevalence of selected impairments, U.S., 1971. *Vital and health statistics,* Series 10, No. 99. DHEW Publication No. (HRA) 75-1526, Washington, DC: U.S. Government Printing Office.

WILLIAMS, P. (1984). *Hearing loss: Information for professionals in the aging network.* NICD/ASHA, Gallaudet College.

Chapter 8

Private Practice Issues

Teresa M. Clark and Darcy Benson

WHAT IS PRIVATE PRACTICE?

Lisa works for an audiologist in San Francisco who has an office downtown. Most of the patients are elderly, hearing-impaired persons who live in retirement communities in the area. Lisa works in this office 4 days a week as a dispensing audiologist. However, after office hours and on weekends, Lisa has her own hearing conservation business. She works mostly with musicians providing diagnostic hearing evaluation, musicians' earplugs and monitoring systems used for live performances.

Michael works in a large otology clinic as the Director of Audiology. He supervises four staff audiologists, one audiology assistant and one clerical support person. The audiology service provides a full range of diagnostic testing and dispenses hearing devices. All audiologists, including Michael, are compensated at a specified annual rate and receive no additional compensation for products they sell. The department does have a budget that must be met. Michael interviews candidates for all positions, but they are also interviewed by the otologist. He does not have final say on who is hired or how revenues generated by the audiology department are spent.

Do either of these clinicians have a private practice in audiology? Most would agree that Lisa does indeed have a private practice, albeit an unconventional one. It is questionable whether Michael has a private practice. He has no ownership in the practice; he lacks management responsibility for financial, personnel, and other practice decisions; he does not benefit from practice growth; he is not the ultimate decision maker; and he is not responsible for the final outcome of the department.

This chapter explores the question of what constitutes private practice, along with a multitude of general issues related to private practice. The chapter is directed toward audiologists considering the idea of going into private practice who need general information about what private practice entails. Those clinicians already engaged in private practice know these issues all too well. The other chapters in this volume deal with specific areas of practice management on a more detailed level. It is hoped that this chapter will provide a global view of private practice issues and serve as a springboard to an understanding of the importance of the information found elsewhere in this volume.

The chapter is divided into several sections that address many different issues facing the private practitioner. It begins with a definition of private practice and a discussion of the development of the underlying values and goals of private practice. Different ways of acquiring practices and the necessary resources required to purchase and run a practice are addressed. How to create an image and to develop and secure a good reputation follow. More concrete topics are explored when addressing equipment needs, patient referrals, and what organization

Audiology: Practice Management. Edited by Hosford-Dunn, Roeser, and Valente. Thieme Medical Publishers, Inc., New York © 2000

systems are necessary for running a private practice. Further sections examine the necessary functions of practice management and who actually performs these functions. Business aspects are found in the sections that discuss establishing relationships with vendors, managing the practice's money, and introducing new sources of revenue. The chapter concludes with a review of current and future trends in private practice.

WHAT IS THE DEFINITION OF PRIVATE PRACTICE?

The roots of audiology private practice are in the medical model of private practice. Audiology private practice is often a unique melding of a service practice that provides diagnostic and rehabilitative services and a retail establishment that sells products. The audiologist works as the healthcare provider rendering services to the patients of the practice, and in many cases selling products that improve hearing. Front office personnel, who take phone calls, schedule appointments, and accept payment for services and products, commonly run such offices.

Some defining parameters are common to all private practices. A private practice is an entity, an independent institution, that allows the healthcare practitioner (i.e., the audiologist) to provide services for his or her population (i.e., persons with hearing loss) and receive direct payment for these services. It is a combination of both a professional enterprise and a business enterprise. The owner of a private practice is investing his or her own time and money, carries the power of decision making without outside intervention, and has ultimate responsibility for the enterprise. The enterprise shows that the owner is not only an autonomous professional but also an autonomous businessperson. No one else shoulders the burden; the owner is the bottom line.

The most common practice is the hearing center that provides diagnostic hearing evaluations aimed primarily at the hearing-impaired individual who needs or is interested in amplification systems or rehabilitative services. Many offices also provide a wide range of diagnostic services to support

> ### CONTROVERSIAL POINT
>
> Private practice may take many forms; however, audiologists who are self-employed are not necessarily in private practice. Audiologists who contract their services, but do not have an active patient following of their own, a monetary investment in a practice or any decision-making authority, do not have a private practice. They are self-employed contractors but do not have a "private practice" per se.

medical doctors in the area and perhaps even specialized diagnostic services for evaluation of the central auditory system. A smaller number of practices provide diagnostic services only. Some audiologists are partnered with medical doctors sharing in the costs and profits derived from the services and products the audiologist provides. A recent survey in *Audiology Express* (1998) shows the breakdown of audiologists by setting, with 31% of the survey respondents being in a private audiology practice (see Fig. 8–1).

Like Lisa, described in the beginning of the chapter, private practice audiologists are looking outside the conventional sector for ways to expand their markets by providing services to the population at large. They are exploring the world of recreational audiology, providing services not only to the music industry but also to individuals whose recreational activities put them at risk for hearing impairment (e.g., skeet shooters, hunters). These professionals also provide services to individuals that might need communication products (e.g., monitors for security personnel, monitors for anchorpersons). The area of hearing conservation for industry provides another avenue for audiologists to expand into the business world.

Other audiologists augment their practice by engaging in clinical research projects with manufacturers in the hearing healthcare industry. In addition, they may act as trainers, introducing concepts underlying new products to audiologists

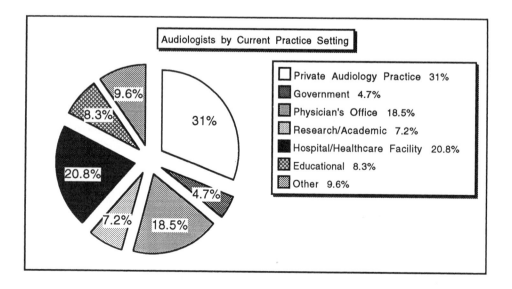

Figure 8–1 Audiologists by Current Practice Setting. (From *Audiology Express*, 4(1); June 1998.)

across the country or world. Some also are sales consultants for the hearing healthcare industry on a part-time basis.

Thus the world of private practice offers the audiologist a wide variety of different settings to provide services and products for the hearing-impaired. These can be carried out in a multitude of ways. In fact, probably as many different private practice settings exist as do audiologists in private practice.

WHAT ARE THE CORE IDEOLOGY, GOALS, AND LONG-TERM VISION OF A PRIVATE PRACTICE?

Certain principles are inherent in successful private practice. As with any business, a private practice must have a core ideology to have long-term success. In an excellent article Collins and Porras (1996) expound on the concepts of core ideology that "defines the enduring character of an organization" because it is the "glue that holds an organization together through time" (p. 66). The core ideology of the practice should not change over time because it is a reflection of the values of the owner (Table 8–1).

Intrinsic to the core ideology is the practice's core values and core purpose. The core values are, as stated by Collins and Porris (1996), the practice's "small set of timeless guiding principles," the "essential and enduring tenets" of the practice. The core purpose is the practice's "reason for being." No matter how large or small the practice, the core values and core purpose must be outlined and understood, ideally by all who are involved with the practice.

From the core values and core purpose the envisioned future of the practice can be outlined. The future includes the goals of the practice and its long-term vision. The goals should succinctly articulate what the private practice owner hopes to accomplish and should be, as explained by Collins and Porras (1996), "clear and compelling . . . the focal point of effort . . . a catalyst for team spirit" (p. 73). The goals may also include the mechanisms that will be used to reach the goals.

They should be clear so that the practice can determine when it has achieved its goals. The goals of the practice may be influenced by many internal and external factors, and, in contrast to core ideology, may change over time as goals are reached. The long-term vision may initially be difficult to define but should include the "dreams, hopes, and aspirations" of the owner. An example of core ideology, goals, and vision can be found in Table 8–1.

The professional expertise and preferences of the owner and, in some cases, the employees will influence the goals. Questions such as the following should be answered: "Is the owner's expertise primarily in diagnostic services or hearing rehabilitation through the fitting of hearing devices?" "Will evoked potential testing or electronystagmography be a diagnostic service of the practice?" "Does the owner prefer to serve a broad age range or to focus specifically on children or adults?"

The physical constraints of the practice, such as location, space and equipment, will affect its goals. Diagnostic services are influenced by how much room is available for specialized diagnostic equipment. The number of patients that can be seen is determined by how many treatment rooms are available. The ability to serve multiple handicapped patients is affected by how accessible the practice is from the street.

The populations the owner wishes to serve and how they are served affect where the private practice is located. Practices whose primary goal is to provide diagnostic audiological services should be established in locations that have a large physician base for referrals. A practice whose goal is to serve children should be located in a community of young families or near a local children's hospital. Offices that want to dispense hearing devices to the geriatric community should locate near retirement communities.

It is the core ideology and goals of a private practice that establish the practice's uniqueness. The practice takes on a persona of its own, reflecting the personality and values of the owner. The core ideology is translated to the support and professional staff and is reflected in their interaction with the patients and in the day-to-day operation of the office. It is this

TABLE 8–1 An example of core ideology, goals, and vision

SAMPLE CORE IDEOLOGY, GOALS, AND VISION
CORE VALUES
Service to the patient above all else
Broadest choice in solutions for the hearing impaired
Excellence in reputation
Highest Integrity
CORE PURPOSE
To improve the quality of life for the hearing impaired through communication solutions
To provide excellence in the delivery of diagnostic services
GOALS
To have employee policies written down in an employee handbook
To have gross receipts of 500K in 3 years
To add evoked potential testing capabilities next year
LONG-TERM VISION
To have three locations in the county within 5 years
To have our business name come to mind immediately when someone says, "hearing aids"

individuality that separates competitive practices from each other and sometimes even branch offices from one another. The services provided by various offices may be similar, but the persona of the offices may be very different. These factors related to core ideology could determine the success of a private practice because the people in the community ultimately will decide which practices are most suited to their needs.

The goals of a successful practice also may change over time. As the practitioners broaden their skill levels and as more capital is available for equipment purchases, other services may be added. The constant changes in managed care in the United States also alter the kinds of services and products provided, thus impacting the practice's goals. In a field that is so closely tied to advances in technology, rapid technological changes provide new ways to address problems, thereby influencing the practice's goals.

A shift in interest areas may also contribute to a change in goals. Some private practice owners have developed a strong interest in business solutions and/or marketing methods. Methods that have worked well for them are repackaged and marketed to other colleagues. These ancillary business activities are carried out within the boundaries of the private practice, providing a new source of revenue. Other owners have become cogent negotiators in the managed care arena and have contracted their time in assisting other colleagues in obtaining managed care contracts.

Each community has its own unique blend of people and needs. The community in which the practice is established affects the goals of the practice by influencing what the practice does and does not offer. Practices located in poor urban neighborhoods must consider taking third-party reimbursement such as Medicaid to serve their community better. Providing a hearing conservation program might be considered in areas with large factories.

Not only does the community shape the private practice goals, but also the practice becomes a part of the communities that it serves. The owner, as audiologist, becomes a part of the medical and allied health communities by providing audiology services at physician offices, in hospitals, and in nursing home facilities. The owner, as professional colleague, may belong to local, regional, and state professional audiology organizations and as an audiology advocate may affect local and state legislation. The owner, as a businessperson, becomes part of the business community and may join the local chamber of commerce, the Better Business Bureau, and other civic groups such as the Rotary club. Joining business and civic groups serves more than one purpose. By establishing a solid relationship with the community, the owner demonstrates support for the community. This can help in establishing relationships with other businesses such as the local insurance agent, the banking institutions, and the local newspaper. The patients of the practice will have a high level of confidence that the owner is a reputable businessperson. In addition, contact with other business people can be a valuable source for referrals to the practice.

Any private practice is a blend of providing professional services and making a living by running a business. Both endeavors must be considered high priorities. An audiologist may provide high-quality professional care, but if equal attention is not paid to the business operation of the practice, the success of the practice is jeopardized. Private

practice audiologists who dispense hearing devices must be aware of the difficulty in striking a balance between operating a retail establishment and maintaining a professional practice. Is the audiologist a seller of products that create a high level of customer satisfaction and a provider of good customer service, or is he or she a professional making judgments and recommendations, with less regard for the preferences of the patient?

CONTROVERSIAL POINT

A male patient comes into the office and has a moderate-to-severe sloping sensorineural hearing loss. The audiologist recommends binaural behind-the-ear (BTE) hearing devices. The patient indicates that he only will consider completely-in-the-canal (CIC) devices because of cosmetic concerns and only can afford one hearing aid. Does the audiologist stand by his or her recommendation and turn the patient away or fit the patient with a monaural CIC, realizing that the benefit to the patient may be minimal at best?

Sound business practices, patient preferences, and professional goals can sometimes be at variance. A clear understanding of the practice ideology, goals, and vision is imperative to bring all these activities into harmony. (Further discussion of professional ethics can be found in Chapters 3 and 9.)

A successful audiology practice should have a clearly articulated outline of how its business activities are envisioned and how they are to be carried out, known as a business plan. The business plan is, most commonly, a written document that includes the core ideology, goals, and long-term vision of a practice, among other things. The business plan is a concise description of the practice and includes the following items: the general concept of the practice, with an outline of the services and the products that will be provided, an analysis of the target market and the population to be served, a marketing plan, an outline of operations, a description of the short-term goals and long-term vision, a financial analysis with financial projections, a risk assessment, and an overall schedule. (A thorough discussion of the writing of a business plan can be found in Chapter 14.)

HOW DO YOU BEGIN PRIVATE PRACTICE AND WHAT RESOURCES ARE NECESSARY?

Many ways exist to begin private practice. The approach chosen often is related to real or perceived financial constraints. A common way is to start from scratch. Some audiologists do this by hanging out a shingle, assembling all the necessary tools of the trade (or at least the bare minimum), and developing a patient base over a period of time. Others initiate partnerships with other audiologists, otolaryngologists, or other healthcare professionals, splitting the cost of equipment and space and revenues for guaranteed referrals. A less common way is to inherit a practice from a family member. Often a person enters the hearing healthcare field as a hearing aid dispenser and encourages a son or daughter to obtain an audiology degree and take over the family business.

Over the last decade many audiologists who wished to acquire a private practice found that buying an existing practice was an easier path by providing an instant patient base and immediate revenue (so-called "turnkey business"). Many of the businesses purchased were not audiology practices but hearing aid practices founded by hearing aid dispensers who were trained to fit and sell hearing aids. Another relatively recent model is to become a "junior partner" in an established practice, with a partnership buy-in over time.

Thus the primary ways to get into private practice are to start on one's own, to purchase one, or to inherit one. In purchasing a practice, it is wise to enlist the services of an attorney and accountant to assist in formulating the purchase price of the business and in negotiating the terms and conditions to be set forth in the purchase agreement. After the sale is completed, the attorney and an accountant will also advise the new owner or owners on setting up the business structure of the practice, whether it is to be a sole proprietorship, a partnership, or a corporation. A thorough discussion of purchasing a private practice can be found in a text by Hosford-Dunn et al (1995).

Regardless of the purchase approach, many resources are required. If one starts one's own business, capital must be available to purchase office and diagnostic equipment, furniture, pay rent, buy products for retail sale (if applicable), and have enough cash on hand to run the business. In addition, in most instances, it may take a relatively long period of time before the business is profitable enough to support the owner and any other ancillary staff. Therefore some outside capital (e.g., from personal savings, personal loans, loans from financial institutions) is needed as the business is growing.

Purchasing an existing business obviously requires more capital. In the best case scenario, personal funds are available, at least for a down payment on the business and for minimum operating capital. Business and personal loans are a common source of capital for a new business. With a business already in place, it is much easier to draw off a modest amount for personal income to survive during the initial years. This is true only if debts from loans or accumulated taxes are not too burdensome. (Refer to Chapters 15 and 16 for a detailed discussion of the financial aspects of private practice.)

In addition to the financial outlay in purchasing or starting a small business, high demands on the owner's physical and emotional resources are also present. Regardless of whether one is starting or purchasing a practice, unless extensive financial resources are available, many jobs and tasks that are not in the traditional job description of an "audiologist" will fall to the audiologist because he or she is the owner. Work hours will number many more per week than the hours of most salaried professionals. The challenges of private practice require energy, tenacity, a willingness to learn new information, and an openness to develop new skills.

Usually, the new owner of a private practice is simultaneously in charge of many different areas. Being director of audiology may be a familiar role, but the owner is now also the director of finance, human resources, information systems, sales and marketing, operations, organizational systems, professional services, and facility maintenance. The different roles the audiologist, as private practice owner, must assume are shown in Figure 8–2.

If a turnkey business is purchased, the first day the practice is open the owner starts seeing patients and suddenly assumes all the additional responsibilities. Trying to see patients in a new work environment, setting up new accounts, and sorting through belongings left behind by the previous owner are daunting tasks. However, trying to get up to speed on all of these other activities is simply overwhelming. Never are there enough hours in day; seldom does one feel that headway is being made on the tasks at hand. Most new private practitioners eat, sleep, and breathe their businesses, often at the expense of their health and personal relationships. Trying to manage stress can become a major issue. Burnout is often cited anecdotally as a major reason for selling practices.

The stress that the private practitioners shoulder is not different from the stresses for any small business. Unfortunately, most audiologists are poorly prepared for the tasks ahead of them in operating a business. They receive little or no business training and that which they did receive still barely touches the broad scope of knowledge and skill needed to run a good solid practice. Starting a practice from scratch can provide some relief because the first several years can be slow and there is time to learn during office hours. However, the stress created from trying to grow a new business and the inherent

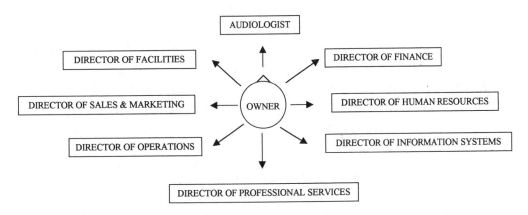

Figure 8–2   The different roles the audiologist, as private practice owner, must assume.

financial burdens create a different type of all-consuming passion. Core ideology, goals, and long-term vision are all important as touchstones during the developing years.

HOW DO YOU CREATE AN IMAGE AND REPUTATION IN PRIVATE PRACTICE?

The core ideology, goals, and long-term vision of a private practice define the practice, but their implementation imparts to the community a certain image of the owner and an image of the practice. Even as practice goals are modified, the image of the practice should remain constant.

It is important for the owner to identify early in the development of the practice how he or she wishes the practice to be perceived by the community. If the owner wants to attract a certain clientele, the corresponding image needs to be created in the minds of both the lay community and the professional community. Image is largely about who the owner is, who he or she feels comfortable serving, and in what capacities he or she provides these services. However, image translates into tangible items as well. The appearance of the marketing materials, the yellow pages ad, the newspaper ads, and the office newsletter all should be consistent with the image the owner wants the community to hold. For example, the practice's stationery and business cards should convey a clear image of the practice to the community. Figure 8–3 illustrates ways of presenting a consistent image through the use of a logo on printed materials. In addition, the location of the office, the sign on the building, the physical layout, and the office furnishing all contribute to the perception of the practice.

Of perhaps greater importance are the intangible items that imprint the practice's image in the mind of the patients and the referral sources. Support staff must have a clear understanding of the image the practice is trying to portray because they have the greatest direct contact with the community. It is imperative that these individuals comport themselves in a manner consistent with the office image. Professional staff must also have a clear idea of the community's perception of the office. If an employee conducts himself or herself in a manner that is inconsistent with the image the owner wishes to portray, the efforts of the owner are undermined and a different image of the practice is created.

Central to the idea of creating an image in any private practice is the perception of competence. Competence is reflected not only in high levels of patient satisfaction and in the professional delivery of services but also in the efficient operation of the entire office. This perception runs from front office scheduling through to the back office bookkeeping functions. An aura of competence translates into patient confidence and trust in the services of the practice in general. For the professional community, being prompt in the return of phone calls, sending reports in a timely manner, and sending thank you letters, all help to create confidence in the practice. Creating a perception of competence generally develops over time through repeated contacts with patients and referral sources.

Fundamental to creating a positive image to the patients and the community is the concept of quality and Continuous

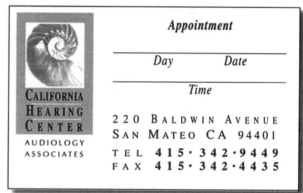

Figure 8–3 Sample patient appointment card and ads showing a consistent use of the practice logo.

Quality Improvement (CQI). CQI requires the practice and clinician go beyond the expected and continually strive for higher levels of patient care. (Chapter 4 addresses this important issue in detail.)

Equally important is the practice of good etiquette, which generates the perception of respect and compassion for the patients who are served. The practice can solidify a perception of confidence by being accessible to patients, being flexible with appointment times, and seeing patients on time.

WHAT EQUIPMENT DO YOU NEED FOR PRIVATE PRACTICE?

The services a private practice provides determines the type of equipment required to run the practice. A practice that focuses primarily on hearing aid dispensing needs an electroacoustic analyzer but does not need sophisticated diagnostic testing equipment. A practice that focuses primarily on diagnostics does not need a hearing aid repair laboratory. A practice that contracts with OSHA-regulated industries to provide hearing conservation programs may need portable equipment. In choosing the equipment for the practice the owner must keep in mind the goals of the practice.

Other factors must be examined. Does the professional staff have the expertise to use the equipment that is needed for that service? Is the office able to bill for the services that the instrumentation performs? Does the practice have the patient base and/or the referral sources to bring in the revenue to pay for the purchase of the equipment?

PITFALL

An owner of a private practice that provides primarily hearing aid services notices that only one facility in the area is doing evoked potential testing and that facility has a several week backup for scheduled testing. The owner concludes that he or she should purchase an evoked potentials unit and add this service to the practice. Even though this looks inviting, underlying stumbling blocks, such as billing and physician referrals, must be considered. Unlike hearing instrument purchases, patients will not pay for these diagnostic services out-of-pocket. Managed care constraints may dictate that the patient cannot be seen at the owner's practice. In addition, the referring physicians may have loyalties to the hospital clinics and refer all special testing to them. The purchase of the equipment cannot be supported.

Clinical and Office Equipment

The most obvious equipment that is needed for a private audiology practice is the basic diagnostic equipment: the audiometer and the sound room. Other basic diagnostic equipment to consider includes insert earphones, a tympanometer or immittance bridge, and a sound-field system. If the audiologist plans to include cerumen management in his or her scope of practice, basic cerumen removal instruments and equipment and infection control supplies are needed (see Chapter 12).

For practices that dispense hearing aids, the appropriate equipment must be obtained. This may include an electroacoustic analyzer, a computer for programming hearing devices, a small but well-equipped repair laboratory, and a stock of new and loaner hearing devices. Practices that provide a broad range of diagnostic services should have an evoked potential system, otoacoustic emissions testing equipment, and/or electronystagmography instrumentation.

General office equipment is also required. The telephone system should meet current office needs and be capable of expansion as the business grows. Telephones should be telecoil compatible, especially if the practice dispenses hearing devices. If the practice serves the deaf population, a TDD is recommended for contacting patients and scheduling appointments. The practice will also need other office equipment: a copy machine, a fax machine, calculators, adding

machines, and perhaps even a typewriter for insurance and other preprinted forms. A label maker, although not imperative, is handy for organizing a practice's hearing aid repair laboratory that requires the storage of many small items, such as earhooks, tubing, and vent tubes.

Computers are now a necessary component of a successful business. They help the business efficiently manage the multitude of data that is generated by the business, thereby allowing more work to be accomplished in less time. A number of decisions must be made in selecting computer systems. One decision is to select the computer hardware. When choosing between IBM compatible PCs or the Apple Macintosh system, the owner must look carefully at available software. At present, more software is available on IBM compatible PCs for audiology-related activities (e.g., software-based diagnostic test equipment, hearing aid fitting systems) than there is on the Apple Macintosh systems. This, in and of itself, is a determining factor in the purchase of computer hardware. (Refer to Chapters 19 and 20 for discussions of computer hardware and software.) Another decision is to determine how many computers are needed and whether they should be networked. Networking increases efficiency and decreases the need for duplicated pieces of hardware but requires more computer knowledge and maintenance.

The software for each of the office functions must also be selected. Software programs can be used for bookkeeping and accounting functions. Hearing aid office management software systems allow tracking of the patients' hearing devices. Database software programs provide a means of keeping track of the patients of the practice and can be used for marketing programs. Hearing aid fitting systems are used for the fitting of computer-programmable hearing devices. Software-based audiological diagnostic programs (e.g., evoked potential testing) facilitate and automate diagnostic measures. Drawing programs are useful for creating forms and marketing materials. Word processing programs are necessary for correspondence and general office communication. Internet services are becoming increasingly important, providing E-mail services and access to Web sites. If the computers are networked, the use of one software system that combines many of the various software functions can be considered. A further discussion regarding computer software and its relationship to the organizational systems of the office will follow later in this chapter. (Refer to Chapter 20 for a more detailed discussion of information systems.)

It can be overwhelming for the private practice owner to itemize the equipment necessary for a private audiology practice and to compute the cost of such equipment. Clearly certain pieces of equipment are necessary to any audiology practice. Other pieces may be optional and may be purchased at a later date. How the equipment is acquired and when it is acquired depends greatly on cash flow.

Methods of Purchasing Equipment

Different ways exist to purchase equipment, and some help to decrease the equipment costs up front. Buying used equipment can substantially decrease the cost of the equipment and the start-up costs of the business. Leasing equipment can be attractive; however, the long-term costs of the lease must be compared with the actual purchase price of the equipment. A special equipment purchase program from the practice's vendors, known as a "co-op" program, is also possible. Some hearing aid manufacturers have co-op programs where equipment is provided at no charge in exchange for a contract to buy a certain number of hearing devices over a specified period of time for a set price. Again, the overall costs of such contracts must be considered. Hearing aids bought through such arrangements often are not subject to volume discounts, and the audiologist ends up paying more for the equipment by losing volume discounts than if the equipment were purchased outright. The contract also ties the audiologist to one particular product over a long period of time. Last, in a time when hearing aid technologies change frequently, it is prudent to weigh this consideration before entering into a co-op relationship. As long as the terms of the agreement are understood, this arrangement may work well when capital expenditures for equipment purchases are limited. (Refer to Chapter 9 for ethics considerations associated with equipment purchase and Chapter 13 for additional information on equipment.)

Many other books and journal articles provide a detailed list of the instrumentation needed for a private practice. An excellent source is a text by Hosford-Dunn et al (1995), which discusses whether to purchase new or used equipment and provides a summary of general equipment that may be needed.

WHAT ORGANIZATIONAL SYSTEMS ARE NECESSARY FOR RUNNING A PRIVATE PRACTICE?

No office runs efficiently or effectively without proper organizational systems in place. The office organizational systems are the framework of the practice, ultimately affecting every aspect of the practice. In addition, the way an office is organized has a great impact on the image of the practice, because a well-run office contributes positively to its professionalism.

Familiarity with organization systems and their impact on the operation of a private practice is an important component to running a private practice. Inappropriate organizational systems hinder practice growth, whereas the appropriate organization systems facilitate growth. Implementation of proper organization systems is one of the most important components of an efficiently run, successful business.

Audiologists who are new to private practice may overlook the importance of appropriate organizational systems but will quickly gain appreciation of these systems as their practice grows. It is helpful if the audiologist has had experience with the ins and outs of organizational systems before setting up shop. Systems that work well for a small, single office, sole proprietorship with one or two support personnel are grossly inadequate for a multiple-office corporation with numerous professional and nonprofessional staff.

Some of the most important organizational systems are scheduling, patient database, patient recall, patient records, hearing aid tracking, billing/finance, and purchasing. In constructing the systems, the audiologist must answer questions such as the following: How are patients to be scheduled? How long should each appointment be? How will walk-ins

be handled? When should recall letters be sent out? How will hearing aid repairs be tracked? How will auditory brain stem response test results be reported? Who orders supplies? Who orders equipment? How will collections be handled?

Organizational systems are generally interdependent. In a well-run practice these systems are conjoined to ensure that patients, goods, and money flow through the practice with the greatest efficiency.

Figure 8–4 shows an example of an intraoffice form ("SuperSheet") that ties together many of the office systems (e.g., scheduling, ordering, computer data entry).

The SuperSheet serves as an instruction sheet between the audiologist and the support personnel. The idea is for the form to accompany the patient chart when the patient is seen in the office. Each box on the form represents one or two information systems. The audiologist checks the appropriate boxes for the patient on a given visit. The support staff follow the audiologist's instructions as shown on the form and initial the boxes when the actions have been completed. For example, a patient is seen for a hearing device consultation and purchases a BTE hearing device. The audiologist completes the SuperSheet form, as follows:

1. The "Hac Data" box with the date of the first visit, last hearing test, last office visit, client category ("Cli Cat") of hearing impairment, and the referral category ("Cli Ref Cat"). In addition, the referral source is specified and dated. This information is subsequently entered into the office patient database.

2. The "Scheduling" box indicating the type of appointment(s) to be scheduled, at what interval(s), and with which audiologist.

3. The "Front Desk" box indicating whether payment is required and other front office actions needed.

4. The "Ordering and Other Requests" box for ordering the hearing device and obtaining medical clearance.

Using this type of flowsheet to link office systems helps to ensure that important information is transmitted between the staff, appropriate action is taken, and hearing devices are tracked. All office personnel are trained in the use of the form; therefore little or no verbal exchange is needed when it is handed off from person to person. Of course, this system only works if everyone completes the form correctly and executes the requests appropriately. When errors occur, the cause of the problem can be tracked more easily. Having this type of organizational framework in place conveys a sense of professionalism to the patient and inspires confidence in the practice.

In addition to defining the practice's organizational systems, one must decide whether these systems will be carried out with computers, manually, or through a combination of manual and computer systems. One may prefer to use a traditional schedule book for patient appointments and to track hearing aid repairs, remakes, and new orders using pen and paper. Office supplies, hearing aids, and equipment may be purchased and tracked without a defined purchase order system. Accounts receivable may be recorded with a paper day sheet. These manual systems, however, will break down as the number of patients increases, as more audiologists are added to the staff, as the number of hearing aids to track grows, and as the number of services expands.

SuperSheet   (V 05.98)

Name: _____   Date: _____   Clinician: ☐ DB ☐ TMC ☐ SB ☐ KH

SCHEDULING

Type of Visit: When: Audiologist:

☐ BAB   ☐ ASAP   ☐ DB
☐ HDC   ☐ 1 week   ☐ TMC
☐ HDF   ☐ 2 weeks   ☐ SB
☐ HDF & EMF   ☐ 3 weeks   ☐ KH
☐ EMF or SMF   ☐ 4 weeks   ☐ _____
☐ F2   ☐ within 30 days
☐ F2 & AT
☐ 2 appts: HDF..........date_____
              & F2/AT.........date_____
☐ 2 appts: HDF/EMF...date_____
              & F2/AT.........date_____

☐ HDR (Appt)   ☐ Get loaner from patient
☐ Pick up
☐ Appt or pick up (patient's choice)
☐ Mail: UPS Ground ___ Airborne ___ FedEx___ US Mail ___

FRONT DESK

HDC Visit
☐ Take deposit payment
☐ 1 copy of Purchase Agreement (for Patient)

HDF Visit
☐ Take payment on account
☐ 2 copies of Purchase Agreement (Patient & SuperSheet)
☐ Enter devices into Handwritten Log Book

ORDERING & OTHER REQUESTS

☐ Order BTE hearing device: patient___   stock___
          Ear: right____   left____
    Make/Model: _____
          Color: _____
      Earhook: screw___ ball joint___   NA___
Remote control: _____
       MediCal: yes____   no____

☐ Fax or mail Med Clearance & envelope to: _____

HEARING DEVICE RETURNS

☐ "Delete Aid"   R: _____
  "Delete Earmold" L: _____
                    RC: _____

☐ Handwritten Log Book, cross off, check "Returned"
☐ Credit account on Superbill
☐ Change Client Category to _____

HAC DATA

FIRST VISIT _____
LAST HEARING TEST _____
LAST OFFICE VISIT _____

CLI CAT
        ☐ LAV   ☐ LN1   ☐ LA1
        ☐ LNO   ☐ LN2   ☐ LA2
        ☐ LAN   ☐ LN3   ☐ LA3
        ☐ EML   ☐ LN4   ☐ LA4
        ☐ CHI   ☐ LN5   ☐ LA5
                 ☐ LN6   ☐ LA6

CLI REF CAT
        ☐ APT   ☐ KAR   ☐ PHY
        ☐ CEI   ☐ KAS   ☐ REH
        ☐ CEP   ☐ MAL   ☐ MAN
        ☐ CON   ☐ NEC   ☐ RPT
        ☐ ENT   ☐ NWS   ☐ WAL
        ☐ HEA   ☐ OTH   ☐ YEL
        ☐ INS   ☐ PEN   ☐ AUD

REFERRED BY _____
DATE REFERRED _____

☐ Change CLI CAT to: _____

AIDS

☐ Aid Fit
    R: BTE__ ITE__ ITC__ CIC__
    L: BTE__ ITE__ ITC__ CIC__
    RC: ____
    Battery: R:_____ L:_____ RC:____
    Warranty Exp: _____ (year)

☐ Earmold Fit   R___ L___
☐ Repair Fit
    R _____
    L _____
    RC _____

☐ Aid Complete   R___   L___ RC___
    R _____
    L _____
    RC _____

RECALL & LETTERS

RECALL DATE ___ / ___ / ___
        ☐ BAB   ☐ YCK   ☐ ICK

TYFR Letter: Send to _____
        (with 8-pack of batteries)

Figure 8–4 An example of an office form that ties together several office systems.

The use of computer programs allows greater efficiency in the running of the organizational systems of the practice. One may decide to use an off-the-shelf program available at a local computer store for some systems. As examples, Quicken and QuickBooks are popular application programs for finance and are available for either the IBM-compatible PC or Apple Macintosh systems. (See Chapter 15 for examples of Quick Books applications to audiology practices.) FileMaker Pro is a comprehensive database application that can be customized to the practice's own patient database requirements. Numerous scheduling programs are also available for keeping track of meetings and patient appointments.

An alternative to the use of these off-the-shelf programs is an integrated office management software program. These special-purpose application programs are designed specifically for the audiology/hearing aid private practice and combine many, if not all, of the necessary organizational systems into one computer application. Some of them have been designed by and are available through independent software companies. In addition, several of the hearing device manufacturers offer proprietary programs for private practice offices. Offices that specialize in industrial audiology have the option of using software specifically designed for industrial audiology. For a list of software applications for industrial audiology, see Chapter 20, Table 20–4. Regardless of which type of private practice one has, the greatest efficiency in managing the organizational systems of the office comes with the use of an integrated office management software program.

Although many organizational systems are important to a private practice, patient records usually form the core of clinical information and care. Therefore it is of great importance that patient charts have a standardized organizational format for easy access to clinical information. Likewise, it is mandatory that a handling system is implemented and adhered to by all staff to enable quick access to all patient records.

WHAT FUNCTIONS ARE NECESSARY IN PRIVATE PRACTICE AND WHO PERFORMS THEM?

All private practices have a variety of tasks that must be carried out. When practices are young, the owners usually do much of the work, seeing patients and running the practice with minimal support personnel. As practices grow, more staff is added to assume some of the owners' responsibilities. Owners are typically the primary revenue generators, and they must weigh the costs of additional staff versus the cost of lost revenues if they continue to divide their time by running their offices themselves with little support staff.

Front Office Staff

In most established private practices, front office personnel perform the daily functions of running the office. These responsibilities, which are traditionally associated with a "receptionist," include answering the phone, scheduling patient appointments, greeting patients, assembling patient charts, and having patients complete appropriate in-office documents. Front office personnel also maintain patient records by filing pertinent information in the charts and storing charts appropriately. They typically input patient information into the computer database and keep the databases updated with changes in patient information. In addition, front office staff frequently handles over-the-counter sales of small items such as hearing aid batteries.

One of the most important and detail-oriented responsibilities of the front office is tracking the inflow and outflow of all resale items in the office, including new earmolds, hearing aids, accessories, batteries, and assistive listening devices. This is an especially important task in offices that dispense hearing aids: new orders and repairs need to be placed, tracked, received, logged-in; patients contacted; and devices delivered. It is critical that all hearing aid orders get to and from the manufacturer expeditiously and that their whereabouts are tracked continually. Valuable time is lost if the tracking system is not efficient. When new hearing devices are ordered, patients should be given a realistic expectation of when they will be ready. For example, in some offices, appointments are scheduled in advance with an estimate of when the devices will arrive. If devices are not received on time, valuable office time and patient time is wasted, because

the appointment must be cancelled. The patients are inconvenienced because the hearing devices are not ready and may be disappointed or angry that the appointment is rescheduled. This reflects poorly on the front desk and on the entire office and shows lack of professionalism.

Shipping and receiving functions are often part of the receptionist's job description. During the course of each day, products will arrive and leave the office through the mail, small parcel service, or overnight air express service. Products leaving the office have to be packaged, logged out, and prepared for handling by one of these methods. Incoming products must be received, unpacked, logged in, priced, and stored. Some products require testing and patients may need to be contacted.

Front office personnel are often responsible for tracking salable inventory, because they are continually handling the products that come in and out of the office. They may also be in charge of maintaining general office supplies such as copy paper, pens and pencils, and forms.

Because many prospective patients are unfamiliar with audiologists, the front office staff serves in a de facto patient relations capacity, providing information to the public about audiologists and about the nature of different audiological test procedures. They may give patients basic information about the different styles and types of hearing devices and encourage hearing aid shoppers to schedule appointments. Front office staff quiet nerves, calm down disgruntled customers, and provide a friendly smile to timid newcomers.

PEARL

A receptionist may be highly skilled but is shy or has difficulty engaging patients in light conversation. This characteristic may be perceived as unfriendliness and indifference by patients who are new to the office. The patients' perceptions of the office are created by their initial interactions with the front office staff. The receptionist should create a sense of comfort and confidence by showing an interest in the patients, by showing understanding, and by being compassionate. A friendly smile goes a long way.

In some offices, front office staff act as hearing aid technicians: troubleshooting basic hearing aid problems, checking batteries, cleaning earmolds, changing tubing, and sometimes performing simple in-house repairs such as replacing battery doors. The front office staff may also collect payments from patients when the appointments are completed and, in some offices, carry out some of the billing.

Additional Support Staff and Services

As the practice grows, additional support staff and services can be added. An office manager can be a valuable addition to a private practice, providing a variety of services such as managing patient accounts, handling third-party billing, supervising front office staff, and serving as administrative assistant to the owner. A private practice may also have a bookkeeper to carry out the bookkeeping functions of the practice or use an outside bookkeeping service. Often, several people in the office share the bookkeeping tasks. For example, front office staff may collect patient payments, the office manager may do the third-party billing and send out patient statements, the bookkeeper may keep track of the payables and receivables, and the owner may pay the bills and take care of banking transactions.

A private practice also needs clerical services. Most small offices have the front office staff or office manager provide the clerical services needed for general office correspondence. Larger practices may use the services of a transcriptionist for the preparation of chart notes and correspondence with referral sources and patients. The need for this type of service varies a great deal from office to office. With office computerization, many professionals handle word processing work themselves.

Outside Consultants

Most small business owners use the services of an accountant to prepare quarterly and annual financial statements and prepare annual income tax returns. Professional accounting services can be especially helpful in providing an understanding of potential tax liabilities and consequences of business decisions and events (see Chapter 15).

Private practices may also hire outside consultants for a variety of needs such as information technology services for computer maintenance and upkeep, mailing-house services for marketing materials, printing services for designing and printing forms and other documents, and legal services for legal counsel (see Chapter 14).

Professional Staff

Larger private practices have a staff of audiologists to provide the services of the practice in addition to the owner; some hire and supervise clinical fellows in audiology and accept audiology students during their intern programs. Some offices have certified or licensed "audiology assistants" to help with test-assisting for diagnostics and a variety of other functions as well. These positions can be full-time, part-time, or on a contract basis.

Human Resource Management

In most practices hiring of both professional and nonprofessional staff is required to complete all the functions needed in private practice. Hiring and managing people is one of the most baffling activities many private practice owners will encounter. Audiologists typically have little training in the area of hiring and managing people.

Hiring competent personnel is difficult at best. It is important to find someone who has the skills required but also someone who can connect with the core ideology and goals of the practice. It is of equal importance to find an individual with the personality type that suits the position for which they have been hired. Most practices want to hire good team players and staff who will stay with them for a reasonable period of time. Finding the right person requires patience and takes time. It generally involves reviewing a large number of resumes and conducting numerous in-depth interviews to find the person that most closely fits the owner's criteria. The

up-front effort may be worth it, however, because hasty hiring can result in choosing an individual that is not a good fit for the position. The owner may be faced, often for the first time, with the unfortunate task of letting people go soon after they are hired. It is an uncomfortable responsibility at best.

Depending on the position, employee searches often start with newspaper advertisements, announcements at local professional meetings, or through professional newsletters. Frequently, networking provides the best candidates for open positions. Family members and friends or family members of employees are also sources that can yield good candidates. (A detailed discussion of human resources can be found in Chapter 6.)

For small practices with one or two staff members, policies and procedures are usually unwritten and are decided on an as-needed basis. As practices grow, it is necessary and highly desirable to record office policies in an employee handbook. Each employee should receive, read, and review the policies with the practice owner or manager. A comprehensive employee handbook makes the policies of the office clear, thereby resolving questions early and thwarting problems that would arise if policies varied for different employees. Office policies should be consistent with state and federal laws and labor codes.

Performance reviews should be performed regularly, typically annually. This gives the employer the opportunity to discuss with the employees their progress in their job performance and to reward employees for a job well done by increasing their compensation. Most employees welcome performance reviews because they provide feedback to them on their performance, channel their energy, and stimulate their growth.

Motivated employees enjoy attending outside classes, seminars, or conferences where they can hone their skills and come in contact with their peers in similar positions. It is surprising and gratifying how much most individuals value these benefits, especially those in nonprofessional positions. Asking employees to attend outside classes sends a clear sign from the employers that they are making an investment in their employees. In most cases such investments benefit everyone involved: the employees usually recognize the investment and are flattered by the employers' commitment to them; the employers gain happier and more highly skilled employees. This type of investment also engenders employee loyalty, a highly prized commodity in the world of small business.

WHAT ARE YOUR PRACTICE PROTOCOLS AND WHY DO YOU NEED THEM?

Much of this chapter is related to business aspects of private practice. But how does the owner manage the way audiology is practiced within the context of private practice? Not only should the basic tenets of audiology be kept clearly in mind as professional tasks are carried out, but systems must be put in place to ensure that the way they are carried out is consistent, regardless of who does the job. This is not just about quality assurance but also about continuity of care. Establishing practice protocols resolves many of the issues associated with the practice of one's profession in the context of private practice. (For a discussion of quality assurance, refer to Chapter 4.)

Protocols should be developed with several goals in mind. They should be consistent with the core ideology, goals, and vision of the practice. Protocols establish continuity of care by specifying what information needs to be obtained during each procedure and by outlining the minimum data requirements necessary to indicate the procedure has been performed correctly and accurately. Protocols establish a level of efficiency by assigning a time frame and billing codes for each procedure. Protocols can give support in preparing clinical reports. This is especially true if templates or checklists are used to create the reports. A further discussion of the use of templates or checklists can be found in Gardner and Stone (1998).

Protocols should give the clinician guidance in providing care. They can be thought of as a means to an end by providing the framework for achieving the goals intrinsic to each patient consultation, evaluation, and rehabilitation plan. The goals are tied to the immediate patient problems and the proposed short-term and long-term solutions. They should be aimed at guaranteeing that each patient receives consultation, evaluation, and/or rehabilitation procedures that provide results that can be tracked over time and that stand the test of validity and reliability. For example, outcome measures should be included in the protocols to determine whether the solutions applied have true validity (see Chapter 5). Protocols should also ensure high test/retest reliability.

Protocols help clinicians evaluate data quickly. They also provide guidance to the clinician when questions arise or problems occur. Protocols and their attendant forms can also provide a ready-made paper trail for the owner or managing audiologist to document patient encounters.

The educational and clinical background of the owner (or managing audiologist) and the clinicians on staff will be reflected in the protocols. The protocols should also be in line with the current standards of care. Although protocols are in place to ensure continuity, they should be flexible enough to allow for variations in patient populations (e.g., non-English speaking patients). Clinicians will also add and subtract from protocols on the basis of their own experiences and biases. In some instances alternate protocols may exist for the same procedures, as long as each protocol is consistent with current professional practices. Although slight variations may be allowed, the protocols must be clearly defined (i.e., written) and followed by all clinicians.

In this age of managed care protocols and associated outcome measures are beginning to take on greater importance.

protocols and that have outcome measures in place. Outcome measures assess benefit, generally by employing some type of pre-evaluation and post-evaluation assessment and, thus, are touted as indicators of patient satisfaction. Whether this is true or not, managed care companies are looking for these tools to be in place before they award managed care contracts.

An important aside to the discussion of protocols in audiology practice is the issue of infection control. Infection control protocols rarely have been implemented in audiology private practice until recently. The initiative for developing this type of protocol has come from heightened awareness of bloodborne pathogens such as human immunodeficiency virus-1 and hepatitis B. Audiologists who work closely with the public are also exposed to a variety of infectious diseases that are transferred by way of mucus, saliva, and the air. In addition, over the past several years many audiologists, have included cerumen management within the scope of their practice, thus increasing the possibility of coming into contact with bloodborne pathogens. For further discussion, see Chapter 11. An excellent source for developing an appropriate infection control protocol can be found in a text by Kemp et al (1996).

The development and implementation of protocols is clearly not a task unto itself. It is closely tied to quality assurance, continuity of care, billing, office efficiency, professional development, and patient satisfaction. Determining what procedures should have established protocols and the specific content of those protocols will affect how professional work is carried out along many dimensions.

In addition to protocols, other information-based mechanisms ensure appropriate patient care throughout the consultation, evaluation, and rehabilitative processes. Many private practices provide new patients with information packets that describe the nature of the evaluation and rehabilitative processes. Diagnostic procedures are sometimes daunting to the patient. Knowing about the procedures can allay fears and make patients relax during testing, allowing for better test results. It is essential that patients and families embarking on habilitative or rehabilitative paths have a basic understanding of hearing loss and how it affects communication. Providing such information makes it easier for the patient to comply with directives during diagnostic and therapeutic procedures. It also facilitates the development of a trust relationship, increasing the likelihood of a positive outcome for the patient.

PITFALL

Many testing protocols in private practice are trimmed to the bone in an effort to save time, contain costs, and guarantee payment from third-party payers. When trying to provide the best patient care in the most abbreviated manner possible, private practice audiologists find themselves in a battle similar to that faced by physicians. It is not always possible to win the battle without casualties.

PEARL

If an existing patient refers a friend or family member to the practice, go out of the way to thank him or her personally. A handwritten note, a phone call, or a package of batteries gives the patient a positive feeling about the office. The patient will refer to the practice again.

Savvy managed care companies are more likely to award managed care contracts to practices that have clearly defined

Some private practices send out questionnaires to patients asking them a variety of questions about the office and about their satisfaction levels. This type of inquiry provides insight regarding the kind of care that patients perceive they have received, the setting in which it was received, and other observations about the practice and staff. Solicited constructive criticism allows for growth of any private practice and ultimately results in providing better patient care.

HOW DO YOU GET PATIENTS?

Patients will come from a variety of different sources, depending on the type of practice. In the past and still today the most common referral source for new and established private practices is the local ear, nose, and throat physician. Practices that have been in business for many years, even if under different ownership, also have a built-in referral system from their existing patient base. This referral system provides not only word-of-mouth referrals to others in the community but also repeat business from returning patients.

The patient base is especially important for hearing aid practices. Most hearing instrument users require continued follow-up care over many years. Newsletters and other direct mail pieces keep patients abreast of new developments, therapies, and advances in hearing aid technologies. The practice's patient base, through word-of-mouth referrals and repeat business, may constitute the bulk of the revenues of the practice.

Private practice owners must always look for ways to increase their patient base (see Chapter 7). Actively marketing to the existing referral sources and recruiting new referral sources provides for an ever-growing practice. Marketing to a broader segment of the medical community beyond the otolaryngologist can expand the practice's patient base. Increasingly, pediatricians, family practice doctors, internists, cardiologists, neurologists, and gerontologists are the physician specialties that commonly refer to an audiology practice. In managed care environments these primary care and specialty providers gain special importance as direct referral sources. Physician referrals are especially important for a diagnostic practice.

Outside contracts with residential communities and/or nursing homes is another avenue for patient referrals. Providing in-services in the community increases name recognition of the practice and establishes the owner as the expert within the community. Being perceived as the expert

---

PEARL

In any professional community it is considered proper protocol to refer a patient back to the original referral source if the patient needs the care of that specific healthcare provider again. Working in a professional community demands that the protocols of that community be learned and followed to garner respect not only from the other professionals in that community but also from one's patients and peers. For a further discussion of this and the problem of "stealing" patients see Stach (1998).

---

typically ensures more referrals. Business contacts in the community through local business meetings, service clubs, or through organizations, such as the Better Business Bureau or chamber of commerce, can also provide the occasional referral.

Office employees may also generate referral to the practice because they generally are part of the local community and have ties to organizations that the owner may not. Knowledgeable and enthusiastic employees are often eager to refer patients to the office and can be a valuable source of word-of-mouth referrals.

Without referrals, any private practice will flounder; therefore it is good practice to acknowledge any and all referrals. In the case of direct referrals from healthcare professionals, it is customary to thank the professional for the referral in a letter or report referencing the patient. With patient referrals, phone calls or thank you letters are appropriate.

PEARL

Patients who are happy with the care they have received may refer others to the practice. However, patients who feel that good care has not been provided or that a wrong has been done will often go out of their way to let others know about their negative experience. Thus it is very important to try to pacify disgruntled patients, even if they are wrong in their complaints.

HOW DO YOU INTRODUCE NEW SOURCES OF REVENUE?

Revenue from Patient Services and Sales

As a practice grows, more and more individuals in the community become aware of the expertise the owner and staff offer, and greater opportunities for expansion arise. For many practices, this leads to establishing outside contracts with other facilities. In some communities the most common outside contract is providing audiological support for local otolaryngology offices. This type of arrangement will bring in more revenue dollars from diagnostic testing done at the physician site. However, the primary increase in revenue is often in the form of the physicians' referrals to the audiology private practice for hearing aid services. Such arrangements require monitoring to ensure the arrangement is profitable. If too much time is spent away from the practice, the revenues that are brought in may be less than the revenues that would be generated if the clinician took care of the practice's own patients. If the physician makes many referrals to the practice, it is probably worth the time spent in the physician's office.

Other common forms of outside revenue are from nursing home and senior residential communities that may want services provided at their facility using the practice's portable equipment. Many caveats exist with regard to providing nursing home care. These types of contracts require tight organization on the part of the nursing home facility and clear guidelines from the managing audiologist regarding the practice's requirements for providing services on-site. For these visits to be profitable, it is important that several patients be scheduled together and that the schedule be as efficient as possible. Patients should receive otoscopic examinations before the audiologist's visit and have excessive cerumen removed so that hearing evaluations can be carried out and ear impressions can be made. If rehabilitative services and products are provided, it is mandatory to arrange in-service training to the nursing home staff in addition to counseling and support to the patients, thus ensuring successful rehabilitative outcomes. Reimbursement for some services may be difficult to obtain. Billing issues must be ironed out before administering services and products.

Public health agencies and governmental programs such as Medicare, Medicaid, State Children's Services, and Vocational Rehabilitation Services may contract with audiologists to provide hearing healthcare for the program recipients. Service may include hearing screening, hearing evaluation, hearing aid consultation, hearing aid fitting, follow-up, and counseling and training. Typically, this type of contract will bring in revenue but at a contract rate far below what is billed to private pay patients. Billing and collecting can be time-consuming and expensive. Therefore resources that are expended for services and products that bring in limited revenue must be weighed against seeing fewer patients but at a standard rate of reimbursement.

Revenues can be increased if private practices provide hearing conservation services, including establishing or maintaining programs for industry or school systems. Recreational audiology lends itself to this type of outside consultation as well. Trap shooters and musicians need hearing protection. Commercial and recreational pilots need molds for communications, as do news commentators and security personnel. Indeed, a few audiologists have structured their private practices almost exclusively on recreational audiology or industrial audiology.

Revenues can also be increased by becoming a provider for managed care organizations and preferred provider organizations (PPOs). Audiologists obtain these contracts through their individual practice, but more often through some type of common group, such as an individual practice association (IPA). Chapters 17 and 18 discuss the role of managed care in private practice.

Obviously, marketing efforts will also provide a mechanism for increasing revenue in a private practice. Hearing aid practices routinely market to the patients in their own database by sending fliers and informational newsletters. Advertising to the general hearing impaired population through the local newspaper and television and/or radio stations can bring in new patients. Lectures at service organizations and professional or civic groups can increase confidence in the practice, resulting in more referrals. (Chapter 7 is devoted to marketing, and details marketing approaches that can be used.)

Revenues from Outside Consulting and Contracting

For other audiologists in private practice, outside contracting with hearing aid manufacturers and/or equipment manufacturers can bring in additional revenues to the practice. Some audiologists are hired to train others to fit and use the manufacturer's products. Other audiologists act as part-time regional sales managers for these companies, providing equipment information and support to the audiologists using the products. Acting as a consultant to a hearing aid company or equipment manufacturer may entail doing clinical research on new products, assisting in new product development, interacting with engineers, and providing general audiological support. These types of relationships can be very advantageous to the audiology field at large. Clinicians who handle products or use equipment have a mechanism, through their consulting contracts, to provide direct input to companies that design their products. It also brings them in direct contact with other audiologists who use the products.

SPECIAL CONSIDERATION

Some outside contractual arrangements may bring up ethical considerations. Professional and personal ethics should govern the audiologists' decision-making process when providing patient care and guide them in the provision of audiological services and products. Disclosing to the patients the nature of the outside relationships will avert potential questions and concerns.

Because the private practice venue allows for more autonomy than many other clinical positions, audiologists in private practice who find their "passion" in a certain area of work are able to parlay this proclivity into new sources of revenue. New talents may be tapped within the context of running their business, and new sources of revenue may be created. For example, some private practitioners bring in additional revenues by developing marketing materials or practice-management products for other private practices to purchase and use. Others develop accessories that they manufacture and sell to other audiologists. Still others have gone on to develop an altogether different business on the basis of the needs of their own private practice and on the practices of others (e.g., sponsoring or arranging continuing education events and products).

Private practice challenges an audiologist not only as a professional but also as an individual. It serves as an important mechanism for professional and personal growth. The audiologist, as business owner, rubs shoulders with people of different disciplines and establishes new relationships with them. Business relationships may develop with other businesses. Business relationships may develop with patients who also are in business. The small business owner's frame of reference is broadened. A private practice, in this day and age, can be a very dynamic entity. It allows managing audiologists to touch on tasks, disciplines, and fields in which they have little or no experience. Initiation into this domain can be overwhelming at times but also an exciting and exhilarating touchstone for exploring the world anew.

HOW DO YOU MANAGE THE BUSINESS ASPECTS OF YOUR PRACTICE?

An audiologist venturing into private practice has little preparation for managing the business aspects of the practice. Audiologists receive formal education in audiology and professional experience in clinical services or research but no training or experience in business and management. Typically, they do not take business classes as part of their bachelor's or master's programs, and most clinical positions in audiology do not expose them to the business aspects of the clinic. How then, does the new private practice owner learn the language of business?

Once the business has been purchased and the basic business structure put into place (e.g., sole proprietorship, partnership, corporation) the audiologist must learn how to manage the financial aspects of the practice. For some, it is with on-the-job training; for others, on-the-job training supplemented with business classes at a local community college. Hiring a competent bookkeeper is essential if the audiologist does not have any prior experience in business.

PITFALL

Although some audiologists do their books themselves, they must weigh the cost of a bookkeeper with the price of doing their own books. This may include the cost of errors caused by lack of bookkeeping knowledge, the potential loss of revenue if the books are done during open business hours, and personal time constraints if they are done after business hours.

Regardless of who actually does the bookkeeping, the audiologist, as owner, must have an understanding of basic bookkeeping and accounting. Managing the assets and liabilities of the business requires an understanding of cash flow (receipts and disbursements), accounts receivable, accounts payable, cost of goods, inventory, depreciation, and collections. Understanding quarterly tax filings and putting away funds for business taxes is fundamental to running a business. Sound business practices must be established from the beginning. For example, collecting for services at the time of visit helps maintain positive cash flow, as does the timely billing of third-party payers. Positive cash flow allows for on-time payments of vendor accounts and the maintenance of good credit.

A professional accountant typically does periodic financial analyses of the business. It is important for private practice owners to find an accountant whose expertise they trust and with whom they have a good working relationship. Fleury (1992) describes the problems that can occur when the client and accountant do not have a good line of communication, what he describes as an "accountant/client gap." He states, "the accountant/client gap is the perceptual difference between what the small business owners think they are buying in accounting services and what the accountant is trained

to provide." A clear understanding of what the client expects from the accountant and what the accountant expects of the of the client is imperative.

PEARL

A good owner/accountant relationship can be a key ingredient to the success of a young business. The owner may put a lot of faith in the accountant, because the owner is not yet business savvy. The accountant's job, however, depends on the owner providing business documents that are complete and timely. The accountant's financial statements and advice are only as good as the data from which they are generated. A good accountant will provide document templates to guide the business novice.

The accountant prepares two main financial statements, the income statement (a summary of income and expenses over a specified period of time) and, for accrual-based businesses, the balance sheet (a summary of the assets and liabilities of the business at a specified point in time). Ideally, the accountant assists in interpreting financial statements, gives advice regarding the financial status of the business, and provides an understanding of how various financial decisions affect the tax liability of the business.

Taxation issues are often a bit of a conundrum to the new small business owner. It is also one of the issues that can cause the demise of a practice that is bringing in revenue and is profitable. Many small business owners learn about business and personal taxation through a baptism of fire if they are lucky enough to survive it. It is imperative that bookkeeping information be forwarded to the accountant in a timely manner to ascertain the tax liabilities of the business, the dates they are due, and to budget appropriately.

Without a rudimentary knowledge of these basic accounting and bookkeeping principles, the owner is not in a position to make critical decisions regarding the finances of the practice. Questions such as the following must be answered: Is the business profitable? What is the break-even point? Should expenses be reduced? Should prices be increased? Is the cost of goods percentage relative to revenue acceptable? Is there a cash flow problem? Should equipment be purchased this year or next? These decisions will have a direct impact on the financial health of the partnership or corporation and will affect its tax liability. Although it is the bookkeeper who prepares the books and the accountant who does the financial analysis and gives advice, it is the owner who must make the bottom-line financial decisions. These financial decisions cannot, and should not, be made by anyone but the owner.

The owner may also want to enlist the services of a professional financial planner or licensed investment advisor who can assist him or her in managing the investments of the business and in financial planning. This may include establishing and managing pension/profit-sharing accounts, money market and mutual funds, stock accounts, and personal financial planning. A financial planner can be of great assistance in helping the practice achieve its financial goals. (Detailed discussion of the managerial accounting financial aspects of private practice can be found in Chapters 15 and 16.)

HOW DO YOU ESTABLISH RELATIONSHIPS WITH VENDORS?

In most small business it is necessary to establish relationships with wholesalers and retailers. In an audiology practice, office supplies and accessories are needed for conducting evaluations (e.g., electrodes, insert earphone disposable tips). If hearing aids and assistive listening devices are dispensed, it is necessary to establish relationships with a variety of hearing aid manufacturers, companies that carry hearing aid accessories, battery suppliers, and companies that specialize in assistive listening devices.

Most vendors require a credit application before entering into a business relationship with the practice. The credit application asks for banking information and credit references from other vendors. For a newly established business, it is prudent to establish a few initial relationships to prove that the practice is solvent enough to pay its bills in a timely manner. These vendors can serve as references to increase the practice's credit pool. Typically, it is easier to establish accounts with larger hearing aid companies than with smaller businesses, businesses whose cash flow is at the mercy of small practices.

For audiologists who dispense, it is wise to limit the number of manufacturers that fabricate products for the practice and companies from which the practice places orders. This is advantageous for several reasons. Special considerations are often needed for certain patients and a close working relationship helps secure the consideration with ease. Of equal importance is to manage effectively the profit margin on products sold. Profit margins naturally increase when higher numbers of products are purchased from a single vendor because of quantity discounts. Buying with quantity discounts applies to all types of products be they hearing aids or tubes of electrode paste. In addition, it is easier for the audiologist to attain familiarity with products if the number of product lines used is limited. Because of this, many dispensing audiologists try to purchase hearing aids from a few companies that have a full line of instruments (e.g., conventional, analog programmable, and digital hearing devices). The practice can then offer patients the highest quality instruments at the best price point for all concerned.

A vendor's customer service can be as important as quantity discounts. Companies that provide good products at reasonable prices, but have very poor turnaround time for new orders and repairs, may not be worth the money saved in product pricing. Equally, if not more important is the manufacturer's quality control. Although patients may acknowledge that the audiologist is the middleman for hearing aids, when products are faulty the finger of blame is pointed at the audiologist. Thus high customer satisfaction will be realized if the practice uses vendors with fast turnaround time and reliable products, even if they cost a few dollars more. The old adage "you get what you pay for" holds true in this case.

In working with hearing aid manufacturers, the practice is doing more than just ordering products from vendors. Many manufacturers are interested helping businesses increase hearing aid sales by providing marketing support. This support often comes in the form of advertising dollars and human resources (i.e., manufacturer sales representatives). For example, as new hearing aid technologies come onto the market, the manufacturer and private practice owner want to make the products known to the public at large. This is done through direct mail, seminars, open houses, newspaper advertisements, and television and radio advertising. Sometimes, the vendor will offset the costs of such marketing activities—when their products are promoted—by paying part or all of a newspaper ad or announcement. At other times, the manufacturer may help the practice host a public information seminar or open house by advertising the activity and by sending a company representative to the practice to provide first-hand information about the new products. Because the manufacturer and practice are promoting the same products together, they are forming a strategic alliance. Such alliance comes at a cost to the dispenser, generally as a commitment to purchase a specified quantity of the manufacturer's products over a given period of time at a set cost.

> ### PITFALL
> Marketing support from hearing aid manufacturers may look attractive on the surface; however, it may not be a wise business decision in the long term. It is important for the owner to have a full understanding of the manufacturers' terms and conditions, because they may require a commitment to purchase more products than the practice can realistically use and the cost over time may be higher than is reasonable.

WHAT ARE THE FUTURE TRENDS IN PRIVATE PRACTICE?

The traditional model of private practice, which this chapter addresses, is the "independent" private practice, with one or several locations. The practice is run and managed by an audiologist, who is the owner, and a professional staff of audiologists who, along with the owner, provide the services of the practice. In the latter part of 1990s we have seen the emergence of new structures for private practice, specifically the IPA and the practice management company. A reemergence of the retail organization model has also occurred. The state of managed care is responsible for bringing about many of these entities. Because managed care companies prefer to award contracts to practices that have multiple offices throughout a specific geographical region, it is forcing private practice audiologists to change the way they practice and to find avenues for getting and keeping these contracts, which can be quite lucrative in some cases. This can mean expanding the number of locations of the practice to better serve the geographical region or to form a group with other practices within the region.

Specialty IPAs are formed to allow private practice owners to band together in an effort to obtain managed care contracts. IPA arrangements are generally short-term, nonbinding, and of minimal risk to the owner. Little outside support and minimal interference are present with the way the practices are run. A few audiology PPOs have grown up alongside the IPAs. These are regional or national networks of audiologists that, typically, cost very little to join. The PPOs group together audiology practices loosely to reap the benefits of obtaining managed care contracts. This allows managed care companies to contract with one IPA or PPO in a specific region and not to have to contract with a multitude of small practices. This also allows the managed care group to negotiate pricing for services and products.

As managed care companies have shown, the costs of healthcare can be cut and profits increased. Enterprising individuals have looked to form new companies within the managed care arena, companies that consist of individual private practices grouped together to obtain managed care contracts. These practice management companies, known as "consolidators," have already created a dramatic change in physician private practices and are now including other healthcare disciplines. Their goal is to increase profits not only by negotiating managed care contracts but also by increasing the efficiency of professional practices and bringing the acumen of big business to the day-to-day operation of these practices.

Independent audiology private practices also align with each other by forming an affiliation with a practice management company. In some instances the practice management company buys out the practice owner, but the owner stays on for a specified period of time as an employee to manage the practice or to see patients. In other instances the model is somewhat of a partnership where the practice management company purchases the assets of the practice, but the owner retains ownership and the right to sell the practice. In this case the practice management company pays the owner a set salary negotiated at the time of buy-in plus a lump-sum payment or stock options in the company. Thereafter the profits of the practice are split, in some ratio, between the management company and the practice. They also may request a long-term commitment on the order of 20 or so years. Several of these practice management companies are publicly held, with stockholders hoping they will be extremely profitable.

The private practice owner who has partnered with a practice management company typically has a mix of clinical and administrative responsibilities. The owner focuses more on providing care to patients and less on the operation of the practice as a business. The practice management company usually trains personnel, provides accounting and bookkeeping services, provides the office's computer information systems, which are linked to the cooperate office, and gives out detailed financial information to the practice on a monthly basis. They also create marketing programs for the practice, make capital available for the purchase of new equipment, and provide general practice support. Other opportunities may also be available for audiologists to open new practices or to buy practices from within the group.

Franchise organizations have also begun to grow in response to managed care and are founded more on a traditional retail model. Generally, the locations are totally owned by the franchise corporation. Some franchise groups purchase existing businesses, whereas others start new practices in multiple locations. When a private practice is bought out, the owners get a lump sum payment and often stock options. In some instances owners make long-term commitments to the franchise company; however, they typically retain no ownership in their former practice. Some owners sell out without any commitment to the franchise organization. If the practitioners remain, they do so as an employee of the organization. The franchise organization sets the monetary goals and achieves them by purchasing in quantity, by having central accounting, by cost control, and through marketing.

Will the traditional model for audiology private practice endure? Some interesting views exist. Bernstein (1997) indicates that he foresees the small, independent audiology private practice, as well as others, completely disappearing within 10 years. The practice management companies will dominate, building on economies of scale. They will begin by purchasing the large, multilocation private practices, what he calls the "dream practices." Regional and national practice management companies will, in turn, buy out the local practice management companies. Because of their large size, the large practice management companies will be able to negotiate managed care contracts more easily. Their marketing activities will be well coordinated and better funded.

Conversely, the remaining practices will see their share of the local market dwindle and will be left to flounder, because Bernstein sees little chance for them to compete with the practice management companies. Being small and independent, they are at a great disadvantage in negotiating managed care contracts, in competing with the well-coordinated and well-funded marketing activities of the practice management groups, and in keeping prices for goods and services competitive.

Bernstein states that the practice management company's "profit margins are so much greater because of their better buying power that they can give tremendous discounts." He states, "the economic fundamentals" of the practice management groups "are so strong that they can't be bucked." He urges audiologists in private practice to build their practices into large dream practices to make them attractive for buyouts by the practice management consolidators. Smaller independent practices should take over other small practices to grow large, grooming themselves to be bought out by the practice management companies. These dream practices will thrive in their new form.

At this writing, these new practice forms are beginning to emerge. Recently, Sonus Corp., currently one of the largest operators of audiology clinics in the United States and Canada, acquired Hear P.O., a management company that operates a national preferred provider network for hearing healthcare professionals. According to an August 1998 press release, in joining forces these corporations have formed the first ever national audiology health network providing multiple benefits to the 1000 Hear P.O. affiliates, 90+ Sonus-owned clinics, and 388 managed care contracts. Hear P.O. affiliates now have access to the Sonus buying group that may translate into significant savings to the affiliates. Sonus is also launching a franchise licensing program in a number of states and plans to have offices in all 50 states.

For many audiologists in private practice, these dramatic changes inspire fear and foreboding. Many are in private practice because they enjoy the autonomy that it affords them, and they recognize the unique professional and personal challenges that are offered in the private practice arena.

Private practice in audiology has not been in existence for many years. Perhaps its days are numbered, at least in the traditional model. The pressures of new healthcare trends and the demands of consumers are effecting changes in the marketplace. They can easily revolutionize an industry. Many changes are afoot. The wise private practice owner will not stick his or her head in the sand but will be ever vigilant in attending to future trends.

REFERENCES

BERNSTEIN, A. (1997). *The Dream practice: The practice builder association's system for growing your practice "by-the-numbers."* Presentation at the annual conference of the Academy of Dispensing Audiologists, Orlando, FL.

COLLINS, J.C., & PORRAS, J.I. (1996). Building your company's vision. *Harvard Business Review,* (Sept.-Oct. 1996); 65–77.

FLEURY, R.E. (1992). Preventing business failure. In: *The small business survival guide* (pp. 21–23). Naperville, IL: Sourcebooks Trade.

GARDNER, H.J., & STONE, M.T. (1998). To save time and labor, consider these audiological report checklists. *The Hearing Journal, 51*(10);86–89.

HOSFORD-DUNN, H., DUNN, D.R., & HARFORD, E.R. (1995). Creating the office. In: *Audiology business and practice management.* San Diego, CA: Singular Publishing Group, Inc.

KEMP, R.J., ROESER, R.J., PEARSON, D.W., & BALLACHANDA, B.B. (1996). *Infection control* (pp. 39–59). Chesterfield, MO: Oaktree Products, Inc.

STACH, B. (1998). *Clinical audiology: An introduction.* Reporting and referring. San Diego, CA: Singular Publishing Group, Inc.

Chapter 9

Ethics in Professional Practice

Jodell Newman-Ryan and T. Newell Decker

Outline

A long habit of not thinking a thing wrong gives it the superficial appearance of being right.

Thomas Paine (1739–1809)

The late 1990s brought many ethical dilemmas to the attention of the average American, particularly litigation against the tobacco industry, cloning, and partial birth abortions. Even conflict of professional interest received considerable publicity in the case of the American Medical Association (AMA) wishing to allow the AMA official seal on several Sunbeam Corporation medical products. Public outcry resulted in abandoning the idea less than 10 days after it was announced. Integrity of researchers was questioned when Francis Collins, director of the National Center for Human Genome Research (NCHGR) at the National Institutes of Health (NIH), admitted that a junior researcher "faked" data in five papers.

The practice of audiology has escaped some public scrutiny, but the growing use of technology, the expanding scope of practice, and the trend of business practices becoming a greater part of the profile of audiology will produce an ever-increasing number of ethical conflicts (Helmick, 1994). Some of these will become public, as in the Food and Drug Administration investigations into hearing aid sales practices. Are audiologists prepared to make ethical decisions in the professional predicaments in which they may find themselves?

Although Seymour suggested that each professional has the responsibility to educate and prepare students to think about relevant ethical issues by way of curriculum offerings (Seymour, 1990, p. 93), entry-level audiologists are not adequately prepared to offer this protection according to Resnick (1993). Resnick (1993) found that information about professional ethics is covered primarily in elective offerings, and even the newly proposed American Speech-Language-Hearing Association (ASHA) certification standards are vague in reference to curricular requirements, stating only that "the applicant must have knowledge of professional codes of ethics and credentialing" (Audiology Standards, Standard IV-B, Foundations of Practice, item B1; ASHA Leader, 1997a). The American Academy of Audiology (AAA) proposed standards for the doctorate of audiology (Au.D.) degree that include, as two of the 18 basic knowledge areas considered necessary for audiological evaluation and treatment, the following requirements: (1) ethics in healthcare delivery; and (2) professional codes of ethics (AAA, 1997a); but again, details are lacking in how to achieve these competencies.

Some evidence exists that audiologists are aware that they need more training in making ethical decisions. A recent survey by ASHA's Council on Professional Ethics and the Research Division described by Buie (1997) found that about one third of the respondents reported that they had no training as undergraduate students and more than a quarter said they had no training in ethics as graduate students. Self-study was the most frequently reported vehicle for ethics training in postgraduate education (27%) followed by in-services or other seminars within the employment setting (21%) in the profession of audiology (or speech-language pathology). On average, 3.7 clock hours of ethics training were reported.

Furthermore, ethics seldom is formally discussed at audiological conferences. Yet, although formal training in making ethical decisions appears lacking, many current events, such as entitlement, the decision by the American Speech-Language-Hearing Association (ASHA) to move the 1995 convention site, efficacy of auditory integration training with

Audiology: Practice Management. Edited by Hosford-Dunn, Roeser, and Valente. Thieme Medical Publishers, Inc., New York © 2000

children who are autistic, the debate over Miss America Heather Whitestone's voicing/signing abilities, and the use of incentives from hearing aid manufacturers, serve as reminders to audiologists of the importance of ethics in many professional issues. The controversy surrounding issues such as universal newborn hearing screening demonstrates the difficulty audiologists experience in openly debating and discussing such emotionally laden value matters.

The overriding principle behind this chapter is to build a socially responsible profession, with specific goals including the following:

1. Providing definitions and an overview of key concepts relating to ethical, moral, and legal issues

2. Developing analytical skills in relation to ethical decision making

3. Improving ethical awareness

4. Demonstrating, through examples and case studies, application of ethical principles related to professional issues

5. Motivating audiologists to investigate ethical issues further

THE RELATIONSHIPS BETWEEN ETHICAL, MORAL, AND LEGAL ISSUES

Values (Latin, to be of worth) are concepts or ideals that give meaning to one's life and provide a framework for one's decisions and actions (Catalano, 1991). Value conflicts arise when events force one to act against one's beliefs. Value conflicts can be defined as incompatibilities or inconsistencies in beliefs, ideals, or concepts that arise within an individual when faced with opposing choices of action or between an individual and an institution when they hold opposing concepts of expected actions (Catalano, 1991). Similarly, a dilemma is a situation requiring a choice between what seem to be two equally desirable or undesirable alternatives (Benjamin & Curtis, 1986). A formal study of approaches to decide systematically what should be done in a given situation (or how to resolve a value conflict or a dilemma in which each alternative course of action can be justified) is ethical theory.

Ethics, as a Western civilization discipline, can be traced to Socrates. According to Christians et al (1987), the original meaning of *eethos* (Greek) was "sent," "haunt," "abode," "accustomed dwelling place;" that is, the place from which we proceed, from which we start out, the "home base." From *eethos* is derived *eethikos* meaning "of or for morals." This word came to represent the systematic study of the principles that ought to underlie behavior in the Greek philosophical tradition; "beliefs that guide life." The Latin noun *mos* (pl. *mores*) and the adjective *moralis* signify a way, manner, or customary behavior. Compared with the Greeks, the Romans were less attentive to the inner disposition, the hidden roots of conduct, and the basic principles of behavior than they were to its external pattern. In current English-language use, morals refer to the standards of right and wrong that one learns through socialization (sometimes based on religious beliefs) and ethics to a basic system of principles. In summary, modern use of the word "ethics" implies a discipline of accepted standards of conduct and moral judgment that

determine right and wrong courses of action, an attempt to formulate and justify systematic responses to the following question: What, all things considered, ought to be done in a given situation?

The predominant method to impose moral values has been to devise laws. Laws are rules of social conduct designed to prevent the actions of one party from infringing on the rights of another party (Catalano, 1991). One principle, which differentiates legal issues from moral and ethical ones, is that only laws are enforceable. Ethical issues are only enforceable to the extent that they are codified and agreed to by a group or a professional society.

PEARL

Failing to follow the Code of Ethics puts patients in jeopardy because they are not receiving appropriate services. It puts our colleagues in jeopardy because it reflects badly on everyone in the professions (Nancy Swigart, 1998).

Ethical Theories

Deontology: Rule-Based and Duty-Based Theories

Deontology (Greek, what is due) is a theory of ethical decision making based on a set of unchanging and absolute principles derived from universal values at the heart of all major religions (i.e., the morals or rules that govern the resolution of ethical dilemmas). Deontology attempts to determine what is right or wrong on the basis of one's duty or obligation to act rather than on the action's consequences (Catalano, 1991). Examples of such theories are those based on (1) a duty to obey a deity's supposed will as expressed, for example, in the Ten Commandments; (2) the works of Immanuel Kant (1734–1804), especially the categorical imperative: "Act only on that maxim that you can will to be a universal law;" and (3) the traditional medical morality rooted in the do's and don'ts of the Hippocratic tradition (such as "do no harm"). A person has a moral duty to carry out or refrain from a certain action if and only if the framework includes a rule or principle requiring or forbidding that type of action (Benjamin & Curtis, 1986). The major limitation of duty-based theories is obvious: inflexibility in situations in which duties or obligations may conflict.

Teleology: Consequence-Based Theories

Teleology (Greek, *telos* = end, completion) is a theory of ethical decision making that determines right or wrong on the basis of an action's consequences. The principle of utility, or usefulness, is the basis for teleology. Utilitarianism holds that the rightness or wrongness of an act is always a function of the extent to which its being performed or its being omitted will contribute to the goal of maximizing the overall good, which may be construed as the total or average happiness or welfare (Benjamin & Curtis, 1986) (i.e., useful acts bring about good, and useless acts bring about harm). Proponents of utilitarianism include David Hume (1711–1776), Jeremy Bentham (1748–1832), and John Stuart Mill (1806–1873). Notice that duty-based theories hold that right actions are not determined exclusively by the production of good consequences; the concepts of "right" and "good" are exclusive in nonutilitarian theories. Teleology has no strict principles, moral codes, or rules to determine conduct in particular situations. The limitations of consequence-based theories are obvious also: Determining the "greatest good" is highly subjective and can result in inconsistent decisions, and the consequences of an act cannot be predicted with assurance in each case.

WHAT ARE PROFESSIONAL ETHICS?

Professional ethics are systems of conduct developed to guide the practice of a specific discipline. "Professionals," from the Latin *professio* meaning a public oath of fealty, or turning over one's loyalty to another, are distinguished from workers by the following three essential features (adapted from Resnick, 1991):

1. By achieving certification and/or licensure, a professional obtains a special monopoly over the right to provide certain services.

2. Professionals have a defined scope of practice, deviations from which may violate the law.

3. Professionals comply with a clearly articulated set of values, or code of ethics. Those professionals who do not comply face sanction as severe as the loss of credentials necessary to engage in the practice of the profession.

PEARL

As our profession seeks more autonomy, it is becoming even more important for us to discuss ethical problems. For one thing, discussions of appropriate behavior prepare us for situations that we may encounter in the future. Moreover, these discussions are also important to our profession in determining for ourselves which direction to go. If we don't decide what is "right" or "appropriate," the public or . . . the legal system will make those decisions for us (Metz, 1997, p. 10).

The medical profession began to regulate conduct at least as early as the fifth century BC through the Hippocratic Corpus currently reflected as an oath in which physicians pledge to apply measures only for the *benefit* of their patients according to their ability and judgment: "As to disease, make a habit of two things—to help, or at least to do no harm" (Jones, 1923). In recent times, self-regulation has come under public scrutiny, as evidenced by the Nuremberg Code (World Medical Association, 1956). This code was developed as a result of the medical atrocities discovered during the Nuremberg trials after World War II and abandons the older notion that human subjects of research should be protected *solely* by the commitment of the professional because German physicians demonstrated they could not "police" themselves. This same concept is found in the "Patient's Bill of Rights" of the American

Hospital Association (AHA, 1973). In 1969 the Joint Commission on Accreditation of Hospitals issued a policy document that scarcely mentioned problems of patients, so various consumer groups asked the commission to redraft the document with closer attention to the needs and perspectives of patients. The AHA then began to debate the issue of patients' rights and adopted its Bill of Rights in late 1972 (published in 1973). This document contains a potentially revolutionary departure from conventional Hippocratic tradition because the physician is required, by claim of right, to incorporate patients into the decision-making process and to recognize the rights of patients to make authoritative decisions (see Appendix). In effect, patients' rights of autonomy are given formal recognition (Beauchamp & Childress, 1989).

Healthcare Rights

Rights are claims possessed by individuals; they require that others not interfere with their exercise of them or that they provide the rightholder with something he or she wants or needs (Benjamin & Curtis, 1986). Rights can originate from natural law, such as the right to live, or from legal assignment by the government, such as those rights of privacy and liberty that are guaranteed by the U.S. Constitution (Catalano, 1991). Long absent in the audiology literature, the concept of "rights" has surfaced recently in a variety of ways. See, for example, Dr. James Jerger's commentary in *Audiology Today* (January/February, 1997), in which he argued that universal hearing screening is justified on the basis that "the gift of language is one of the fundamental human rights of every child."

To examine principles influencing healthcare ethics in more detail, consider the following rights:

Autonomy
Justice
Beneficence
Informed consent
Confidentiality

"Autonomy" refers to the right to make decisions about one's self, and "justice" refers to the obligation to be fair to all people. Beneficence refers to *doing* good for patients (as opposed to "benevolence" or simply *wishing* for the patient's good) and not harm (which may include the prevention of harm and removal of harmful conditions according to Beauchamp and Childress, 1989).

On the surface, it is difficult to find fault with these rights, but closer inspection reveals some conflicts. For example, healthcare professionals believe that patients expect professionals to "take care of them," that patients expect to benefit from the expertise of the professionals. The argument proposes that a professional has superior training, knowledge, and insight and is in an authoritative position to determine what is in the patient's best interests (Beauchamp & Childress, 1989). Accordingly, audiologists often tell patients what *they* want patients to do, whether dictating which diagnostic tests to administer or which hearing aids are appropriate. Typically, these decisions are made without significant input from the patient and violate the right to autonomy by proposing that professional beneficence can legitimately take precedence over respect for the patient's autonomy (Beauchamp & Childress, 1989). Consider the term *paternalism* meaning, generally, that an adult is being treated as if he or she were a child by persons acting as if they had the authority and concern of a parent (Benjamin & Curtis, 1986). Paternalism can be a positive force, such as healthcare professionals making decisions in emergencies, or a negative force, such as in justification for particular acts of manipulation or coercion on the part of healthcare professionals. Like the parent, the healthcare professional will claim to be acting on the behalf, although not at the behest, of the patient; like the child, the patient is presumed unable to appreciate the connection between the healthcare professional's behavior and his or her own welfare (see Childress, 1979, for more information).

So, increasingly, healthcare professionals are considering patient's "rights" in professional decisions. Audiologists might counter that they do not force patients to act in a certain way, they merely *persuade* patients to act in their own best interests. Rational persuasion consists of appealing to another person's rational capacities to influence his or her behavior. Manipulation has a more negative connotation (although, interestingly, it is derived from the same root, for *handle*, as "management") and is a mode of altering another's beliefs or behavior by subverting or bypassing his or her rational capacities. Deception is a form of manipulation, and manipulation, like coercion and rational persuasion, is a way of inducing others to do what one wants them to do. Obviously, the ability of an audiologist to influence a patient's behavior is more complicated, when comparing these different "rights," than one might imagine at first glance.

Interestingly, the right to autonomy could be applied to professionals as well. An audiologist, as a *person*, has the right to function autonomously as does every other person. Every person can demand that he or she be recognized as a person worthy of dignity and respect with the right to act autonomously and to make justifiable claims on others for these general rights (Benjamin & Curtis, 1986). Collaboration implicitly assumes that healthcare professionals are morally autonomous or self-determining (Benjamin & Curtis, 1986). What is the appropriate course of action when an audiologist disagrees with another audiologist's actions? Or with another professional's actions? Or if an audiologist thinks that a physician is following an unsafe practice? The expansion of knowledge, together with recent technological and social changes, has necessitated redefinitions of the scope of audiological practice and contributed to tensions in audiologist-physician relationships and relationships with other professionals in many areas such as vestibular rehabilitation and cerumen management.

Another conflict is evident when examining the "right" to audiological services. A lack of equal access to healthcare exists for all individuals because of the inability of some to pay for it. Healthcare can be considered a *right* or a *privilege*, and there is justification for each viewpoint. Because of burgeoning demands for expensive medical care and the need to contain the costs of healthcare, cost-effectiveness analysis (CEA) and benefit-cost or cost-benefit analysis (CBA) are two controversial tools of formal analysis increasingly used in decision making about societal policies regarding health (Beauchamp & Childress, 1989). Critics claim that these methods are not sufficiently comprehensive to include all relevant values and options, that they are often subjective and biased, and that they are sometimes ad hoc rather than derived from a general and defensible theory.

CONTROVERSIAL POINT

"Is the term clinical business an oxymoron? Can patient health be consistent with the standards of business? *Alternatively*, can a clinical business play by two different sets of rules—business and professional?

As a patient, I would wish for decisions about my health to be made without regard to profit. . . . Despite my high demands, I expect that even my physician will make a profit—but not at the expense of my health" (Metz, 1997, p. 16).

A relatively recent "right" is that of "informed consent:" the patient's uncoerced permission to have a test or procedure performed after having been given complete information about the test or procedure, other options, and potential consequences of all choices (Catalano, 1991). This idea gained momentum, as mentioned earlier, from evidence presented at the Nuremberg trials. This concept appears in many healthcare professionals codes of ethics and in the Patient's Bill of Rights (see Appendix), which states that informed consent must be obtained before the start of any procedures and/or treatment and the information needed to make this "informed" decision should include details of the specific procedure and/or treatment and the medically significant risks involved. Consider the following violation of the right to informed consent as described by Beauchamp and Childress (1989):

Case of Mohr v. Williams: A physician obtained a patient's consent to an operation on the patient's right ear. In the course of the procedure the physician determined that the *left* ear was actually the one that needed surgery and operated on it instead. A court found that the physician should have obtained the patient's consent to the surgery on the left ear because express consent to a *particular* surgery is required. If a physician advises a patient to submit to a particular operation and the patient weighs the dangers and risks incident to its performance and finally consents, the patient thereby, in effect, enters into a contract authorizing the physician to operate to the extent of the consent given, but no further.

PEARL

Always consider patients' rights in making clinical decisions.

It is sometimes argued that most patients and subjects cannot comprehend enough information or appreciate its relevance sufficiently to make decisions about medical care or participation in research (see for example, Ingelfinger 1972, 1980; Mulford, 1967). The term *competence*, or decision-making capacity, is used in biomedical contexts in which both physical and mental conditions can render patients and subjects incapable, in psychological fact or in law, of adequate decision making (Beauchamp & Childress, 1989). Competence functions as a factor to distinguish between persons from whom decisions should be solicited and those from whom they need not or should not be solicited on the basis of whether that person can make reasonable decisions based on rational reasons. Difficulties arise, however, because competence varies along a continuum, but for practical and policy reasons cutoffs on this continuum are needed, so that any person below a certain level of abilities will be treated as incompetent (Beauchamp & Childress, 1989). Are audiologists in a position to judge the mental competence of patients when signing consent forms, contracts to purchase hearing instruments, and so forth?

Another right is that of confidentiality. Both the American Academy of Audiology (AAA) and the American Speech-Language-Hearing Association (ASHA) stipulate in their codes of ethics that audiologists must maintain the confidentiality of the information pertaining to patients. What is left unstated is who else might be bound by that duty, and the precise definition of "confidentiality." For example, an audiologist tests a child and the next week receives a telephone call from a teacher at ABC Learning Center. The teacher says, "Ms. X [the child's mother] wanted me to call you regarding her child. What can you tell me about this child?" The obvious answer is "nothing" unless the child's mother specifically already has allowed the audiologist to release information to that particular teacher. But what if the teacher calls and reaches a secretary? Again, consider the difference between a professional and other workers. Although the *audiologist* has a responsibility to maintain confidentiality, the *secretary* is not bound by the same code. Although recommendations exist for secretaries (for example, a 1943 book by Bredow states that "the fiduciary relationship that exists between doctor and patient also covers secretarial contacts in the medical office"), they are not *bound* by a code of ethics or licensure laws. Is the audiologist, as a supervisor, responsible for ensuring confidentiality in the entire practice? If so, is that responsibility a moral responsibility, an ethical responsibility, and/or a legal responsibility? Employer liability refers to employers' responsibility for actions committed by their employees while on the job and emanates from the legal doctrine of *respondeat superior* ("let the master answer;" Catalano, 1991). Writing expectations regarding behavior into employee contracts might assist with delineating responsibilities to individuals who may not have the same understanding of confidentiality as the "professional."

Although the concept of confidentiality is publicly acknowledged by professionals, some propose that it is widely ignored and violated in practice. Ubel et al (1995) sent researchers to ride elevators in Pittsburgh hospitals and to note remarks they found inappropriate. In 259 elevator rides, the researchers found that approximately 14% of the conversations threatened patient privacy, raised questions about quality of care, or included derogatory comments about patients. When individuals sign forms saying that only those professionals directly involved in their care will have access to private information, do they know the identities of those professionals? For instance, Siegler (1982) has argued that confidentiality is compromised systematically in the course of routine medical care. He presented the case of a patient who became concerned about the number of people who appeared to have access to his record and threatened to leave the

hospital prematurely unless the hospital would guarantee confidentiality. On inquiry, Siegler discovered that many more people than he had suspected had legitimate needs and responsibilities to examine the patient's chart. When he informed the patient of the number (approximately 75), he assured the patient that "these people were all involved in providing or supporting his health-care services" but the patient retorted, "perhaps you should tell me just what you people mean by `confidentiality.'"

Many audiologists may be violating the confidentiality of their patients according to a recent survey by ASHA's Council on Professional Ethics and the Research Division described by Buie (1997). Most clinicians (86%) deal with ethical dilemmas by discussing them with a colleague. This approach is followed by discussing the situation with a care team (75%). A large number of respondents said they discussed such dilemmas with nonprofessional friends or family (47%).

Returning to the concept of ethical, moral, and legal issues, but now specifically in regard to professional ethics, professional morality, and professional legality, consider Figure 9–1, which schematically illustrates the interrelationship among illegal, unethical, and malpractice transgressions. For example, deceptive advertising may not be illegal or amoral but is unethical (Resnick, 1993).

METHODS FOR MAKING ETHICAL DECISIONS

As strongly argued by Resnick (1993), professionals have a responsibility to think about ethics and issues relevant to ethics such as social ethics, business ethics, bioethics, and professional ethics. Scientific knowledge has been expanding and continues to expand at an exponential rate, and many new

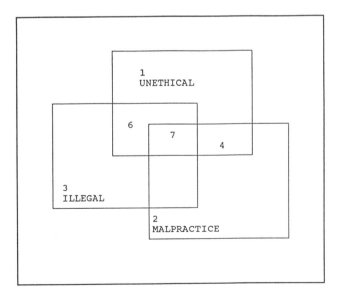

Figure 9–1 Diagrammatic presentation of the relationship among sanctioned conducts. Behavior can be either unethical (1), malpractice (2), or illegal (3). Area overlap indicates conduct can also be unethical and malpractice (4), malpractice and illegal (5), illegal and unethical (6), or all three (7), unethical, illegal and malpractice.

technologies come into use before their ethical implications have been fully explored (Creager, 1980), making it essential to explore beliefs about science and technology. Audiologists must be aware of their own value systems, acknowledge that patients may have different ones, respect those differences, and make necessary adjustments (Luterman, 1979).

PEARL

"Decision-making comfort"—If I carry out this decision, will I be comfortable in telling family members about it? Would I advocate my behavior as an example to my children? Is this the decision that a wise person would make? Can I live with myself after making the decisions?

Cognitive ability does not automatically provide people with the ability to understand their own values and to find solutions to values problems (Harmin et al, 1973); future professionals and practicing professionals need to be *taught* to evaluate alternatives to successfully manage problems resulting from ethical quandaries. Unfortunately, the study of ethics requires careful and extended deliberation and discussions, whereas clinical settings tend to emphasize opposing qualities such the ability to make rapid decisions in the face of daily crises. The rush of events forces us to make ethical decisions by reflex more than by reflection (Christians et al, 1987). By careful consideration of the following issues and completing the suggested activities, audiologists should be able to make these decisions more automatically.

Ethical Decision-Making Models

Seymour (1994) proposed a model (Table 9–1) to assist with identification and resolution of ethical dilemmas.

Another technique for uncovering the important steps in moral reasoning is the Potter box (Fig. 9–2). Potter (1965, 1972) formulated a model of moral reasoning (see Christians et al, 1987, p. 3).

Potter explains the process in the following manner:

Step one—Definition: Determining and obtaining relevant factual information.

Step two—Values: Expose values, draw relevant distinctions between values, and debate underlying values (or construct an argument). The word *argument,* in the logician's sense, is a set of reasons or premises together with a claim or conclusion that they are intended to support. Having identified an ethical issue, the next step is to construct and evaluate arguments for and against various positions.

Step three—Principles: Such as those espoused in a code of ethics. For example, respecting confidentiality.

Step four—Loyalties: allegiance; to whom is duty owed? To a company? To the profession? To a particular patient? To the family? To the community? To society?

The line of decision making that is followed has its final meaning in the social context (Christians et al, 1987, p. 19).

TABLE 9–1   Seymour model

Identification and resolution of ethical dilemmas

What is the problem/conflict/dilemma?
  Is it a professional violation?
  Is it a legal violation?
  Is it both?

What values are in conflict?
  Under the circumstances, what is of most value?
  Will feelings interfere with judgment?

What evidence is available for objective consideration?
  What parties are involved?
  Have all parties been heard and all evidence considered?
  Whose evidence is most convincing/believable?
  Is there consistency in the evidence?
  Has all available evidence been considered?
  What is acceptable practice in this situation?

What action(s) can be taken or recommended?
  Would outside consultation be beneficial?
  Define social, cultural, or political impact(s) consequent to potential actions
  Identify long-term and short-term impact(s) consequent to potential action(s)
  Test each potential action for fairness
  Will the decision be fair to all involved?

How will the decision impact the present and future?
  How will the decision affect morale of parties involved?
  How will the decision change how I feel about myself as a person and as a professional?
  How will the decision improve or deteriorate present and future operations?

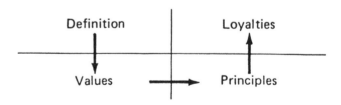

Figure 9–2   The Potter box.

PEARL

Ethical decisions are often not self-evident. Time permitting, gather insights from others who might be stakeholders in the decision.

Ways of Exploring Values

In both models an early step in making an ethical decision is clarifying values: "know thyself." One's personal value system should be reviewed. The influences of religion, cultural beliefs, and personal experiences should be explored to understand one's comfort with specific ethical issues. According to Raths et al (1966), great diversity exists among people in the clarity of their values: some have clearly defined values and live

Example 1: ASHA Legislative Council 7-94 resolution: "Clarify the Association's position regarding membership in organizations that practice discrimination by members holding elected office, staff position, or appointment" (ASHA, 1994b).

"What I do on my own time is my own business."

"Everything I do affects my profession."

Points to consider (as suggested by Resnick, 1993): the financial constraints involved in investigations, the right to privacy, and the voluntary nature of most ASHA positions.

Example 2: The use of nonhuman animals in hearing research:

All life is sacred; no invasive animal research.

Animal experiments should be unregulated.

Points to consider: animal sensitivity to pain, cost/benefit ratios, and the relevance of nonhuman animal models to human communication.

Example 3: Healthcare reform:

Complete government control over healthcare.

No government involvement in healthcare.

Example 4: Genetic engineering:

Examine how to eliminate forms of hereditary deafness.

Individuals have full reproductive rights.

Example 5: Bonuses from manufacturers:

Bonuses always conflict with professional decisions.

Bonuses never influence professional decisions.

Figure 9–3 Values continuum examples.

purposefully while fostering changes in positive and constructive ways, whereas others may suffer from a confusion of values and exhibit apathy, uncertainty, and inconsistency. They defined a value as something that is important in human existence and that meets the following criteria: is freely chosen from among alternatives, is chosen after thoughtful consideration of the consequences of each alternative, is publicly affirmed, is acted on, and persists as a consistent pattern in life (Raths et al, 1966).

> **PEARL**
>
> **About things on which the public thinks long, it commonly attains to think right.**
> **Samuel Johnson, 1709–1784**

The values-clarification approach, as defined by Simon et al (1972), does not aim to instill any particular set of values but rather to help learners use the processes of valuing in their own lives to discover cognitive and personal meanings for themselves and to apply these valuing processes to already formed beliefs and behavior patterns and to those still emerging. The process involves learning to weigh the pros and cons and the consequences of the various alternatives.

Because all alternatives are not equally viable, the next step after clarifying values is to rank the values. Kieffer (1979)

> **PEARL**
>
> **Always let your conscience be your guide. (*"The Adventures of Pinocchio"* by Carlo Collodi, 1883)**

offered suggestions for ranking values: (1) state the problem; (2) determine the possible courses of action; (3) state the values or moral judgments involved in each course of action; (4) rank-order the values; and (5) decide the course of action most consistent with the highest ranking values.

Finally, self-assess after values clarification; the real "clarification" part (Harmin et al, 1973). Ask oneself what was learned that was important, what beliefs changed or became firmer, and how one might change any behavior as a result of the experiences.

Suggested Activities Using a Values Continuum

A values continuum can be an exercise in which individuals consider the issue and then place a mark on the line that best represents their opinions, beliefs, attitudes, behaviors, and so forth. Then they should consider why they made those decisions and what, if anything, could make them move to a different place along the continuum (Fig. 9–3).

Suggested Activities Using Debates or Arguments

After completing the values continua just discussed, the reader may wish to consider arguments for the following issues:

Issue 1: Cochlear implantation in children. One side could support the absolute right of parents to choose what they think is right for their children, whereas the other side could support the rights of the children to self-determine their treatment. A related debate is the classic "manual" versus "oral/aural" controversy.

Issue 2: The rights of businesses to produce products to sell versus the rights of consumers to be protected from exaggerated advertising claims (for example, "Whisper XL™"). Similarly, provide support for the rights of society to be spared the costs incurred by personal behavior it considers "reckless" (such as traumatic brain injury treatment costs for persons not wearing seat belts or helmets) versus individual freedoms. Noise abatement arguments involve many of the same issues. Points to consider: personal freedom, right to privacy, government intervention, funding issues, employment opportunities, and the psychology of advertising.

Issue 3: The issues surrounding moving the 1995 ASHA convention site. Pertinent background information includes the legislative council resolution stating that ASHA conventions shall be held in cities that do not have laws, policies, or ordinances that conflict with the nondiscriminatory clauses of the ASHA Bylaws and Code of Ethics pertaining to race or ethnicity, national origin, religion, age, gender, disability, or sexual orientation. ASHA ruled that Cincinnati violated this code by removing protection from discrimination (ASHA, 1994a). Other multicultural issues for debate might include culturally biased versus culturally unbiased assessment and affirmative action.

Issue 4: Cost/benefit ratios and definitions of "risk" in terms of universal hearing screening, vaccinations (particularly for rubella), noise abatement, and so forth.

Other Suggested Activities and Thought-Provoking Issues

Audiologists are asked to assist in the determination of brain death by performing and interpreting auditory-evoked potential tests. They may need to explore their attitudes about death to accomplish these tasks effectively. Gravely ill persons are encountered infrequently during typical practicum experiences, but feelings and attitudes toward death could be explored as preparation for future professional activities. Other similar topics to consider: euthanasia (including the Oregon "Death with Dignity Act" governing physician-assisted suicide) and issues surrounding using evoked potentials as a way to determine brain death.

To develop skills of determining authors' biases, code articles with pluses or minuses, indicating what the writer is for (plus) or against (minus) or to indicate when they agree (plus) and disagree (minus) with the author. Suggested topics include recent articles discussing the merits of the Au.D. degree, using support personnel, providing auditory integration training therapy, and requiring universal newborn screening.

Investigate a local hospital's ethics committee. What professionals are invited into the committee? What issues confront them? How do they investigate charges of ethical misconduct?

Consider the case of a child identified as having a hearing loss at 3 years of age (which appeared as an ethics roundtable discussion in ASHA, 1997b; and on the ASHA Web site). Amplification is recommended, but the mother has not obtained hearing aids 9 months later. When asked why, she replies, "I'm not sure I want the child to wear hearing aids; I think he'll outgrow this."

Who is/are the patient(s)? What are the rights of (1) the child, (2) the mother, (3) other family members, (4) the community, (5) society?

Is culture a consideration in this case? Could there be cultural and/or religious reasons that would justify the mother's actions?

Is there a conflict between the obligation of the audiologist to provide the child with the best possible care and the family's right to self-determination?

Is there a conflict between a child's right to treatment and the family's right to refuse treatment?

Does the degree of hearing loss matter? In other words, would the audiologist's values and/or actions be different for a child in this situation who has a mild hearing loss versus a child who has a severe hearing loss?

Does it matter whether the mother has agreed to other therapeutic approaches for the child? In other words, would the audiologist's values and/or actions be different if the mother had enrolled the child in a preschool total communication program instead of taking no action?

Is there sufficient evidence that the mother understands the recommendation? Has the information been presented to her in such a way that she comprehends the material and is cognizant of the risks?

Is there sufficient evidence (educational, psychosocial, vocational) to prove that amplification is needed? If so, is that evidence made available to family members in a way they can understand?

Does it matter *why* the mother has not obtained hearing aids for the child? Are there justifiable reasons such as financial constraints, inability to find transportation, and so forth?

Could this situation be considered abuse? If so, is there an ethical, moral, and/or legal obligation to contact child protective services? Are there any risks in doing so? The United States Congress passed amendments to the Child Abuse and Treatment Act (1984) that defined child abuse as the "withholding of medically indicated treatment" from children. Courts have often allowed Jehovah's Witnesses to reject blood transfusions for themselves, while refusing to allow them to reject medically necessary blood transfusions for their children. In some cases parents may be charged with child neglect if they fail to seek or permit highly desirable medical treatment, even if the treatment is not necessary to save the child's life (see Beauchamp & Childress, 1989; Sampson, 1970).

CODES OF ETHICS AND THEIR APPLICATION

The words *ethics* and *ethical* can be used and interpreted in a variety of ways, depending on who is using them and the context of the discussion in which they are used.

"Take your car to Joe down at Sam's Body Shop, 'cause he is a really ethical guy!"

"If you want a really ethical legal opinion, go see Rachael Smith at Smith, Falmouth and Spiker."

Judging from the court of public opinion, both of these folks have well-developed ethics. But are they the same kinds of ethics? Are the codes of ethics by which these people operate similar? The answer in both cases is "probably not." Even though both the above individuals have a well-developed sense of ethics, the base from which their codes flow is, most likely, not similar.

CONTROVERSIAL POINT

"Standard practice" is often a term used to describe what one thinks is ethical on the basis of a subjective belief that "everyone else is doing it." Codes of ethics are written and agreed to by the membership of an organization, and until those codes are altered they *are* the accepted rules of practice no matter what one may think might be the "standard practice."

Ethical decision making is based on ethical codes that serve as guidelines for the profession (Catalano, 1991). A code of ethics is a series of statements setting forth the values of an organization through a listing of its principles (Konold, 1978) and typically is accompanied by an array of sanctions, or punishments, to be meted out for proven violations of the code. The principles are achieved when practitioners of the profession comply with a set of rules that provide the minimum standards and behavioral expectations necessary to support the principles (Resnick, 1993). Joe may be an honest mechanic and fundamentally interested in doing right by his customer, but it is doubtful that he is a member of any organization that made him *swear* to abide by a formalized code of ethics when he joined the organization. Furthermore, should he commit an ethical slip, it is unlikely that he would be called before an ethical practices board. Such would not be the case with attorney Smith. The American Bar Association provides lawyers with guidance on a wide variety of potential ethical dilemmas. The Bar Association's code of ethics is written down and Smith is sworn to uphold it under penalty of sanction.

Ethical codes for healthcare professions outline the healthcare provider's responsibilities to the patient, to the employer, and to society. According to Benjamin and Curtis (1986), codes of professional ethics are often a mixture of creeds and commandments. As creeds, they affirm professional regard for high ideals of conduct and personally commit members of the profession to honor them, thus constituting a sort of oath of professional office. As sets of commandments, codes of professional ethics have two principal functions: (1) they provide an enforceable standard of minimally decent conduct that allows the profession to discipline those who clearly fall below the minimal standard; and (2) they indicate in general terms some of the ethical considerations professionals must take into account in deciding on conduct.

If the code is to be simple, comprehensive, and acceptable to all professionals within the practice, it will be so abstract and general that it cannot, without significant interpretation, be applied to many specific problems (Benjamin & Curtis, 1986). Yet, on the other hand, a very specific code aimed at anticipating all the moral problems that can arise will be (1) controversial, (2) overly lengthy, and (3) by nature incomplete because all possible scenarios can never be anticipated. Therefore neither a brief, simple code nor a long, detailed one will offer both clear guidance and attain widespread acceptance (Benjamin & Curtis, 1986).

Generally, codes of ethics are developed by an organization for the following purposes (Catalano, 1991; Resnick, 1993):

1. To maintain professional goals and standards by improving/preserving/monitoring the behavior of organization members.

2. To improve/protect public perception of the organization by establishing boundaries for professional accountability.

3. To develop and evaluate new professional practices and to re-evaluate existing ones.

4. To provide the basis for membership in the organization.

The AAA and ASHA have well-developed ethical codes. Both of these codes may be seen in their entirety in Appendix I of this volume. Although these codes differ from each other in form, the content is remarkably similar. Both consist of a series of ethical "principles" that range from admonitions regarding the welfare of persons served to those regarding the provision of accurate information regarding conditions treated and the abilities of the person giving the service. In both of the codes the ethical principles are followed by a set of ethical "proscriptions" that serve to elaborate the expected behavior of the professional. Each code contains an expectation for obedience to the principles and a set of procedures for dealing with infractions of the codes. Note that both AAA

and ASHA codes are paternalistic and ignore the modern trend expressed in codes of some other professions to allow for input from the *consumer* (Resnick, 1993).

Before attempting to apply a professional ethics code to specific cases, it might be helpful to discuss each of the principles of the Code of Ethics of the American Academy of Audiology. It is not fundamentally different from the much older Code of ASHA and in doing so one can obtain an understanding of what the profession of audiology thinks is important for its members in their interactions with each other and the public.

Principle 1: Members shall provide professional services with honesty and compassion and shall respect the dignity, worth, and rights of those served.

This is a far-reaching principle that speaks to the need for audiologists to provide their services to those who need them without considerations that are unjustifiable or irrelevant to the needs of the patient. It also speaks to the need for maintaining confidentiality when dealing with patients and for the need for respect for basic human rights.

Principle 2: Members shall maintain high standards of professional competence in rendering services, providing only those professional services for which they are qualified by education and experience.

This principle appears to speak to the level of education, certification, and expertise of the audiologist. It also speaks to the need for the audiologist to exercise caution in the delivery of services (do no harm) and to provide services without regard to gender, race, religion, national origin, sexual preference, or general health. In addition, the principle calls for the audiology employer to provide careful supervision of those to whom work is delegated. Central to the principle is the recognition of the need for continuing education. It would be difficult to "maintain high standards of professional competence" in an ever-changing world without regular educational upgrading. Furthermore, as scope of practice expands, the audiologist must make careful decisions about what he or she is willing to take on in everyday practice. The Certificate of Clinical Competence from ASHA is only intended to ensure that the audiologist is capable of providing basic clinical services and not to be a carte blanche for all clinical practice.

PEARL

Be willing to admit lack of knowledge or expertise and seek guidance when necessary to minimize potentially poor clinical decisions, including potential violations of good ethical practice.

The principle also speaks to a fundamental need to maintain the trust of the public in our referral procedures. For example, a central tenet in the delivery of professional services is that one shall not accept benefits of items of personal value for receiving or making referrals. Conflict of interest, whether perceived or actual, is to be avoided at all costs. Fundamental to our continuation as a profession is the trust of the public. Once lost it is difficult if not impossible to recover. The audiologist must examine his or her actions in this regard in the cold light of what the Code of Ethics has to say. An audiologist's subjective belief that his or her professional judgment to use a particular manufacturer's item is unaffected by an incentive plan provided by the manufacturer is not a compelling argument. If subjective belief in one's motives were sufficient, objective ethical codes for professional behavior could never be enforced. The reality of the situation is that individuals cannot always sort out their motives, and the best professional practice would be to avoid situations that may cause the patient to think that economic gain might be more important than the patient's welfare. Whenever an audiologist receives something of substantial value from a vendor, simply as a result of having ordered from that vendor, the potential for distortion of clinical judgment, clinician/patient relationships, and an ethical conflict is present.

> ## CONTROVERSIAL POINT
>
> **A group of audiologists practicing in a hospital setting wish to have a video otoscopy unit. Appeals to the hospital administration are not fruitful. The Primx Co. comes forward with an interesting offer: Primx will supply the piece of instrumentation in return for a guarantee of a certain number of hearing instrument purchases from them over the next 5 years.**
>
> **Those involved in the industry are quite skillful at making appeals on the basis of scientific information, personal contact, and economic incentives. No matter how this group of audiologists might feel about their ability to conduct their profession in an unbiased fashion over the next 5 years, the practice cannot help but be influenced by this economic relationship. Obviously, financial entanglements that can be misconstrued by the public and provide for hidden influences on audiologist/patient relationships should be carefully evaluated.**

Principle 3: Members shall maintain the confidentiality of the information and records of those receiving services.

Unless required by law, patient records should remain closed to all but those providing the service. Patients should never be discussed in any environment where the conversation is likely to be overheard. Those persons responsible for the supervision and training of student clinicians must make every effort to inculcate this aspect of professionalism.

Principle 4: Members shall provide only services and products that are in the best interest of those served.

This principle, like principle 3, also requires that persons not exploit persons served for any reason and that the professional not engage in any activities that might be construed as a conflict of interest or appear as a conflict of interest. The

principle also guides the billing behavior of those who are reimbursed by third-party payers.

> ## CONTROVERSIAL POINT
>
> **When service charges are not itemized in a detailed manner, there is room for "bundling" of costs. Although this saves time, is it ethical to consumers? Should a full accounting be made of all individual charges, even if some of those charges are not covered by third-party payers? Or is it better to apply an "umbrella" charge instead of detailing the actual cost the audiologist paid for the hearing aid to the manufacturer, an hourly charge for counseling, fees for real-ear measurement, the impression-taking charge, mailing charges, etc?**

Principle 5: Members shall provide accurate information about the nature and management of communicative disorders and about the services and products offered.

This principle indicates that, within reason, the service provider should fully disclose the nature of the disorder and the treatment suggested. Providers of services must not guarantee results nor must they twist available scientific information to suit their needs. For example, conflicting evidence exists in the literature that the use of two hearing aids is better than the use of one. Nevertheless, it is unethical for an audiologist to deliberately quote this information in such a manner that it would serve to scare the public into the use of two hearing aids.

In addition, principle 5 also provides guidance for those engaged in teaching and research. Freedom of choice to participate and full disclosure of the research is vital. In a teaching situation the dignity of the patient being observed must be preserved at all times.

Principle 6: Members shall comply with the ethical standards of the Academy with regard to public statements.

Once again, the principle admonishes us to be careful about the claims that we make about our products and our services. Furthermore, we are not to make claims about our education that are unfounded or to use degrees that we have not earned from accredited institutions of higher education or degrees that have not been earned in audiology or a closely related discipline.

Principle 7: Members shall honor their responsibilities to the public and to professional colleagues.

The principle reminds us of the fiduciary trust that we have with the public and warns us against any activity that might break that trust.

Principle 8: Members shall uphold the dignity of the profession and freely accept the Academy's self-imposed standards.

The Code of Ethics of the Academy is a part of the membership application to the Academy. Each new member signs this Code and thereby agrees to abide by it. Should it happen that aspects of the Code exist that a person does not agree with or does not intend to follow, membership in the organization ought to be avoided. The Code of Ethics represents the standards by which all members of the Academy have agreed to abide. Members are specifically advised that they must cooperate with the Ethical Practices Board on all matters pertaining to the Code and that they have a duty to report any individuals that may be operating outside of the Code of Ethics.

Beyond the code of ethics of any particular national organization, other more local entities make claims on the ethical practice of the professional.

State Associations

In the case of both AAA and ASHA a provision allows state affiliate chapters of the parent organization. Each state affiliate is expected to follow a series of chartering steps and included among those is the establishment of a code of ethics that is exactly the same as that of the national organization.

Certification and Licensure Boards

Certification and licensure are means of regulating healthcare professions and declaring and legitimizing professional expertise. Certification is a professional credential that has no legal status unless defined in an audiology practice act such as state licensure. Licensure is the method the state uses to establish a minimum level of competency for healthcare practitioners (Catalano, 1991). State audiology practice acts (licensure) contain a set of common elements such as the following:

1. A definition of professional audiology and its scope of practice; an outline of the activities a licensed audiologist may legally perform within that state.

2. Requirements for licensure (including personal characteristics, educational requirements, passing score on the licensing examination, and citizenship) and possible exemptions from state licensure laws.

3. Requirements for relicensure, including those for voluntary or mandatory continuing education.

4. Definitions of reciprocity to recognize the equivalence of another state's license and board.

5. Means for disciplinary actions and requirements for due process of violations of the practice act, including private reprimand or warning, public reprimand, probation, suspension of license, refusal to renew license, and license revocation.

6. Criteria for creating the state board and for designating members to serve on the board.

7. Penalties for practicing without a license.

In addition to state licensure, individual institutions, such as hospitals, may adopt policy manuals. An institution's manual of policies and procedures specifies the permissible scope of practice for different professionals within a given setting in that institution; this scope of practice may be more narrow than (but cannot exceed) that described by the state practice act for each individual profession.

ETHICAL PRACTICES BOARDS

Ethical practices boards (EPBs) or institutional ethics committees can be useful in monitoring activities of professionals and in helping the public and professionals address critical ethical dilemmas in healthcare (Benjamin & Curtis, 1986).

Most professional organizations have bodies in whom they invest the responsibility to adjudicate all matters related to the ethical practice of the profession. Both the ASHA and the AAA have such bodies. Membership on these boards is normally voluntary and made up of members who express an interest in serving in such a capacity. Appointments to the EPB of the AAA are made by the Board of Directors (BOD) of the Association on recommendation of the current Chair of the EPB.

The fundamental task of the ethics board is to interpret the code of ethics of the organization in a manner that is uniform and unbiased across the membership. Often this is a difficult task given that each person brings to the board a certain personal "slant" on the ethical rules. Nevertheless, each case is reviewed on its own merits, and in difficult cases the board acts collectively and issues a unanimous opinion.

To ensure that the board acts in an unbiased and uniform fashion, normally a set of formalized procedures will be used for dealing with complaints. In some older professional organizations such as the American Psychological Association (APA) the procedural rules are lengthy and couched in a good bit of legal jargon. The procedural rules for the ASHA and AAA ethics boards are simpler. The reader might wish to visit the Web site for the APA Ethical Practice Board at *http://www.apa.org/ethics/rules.html* for a look at such a set of procedures.

Normally, the process of filing a complaint originates with a member who believes that another member has broken with the Code. This process, however, does not always have to be the case. The EPB may, in fact, act on its own initiative in what is known as a *sua sponte* (Latin, of one's own accord; unsolicited) complaint. When a member makes a complaint, the EPB will normally ask that the complainant sign a waiver of confidentiality statement. This is done to accomplish a very basic tenet of the American justice system, namely that the accused (respondent) has a right to know the identity of the accuser. In all cases the name of the complainant is kept confidential and made known to the accused only if specifically asked. Should the complainant not wish his or her name to be made known and should the EPB believe that the alleged infraction is significant enough to warrant investigation, it may go forward acting *sua sponte*.

After the initiation of a complaint, the EPB will assign a case number to the complaint. After that, a letter is written to the person alleged to have made the infraction wherein the specific complaint and the section of the code applicable is referenced. The respondent is given a reasonable period of time in which to respond. After the response, the EPB will deliberate and either determine that additional information needs to be gathered or make a determination as to whether the infraction was committed and, if so, what punishment (sanction) should be applied. Where the ASHA EPB is concerned, this level of the process is called the "initial determination" and allows the respondent to prepare for a "further consideration hearing." The further consideration stage allows the respondent time to prepare a statement that clarifies any misunderstandings or to make a case for a lesser sanction. AAA does not make use of the further consideration phase of the process but instead allows the respondent to appeal directly to the BOD within 30 days of the notification of the EPB ruling on the matter. The appeal must be based on either a procedural issue or on the belief that the sanction was excessive for the infraction committed. Decisions of the BOD are final.

EPBs have various levels of response to infractions of their codes. The AAA allows for four different sanctions: reprimand, cease and desist, suspension of membership, revocation of membership.

Reprimand is the minimum level of punishment and consists of a reminder of the section of the Code that had been violated and perhaps some education on the topic. Knowledge of the notification of the violation and the sanction are restricted to the member and the EPB.

Cease and desist is the next level of sanction and requires that the member sign a cease and desist order. The order specifies the type of violation, and by signing the member agrees not to continue the offending behavior. Knowledge of the cease and desist order is only between the member and the EPB. On a two-thirds agreement of the BOD, however, the sanction may be reported in an official publication of the Organization.

Suspension of membership may range from a minimum of 6 months to a maximum of 12 months. During the period of the suspension the violator may not participate in any official functions of the Academy. At this level, notification of the violation and the sanction is made to the respondent, the complainant, and the membership of the academy through one of its official publications. Notification of the violation and the sanction may be extended to others as determined by the EPB. Often this option is used in notifying the licensing board in the respondent's state, the EPB of ASHA, and/or the EPB of the State Association.

Revocation of membership is considered the ultimate punishment for violation of the Code of Ethics. All actions associated with the suspension of membership are followed in the case of revocation. The member has the right to reapply for membership 1 year after the revocation but is not guaranteed reinstatement.

Records of all EPB actions are kept in a central location and maintained in a secure fashion. Confidentiality is maintained in all EPB discussions, correspondence, and communication. No member of the EPB may give access to or speak independently about EPB activities unless given specific permission to do so by the remaining members of the EPB.

CASE STUDIES AND POSITIONS

Identifying the ethical issues of a given situation is not always self-evident; thus analysis of actual and hypothetical cases can be a primary tool for firing the moral imagination (Christians et al, 1987) and sharpening ethical decision-making skills. The following cases present ethical dilemmas that typically confront practicing audiologists. The reader may wish to consult the book entitled *Ethical Practices in Speech-Language Pathology and Audiology: Case Studies* by Pannbacker et al (1996) for additional information.

Special Case Studies

Several types of ethics infractions seem to be more common than others and, perhaps, bear some additional discussion. These infractions involve the use of degrees, criminal behavior, and conflict of interest. We include case studies after each of these to illustrate the process of ethics violation adjudication.

Use of Degrees

Principle 6 of the Code states that "Members shall comply with the ethical standards of the Academy with regard to public statements." Rule 6a is intended to elaborate this principle and states that "Individuals shall not misrepresent their educational degrees, training, credentials, or competence. Only degrees earned from regionally accredited institutions in which training was obtained in audiology, or a directly related discipline, may be used in public statements concerning professional services."

Degrees from accredited institutions are those obtained from postsecondary educational institutions accredited by regional accrediting agencies recognized by the United States Department of Education or the Council On Post-Secondary Accreditation. The North Central Association of Colleges and Schools and the Western Association of Schools and Colleges are examples of such accrediting agencies.

Normally, the EPB will presume that degrees granted by programs departments or institutions that do not hold regional accreditation at the time the degree is awarded are not equivalent unless and until the individual degree holder submits evidence that the requirements for the degree meet the minimal standards specified for the required regional accreditation.

The EPB is aware that graduate degrees are granted in an array of disciplines that add to the understanding of normal and disordered communicative ability. The Board believes, however, that risks of misrepresentation exist when doctoral degrees granted in disciplines unrelated to audiology are used in public announcements that are connected to the practice of audiology.

The Board is also aware of entities in the United States and in other countries that award nonstandard advanced degrees for qualifications consisting of little more than proof of work experience and submission of a narrative summary describing participation in the professional field. The EPB takes the position that the public use of nonstandard doctoral degrees by members of the American Academy of Audiology in connection with their practice is, at the very minimum, misleading to the consumer of professional services.

To be in compliance with the Code of Ethics, Academy members who use their degrees in public statements may only use graduate degrees earned from regionally accredited institutions in which training was obtained in audiology (or a directly related discipline). Public statements are usually taken to include such items as stationery, business cards, catalogs, advertisements (including telephone directory listings), directories, programs, announcements, marketing materials, signs, or other published materials where members are identified for professional purpose.

Case 1

A well-known audiologist is reported to the EPB for using the title Ph.D. in conjunction with a professional presentation on hearing at a regional conference on hearing loss. The complaint alleged that the Ph.D. was acquired from an institution that was not "regionally accredited."

Resolution

The Board investigated the complaint asking the audiologist to supply the details of the degree. It was determined that the person graduated from an institution that was not regionally accredited. Shortly thereafter, however, the institution did receive accreditation.

The Board deliberated and found the respondent to be in violation of Principle 6: Rule 6a. The Board found no evidence that the violation had an impact on quality of service. The degree was in audiology so no public deception was involved. The rule clearly states, however, that degrees must be earned from regionally accredited institutions. The sanction was reprimand. Of course, implicit in the Board's action was an understanding that the individual involved would voluntarily cease and desist in the use of this degree designator in all public statements related to the profession.

Case 2

An audiologist is reported to the EPB for displaying a doctoral title on the office door that is alleged not to have been earned.

Resolution

The Board investigated the complaint asking the audiologist to supply the details of the degree. It was determined that the person was granted the degree by a private credentialing organization and that it was not an advanced degree obtained by graduating from a regionally accredited institution.

The EPB sent a cease and desist order to the member and pointed out the use of an unearned degree is a violation of Principle 6: Rule 6a of the Code of Ethics. The member failed to acknowledge the Board's request and continued to use the degree in conjunction with professional practice. After further consideration, the EPB recommended to the BOD that the person's membership in the Academy be terminated. This action was taken, the member's name was published in *Audiology Today*, and the licensing board of the state in which this person resided was also notified.

Criminal Behavior

In his book on ethics, Resnick points out that one of the most difficult things for ethics committees to deal with is the fact that not every "transgression by a professional is a professional transgression" (Resnick, 1993). By this he means that ethics committees must understand that human behavior might be judged on either legal, moral, or ethical bases. Transgressions that are unethical may not be immoral or illegal. Some sorts of illegal behavior are not judged to be unethical. On the other hand transgressions may be both unethical and illegal. When does illegal behavior become actionable under a code of ethics? One reasonable answer might be "when the illegal activity begins to reflect upon the dignity of the profession."

Principle 8 states that "Members shall uphold the dignity of the professions and freely accept the Academy's self-imposed standards." These standards indicate that a member will not engage in dishonest or illegal conduct that might adversely reflect on the profession. Certainly, some types of illegal behavior probably would not raise the eyebrows of an

ethics committee (e.g., running a red light, failure to pay child support, or cheating at cards). But what of convictions for major felonies? Would we be comfortable calling someone a colleague who had been convicted for rape, murder, or Medicaid fraud?

Case 1

It is brought to the attention of the EPB that an audiologist (a member in good standing) is currently serving time in a state penitentiary for the attempted murder of the member's spouse. Is this the type of behavior that should result in termination of membership?

Resolution

The EPB requested copies of the conviction records of this person to validate the complaint. In addition, the member was allowed to write a letter of explanation to the EPB. After consideration, the EPB found the member to be in violation of Principle 8: Rule 8b of the Code of Ethics. Membership in the Academy was terminated.

Case 2

A complaint was filed with the EPB regarding the advertising of a member in private practice. The complaint alleged that the advertisements indicated that the use of two hearing aids was always better than the use of one. In addition the ad emphasized that if two hearing aids were not used, a strong likelihood existed that the hearing on the unaided ear would be damaged.

Resolution

The EPB considered the case and looked carefully at both the wording of the ad and the form of the ad. The form of the ad with its bold type was not considered in good taste, but that alone did not make it outside the bounds of ethical practice. The wording of the ad was another matter. Certainly evidence exists in the scientific literature that binaural hearing aids are often an advantage over monaural but are they "always better?" Research literature also indicates that some deterioration might result from sensory deprivation. But is this literature strong enough to be presented in an unequivocal manner in a public announcement?

After deliberation, the EPB found that the ad violated Principle 6: Rule 6a of the Code of Ethics. "Individual's public statements about professional services and products shall not contain representations or claims that are false, misleading, or deceptive." The sanction in this case was reprimand.

Conflict of Interest

Issues involving conflict of interest are very difficult to manage because they include both actual conflict of interest and the appearance of conflict of interest. Admonitions against conflict of interest appear in several places within the Code. For example, Principle 4: Rule 4c indicates that "Individuals shall not participate in activities that constitute a conflict of professional interest." Principle 7: Rule 7a indicates that "Individuals shall not use professional or commercial affiliations in any way that would mislead or limit services to persons served professionally. In addition, the EPB has published a position statement called "Conflicts of Professional Interest" (AAA Ethical Practices Board, March/April, 1997a) in which the position of the Academy with respect to conflict of interest and the appearance of conflict of interest are discussed.

For audiologists, the relationship between the practitioner and the product provider seem to be the largest source for potential conflict of interest. However, Resnick (1993) details several others as ". . . practitioner ownership in a commercial

> ## PITFALL
>
> Conflicts of interest involve public trust of professionals. Conflicts of interest not only injure particular patients but also may damage a whole profession by altering public trust.

venture with the potential for abuse, compensation systems based upon quotas, selling the product prescribed, fee splitting, contractual group practice arrangements. . ."

Most people do not think that they are engaged in any activities that have conflict-of-interest overtones. A practitioner's subjective belief of his or her innocence, however, is not enough. Were it true, there would be no need for several hundred years of ethics codes in various professions. The simple fact is that humans are easily drawn into situations that, at the very least, have the appearance of conflict of interest. Appearance is certainly enough to give a profession a black eye with a public that does not often care about the cold facts.

Many professional organizations have position papers dealing with conflict of interest. In some of those papers the guidelines are quite specific and in others much more vague. Perhaps it would be instructive to borrow from some of those papers and cast the guidance offered into the light of audiology practice. This guidance applies to many commonly occurring situations in a variety of professional practice environments. The guidelines are only representative and readers are encouraged to consider their own practice environment in the general context of conflict of interest.

> ## PEARL
>
> The Healthcare Quality Improvement Act of 1986 was passed to address physicians who were biased toward their own self-interests. Audiologists who dispense hearing aids are at risk for a similar ethical lapse (Woods, 1995, p. 373).

Gifts

Audiologists should not accept cash gifts, gifts of significant value that are not primarily for the benefit of persons being served professionally, gifts of any nature that are not appropriate to the audiologist's professional practice, or gifts with "strings attached." The test for acceptability of gifts is twofold. First, the audiologist should ask "would I have any hesitation about disclosing this gift to my patients?" and furthermore, "would my patients have any suspicion that this gift might bias my approach to their treatment?" Second, the audiologist must ask if the acceptance of the gift would bring on any public perception of conflict of interest. Appearance of conflict of interest is surely as important as actual conflict of interest.

Honoraria and Expenses (e.g., Travel, Lodging, Meals, Preparation)

Audiologists may accept these types of remuneration when they are providing actual consultative services or when they are invited speakers at professional conferences or public meetings.

Subsidies

Workshop or conference sponsors may accept monies and support from professionally related commercial enterprises to help underwrite the costs of continuing education events, as long as such support is fully disclosed to conference participants and does not bias or give the appearance of the potential to bias in the professional judgment or practice or speakers or sponsors. In the case of subsidies to individual practitioners such as loans for equipment or outright provision of equipment, the audiologist must ask the same questions that were suggested under Gifts. Once again, it needs to be stated that the audiologist's subjective belief that his or her professional judgment is unaffected by an incentive plan provided by the manufacturer is not a compelling argument. The decision to provide a particular manufacturer's item, to participate in a particular manufacturer's loan program, or to accept the provision of certain equipment from a manufacturer is a serious ethical issue and must be evaluated against the profession's agreed-on code of ethics.

Scholarships or Educational Funds

These types of financial arrangements should be structured in such a way that selection of recipients is made by the academic institution in the case of students, the sponsor in the case of a conference, or an independent panel of judges where that approach might serve the best interest of the profession.

"Self-Dealing"

Audiologists should avoid purchasing equipment from, or entering into contract negotiations with, organizations in which they have financial interests, or make full and timely disclosure of any self-dealing that occurs in situations in which self-dealing is unavoidable. Once again the intent of this guideline is to prevent the situation where the public might perceive an element of conflict of interest and lose trust in the profession.

> ## PITFALL
>
> Volume discounts: In general, one's patients expect that a profit will be made. However, that profit should not be made at the expense of unencumbered clinical decision making and not at the expense of the patients' hearing healthcare.

Referrals

Audiologists working in a professional setting should not refer patients exclusively to themselves in another professional setting or distribute available resources in a manner that is unfair or gives the appearance of being unfair.

Research and Administration

Audiologists engaged in research or administration should maintain "arms-length" relations with sponsors. They should avoid benefiting, or appearing to benefit, from sponsors by using institutional resources inappropriately or withholding research or clinical treatment data from the public or other interested professionals.

Additional Illustrative Cases

In the following section we offer an extensive list of cases that illustrate many of the principles of both the codes of ethics of AAA and/or ASHA. In addition, we offer the reader suggestions for background information and points to consider when reflecting on these ethical decisions.

Cases Related to American Academy of Audiology Code of Ethics Principle 1

Case 1: Possible discrimination on the basis of sexual orientation

An employee in an infectious disease specialist's office calls a hospital-based audiology department to schedule audiometric monitoring because ototoxic medications will be administered next week to an individual who is HIV positive. The response is that the audiology department does not perform those types of tests.

Suggestions

1. Consult AAA's Code of Ethics, especially Principle 1, Rule 1a; Principle 2, Rule 2c.

2. Consult ASHA's Code of Ethics, especially Principle I, Rule C.

3. Revise the department's protocol on ototoxic monitoring.

4. Review the department's procedures on universal precautions and contact someone to give an inservice on universal precautions if necessary.

5. Invite speakers from local groups (such as lesbian/gay organizations) to talk to employees of the audiology department.

Case 2: Incorrect diagnosis; need for referral

An adult patient is seen for a hearing evaluation. The patient reports that she was diagnosed with an "inner ear" hearing loss by another audiologist and provides an audiogram and report by the other audiologist. The patient cries frequently throughout the interview and the evaluation. She lists a variety of psychotropic medications (mostly antianxiety) that she is taking currently and admits being under the care of a psychiatrist but says that she is required to see the psychiatrist only once per year. Current test results show normal hearing, but the patient displayed behaviors consistent with a nonorganic hearing loss (inconsistency, facial expressions indicating straining to hear, and so forth).

Points to Consider

1. Should the audiologist present the test results in such a way that the patient is told she does *not* have a hearing loss?

2. This patient shows significant evidence that she is "upset." If this patient later harms herself, is the audiologist liable? Is the psychiatrist liable because visits are scheduled too infrequently? Should the audiologist contact the psychiatrist and report the patient's behavior or is this a violation of confidentiality? Should the audiologist not discuss the current findings with the patient and allow the patient to leave believing she has a hearing loss so as not to "upset" her further?

Suggestions

1. Consult AAA's Code of Ethics, especially Principle 1; Principle 2, Rule 2a; Principle 5, Rule 5a.

2. Consult ASHA's Code of Ethics, especially Principle I, Rules B, D, and I.

Cases related to American Academy of Audiology Code of Ethics Principle 2

Case 3: Internet posting of advice

The following is adapted from a 1997 posting on an open (i.e., not just for professionals) ListServe by a person identified as an audiologist:

> My own experience is that saltwater nosedrops have "cured" 6 years of persistent negative middle-ear pressure in my child. Nosedrops after school and at bedtime are the solution. Additionally, I now have 3 patients with several years of episodic negative and absent middle-ear pressure who have returned to normal with saline nosedrops.

Points to Consider

1. Is this posting a retelling of personal experience and the experience of patients or are readers being medically advised? If this is advice, is it within an audiologist's scope of practice?

2. Would it matter if this advice were given to one patient face-to-face instead of countless individuals who happen to access it over the Internet?

Suggestions

1. Consult AAA's Code of Ethics, especially Principle 2.

2. Consult ASHA's Code of Ethics, especially Principle I, Rule A; Principle II, Rule B; and Principle III, Rules A and B.

Case 4: Possibility of battery (abuse)

A middle-aged female has gone to the same audiologist for many years. She has a long-standing mild-to-moderate sensorineural hearing loss and wears bilateral hearing aids. She suddenly presents with a tympanic membrane perforation that she says resulted from using "a ballpoint pen to scratch" her ear. The audiologist refers the patient to a local otolaryngologist for treatment. Two months later she returns, and otoscopic inspection reveals that the perforation has healed. The audiologist performs immittance testing to be more certain and finds results consistent with an overly compliant middle ear system (previous testing had always shown compliance to be within normal limits). During questioning the patient says "I guess that Q-tip really went too far into my ear." Noting the inconsistency in her story, the audiologist continues to question her and she begins to cry and leaves the office. The audiologist suspects battery in this case.

Points to Consider

1. Does the audiologist have a responsibility to refer this patient to the police? To protective services? To a social welfare agency?

2. Would the audiologist's responsibility differ if the patient were a child instead of an adult?

Suggestions

1. Consult AAA's Code of Ethics, especially Principle 2, Rule 2a; Principle 3, Rule 3a.
2. Consult ASHA's Code of Ethics, especially Principle I, Rules B and I.

Case 5: Self-referrals/Possible conflict of interest

An audiologist works part-time at two different sites: one site includes hearing aid dispensing services, and the other does not. The audiologist refers patients from the nondispensing site to the other site.

Points to Consider

1. Is a "benefit" clearly defined in AAA Code of Ethics, Rule 2a? As Resnick (1993) questions, if a referral source is happy with an audiologist's work and recommends this audiologist to another practitioner who then sends that audiologist referrals, is that not a benefit received from the original referral source?
2. Consider a similar scenario in which hearing aids are dispensed at both sites, but the audiologist only receives commission at one site. Is it ethical to send more patients to that site instead of equally to both?

Suggestions

1. Consult AAA's Code of Ethics, especially Principle 2, Rule 2a; Principle 4, Rule 4c.
2. Consult ASHA's Code of Ethics, especially Principle I, Rule B; Principle III, Rule B.
3. Always refer to multiple sites.

Case 6: Possible failure to refer

An audiologist sees a patient with a recent-onset unilateral hearing loss and vertigo.

Points to Consider

1. Must the audiologist refer the patient to a physician?
2. Must the audiologist recommend that the patient see a physician *only* if the patient is interested in purchasing hearing aids?
3. What are the audiologist's responsibilities if the patient's HMO primary-care physician clears the patient for amplification without first sending the patient to a specialist?
4. Is the age of the patient a determining factor?

Suggestions

1. Consult AAA's Code of Ethics, especially Principle 2, Rule 2a.
2. Consult ASHA's Code of Ethics, especially Principle I, Rules A and B.
3. Review the Federal Food, Drug, and Cosmetic Act (Food and Drug Administration, 1977) regulations for fitting hearing aids.

Case 7: Possible substance abuse

An audiologist consumes three alcoholic drinks within an hour's time at a farewell luncheon for a coworker and then reports to work for the afternoon.

Points to Consider

1. Is this a one-time occurrence or a common pattern of behavior?
2. Will the audiologist be seeing patients for the afternoon?

Suggestions

1. Consult AAA's Code of Ethics, especially Principle 2, Rule 2b.
2. Consult ASHA's Code of Ethics, especially Principle I, Rules A and L; Principle IV, Rule B.
3. The audiologist should seek professional assistance for substance abuse if this is a pattern of behavior.
4. Arrange all social activities after work to prevent this behavior from occurring.

Case 8: Cerumen management and scope of practice issues

An audiologist is in private practice in the same office building as an otolaryngologist. The audiologist typically refers patients to the otolaryngologist for cerumen removal. After noticing that the patients did not return, the audiologist learns that the otolaryngologist's office is now dispensing hearing aids. Should the audiologist begin performing cerumen removal?

Points to Consider

1. Is the audiologist trained to remove cerumen?
2. Is cerumen removal an accepted practice for audiologists in the state in which the audiologist practices?
3. If the audiologist performs cerumen removal on many patients (and hence does not refer as often to the otolaryngologist), will the otolaryngologist continue to see cases that are outside the audiologist's scope of practice, such as when pus or blood is evident in the external auditory meatus? If not, how will the audiologist cultivate another referral source?
4. Does the audiologist's liability insurance cover cerumen removal?

Suggestions

1. Consult AAA's Code of Ethics, especially Principle 2, Rule 2b.
2. Consult ASHA's Code of Ethics, especially Principle II, Rule B.
3. Audiologists should formally learn how to remove cerumen by attending a course, reading information, performing the operation under supervision, and so forth.
4. Audiologists should verify that cerumen removal is covered by contacting the appropriate insurance companies and licensure boards before beginning this practice.

Case 9: Universal precautions

A parent asks the audiologist whether toys in the waiting room have been disinfected. The audiologist is unsure.

Suggestions

1. Consult AAA's Code of Ethics, especially Principle 2, Rule 2b.
2. Consult ASHA's Code of Ethics, especially Principle I.
3. Review universal precautions and set up a protocol for adhering to them.
4. Educate *all* staff members about universal precautions.
5. Educate all patients about universal precautions.

Case 10: Use of support personnel

The following letter was sent to an audiologist from a person requesting employment:

I work as an Audiologist Assistant at _____ Otolaryngology Group in [city, state]. I feel as if I have earned a great deal of hands-on experience in all aspects of audiology while at this position. I currently perform all diagnostic testing for the practice including: ABRs, ENGs, ECoGs, and posturographys. I also assist in two-tester hearing evaluations and hearing aid fittings. I am very pleased with this work experience but find myself needing to move to [new city, state] and am interested in employment. Please contact me if I can assist you in your practice.

Points to Consider

1. Is an audiologist supervising this "audiology assistant?"
2. If so, has the audiologist supervised appropriately?
3. If there is no supervising audiologist, can the assistant *ethically* perform these duties under supervision of a physician?
4. If there is no supervising audiologist, can the assistant *legally* perform these duties under supervision of a physician?

Suggestions

1. Consult AAA's Code of Ethics, especially Principle 2, Rule 2d.
2. Consult ASHA's Code of Ethics, especially Principle I; Principle II, Rules A, B, D, and E.
3. Verify state licensure laws regarding the audiology scope of practice and the audiology assistant scope of practice.
4. Consult recent professional publications regarding the scope of practice for audiology assistants.

Case 11: Continuing education

An audiologist lives in a state where continuing education is not required for relicensure.

Points to Consider

1. Even though not required, is there a responsibility for professionals to maintain familiarity with current developments in the profession?
2. If so, should any audiologists be exempt from this responsibility? If so, for whom should exceptions be made?

Suggestions

1. Consult AAA's Code of Ethics, especially Principle 2, Rule 2f.
2. Consult ASHA's Code of Ethics, especially Principle II, Rule C.

Cases Related to American Academy of Audiology Code of Ethics Principle 3

Case 12: Possible failure to obtain proper consent and possible failure to maintain confidentiality

An audiologist investigated the effects of unilateral hearing loss in middle-school–aged children by obtaining data (test scores) from clinical files. The results showed that these children were much more likely than normal-hearing children to be enrolled in remedial reading programs. The study was published in a professional journal and publicized in the local newspaper. One family read the article and called the clinic to see whether information about their child had been used in the study. They were told that their child was included in the study but that no names appeared in the research journal article (or the newspaper article). They still filed a complaint because they were not notified before their child's chart was examined.

Points to Consider

1. Is AAA Code of Ethics Principle 3 clear regarding the records of those who have *already* received services (Resnick, 1993)?
2. Should audiologists assume that patients and their families understand who has access to their files and under what circumstances?
3. Are consent forms written in such a way that *all* patients can truly understand the materials, including those for whom English is a second language and those who have reduced language abilities (whether from low intelligence, profound deafness, dementia, traumatic brain injury, and so forth)?
4. What changes, if any, in conduct are expected when the audiologist changes roles from "clinician" to "researcher" and the patient changes roles from "patient" to "subject?" McCarthy and Peach (1993) suggest asking questions such as: Should the "patient" who is now a "subject" be charged for services? Are tests administered to this patient/subject that are part of the research battery but not part of a routine clinical evaluation battery? Is the ultimate goal of treatment better patient outcome or answers to a research question?

Suggestions

1. Consult AAA's Code of Ethics, especially Principle 3, Rule 3a; Principle 5, Rule 5c.
2. Consult ASHA's Code of Ethics, especially Principle I, Rules I and K.
3. Ensure that informed consent is obtained from patients and/or their families.
4. Ensure that the consent form is written in language that the family understands; use interpreters if necessary.
5. Ensure that the consent form includes all foreseeable uses of the patient's data.
6. If use of the patient's data changes, renew the consent form.
7. Review procedures for maintaining patient confidentiality.

Case 13: Possible breach of confidentiality

A graduate student in special education who has a moderate-to-severe hearing loss enrolled in the university's aural rehabilitation program. This student enrolled in some classes in the department of communicative disorders and so happened to be in the graduate student workroom and found a portion of a clinic report, bearing the student's name, on top of the recycled paper bin. The student complained to the clinic director and department chair.

Suggestions

1. Consult AAA's Code of Ethics, especially Principle 3, Rule 3a.
2. Consult ASHA's Code of Ethics, especially Principle I, Rule I.
3. Review procedures to protect patient confidentiality and to obtain informed consent.

CONTROVERSIAL POINT

Clinicians use volume discounts to lower their wholesale price for hearing aids.

1. **This practice could be considered as *ethical* if, for example, the difference in price is used to enhance services such as providing services to patients who are unable to pay or to cover counseling services (as a practitioner's "time" is often not billable directly).**

2. **This practice could be considered as *unethical* if the audiologist does not directly pass on the savings to patients, violating the principle of charging only for services rendered. Note that the clinician's definition of "services" may dictate the course of action in this case.**

3. **This practice could be *illegal* if, for example, the audiologist does not report the cost savings to third-party payers (see Case 14). State and federal laws on pricing are numerous and complicated (Hosford-Dunn et al, 1995).**

Cases Related to American Academy of Audiology Code of Ethics Principle 4

Case 14: Possible billing improprieties

An audiologist who receives a "large quantity" discount for dispensing the hearing aids of a certain manufacturer bills Medicaid for those patients fit with these hearing aids. The audiologist does not, however, pass the discount savings on to Medicaid. Does this represent fraud?

Suggestions

1. Consult AAA's Code of Ethics, especially Principle 4, Rule 4b.
2. Consult ASHA's Code of Ethics, especially Principle I, Rule J; Principle IV, Rule B.
3. Consult local/state Medicaid guidelines.

Case 15: An audiologist is convicted of embezzling funds from the accounts of a state association, resulting in a fine and a prison term.

Point to consider

Is AAA Code of Ethics Rule 8b clear regarding the *legal* conduct that adversely reflects on the profession (Resnick, 1993)?

Suggestions

1. Consult AAA's Code of Ethics, especially Principle 1; Principle 8, Rule 8b.
2. Consult ASHA's Code of Ethics, especially Principle IV, Rule B.

Cases Related to American Academy of Audiology Code of Ethics Principle 5

Case 16: Questionable professional practices

An audiologist includes auditory integration therapy (AIT) in a rehabilitation services pamphlet.

Points to Consider

1. Is there evidence to support the efficacy of this procedure?
2. Are the patients/families charged full price for this therapy or is there a reduced charge because it is considered "experimental?"
3. Are there additional therapies provided to each patient who receives AIT or is AIT sometimes the exclusive treatment?
4. Consult articles such as McCartny and Peach (1993).

Suggestions

1. Consult AAA's Code of Ethics, especially Principle 5, Rule 5b.
2. Consult ASHA's Code of Ethics, especially Principle I, Rules D, E, and F; Principle III, Rules C, D, and E.
3. Consult AAA Position Paper on Auditory Integration Training.
4. Consult articles such as McCartny and Peach (1993).

Case 17: Questionable advertising practices

An advertisement is published showing an audiologist dressed in a full length white coat. Elsewhere in the ad there is an indication that "Dr." so-and-so is on the staff at a local hospital and would be happy to see patients for hearing evaluation at that facility.

Points to Consider

1. At what point does incomplete or inaccurate information move into the realm of deceptive and misleading advertising?
2. By whose definition is "accurate information" judged in Principle 5 (Resnick, 1993)?

Suggestions

1. Consult AAA's Code of Ethics, especially Principle 5, Rules 5a and 5b.
2. Consult ASHA's Code of Ethics, especially Principle I, Rules A, D, E, and J; Principle III, Rules C, D, and E; Principle IV, Rule B.

Cases Related to American Academy of Audiology Code of Ethics Principle 6

Case 18: Questionable use of credentials

An audiologist purchases the Au.D. credential and subsequently begins to sign all correspondence as Dr. X and tells all patients to refer to him/her as Dr. X.

Points to Consider

1. Individuals who use the entitled Au.D. credential insist that it is earned by virtue of numbers of years spent in

practice. Furthermore, they contend that the process of "earned entitlement" is a legitimate process involving peer review of credentials.

2. Others contend that the credential is fraudulent. For example consider the following statement made by Resnick (1993): "There is growing concern that individuals intent on being called *doctor* are enrolling in nonaccredited doctoral degree programs, mail-order degree mills, or obtaining a doctoral degree in a major area unrelated to the management of communicative disorders. Individuals who sport degrees of this type are willfully misleading the public, are being deceptive, and may be found guilty of violating the public trust" (Resnick, 1993, p. 140). Is there evidence that use of the credential has misled the public?

3. What is the definition of "misrepresent" in Rule 6a?

4. If another audiologist receives a report from someone using the credential, does that audiologist have an obligation to report the violation according to AAA Code of Ethics Principle 8, Rule 8c?

5. Are audiologists who drop membership from professional organizations because they disagree with the EPB's position (on this issue or any others) behaving professionally? See for example, a letter to the editor of *Audiology Today* entitled "I'm Walking," November/December, 1997, p. 10.

Suggestions

1. Consult AAA's Code of Ethics, especially Principle 6, Rule 6a.

2. Consult ASHA's Code of Ethics, especially, Principle III, Rule A; Principle IV, Rule B.

Cases Related to American Academy of Audiology Code of Ethics Principle 7

Case 19: Misrepresentations of fact to patients and professionals

An audiologist in private practice who has an occasional "guest appearance" in classes at a local university indicates in his advertisement that he is "affiliated" with the university.

Points to Consider

1. Is this a misrepresentation of fact? Is it likely to mislead the public?

2. Are professional colleagues likely to make false assumptions from this type of statement?

Suggestions

1. Consult AAA's Code of Ethics, especially Principle 7, Rule 7a and Rule 7b.

2. Consult ASHA's Code of Ethics, especially Principle III, Rule D.

3. Consult ASHA's position statement on "Public Announcements and Public Statements."

Cases Related to American Academy of Audiology Code of Ethics Principle 8

Case 20: Misrepresentations of fact to patients and professionals

An audiologist serves a substantial number of indigent patients at a clinic. A friend of this audiologist, another audiologist, frequently donates supplies and monies to this clinic.

The first audiologist receives a letter with a check from the second audiologist and the letter is signed "Dr. _____ ." The first audiologist knows that the second does not have a doctorate earned from a regionally accredited institution.

Points to Consider

1. Should the first audiologist confront the second audiologist over the use of the title "doctor"?

2. Should the first audiologist report the second audiologist to the appropriate ethical practice boards?

3. If the first audiologist does not confront the second over the use of the title "doctor" over fear that donations will cease, is the first audiologist in violation of the code of ethics?

Suggestions

1. Consult AAA's Code of Ethics, especially Principle 8, Rule 8c.

2. Consult ASHA's Code of Ethics, especially Principle 4, Rule G.

ADVOCATING FOR CHANGE

Formal instruction in ethical valuing is rare. Currently, audiology practitioners are not required by their certification standards to have formal coursework in the area of ethics. Graduate education programs include few formal courses in this critical area of professional ethics. The need for professionals to understand and appreciate the ethical, moral, and legal strategies that apply in selecting a path to ethically correct and professionally acceptable decisions seems to be a much-needed area for development in the professional arena (Resnick, 1993). This development should be encouraged from at least three fronts: (1) professional accrediting associations could require evidence of formal coursework in ethics (such as through ASHA's Educational Standards Board); (2) individual academic departments independently should consider formal coursework in ethics through their respective curriculum committees as universities consider changes that may be required to implement the Au.D. (or to otherwise expand their audiology curricula); and (3) licensure boards should require evidence of continuing education credits in ethics. In focusing attention on the need for schooling in professional ethics the emphasis must be directed toward methods that develop sensitivity toward ethical thinking to *avoid* problems—not to finding an ethical solution to problems once they have emerged (Resnick, 1993).

SUMMARY

Ethical decision making in healthcare has been influenced by numerous factors, including sociocultural changes, scientific and technological advances, legal issues, and consumer involvement in healthcare (Catalano, 1991). The public's trust in a healthcare profession increases proportionately to the degree in which the profession's members guard and protect the public's interests (Catalano, 1991). In a purely technical sense all professionals are educated to solve problems, thus it is critical that professionals maintain a sensitivity to the need for strong moral, ethical, and legal judgment (Resnick, 1993). Each audiologist has the obligation to confront ethical issues and their implications for personal and professional conduct. Each audiologist also has the duty to address the ethical aspects of audiological practice with patients, colleagues, and students. Institutions have a responsibility to articulate standards for ethical conduct and to see that they are enforced (Gunsalus, 1997).

CONCLUSIONS

The demand for ethical accountability among professions will increase in the future; the professions must respond effectively while they are still in control of their destiny (Resnick, 1993). Ways to achieve ethical accountability argued for in this chapter include demanding the formal teaching of professional ethics to audiology students, analyzing one's own values and belief systems with the goal of integrating theory and practice so that patient welfare is the central guiding principle in *all* professional activities (Christians et al, 1987), practicing within an environment that follows the principles of audiology's Codes of Ethics, and advocating for continuing modification of professional activities as new technologies and developments emerge. Only after professionals solve many of the ethical dilemmas that exist currently can emphasis be directed toward methods that develop sensitivity toward the goal of ethical thinking to avoid problems in the future (Resnick, 1993). The search for cognitive meaning in ethics remains primarily an intellectual exercise, unless, somehow, the meaning carries over into life. Improving analytical skills and raising moral sensitivity are lifelong endeavors, particularly in an ever-changing profession such as audiology.

Appendix
American Hospital Association
A Patient's Bill of Rights

The American Hospital Association presents a Patient's Bill of Rights with the expectation that observance of these rights will contribute to more effective patient care and greater satisfaction for the patient, his physician, and the hospital organization. Further, the Association presents these rights in the expectation that they will be supported by the hospital on behalf of its patients, as an integral part of the healing process. It is recognized that a personal relationship between the physician and the patient is essential for the provision of proper medical care. The traditional physician-patient relationship takes on a new dimension when care is rendered within an organizational structure. Legal precedent has established that the institution itself also has a responsibility to the patient. It is in recognition of these factors that these rights are affirmed.

1. The patient has the right to considerate and respectful care.

2. The patient has the right to obtain from his physician complete current information concerning his diagnosis, treatment, and prognosis in terms the patient can be reasonably expected to understand. When it is not medically advisable to give such information to the patient, the information should be made available to an appropriate person in his behalf. He has the right to know, by name, the physician responsible for coordinating his care.

3. The patient has the right to receive from his physician information necessary to give informed consent prior to the start of any procedure and/or treatment. Except in emergencies, such information for informed consent should include but not necessarily be limited to the specific procedure and/or treatment, the medically significant risks involved, and the probable duration of incapacitation. Where medically significant alternatives for care or treatment exist, or when the patient requests information concerning medical alternatives, the patient has the right to such information. The patient also has the right to know the name of the person responsible for the procedures and/or treatment.

4. The patient has the right to refuse treatment to the extent permitted by law and to be informed of the medical consequences of his action.

5. The patient has the right to every consideration of his privacy concerning his own medical care program. Case discussion, consultation, examination, and treatment are confidential and should be conducted discreetly. Those not directly involved in his care must have the permission of the patient to be present.

6. The patient has the right to expect that all communications and records pertaining to his care should be treated as confidential.

7. The patient has the right to expect that within its capacity a hospital must make reasonable response to the request of a patient for services. The hospital must provide evaluation, service, and/or referral as indicated by the urgency of the case. When medically permissible, a patient may be transferred to another facility only after he has received complete information and explanation concerning the needs for and alternatives to such a transfer. The institution to which the patient is to be transferred must first have accepted the patient for transfer.

8. The patient has the right to obtain information as to any relationship of his hospital to other healthcare and educational institutions insofar as his care is concerned. The patient has the right to obtain information as to the existence of any professional relationships among individuals, by name, who are treating him.

9. The patient has the right to be advised if the hospital proposes to engage in or perform human experimentation affecting his care or treatment. The patient has the right to refuse to participate in such research projects.

10. The patient has the right to expect reasonable continuity of care. He has the right to know in advance what appointment times and physicians are available and where. The patient has the right to expect that the hospital will provide a mechanism whereby he is informed by his physician or a delegate of the physician of the patient's continuing healthcare requirements following discharge.

11. The patient has the right to examine and receive an explanation of his bill regardless of source of payment.

12. The patient has the right to know what hospital rules and regulations apply to his conduct as a patient.

No catalog of rights can guarantee for the patient the kind of treatment he has a right to expect. A hospital has many functions to perform, including the prevention and treatment of disease, the education of both health professionals and patients, and the conduct of clinical research. All these activities must be conducted with an overriding concern for the patient, and, above all, the recognition of his dignity as a human being. Success in achieving this recognition assures success in the defense of the rights of the patient.

Reprinted from AHA (1973), with permission.

REFERENCES

AMERICAN ACADEMY OF AUDIOLOGY. (1991a). *Code of ethics.* Houston, TX: American Academy of Audiology.

AMERICAN ACADEMY OF AUDIOLOGY. (1991b). Code of ethics. *Audiology Today, 3*(1);14–15.

AMERICAN ACADEMY OF AUDIOLOGY COMMITTEE ON PROFESSIONAL EDUCATION. (1997a). AAA Proposed academic and performance standards for the Au.D. degree. *Audiology Today, 9*(1);11.

AMERICAN ACADEMY OF AUDIOLOGY ETHICAL PRACTICES BOARD. (1997b). Conflicts of professional interest. *Audiology Today, 9*(2);26.

AMERICAN HOSPITAL ASSOCIATION. (1973). Statement on a patient's bill of rights. *Hospitals, 47*(Feb.);41.

AMERICAN SPEECH-LANGUAGE-HEARING ASSOCIATION. (1994a). *Code of ethics.* Rockville, MD: American Speech-Language-Hearing Association.

AMERICAN SPEECH-LANGUAGE-HEARING ASSOCIATION. (1994b). Code of ethics. *ASHA, 36*(3), Suppl. 13;1–2.

AMERICAN SPEECH-LANGUAGE-HEARING ASSOCIATION. (1994c). Legislative Council Resolutions. *ASHA, 36*(10);21.

AMERICAN SPEECH-LANGUAGE-HEARING ASSOCIATION. (1997a). Standards and implementation for the Certificate of Clinical Competence in Audiology. *ASHA Leader, 2*(20);7–8.

AMERICAN SPEECH-LANGUAGE-HEARING ASSOCIATION. (1997b). Can a parent refuse hearing aids for her child? Ethics Roundtable. *ASHA, 39*(4);64.

BEAUCHAMP, T.L., & CHILDRESS, J.F. (1989). *Principles of biomedical ethics* (3rd ed.). New York: Oxford University Press.

BENJAMIN, M., & CURTIS, J. (1986). *Ethics in nursing* (2nd ed.). New York: Oxford University Press.

BREDOW, M. (1943). *Handbook for the medical secretary.* New York: McGraw-Hill.

BUIE, J. (1997). Clinical ethics survey shows members grapple with ethical dilemmas. *ASHA Leader, 2*(20);1,3.

CATALANO, J.T. (1991). *Ethical and legal aspects of nursing.* Springhouse, PA: Springhouse Corporation.

CHILD ABUSE PREVENTION AND TREATMENT AND ADOPTION REFORM ACT AMENDMENTS OF 1984 Public Law 98-457,42 U.S.C. 5101 and following (1984). Child Abuse and Neglect Prevention and Treatment Program: Final Rule. *Federal Register 50,* April 15, 1985,14878–14901.

CHILDRESS, J.F. (1979). Paternalism and healthcare. In: W.L. Robison, & M.S. Pritchard. (Eds.), *Medical responsibility* (p. 18). Clifton, NJ: Humana Press.

CHRISTIANS, C.G., ROTZOLL, K.B., & FACKLER, M. (1987). *Media ethics: Cases and moral reasoning* (2nd ed.). New York: Longman.

CREAGER, J.G. (1980). Teaching ethical decision making. In: F.B. Brawer. (Ed.), *New directions for community colleges: Teaching the sciences* (pp. 17–25). San Francisco: Jossey-Bass.

FOOD AND DRUG ADMINISTRATION. (1977). Hearing aid devices—professional and patient labeling and conditions for sale. *Federal Register, 42* (Feb 15);9286–9296.

GUNSALUS, C.K. (1997). Ethics: Sending out the message. *Science, 276*;335.

HARMIN, M., KIRSCHENBAUM, H., & SIMON, S.B. (1973). *Clarifying values through subject matter: Applications for the classroom.* Minneapolis, MN: Winston Press.

HELMICK, J.W. (1994). Ethics and the profession of audiology. *Seminars in Hearing, 15*;190–197.

HOSFORD-DUNN, H., DUNN, D.R., & HARFORD, E.R. (1995). *Audiology business and practice management.* San Diego: Singular.

"I'm Walking." (Letters to the Editor) (1997). *Audiology Today, 9*(6);10.

INGELFINGER, F.J. (1972). Informed (but uneducated) consent. *New England Journal of Medicine, 287*;455–456.

INGELFINGER, F.J. (1980). Arrogance. *New England Journal of Medicine, 303*;1507–1511.

JERGER, J. (1997). Commentary: Universal hearing screening and human rights. *Audiology Today, 9*(1);9.

JONES, W.H.S. (1923). *Hippocrates. Vol. 1. Epidemics 1:11* (p. 165). Cambridge, MA: Harvard University Press.

KIEFFER, G.H. (1979). Can bioethics be taught? *American Biology Teacher, 41*(3);176–181.

KONOLD, D. (1978). *Codes of medical ethics: History.* New York: Free Press.

LUTERMAN, D. (1979). *Counseling parents of hearing-impaired children.* Boston: Little, Brown.

MCCARTHY, P., & PEACH, R.K. (1993). Ethical considerations in clinical research. *Journal of the Academy of Rehabilitative Audiology, 26*;51–56.

METZ, M.J. (1997). Ethical, legal, or moral? "If it feels good...?" *Hearing Journal, 50*(10);10–16.

MOHR V. WILLIAMS, 95 Minn. 261, 104 N.W. 12 (1905), at 15.

MULFORD, R. (1967). Experimentation on human beings. *Stanford Law Review, 20*(November);106.

PANNBACKER, M., MIDDLETON, G.F., & VEKOVIUS, G.T. (1996). *Ethical practices in speech-language pathology and audiology: Case studies.* San Diego: Singular.

POTTER, R.B. (1965). *The structure of certain American Christian responses to the nuclear dilemma 1958–63.* Ph.D. dissertation, Harvard University.

POTTER, R.B. (1972). The logic of moral argument. In: P. Deats (Ed.), *Toward a discipline of social ethics* (pp. 93–114). Boston: Boston University Press.

RATHS, L.E., HARMIN, M., & SIMON, S.B. (1966). *Values and teaching.* Columbus, OH: Merrill.

RESNICK, D.M. (1991). An introduction to ethics. *Audiology Today, 3*(5);13.

RESNICK, D.M. (1993). *Professional ethics for audiologists and speech-language pathologists.* San Diego, CA: Singular.

In re Sampson, 317 NYS 2d. (1970). In: A. Holder. (1975). *Medical Malpractice Law* (p. 17). New York: John Wiley.

SEYMOUR, C.M. (1990). The hunt for absolute goodness. In: *American Speech-Language-Hearing Association Reflections on ethics* (pp. 91–93). Rockville, MD: American-Speech-Language-Hearing Association.

SEYMOUR, C.M. (1994). Ethical considerations. In: R. Lubinski, & C. Frattali (Eds.), *Professional issues in speech-language pathology and audiology* (pp. 61–64). San Diego, CA: Singular.

SIEGLER, M. (1982). Confidentiality in medicine: A decrepit concept. *New England Journal of Medicine, 307*;1518–1521.

SIMON, S.B., HOWE, L.W., & KIRSCHENBAUM, H. (1972). *Values clarification: A handbook of practical strategies for teachers and students.* New York: Dodd, Mead & Co.

SWIGERT, N. (1998). Taking ethics seriously. *ASHA, 40*(3); 11.

UBEL, P., ZELL, M.M., MILLER, D.J., FISCHER, G.S., PETERS-STEFANI, D., & ARNOLD, R.M. (1995). Elevator talk: Observational study of inappropriate comments in a public space. *American Journal of Medicine, 99*(2);190–194.

WOODS, A. (1995). Risk abatement in an audiology practice. In: H. Hosford-Dunn, D.R. Dunn, & E.R. Harford (Eds.), *Audiology business practice management* (pp. 367–394). San Diego: Singular.

WORLD MEDICAL ASSOCIATION. (1956). Declaration of Geneva. *World Medical Journal, 3*(Suppl. 12).

Chapter 10

Preparing the Clinical Report

Stephen Gonzenbach

Written and oral reports are critical to daily management of audiology practices. This chapter discusses clinical reports that can be tailored for individual practice, referral source, and patient needs. The chapter is organized from general to specific: a discussion of professional communications precedes generic analysis of report requirements, followed by numerous sample reports for different applications.

THE IMPORTANCE, INTENT, AND VALUE OF REPORTING

Communication skills hold special significance in the audiology profession, as evidenced by a sampling of certification standards (Table 10–1). "Please describe your communication skills" is a typical interview query in our profession. An audiologist's ability to communicate effectively through oral and written reports is an important factor in determining how his or her professional skill and clinical judgement are assessed by colleagues and patients. In the case of patients that perceived competence translates into the bond of trust that the audiologist develops with the patient—what is often referred to as the "bedside manner."

TABLE 10–1 Selected standards set by ASHA for certification in audiology, effective January 1, 2007

Standard IV-A: Prerequisite Knowledge and Skills
The applicant must have prerequisite skills in oral and written or other forms of communication.

Standard IV-D: Evaluation
D11 Document evaluation procedures and skills
D15 Maintain records in a manner consistent with legal and professional standards
D16 Communicate results and recommendations orally and in writing to the patient and other appropriate individual(s)

Standard IV-E: Treatment
E15 Document treatment procedures and results
E16 Maintain records in a manner consistent with legal and professional standards
E17 Communicate results, recommendations and progress to appropriate individual(s)

From American Speech-Language-Hearing Association (1997).

Audiology: Practice Management. Edited by Hosford-Dunn, Roeser, and Valente. Thieme Medical Publishers, Inc., New York © 2000

The Value of the Spoken Word

Oral communications distill down to what the patient or colleague recalls about the audiologist's presentation of the diagnosis or treatment plan. To a large extent, the professional value of an audiologist's services is judged on the basis of the oral report (Miller & Groher, 1990). Validate this by anecdotal observations and experiences: recall a description of a visit to a physician or other professional practitioner. What factors contributed to the perception of the practitioner's competence? How was trust in that practitioner secured? Was it based on appearances (e.g., spaciousness of the office, receptionist's demeanor) or how much was charged for services? Perhaps these factors contributed to a perceived level of trust or competence, but the interaction the patient had with the service provider made the difference. If the practitioner appeared confident, communicated in words that were easy to understand, and took time to answer questions, it is very likely that the patient developed a trust and confidence in that practitioner. If the patient left the office confused, uncertain, or unsure of what was explained, the patient was more likely to question the practitioner's competence.

PITFALL

Avoid rapid, incomplete, or inappropriate oral communications. They promote confusion and frustration in patients, staff, and referral sources. Exercise as much care in preparing oral communications as you do in preparing a written report. "The purpose is to communicate, not to impress or obfuscate" (Stach, 1998, p. 403).

The Value of the Written Word

SPECIAL CONSIDERATION

Many practice settings cannot function without gaining accreditation or independent review by outside agencies. As examples, ASHA accredits clinical services programs, and the Joint Commission on Accreditation of Healthcare Organizations (JCAHO), accredits medical centers, long-term care facilities, and organized patient care programs. Accreditation review relies heavily on "...medical records, preprinted forms, handwritten notes, and other types of printed documentation..." to demonstrate implementation and compliance with agency standards (JCAHO, 1996). The concept of the review process is clear and can be summed up as "If it isn't documented, it didn't happen."

The written report is the permanent record of the patient contact. It provides more than a diagnosis of a patient's condition or description of what transpired during a patient visit.

The report represents a continuum of professional thought applied to the patient's presenting complaints, and as such, reflects the audiologist's systematic diagnostic skills. In final form, it must clearly and succinctly summarize the lucid and logical thought processes used by the audiologist to reach conclusions, diagnoses, or plans.

CONTROVERSIAL POINT

The use of the term *diagnosis* by an audiologist is not accepted in all circles. Some suggest that the audiologist makes an *assessment*. Offering a diagnosis is often considered the exclusive domain of physicians. The audiologist should select terms with sensitivity to the practice setting.

The report must also be persuasive by demonstrating why specific procedures were performed or are recommended. Cost-conscious patients and third-party payers are concerned about unnecessary tests that contribute little additional information to the assessment or diagnostic process. The report must communicate what procedures were completed and why. If additional tests or procedures are needed, the report must state why they are needed and how they may affect clinical outcome. For example, if pure tone air conduction responses are consistent with bone conduction responses, word recognition scores are symmetrical, and the patient's chief complaint is that he or she is experiencing more trouble following conversations in the past few years, is acoustic immitance necessary? Although a case can be made for either outcome, the important issue will center on the audiologist's ability to logically and briefly support the choice.

Structure is also important for notes in patient charts or medical records. As Kay and Purves (1996) point out, the term *medical record* may imply a record of absolute truth, when in fact it is a repository for different viewpoints, different biases, and varying degrees of completeness. The authors propose that the patient record functions more as a clinical communication in narrative format—as a sort of "story" that focuses and directs the attention of patient and clinician. Over time, notes form a chronology that a reader may follow to develop a picture of a patient's assessment and treatment, which is especially important at follow-up when dealing with patients who are poor historians. Audiologists should adopt a dual perspective in preparing chart notes: an overview of how the report contributes to the "patient's story," coupled with close attention to factual data and observations that are unclouded by personal bias.

PEARL

Third-party payers look for clear evidence of each procedure that was completed. If payment is requested for a procedure that cannot be identified, many payers will likely dismiss the claim or even consider it fraud if a pattern of missing documentation begins to emerge.

The Value of Time

The report must be complete but brief. Is there an ideal length to a report? That depends on the purpose of the report, to whom it is communicated, and the time available to prepare it (Iskowitz, 1998). In institutional medical settings reports are usually brief and direct, documenting a continuum of services provided by multiple providers to a patient by means of the consultation process. In university training settings reports are usually longer, more detailed, and more likely to be released to patients. Under managed care, practitioners are expected to see more patients during the workday, yet the demand for documentation continues or increases. These pressures and expectations drive the length of reports but must not infringe on their quality. A professional is expected to express complete findings, yet those findings must be expressed in a clear, simple, and direct manner. Often, such constraints lead to the development of templates—predefined report formats that may be edited as needed (Stach, 1998) and checklists that almost eliminate the need to add additional information (Gardner & Stone, 1998). Templates and other time management approaches are discussed in a later section of this chapter.

HOW WE LEARN TO REPORT

Despite the importance of reporting, systematic discussions of reporting and report writing are sparse in the audiology literature. A recently published chapter on report writing by Stach (1998), is an example of the limited publications devoted to this topic. Despite a large number of comprehensive texts on audiology and practice management, they do not include report writing as an individual topic (e.g., Butler, 1986; Hosford-Dunn et al, 1995; Jacobson & Northern, 1991; McCollom & Mynders, 1984; Rizzo & Trudeau, 1994; Wood, 1991).

Writing or presenting well are not innate skills but are cultivated over time. All students write or present during their academic training, but the skills associated with preparing a term paper or delivering an oral report are quite different from those associated with writing a diagnostic report or presenting a case in grand rounds. Both require synthesis of information, but expectations for term papers and speeches include length, detail, and research. Expectations for diagnostic reports and case presentations revolve around brevity with a compendium of historical and empirical data.

Formal training in communications is not included in audiology graduate training curricula, although ASHA identifies appropriate course work as including public speaking, grammar, and composition (American Speech-Language-Hearing Association, 1997). Typically, audiology students learn to present cases and write reports in a post-hoc manner, as evidenced by two informal surveys conducted recently by me with audiologists and local training institutes. Only a few audiologists recalled didactic training in which prior reports were reviewed or in which student discussion resulted in a report written by group consensus. In most situations report writing was addressed during the school's clinical training program by the clinic supervisor or coordinator. The usual process was iterative, with students preparing successive draft reports for supervisors' editing and final approval. The process continued in practicum placements, where students encountered different expectations according to setting and individual supervisors. As the process continues throughout training and the clinical fellow experience, the audiologist develops an individual report style reflecting an eclectic format for report preparation. By inference, the process for learning to present cases orally or prepare chart notes is similar but with less feedback from supervisors.

Analysis of this post-hoc training process indicates that much of the graduate instruction in reporting is essentially *intuitive*, guiding students to "know" when to (1) include information and when to delete it, (2) use styles that are situation-appropriate and audience-appropriate, and (3) synthesize data according to purpose of the report. But doing is not always the same as understanding: few of the students queried in the two informal surveys could state consistent purposes for writing reports, nor could they explain what information should be contained in reports. Further study is necessary to determine to what extent these informal observations generalize to audiology training programs and audiology graduates, but to the extent that they do, they underscore a weakness in developing audiologists' communication skills that is not addressed consistently in professional training programs.

What is needed, in addition to the intuitive approach, is a concomitant *deductive* process in which students and clinicians are presented with a clear conceptual framework for preparing reports and documents that are necessary in their daily practices. The conceptual framework needs to teach the fundamentals and goals of a variety of report styles. The remainder of this chapter attempts to sketch a rudimentary framework by using general observations and questions to deduce different report types and providing specific examples of different genre.

THE FRAMEWORK: CONSUMER EXPECTATIONS

An important part of preparing a report is to consider who is receiving or reading the report. Is the consumer a physician, the patient, a family member, an affiliated professional, or a reviewer from an internal quality office or accrediting agency? In some fashion the expectations of the consumer dictate the focus, format, style, and content of the report. For example, a recent contract proposal for audiology services specifically stipulated that "The report must be written in language easily understood by the layman." Clearly, this consumer has a specific expectation of the written report. Contrast that with a different consumer—an otolaryngologist. The otolaryngologist expects a completed audiogram with abbreviated notes in the comments section. The otolaryngologists's report might be confusing to this contract consumer, whereas the contract consumer's report bores or frustrates the otolaryngologist.

The writer or presenter must also prepare on a "need-to-know" basis. Certain historical information is not necessary for all readers. Moreover, patient confidentiality must be maintained. For example, historical information may include the presence of hypertension, diabetes, alcohol abuse, drug abuse, HIV, or other conditions. The audiologist must determine what conditions are pertinent, what value they have in the audiological diagnosis, and what impact they have on the overall plan of action.

Often, audiologists prepare reports for referring ENT physicians with whom they maintain close working relationships. If they generate these reports frequently, audiologists may develop a false sense that all consumers approach the reports with the same knowledge as ENT physicians. This is not typically the case: primary care physicians usually need more information and direction to understand what an audiology report signifies and how it applies to a patient.

How can consumer expectations be determined and addressed? The following factors address some critical concepts for preparing reports.

Identify the Referral Source Type

A referral from an ENT physician is different from the referral of primary care physician. The ENT referral is specific. After an otologic examination, the ENT physician needs an assessment of the patient's hearing ability. Perhaps a history of effusion is noted but not active. The physician needs to determine whether a conductive hearing loss is present. Audiological results may support a surgical or nonsurgical approach to management of the patient's complaints and condition.

Other referrals are more general: A primary care referral requests "hearing test and evaluate for hearing aids;" a self-referred patient complaining that " . . . people just don't talk like they used to. They mumble and swallow their words!"

The ENT physician needs direct clinical data to assist in patient management. The primary care physician expects general diagnostic information and treatment recommendations. The self-referred patient wants simple, direct information and treatment recommendations with minimal technical data and an extra measure of time and understanding.

SPECIAL CONSIDERATION

Audiologists rarely prepare reports specifically for forensic applications, but any documents may become evidence in legal proceedings. Be careful to support findings and document what occurred during testing and treatment of the patient. Many years may elapse between the time of evaluation or treatment and the time that litigation begins. The written record is the only way to recall what happened.

Match Language to the Referral Source Type

If the purpose of the report is to provide direct clinical data to an otologist, use appropriate professional abbreviations and jargon. For example, "Precipitous mild/severe SNHL at 2K and above, AU." Alternately, the same report given to a patient who is coming to terms with hearing loss will describe the diagnosis as "an inner ear type hearing loss in the mid to high frequencies that interferes with speech perception in both ears." Both reports communicate the same findings, but their functions and presentations differ. The former provides the ENT physician direct, concise data that requires no repetition.

The latter informs and educates the patient regarding the results and how those results may affect the patient.

CONTROVERSIAL POINT

The choice of customer-specific language is not cast in stone. In contrast to this chapter's recommendations, Stach (1998) adopts an opposing view: "Reporting of audiometric test results should be done in a clear enough manner that the report can be generally understood, regardless of the nature of the referral source." (p. 404)

Pay Attention to Form and Content

Melding of form with content is the capstone of a good report: it must be substantive *and* neat. A legible, organized, well-written report conveys value and worth to the consumer. Attempting to read an audiogram with scribbled notes at the bottom like the one in Figure 10–1 is a frustrating and discouraging experience. Once deciphered, the data appear valid, but the reader may form a negative perception about the competence of the audiologist. In Figures 10–2A and 10–2B, the data are clear and neat, and the audiogram is easy to read and interpret. The issue of professional competence is not likely to arise unless something in the test data is questionable.

Consider the following criteria as you read or write a report:

- Is it legible? Use a typewriter, word processor, or write clearly.
- Are sentences or phrases grammatically correct?
- Is the meaning clear? A well-written report should not have multiple interpretations.
- Are supporting documents included? Are they correctly labeled and referenced?
- Are data necessary? Do other tests or documents add information to the diagnostic picture or are they just there to imply thoroughness by sheer quantity?

Be certain to keep you written and oral communications clear, concise, and consistent (Stach, 1998).

TYPES OF REPORTS

Audiologists provide services to a wide range of patients with many diverse needs. Patients may need comprehensive assessment, simple screening, or some intermediate evaluation of hearing status. The type of evaluation may involve "site-of-lesion" testing, amplification assessment, or nothing more than a progress note detailing an office visit. Regardless of need or complexity, any interaction must be supported with written documentation and usually with oral summary.

Diagnostic Report

The most common type of report prepared by audiologists, the diagnostic report, usually appears either underneath the audiogram on the same page or may appear as a separate

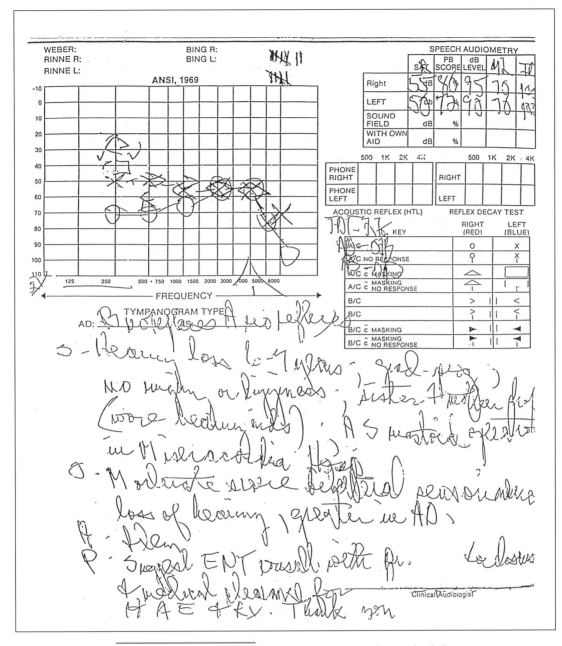

Figure 10–1 A handwritten audiogram report with poor legibility.

report page as an attachment to the audiogram. It is written when a patient is seen for a comprehensive evaluation of peripheral auditory function. This procedure is known by a variety of names (e.g., Comprehensive Audiological Assessment [CAA], Comprehensive Audiological Evaluation [CAE], Audiological Assessment [AA], Diagnostic Hearing Evaluation [DxHE]). Whatever the name, the purpose is to provide a complete description of the patient's hearing sensitivity, word recognition ability, and middle ear function. The audiologist's assessment should provide the following:

- Pertinent history, as needed
- Description of objective test findings

- Assessment of auditory function
- Appropriate recommendations (e.g., medical assessment, amplification needs, management strategies, hearing conservation, and follow-up)

The diagnostic report format applies to special purpose testing as well: hearing aid evaluation, central auditory processing, or site of lesion assessments (e.g., auditory brain stem response, electrocochleography, electronystagmography, oto242 acoustic emissions, or balance tests). Although the purpose of the report varies according to what tests were performed, the report format must include the generic categories bulleted previously.

AUDIOLOGY EXAMINATION
Addendum to VA Form 10-2364

VETERANS HOSPITAL VAMC New York, NY

NAME: DATE SEEN: 03-13-98
SSN: VISIT: CAE AGE: 62 STATUS: OP

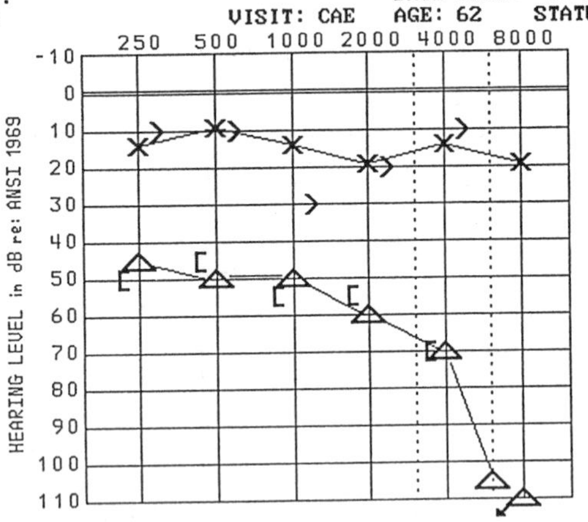

Examiner:

AUDIO SUMMARY

	RIGHT	LEFT
SRT	*55	5
2 Freq	50.0	12.5
3 Freq	53.3	15.0
4 Freq	CNE	CNE
PB Max	44	100
PI-PB	.09	

ACOUSTIC IMMITTANCE

	RIGHT	LEFT
ME Press	+35	+35
St Admit	.80	.70
Type	A	A
Acoustic Reflex (1K)		
Contra	80	80
Ipsi	85	80
Reflex Decay		
500	NEG	NEG
1000	NEG	NEG

SYMBOLS KEY

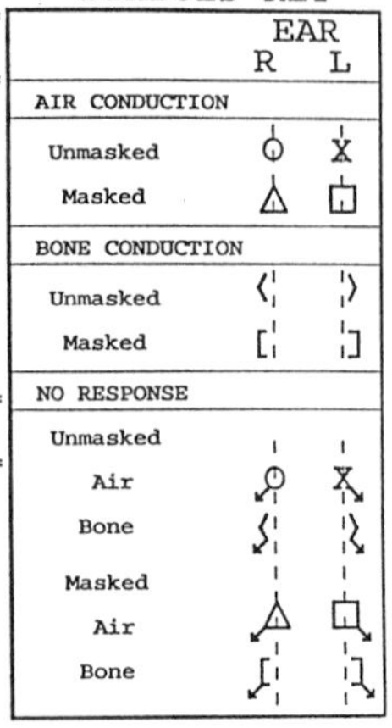

REMARKS:
Type A tympanograms AU. Acoustic reflexes obtained WNL AU with ipsilateral and contralateral stimulation. ARD negative for VIII N. pathology AU.

COMMENTS:
* Masked Responses
SDT per MLV NU6 hlaf-lists.

S: Vet seen for CAE with report of hearing loss AD of 10 year duration, etiology unknown. He denied ear pain and tinnitus AU.
O: Moderate sloping to profound SNHL AD. Hearing WNL AS. Speech discrimination poor AD (44%) and excellent AS (100%).
A: Asymmetrical hearing. SNHL AD. Hearing WNL AS. Otologic evaluation of hearing/speech asymmetry recommended. Hearing aid recommended AD. Vet expressed no interest in amplification.
P: Self-initiated ENT. Annual audio.

SIGNATURE: ______________________

Oct 1989 Computer-generated form created at the VA Medical Center, Little Rock, AR

Figure 10–2A A computer generated audiogram report that is easy to read.

Progress Notes

This is a simple, condensed document that reflects the outcome of a patient contact. As previously discussed, the purpose of the progress note is to provide a summary of the patient's presenting problem(s) and the actions taken to address the problem(s). The progress note is a valuable component of the chronology of patient care and serves to refresh the memory of the audiologist regarding the particulars of care for that patient.

Treatment Plan

This report delineates the goals and objectives that the audiologist sets for the patient. The plan should specify strategies for measuring outcomes (for further information and examples of outcome measurements, see Chapter 5 in this volume). Treatment plans are most appropriate for new hearing aid users, patients with cochlear implants, or patients desiring speech-reading training. Treatment plans usually are encapsulated in the broader diagnostic report or summarized in a progress note. This is one area where audiologists tend to be too brief in reporting. For example, audiologists often fit amplification without providing a structured aural rehabilitation plan, even though the provision of aural rehabilitation may enhance the positive outcomes for new hearing aid patients. Even a simple treatment plan directs the audiologist and the patient to focus on goals and objectives to ensure a successful hearing aid

AUDIOLOGY EXAMINATION
Addendum to VA Form 10-2364

VETERANS HOSPITAL   VAMC New York, NY

NAME:
SSN:

DATE SEEN: 07-28-98
VISIT: CAE   AGE: 89   STATUS: OPT

250 500 1000 2000 4000 8000

HEARING LEVEL in dB re: ANSI 1969

-10 0 10 20 30 40 50 60 70 80 90 100 110

AUDIO SUMMARY

	RIGHT	LEFT
SRT	50	*90
2 Freq	47.5	77.5
3 Freq	53.3	83.3
4 Freq	63.8	86.3
PB Max	48	CNE
PI-PB		

ACOUSTIC IMMITTANCE

	RIGHT	LEFT
ME Press		
St Admit		
Type		
Acoustic Reflex (1K)		
Contra		
Ipsi		
Reflex Decay		
500		
1000		

SYMBOLS KEY

	EAR R	L
AIR CONDUCTION		
Unmasked	O	X
Masked	Δ	□
BONE CONDUCTION		
Unmasked	<	>
Masked	[	]
NO RESPONSE		
Unmasked		
Air		
Bone		
Masked		
Air		
Bone		

Examiner:

REMARKS:

COMMENTS:
* Masked Responses
Pt last seen in 1997. He reported no changes. AD is better than AS and he used a HA in the right only.

RESULTS: Sloping moderate to severe/profound SNHL at 250-8KHZ with poor WR ability (48%) AD. Essentially a gradually sloping severe to profound mixed and SNHL AS with no usable hearing for speech. Today's results were essentially unchanged from those of 1997.

PLAN: Interim Wms. pockettalker, impression for new aid AD. Self initiated retest in 12 months or PRN.

SIGNATURE:

Oct 1989

Computer-generated form created at the
VA Medical Center, Little Rock, AR

Figure 10–2B   A computer generated audiogram report that is easy to read.

fitting. Likewise, planning and setting objectives for patients with cochlear implants allow the patients to learn more about their instruments' capabilities and develop reasonable expectations for achievable listening goals.

Oral Report

To the Patient

When audiologists relate findings and recommendations to a patient, they are reporting. This report is the audiologist's best opportunity to communicate with the patient and the patient's family. The report takes the form of a simple explanation of hearing sensitivity, word recognition, middle ear function, and how these compare with normal auditory function and how they affect the patient's daily listening experiences. Examples, graphs, and reference points (e.g., "normal conversations are in the 40- to 60-dB range on the graph") are useful. The oral version of the report is likely to redescribe and rephrase the results and recommendations on different levels of complexity as the patient processes the information.

To the Referral Source

In a medical setting audiologists may accompany the audigram with an oral report to the referral source, commonly the

ENT physician. Many physicians depend on a brief explanation of the test results before providing follow-up examination and consultation with the patient.

Clinical Rounds

In clinical rounds the audiologist presents an interesting or challenging case to colleagues. The purpose is to guide them to the question or issue at hand to gain peer review and advice. A presenter must be familiar with all material and present it in a clear, concise manner. Little is accomplished unless the presenter communicates effectively and asks the right questions. Perhaps the patient's physical limitations or audiometric configuration make a completely in-the-canal fitting inappropriate, yet he or she demands that type of instrument—what would other audiologists recommend? Perhaps radiographic imaging revealed a vestibular schwannoma that was missed by audiological assessment—why? Discussing a difficult case with peers can be a humbling experience but can lead to further opportunities to learn, improve patient treatment, and modify assessment techniques. For further discussion of the importance of case presentation, see section entitled "Clinical Case Staffing" in Chapter 4 in this volume.

PEARL

Requiring students or trainees to conduct case presentations is an excellent method for improving oral and written communication.

REPORT ELEMENTS AND EXAMPLES

The remainder of the chapter looks at "real world" specifics, detailing four basic elements of reports through a variety of examples for different practice settings. The reports are replete with typical abbreviations and acronyms that are used in medical or audiology practices. Readers should consult Appendix A for definitions of unfamiliar terms.

SOAP Format

The following describes four common elements of a report: **S**ubjective, **O**bjective, **A**ssessment, and **P**lan. These components are emphasized more or less, depending on the intent and venue of the report. Taken together, they form a SOAP format, which

---

SPECIAL CONSIDERATION

Take care in crafting the assessment sentence. More often than not, it is the first and sometimes only component of the SOAP that is read. If another audiologist were provided the same "subjective" and "objective" information, the same assessment should be reached. The assessment cannot imply or conclude an outcome other than what the data supports.

---

is often seen in medical or institutional settings (Northern & English, 1991, p. 69) and is illustrated in Figures 10–3 and 10–4.

- *Subjective:* Lists relevant complaints, historical information, medical/otologic data, and the rationale for the visit. Subjective observations about the patient may be documented here (e.g., "poor historian").
- *Objective:* Describes what was done (procedures) and what was found (results, conditions that existed during testing). Does not state conclusions. The purpose is to provide an understanding of the audiologist's approach to assessment of the presenting complaint(s).
- *Assessment:* Synthesis of subjective and objective information in one or two sentences.
- *Plan:* Relates appropriate next steps that the patient should follow. Documents patient education efforts.

In Figure 10–3 the essentials are present for the "subjective" paragraph: age, gender, race, date and type of service, presenting complaint, otologic, and other relevant history. On the basis of subjective data, it is reasonable to predict a hearing loss as a result of noise exposure and presbycusis.

The objective paragraph in Figure 10–3 contains a chronology of what was completed. No conclusions are made. Reporting SRT/PTA agreement indicates that the audiologist is aware of possible functional components. Reporting the results of an otoscopic inspection is also valuable. The assessment is a direct synthesis of subjective and objective data. Finally, the plan documents patient education, relates the patient's response, and provides the appropriate plan of action, including a recommendation for periodic monitoring.

CONTROVERSIAL POINT

Refrain from diagnosing medical conditions. "Otoscopic inspection indicates possible central perforation of the TM" is preferable to "A central perforation of the TM was observed by otoscopic evaluation." The former is within the scope of audiologists whereas the latter is within the scope of the medical professional. Use objective data from impedance testing to support what was visually suspected (e.g., "CHL likely associated with TM perforation, consistent with abnormally large PV").

Figure 10–4 is a SOAP for an ABR evaluation. Note that formats are similar for the cases in Figures 10–3 and 10–4, but different clinical pictures emerge.

In Figure 10–4 in the subjective section the report of unilateral, sudden hearing loss with tinnitus, corroborated by prior CAE, and the medical history of neurofibromatosis suggest eighth nerve involvement. Hypertension may also contribute to the hearing condition. Objective results are consistent with data reported in the subjective component. Assessment makes it clear that results point to more than a peripheral condition. The plan documents patient education and provides suggested follow-up recommendations.

SUBJ: 72-y/o w/m seen 7/15/98 for CAE. C/o difficulty hearing friends & family, especially in competing noise, x 2-3 years. Denies tinnitus, discharge, vertigo, & imbalance. 27 year hx occupational noise exposure (steelworker) w/o PHP.

OBJ: Tone thresholds WNL through 1 kHz, mild to severe at 1.5 K-4 kHz, recovered to moderate at 8 kHz, AU, w/ no sig a/b gaps. Good SRT/PTA agreement. Good WR ability at 70-dB, HL, AU. Minimal cerumen, AU, by otoscopic inspection.

ASSESS: Mild sloping to severe with recovery to moderate SNHL above 1 kHz, AU, 2° to long-term noise exposure.

PLAN: **1.** Counseled pt re handicapping conditions of his LOH & benefits of binaural amplification.
      2. Per pt request, set appts to obtain medical clearance and RTC for HAE.
      3. Self initiated annual retest or PRN.

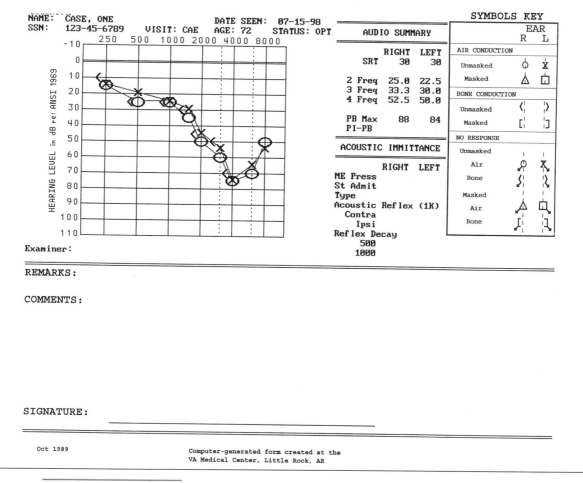

Figure 10–3 SOAP and audiogram for a typical noise-induced hearing loss, recommending amplification.

SUBJ: 52 y/o w/f, referred from Neurology, seen on 7/29/98 for ABR. Pt reports sudden onset hearing loss and tinnitus, AS, x 2 wk. CAE 1 wk ago showed asymmetrical LOH and WR. Denies vertigo, headache, otalgia and canal discharge. Medical Hx remarkable for neurofibromatosis, +HTN, and NIDDM.

OBJ: ABR to suprathreshold click stimuli is WNL, AD, in terms of repeatable absolute and interpeak latencies of waves I, III, and V. Repeatable AS responses showed normal latency wave I, but delayed peak latencies for waves III and V. Interpeak latencies were also delayed and intra-aural wave latency difference is abnormal (.5 ms).

ASSESS: Cannot R/O retrocochlear pathology, AS, due to abnormal ABR in that ear.

PLAN:
1. Pt advised of results and referred back to neurologist, ENT consultation may be considered.
2. CROS amplification described in response to pt's inquiries, but rx further review S/P medical management.
3. Audiological reassessment as medically advised.

AUDIOLOGY EXAMINATION
Addendum to VA Form 10-2364

VETERANS HOSPITAL   VAMC New York, NY

NAME: CASE, TWO   DATE SEEN: 07-15-98
SSN: 234-56-7789   VISIT: CAE   AGE: 52   STATUS: NT

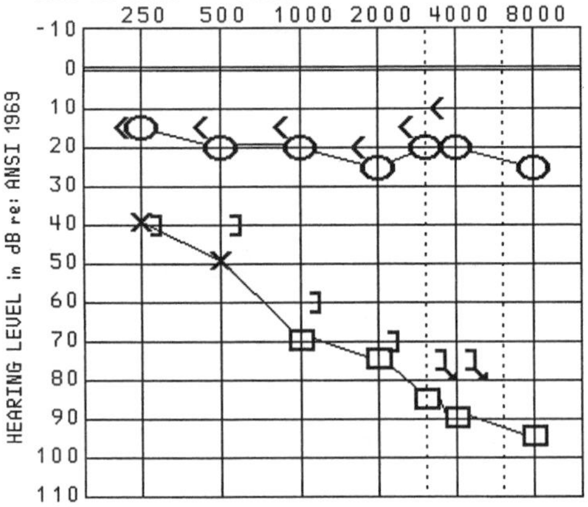

Examiner:

AUDIO SUMMARY

	RIGHT	LEFT
SRT	20	*70
2 Freq	20.0	60.0
3 Freq	21.7	65.0
4 Freq	21.3	80.0
PB Max	100	64
PI-PB		.25

ACOUSTIC IMMITTANCE

	RIGHT	LEFT
ME Press	+30	+65
St Admit	.90	.70
Type	A	A
Acoustic Reflex (1K)		
Contra	105+	105+
Ipsi		
Reflex Decay		
500		
1000		

SYMBOLS KEY

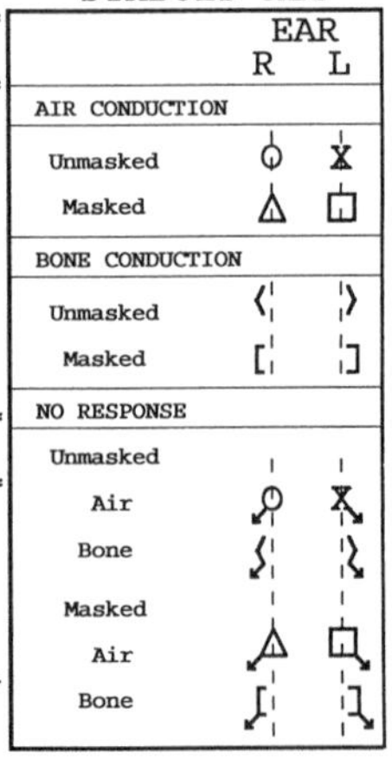

REMARKS:

COMMENTS:

SIGNATURE: ______________________

Oct 1989   Computer-generated form created at the VA Medical Center, Little Rock, AR

Figure 10–4 SOAP and audiogram for retrocochlear workup by means of ABR.

The Necessary and Sufficient Rule

PEARL

Observe the *necessary and sufficient rule*. The report must include data that are relevant to the outcome and leave out data that are not relevant to the outcome. This satisfies the *necessary* requirement. Use caution to omit *only* those data that have no impact on the outcome. Do not try to alter the outcome by selective data omission. This satisfies the *sufficient* requirement.

Subjective elements tend to reiterate what is already well known by referral sources, especially if audiologists work in ENT programs or practices. Likewise, the objective element lends itself to detail that may not be of interest to the reader: audiologists may feel compelled to provide detailed descriptions of procedure (e.g., electrode arrays) or audiometric configuration. Most of this is unnecessary in the report because the audiogram can usually "speak for itself" and much of the important technical information should appear on the test sheet (e.g., Cz-A1). Nonetheless, do not abandon descriptive elements for the sake of brevity or perceived reader interest if data are important to the outcome. The fundamental factor in preparing the report is awareness of what to include and what *not* to include as illustrated in Table 10–2 by two versions of a "subjective" component.

The second subjective version in Table 10–2 covers the salient points and notes problems that may require follow-up by other professionals. An accompanying plan component could state: "Patient agreed to see a social worker regarding concerns he expressed about his family. He also agreed to contact his primary care physician regarding medication concerns."

PEARL

Hearing loss is a sensory deprivation that can affect the whole person. Audiologists must demonstrate sensitivity to the needs and concerns expressed by patients by making reasonable attempts to guide them in appropriate directions for qualified support.

The family and medical concerns expressed by the patient in Table 10–2 are not within the audiologist's scope of practice. However, it is reasonable and perhaps necessary to document that the problem was observed and that appropriate recommendations were made. Failure in this regard may render the report insufficient.

Nowhere is the necessary and sufficient rule more important than in the "assessment", where the audiologist must decide how to describe results and state what is "significant," "unchanged," and so on. A deviation in pure tone responses of ± 5- or 10-dB at one or two frequencies is not evidence of a

SPECIAL CONSIDERATION

The American Academy of Otolaryngology–Head and Neck Surgery (AAO-HNS) has established guidelines that identify audiometric test patterns that require medical referral:

- Average air-borne gap of 15 dB or more at 500, 1000, and 2000 Hz
- Average threshold difference between ears of 15 dB or more at 500, 1000, 2000 and 3000 kHz

significant change. Some patients and more exacting readers may take exception to this. Hence, when normal variation is noted from one test to another, the results are reported as "essentially unchanged" or "no significant changes were observed." This technique provides the audiologist an excellent strategy to avoid spurious arguments over small, but measurable differences.

Modified SOAP Format

Stach (1998) points out that it is not always necessary or desirable to use a full SOAP format. It should be reserved for new patients or settings where a complete report is expected. Use an abbreviated report format that combines subjective and objective elements for established patients, periodic repeat testing, or by agreement with the report's consumer. Although abbreviated, the report must still contain the essential information. Tables 10–3 and 10–4 are examples of abbreviated reports.

The modified SOAP in Table 10–3 provides information on age, gender, race, date and type of service, previous results, pertinent otologic history, and the rationale for testing. The results are direct, with a comparison to previous test data. The plan is simple but includes patient education and reasons for retesting.

Table 10–4 contains two abbreviated reports for a patient who is evaluated and fitted with binaural amplification. Note that the reports describe what was done, document objective results, and establish educational goals for the proposed treatment plan.

Progress Notes

In the daily practice management of patients, progress notes are the basic format used to document the audiologist's activities and interactions with the patient. Recall that a purpose of writing notes is to create an understandable patient story that documents all significant interactions with the provider or clinic. Integrated SOAP formats of the types illustrated in Tables 10–5 and 10–6 support this approach to documentation. In both progress notes documentation describes the patient's complaint or needs indicates the setting and the professional(s) involved in the encounter, shows how the patient was involved in the process, indicates the projected follow-up, and provides a description of the outcome.

The progress note in Table 10–5 describes the reason for the patient's visit, what his apparent learning modality will be, if learning barriers were observed, and established the goals of the class. It is important to state these pieces of information

TABLE 10–2 Example of a subjective component, written first without regard to the "necessary and sufficient" rule, and rewritten in observation of the rule

---

*Violates **Necessary and Sufficient** Rule*

SUBJ: This 88 y/o w/m was seen for CAE on 6/23/98. C/o allergies to varied substances. He described a recent altercation with his landlord over a leaky faucet and other infractions of his lease agreement. He said that communication was sometimes a problem but that he got along. Medical Hx included arthritis, S/P hip replacement, CABG x 4 in 1989 and visual difficulty. He also reported medication noncompliance because he was unable to open the bottles and see which bottles he needed. He asked many questions about unrelated medical conditions and offered a series of statements relating to the overall administration of Medicare. He c/o his sister's inattention to his needs and his children's infrequent contact. Tinnitus was noted as sporadic, whereas vertigo and discharge were denied. He did not perceive a loss of hearing and at the outset of testing, denied a need for hearing aid. He also expressed a need to "Get a move on," because he had other appointments that morning.

*Observes **Necessary and Sufficient** Rule*

SUBJ: 88 y/o w/m, seen for CAE on 6/23/98 denied LOH, but reported occasional communication difficulty and tinnitus. Denied vertigo, ear pain, and discharge. Other medical and otologic Hx unremarkable. Pt expressed several concerns related to family and medical management.

TABLE 10–3 Example of a modified SOAP format combining subjective and objective components and stating assessment in "Results" component

---

57 y/o h/m seen 5/13/98 for repeat CAE. Employed in power generation station in high noise x 15 yr. Previous results (4/25/96) indicated mild SNHFHL above 3 kHz, AU. Patient perceives no change in hearing ability. Otologic Hx continues negative.

RESULTS: Mild SNHFHL above 3 kHz with excellent WR AU. Essentially unchanged from 4/25/96.

PLAN: Amplification is not recommended. Pt. Counseled to continue use of PHP. Self-initiated annual audiometric monitoring or prn.

TABLE 10–4 Modified SOAP format for hearing aid evaluation and hearing aid fitting reports

---

Evaluation Report

67 y/o, b/m, with sloping mild to moderate/severe SNHL, seen for HAE on 4/15/97. MCl = 75-dB HL, AU; UCL = 105 + dB HL, AU. He expressed concern with size of the instrument and the need to wear two aids. Expectations and limitations of amplification were discussed with the patient, as well as size and color options. The need for aural rehabilitation was stressed as an important part of a successful fitting. Impressions were taken.

RESULTS: Patient agreed to try binaural amplification in a CIC style device. Otoscopic inspection indicated WNL conditions after impressions removed.

PLAN: Fitting appointment x 3 weeks. Aural Rehab F/U advised.

Hearing Aid Fitting Report

Mr. S. was seen for a binaural hearing aid fitting on 5/3/97. REM indicated good gain and frequency response, AU. No c/o pain or discomfort with instruments. He was instructed on insertion/removal of devices and batteries. He experienced some trouble manipulating instruments, but was able to handle battery insertion/removal. He was given supportive literature and counseled on use, care, expectations, and limitations of hearing aids.

RESULTS: This appears to be a successful hearing aid fitting. Devices issued were Acme Minis (SN# L98-12324 & R98-56789) using ZA 10 batteries.

PLAN: Patient was enrolled in an aural rehabilitation class to obtain further instruction and practice in insertion/removal of the aids and to address any questions that might arise regarding problem with the instruments. RTC x 2 wks (appt set), or prn. He was advised to discontinue use of the instrument(s) if pain or discomfort developed and contact this clinic right away.

---

because many third-party payers and outside reviewers evaluate patient education on the basis of what is contained in the notes. The progress note described what was done, how the patient participated and what actions for follow-up we recommended consistent with the SOAP format.

A variation of the progress note documents a particular type of contact with a patient (e.g., a walk-in). Documentation of this type of contact adds to the patient's management story by documenting what transpired during the visit. This is especially important in a practice setting in which several staff members may interact with the patient. A patient may forget instructions, recall events differently than the provider, or deny receiving products. In such instances the progress notes from all audiologists or staff members that have worked with the patient are very useful to ensure treatment continuity and consistency in handling the patient.

Table 10–6 describes a scenario that is familiar to experienced dispensing audiologists but always poses a concern for appropriate patient management. In this case a patient walked into the clinic without an appointment, complaining that no one ever showed him how to use his hearing aid. He loudly proclaimed that the clinic did not care about him and gave him an inferior hearing aid. A review of the prior notes indicated that on three previous visits the patient and his attendant were provided with instruction in use, care, and expectations of hearing aids. The notes were consistent in reporting the patient's dexterity and spatial relation problems, manifest in his difficulty with insertion and removal of the low-profile custom instrument. Just as consistently, the note indicated that the patient repeatedly stated to other audiologists that a smaller hearing aid would be a better instrument. The notes documented the education, strategies, and techniques that were used with the patient. One additional note documented that the patient failed to keep his aural rehabilitation class appointment. The audiologist documented the visit as shown in Table 10–6.

TABLE 10–5 Progress note in synthesized SOAP format for the patient fitted previously with amplification, as described in Figure 10–8 reports

Mr. S. was seen on 5/20/97 in a group setting aural rehab class. He is a new hearing aid user with no previous hearing aid experience. He appeared ready to learn and it was assumed that he would learn best with a visual/hearing/doing approach. There were no apparent barriers to learning. The focus of the group was on the care and maintenance of the hearing aid, insertion, removal and testing of hearing aid batteries, and optimizing the use of the aids. Methods included discussion, demonstration, handouts, modeling, and videotape. He demonstrated that he could insert his hearing aids correctly and appeared to grasp the concepts. He successfully inserted and removed the batteries, and inserted and removed his hearing aids without difficulty. He was given patient education materials, a battery tester, and a letter inviting him to attend a second session of aural rehabilitation.

TABLE 10–6 Progress note for a walk-in patient with unresolved complaints

This patient was seen on 7/20/98 as a walk-in with a c/o HA insertion problems. The patient blamed the audiologist for not providing him with a good hearing aid. His home care attendant accompanied him. In view of the patient's documented difficulty with device insertion, the patient and attendant were reinstructed in insertion and removal techniques for the aid. Previous techniques were reinforced and demonstrated. After several attempts, the patient was able to insert the device with less difficulty. Because the attendant was able to handle the process easily, she agreed to take responsibility for daily insertion and removal of the aid. Both were counseled as to strategies to check for proper orientation of the device and placement skills. Both were advised to contact this clinic if additional difficulty was encountered. The patient was again urged to attend an aural rehabilitation class, but he declined. The patient was again advised that given his continuing dexterity difficulty, smaller hearing aids were not appropriate. In addition, he should consider alternative amplification devices in place of hearing aids if dexterity problems continue.

The note in Table 10–6 specifies the presenting complaint, who participated in the visit, what procedures or services were provided, and the outcome of the visit. Also, follow-up recommendations were made. Because of the prior documentation, the audiologist was able to provide consistent treatment and a consistent approach in dealing with the patient. Without clear documentation, patient treatment could be fragmented, resulting in a disjointed treatment plan that is confusing to the patient, the home attendant, and the staff.

EFFICIENCY APPROACHES FOR REPORTING

Electronic Data Management and Communications

Before computerized audiograms, the red/blue pens and carbon paper were audiology staples. Today, audiologists cannot afford to function without some form of electronic record storage and word processing. The ability to quickly access chart notes, merge patient information with report templates, and keep track of hearing aid adjustments is crucial in daily practice. Compared with the traditional method of pulling a chart and handwriting a clinical note, it is much faster and easier to call up a patient record on the computer and add a note documenting services, provider, and procedures at each visit.

In addition to standard office management software, special application programs interface with audiometric equipment and programmable and digital hearing aids. For example, the NOAH program (HIMSA, 1993) is a software platform that contains a database for patient demographics and a journal for note entries. At present NOAH has limited interface capability with audiometric equipment (audiometer, acoustic immittance). It interfaces with a number of hearing aid manufacturer's programming software packages. The NOAH program will automatically generate reports containing a broad variety of this information (see Appendix A), which may be used to supplement chart notes or for communications with referrals sources. The efficacy of electronic data management is clear; however, the intrinsic value of the NOAH program will vary by practice setting. The prudent practitioner must evaluate the data management program to assess whether it meets the needs of his or her practice before committing to an expensive and often limited technical support system.

Traditionally, independent audiology practices send reports by mail to referral sources. This method is slow because of delivery time, inefficient because it is not interactive, and expensive because of stationery and postage costs. A different approach uses a computer-generated cover letter that is faxed to the referral source at the time of the patient's evaluation, along with test results and any additional forms that require signature. This approach is illustrated in Figure 10–5A, where a letter report in modified SOAP format describes the patient whose data are shown in the NOAH reports of Appendix A. In this example, the faxed report would consist of the letter report, audiometric results (pages 2 and 3 of the NOAH report in Appendix A), and the request for medical clearance shown in Figure 10–5B. Many small advantages accrue from this approach:

- The referral source (and any other relevant agencies or professionals) receives the report and data on the day of the examination—often while impressions are setting up in the patient's ears.
- If amplification is recommended, the signed medical clearance is usually faxed back promptly, allowing complete documentation of regulatory requirements well before the patient is fit with amplification.
- The report is printed on standard printer paper—it is not necessary to use expensive letterhead or load the printer with special paper. In the well-networked office the computer-generated report can be faxed directly without ever having to make a "hard copy" of the results.
- The medical clearance form, returned to the office by fax, may be filed directly in the patient's chart.
- In general, busy physicians are pleased to receive "instantaneous" results and also reduce paperwork handling in their office.

CONTROVERSIAL POINT

Some audiologists may object to the use of "canned" statements that might remove individual interpretation from the report. However, standard statements or templates can be edited or modified to clarify information in specific cases.

Templates

All audiology practices develop standard abbreviations such as those listed in Appendix A, as well as standard phrases and formats for report writing. These are commonly referred to as templates or boilerplates. Once developed, prepared forms can save time and ensure that important aspects of audiological assessment and rehabilitation are not overlooked. For example, the cover letter report and medical clearance in Figures 10–5A and 10–5B were generated from templates.

From the previous examples of reports and notes, it is a simple task to create templates for a diagnostic report, hearing aid fitting, or aural rehabilitation class, by highlighting statements that can be checked off when applicable. As has been observed, "Experienced audiologists know that there is a finite number of ways they can describe the outcomes of their various audiometric measures." (Stach, 1998, p. 423). Consider the following example of hearing aid fitting (Table 10–7) in which the words in bold italics are fields to be filled in with appropriate information.

SPECIAL CONSIDERATION

When using templates, "... not all reports can be written using this approach. For example, results on a patient who is exaggerating a hearing loss need to be carefully crafted and do not lend themselves well to this type of automation. Neither do some reports of pediatric testing" (Stach, 1998, p. 427).

```
                          Centerville Audiology & Hearing Aids
                          1 W. Broadway
                          Centerville, NY 11111
                          101-121-1212
                          FAX: 101-511-5111
     Date: 10/15/98
     _____
                          Facsimile Transmission
     _____
     TO: Ann Jones, MD

     Fax #: 123-1234
     _____

     Page 1 of 4

     Dear Dr. Jones,

     Mr. John Smith was seen today for a diagnostic hearing
     evaluation and hearing aid consultation.  He c/o bilateral
     tinnitus and hearing loss.  He denies dizziness, ear pain,
     headache.  30-yr h/o noise exposure (flight line). Neg h/o
     familial hearing loss or middle ear disease.

     Ear canals are clear by otoscopy. Results (see attached) are
     consistent with bilateral cochlear hearing loss secondary to
     noise exposure and presbyacusis.  Middle ear function is WNL
     and there is no empirical evidence of retrocochlear
     involvement.

     Mr. Smith would benefit from binaural amplification and
     expressed an interest in digital technology. These
     instruments were demonstrated today.  Following discussion of
     fitting strategies, expectations, and costs, he decided to
     consult with his wife and set an appointment next week to
     order binaural behind-the-ear digital instruments.

     I appreciate your reviewing attached audiometric results,
     then signing and faxing back the medical clearance, which is
     recommended by the FDA for fitting hearing aids.  Please let
     us know if there are questions or concerns regarding this
     patient.  Thank you.

     Sincerely,


     _____
     (Audiologist's Name, Title)
     (office name)
```

A

```
                          MEDICAL CLEARANCE


     FROM:   Ann Jones, MD
             Medical Plaza
             1 Medical Way, Suite 301
             Centerville, NY 11111

     TO:     Centerville Audiology & Hearing Aids
             1 W. Broadway
             Centerville, NY 11111

     Mr. John Smith (DOB: 01/01/1925) has been medically evaluated
     in my office.  This patient may be considered a candidate for
     amplification bilaterally.


     _____        _____
     Physician Signature                   Date

     FDA Reg. Section 801.421



     Please sign and fax to:  101-511-5111
```

B

Figure 10–5 Example of a fax letter report (**A**) with request for medical clearance (**B**).

TABLE 10–7   Example of a rudimentary template for preparing a hearing aid fitting report

---

Patient name was seen for a hearing fitting on *date*. REM was performed indicating:

☐ Adequate gain and frequency response

☐ Adequate gain but inadequate frequency response

☐ Inadequate gain but good frequency response

☐ Unacceptable gain and frequency response

The patient *was/was not* able to insert and remove the instrument and battery. *She/He* was given supportive documentation. The patient was counseled in use, care, expectations, and limitations of hearing aids. The patient was advised to remove the instrument if pain or discomfort developed and contact the clinic. *She/He* acknowledged *his/her* understanding of these issues. Device(s) issued were *brand name model* with S/N *L* and *R* with *battery type.*

The template in Table 10–7 is simple to use. Because preferences and formats vary by practice, audiologists should choose templates that satisfy the needs of particular practice settings and clerical support. Templates lend themselves to development by means of word processing programs that are standardly available in office management software.

Checklists

A related approach is to use checklists that do not require office automation. The use of checklist–type reporting may be useful in some settings, but care should be taken in using this approach. Electronic data management is the preferred method for capturing, storing, recalling, and managing patient data. Consider that checklist–type reporting can be easily prepared in an electronic format, obviating the need for paper and pencil–type records. Notwithstanding, Gardner and Stone (1998) have published checklist report forms for adult and pediatric diagnostic audiology reports and a hearing aid consultation report. They are reproduced in Appendix B to demonstrate the format and comprehensive contents of these suggested forms.

The authors recommend using the following guidelines to fill out checklist reports:

1. "Reports must be in the audiologist's own handwriting—no need for a computer, word processor, or typewriter.

2. Each form must contain all essential information on a single page.

3. Checkmarks must be used wherever possible and fill-in-the-blank information only when necessary.

4. Abbreviations must always be accompanied by a simple key to their meanings.

5. When clarifications are needed, they are to be entered in the 'Other' or 'Comments' section." (p. 86)

CONCLUSIONS

Effective written and oral reporting are important skills for daily management of audiology patients and practices. Many audiology students who enter the field have little or no formal training in report preparation. A variety of reports are required in audiology practices. These include diagnostic reports; progress notes; treatment plans; and oral presentations to patients, families, and referral sources. Clinical rounds are also an important part of communication in some audiology settings. In all cases audiologists should write or present reports that include the following:

- Are brief and concise
- Integrate form with content
- Avoid personal bias
- Are formulated clearly, with the reader in mind
- Adhere to the "necessary and sufficient" rule

Standard elements of reports are: *S*ubjective, *O*bjective, *A*ssessment, and *P*lan (SOAP). A number of examples are used to illustrate how emphasis on individual SOAP elements varies, depending on the type and purpose of the report. Many of the reports lend themselves to templates or checklists, and examples are provided for these applications. In the future the value of electronic data management and communications is likely to grow in audiology practices because more patient information is collected, stored, and accessed by computers.

ACKNOWLEDGMENT

The program to display and print the computer generated audiograms shown in Figures 10–2A and 10–2B, 10–3, and 10–4 is credited to Kenneth Heard, Ph.D., Chief, Audiology, currently at the Atlanta VA Medical Center.

Appendix A
A NOAH Report

Client Report

Client No.:	0000753
Last Name:	Smith
First Name:	John
Occupation:	retired engineer
Address 1:	1 E. Main St.
Address 2:	
City/State/Zip:	Centerville NY 11111- -
Phone 1/2:	101 101-0111

Birth Date: 1/ 1/25

CENTERVILLE AUDIOLOGY AND HEARING AIDS, INC.
1 W. Broadway
Centerville, NY 1111
(101) 121-1212

Other:

Referral: Centerville Retirement Ctr
Social Security:
Insurance 1: Medicare
Insurance 2:

Physician: Ann Jones, MD

Insurance 1#: 101-01-1010A
Insurance 2#:

Manufacturer:

Hearing Instrument Right:	Hearing Instrument Left:	Remote Control:
Type:	Type:	Type:
No.: #	No.: #	No.: #

Client Report

Client No.: 0000753

Last Name: Smith

First Name: John

Birth Date: 1/ 1/25

**CENTERVILLE AUDIOLOGY
AND HEARING AIDS, INC.**

1 W. Broadway

Centerville, NY 1111

(101) 121-1212

Right:

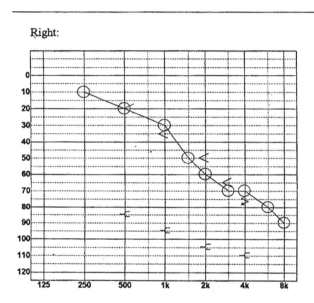

Left:

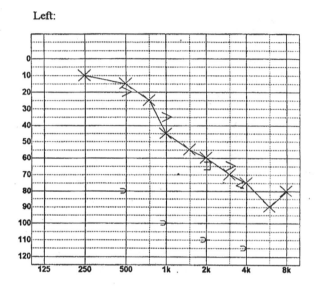

Speech MCL		Speech Reception Threshold						
		Phones					Sound Field	
Right	Left	Right	Mask.Lvl.	Left	Mask.Lvl.	Binaural	Right	Left
dB	dB	dB	dB	dB	dB	dB	dB	dB
70	75	30		35				
Speech UCL				Aided 1:				
95	95			Aided 2:				

Speech Discrimination (Unaided/Aided Comparison)											
Phones						Sound Field					
Right		Mask. Lvl.	Left		Mask. Lvl.	Binaural		Right		Left	
%	dB	dB	%	dB	dB	%	dB	%	dB	%	dB
72	70	50	68	75	55						
				Aided 1:							
				Aided 2:							

Client Report

Client No.: 0000753 Birth Date: 1/ 1/25

Last Name: Smith

First Name: John

**CENTERVILLE AUDIOLOGY
AND HEARING AIDS, INC.**
1 W. Broadway
Centerville, NY 1111
(101) 121-1212

Speech Discrimination in Noise (Unaided/Aided Comparison)																	
Phones						Sound Field											
Right			Left			Binaural			Right			Left					
%	dB	S/N	%	dB	S/N	%	dB	S/N	%	dB	S/N	%	dB	S/N			
			Aided 1:														
			Aided 2:														

Right	Tympanogram	Left
A	Type (A, As, Ad, B, C)	A
1.2	Physical Volume (in cc)	1.4
2.50	ECV, Ear Canal Volume (ml / cc)	2.50
0	Point of Maximum Compliance (daP / mmH$_2$O)	10
1.30	SC, Static Compliance (ml / cc)	1.10

Acoustic Reflex	500 Hz		1000 Hz		2000 Hz		4000 Hz	
	IPSI	CONTR	IPSI	CONTR	IPSI	CONTR	IPSI	CONTR
Probe Right Ear		80	80	100		110		nr
Decay				neg				
Probe Left Ear		85	100	95		105		nr
Decay				neg				

Appendix B
Checklist Report Forms

HUNTINGTON HEARING & SPEECH CENTER
44 Elm Street, Huntington, Long Island, New York 11743-3403 •• Phone (516) 271-6263

- *Audiology Services*
- *Speech, Voice & Language Therapy*
- *Digitally Programmable Hearing Aids*
- *Hearing Conservation Services*

AUDIOLOGICAL EVALUATION On:_____

Name:_____ Gender ☐ M ☐ F DOB (Age):_____ (   )
Ref'd by:_____ Eval'd by:_____ Sup'd by:_____
Last eval'd here (Date_____) Other_____

HISTORY
If prior audiological evaluation elsewhere, where _____ when _____
Reason for testing: ☐ Decreased hearing ☐ Speech delay ☐ Middle ear problem ☐ Other_____
Other Information/Comments·_____
_____

AUDIOLOGICAL RESULTS

Degree of hearing loss:

Right:_____
_____
_____
Left:_____
_____
_____
Bilateral:_____
_____
_____

If hearing loss, type: **R** **L**
  Sensorineural(S) Conductive(C) Mixed(M) ___ ___
Comments:_____
_____
Spch Discr: (see audiog) R____ % L____ % B____ %
Site of Lesion (findings most consistent with): **R** **L**
  Cochlear(C) Retrocochlear(R) . . . . . . ___ ___
  Retrocochlear cannot be ruled out . . . . . . ☐ ☐

Middle ear function: (see tympanogram) . . . **R** **L**
  Normal(N) Stiff(S) Flaccid(F) . . . . . . ___ ___
  Retracted(R) Effusion(E) Wax(W) . . . ___ ___
  PE tube/ TM perforation . . . . ___ ___
  Acoustic Reflexes (1000Hz):
    Present(P) Absent(A) Elevated(E) . ___ ___
  Comments:_____
_____

Comparison to previous findings:
  Same(S) Better(B) Worse(W)
  Pure tones: . . . . ___ ___
  Speech discrimination: . . . . ___ ___
Reliability: ☐ excellent ☐ good ☐ fair ☐ poor
  Comments:_____
_____
_____
_____

RECOMMENDATIONS
❏ Medical/otological consultation to:
  ☐ Check middle ears ☐ Remove cerumen ☐ Assess need for further testing ☐ Clear for amplification
  ☐ Monitor middle ear status with tympanometry ☐ Other_____
❏ Re-evaluate hearing ☐ Annually ☐ After medical consultation/treatment ☐ When fluid has resolved
  ☐ In_____ ☐ Until complete audiogram is obtained ☐ Other_____
❏ Consider: ☐ Central auditory processing evaluation ☐ Assistive listening devices_____
❏ Educational suggestions
❏ Speech and language evaluation ☐ Other _____
❏ Hearing Aid Consultation: ☐ Carried out ☐ Was scheduled ☐ To be scheduled
  ☐ Hearing aid recommendation_____

Comments_____

AUDIO.CHK May 22, 1998

Courtesy of Gardner & Stone (1998).

HUNTINGTON HEARING & SPEECH CENTER

44 Elm Street, Huntington, Long Island, New York 11743-3403 •• Phone (516) 271-6263

- *Audiology Services*
- *Speech, Voice & Language Therapy*

- *Digitally Programmable Hearing Aids*
- *Hearing Conservation Services*

INFANT AUDIOLOGICAL EVALUATION On: _____

Name: _____ Gender ☐ M ☐ F DOB (Age): _____ ( )
Evald by: _____ Supvd by: _____ Last eval'd here: _____
Ref'd by: _____ Accompanied by: _____

HISTORY

If prior evaluation elsewhere, where? _____ when _____
Reason for testing: ☐ Speech/language delay   ☐ Middle ear problem   ☐ Other _____
Other Information / Comments: _____

METHOD

	Sound Field	Earphones	Reliability
☐ Behavioral Audiometry: Speech(S) Tones(T) Noise(N)	___	___	___
☐ Conditioning Orienting Reflex Localization Responses (COR)	___	___	___
☐ Conditioned Play Audiometry	___	___	___
☐ Speech Awareness Threshold	☐	☐	___
☐ Speech Reception Threshold	☐	☐	___

Comments: _____

FINDINGS & CONCLUSIONS

Middle ear function: (see tympanogram) . . . . **R**   **L**
    Normal(N) Stiff(S) Flaccid(F) Retracted(R) Effusion(E) (Wax(W) PE tube(PE) Perf(P) . . . . ___   ___
Acoustic Reflexes (1000Hz):
    Present(P) Absent(A) Elevated(E) . . . . ___   ___
    Comments: _____ ___   ___
Peripheral hearing based on responses to: Speech(S) Tones(T) Noise(N)
    ☐ Binaural hearing appears adequate for speech/language development . . . . ___
    ☐ A _____ hearing loss ☐ cannot be ruled out ☐ is suspected . . . . . ___
        ☐ Impedance findings suggest that if a hearing loss is present it would likely be conductive (middle ear)
    ☐ A unilateral hearing loss
        ☐ Cannot be completely ruled out . . . . ___
        ☐ Is not strongly suspected . . . . ___
    ☐ A high frequency hearing loss cannot be completely ruled out . . . . ___
    ☐ Comments _____ ___

RECOMMENDATIONS

☐ Medical/otological consultation:
    ☐ Check middle ear status   ☐ Remove cerumen   ☐ Assess need for further testing   ☐ Clear for amplification
    ☐ As needed   ☐ Other _____
☐ Monitor middle ear status with tympanometry
☐ Re-evaluate hearing ☐ Annually   ☐ After medical consultation/treatment ☐ When fluid has resolved
    ☐ In _____   ☐ Until definitive results obtained   ☐ ABR/OAE eval   ☐ Other _____
☐ Speech and language evaluation
☐ Other _____
Comments _____

INFAUDIO.CHK May 22 1998

Courtesy of Gardner & Stone (1998).

HUNTINGTON HEARING & SPEECH CENTER

44 Elm Street, Huntington, Long Island, New York 11743-3403 •• Phone (516) 271-6263

- *Audiology Services*
- *Speech, Voice & Language Therapy*

- *Digitally Programmable Hearing Aids*
- *Hearing Conservation Services*

Dear Dr.

   Thank you for referring your patient, _____ seen on _____ for a hearing aid consultation. After reviewing the audiometric data and considering information obtained during the interview, we offered our opinion as to the reasonable options available.

BASED ON THE ENSUING DISCUSSION, we recommended:
☐ No hearing aid use at this time   ☐ Continue use of own hearing aid(s)
Hearing aid use for the ☐ right ☐ left ear(s)
Technology: ☐ Digital ☐ Programmable ☐ Conventional ☐ Other _____
Hearing aid style: ☐ Behind-the-Ear, ☐ In-the-Ear, ☐ In-the-Canal, ☐ Completely-In-the-Canal,
   ☐ BICROS, ☐ CROS, ☐ Other _____
☐ Home auditory training program for high frequency hearing loss
☐ Assistive listening device(s)
   ☐ Telephone amplifier
   ☐ Infra Red listening system for the television
   ☐ Telephone device for the deaf (TDD or TTY)
   ☐ Close captioning
   ☐ FM system
   ☐ Amplified classroom
   ☐ Use of assistive listening strategies (lipreading, slowed rate of speech, preferential seating, etc.)
   ☐ Other_____
☐ Use of tinnitus masker (☐ BTE, ☐ ITE, ☐ bedside ☐ Other_____)
☐ Other _____

AFTER CONSIDERING OUR RECOMMENDATIONS, your patient has decided to:
☐ Have a 30-day trial with _____
   the hearing aid delivery is scheduled for _____
☐ Start with a hearing aid for the ☐ right ☐ left ear and consider a hearing aid for the other ear in the future
☐ Return for a demonstration of digital/digitally programmable instruments
☐ Take our recommendations under advisement, review the literature we have provided and contact us when ready
   We very much appreciate your confidence in us. If there is any way we can be of further service, please call.

                          Very truly yours,

                          _____

PERSONAL NOTE_____

_____

_____

                                              FOLLOWUP.REF May 22, 1998

Courtesy of Gardner & Stone (1998).

Appendix C
Common Abbreviations Used in Audiology Reports

This compilation from several offices and medical settings is not exhaustive; many offices have their own lists of abbreviations. Abbreviations are acceptable in reports as long as they follow conventions within the work setting. Use abbreviations cautiously when reports are generated for nonmedical or institutional settings. For a more complete listing of audiology terms, the reader is referred to the *Comprehensive Dictionary of Audiology: Illustrated* by Stach (1997). For illustrations and explanations of anatomical and audiological terms, also see *Roeser's Audiology Desk Reference* (1996).

Abbreviation	Description
+ or −	Indicator of a *positive* or *negative* condition (e.g., +HTN or −ETOH abuse)
2°	Secondary (e.g., HFSNHL 2° noise exposure)
a/b	Air/bone (e.g., 15 dB a/b gap)
AA	Audiological assessment
ABR	Auditory brain stem response
AD	Right ear
AIDS	Acquired immunodeficiency syndrome
ARD	Acoustic reflex decay
ART	Acoustic reflex threshold
AS	Left ear
ASNHL	Asymmetric sensorineural hearing loss
ASSESS	Assessment
AU	Bilateral
b/f	Black female
b/m	Black male
BSER	Brain stem evoked response
c/o	Complained of
CAA	Comprehensive audiological assessment
CABGxn	Coronary artery bypass graft by *n*, where *n* is the number of arteries grafted
CAE	Comprehensive audiological evaluation
CAP	Central auditory processing
CIC	Completely in the canal hearing aid
CNE	Could not evaluate
CNT	Could not test
CPA	Cerebellopontine angle tumor
CROS	Contralateral routing of signal
CT	Coaxial tomography
CVA	Cerebrovascular accident
dB	Decibel
DPOAE	Distorsion product otoacoustic emission
Dx	Diagnosis
DxHE	Diagnostic hearing evaluation
EAC or EAM	External auditory canal or meatus
ENG	Electronystagmography
ENT	Ears, Nose & Throat
ETOH	Ethanol—referring to use of Alcohol (e.g., +ETOH abuse)
F/U	Follow up
h/f	Hispanic female
h/m	Hispanic male
HA	Hearing aid
HAE	Hearing aid evaluation
HAX	Hearing aid check
HIV	Human immunodeficiency virus
HT	Hearing test
HTN	Hypertension, high blood pressure
Hx	History
Hz	Hertz
IAC or IAM	Internal auditory canal or meatus
IROS	Ipsilateral routing of signal
ITE	In the ear hearing aid
Khz	Kilohertz
LOH	Loss of hearing
MCL	Most comfortable listening level
ME Press	Middle ear pressure
Meds	Medications
MLV	Monitored live voice
MRI	Magnetic resonance imaging
NIDDM	Noninsulin dependent diabetes mellitus
NOAH®	Registered trademark of hearing instrument manufacturers software association (The letters do not represent any other words.)
OAE	Otoacoustic emissions evaluation
OBJ	Objective
PHP	Personal hearing protection
PI-PB	Performance intensity-phonetically balanced— refers to changes in word recognition ability with change in sensation levels
PN	Progress note
PRN	pro re nata— as occasion arises or as needed
PTA	Pure tone average (generally of .5, 1K, and 2kHz)
PVT	Physical volume test
R/O	Rule out
Rehab	Rehabilitation
REM	Real-ear measurement
RTC	Return to clinic

Rx	May represent rehabilitation or medication, context dependent	STAT	To be done immediately
S/P	Status post—often used to refer to patient's condition after a particular incident (e.g., "S/P CVA 2 yrs ago")	SUBJ	Subjective
		TM	Tympanic membrane
		Tx	Treatment plan
		TYMPS	Impedence testing
SDT	Speech detection threshold	UCL	Uncomfortable listening level
SF	sound field	w/f	White female
SNHL	Sensorineural hearing loss	w/m	White male
SOAP	Report writing format standing for **s**ubjective, **o**bjective, **a**ssessment, **p**lan	WNL	Within normal limits
		WR	Word recognition ability
SOL	Site of lesion	y/o	Year old
ST	Spondee threshold	ZA	Zinc air: refers to battery composition type
St Admit	Static admittance		

REFERENCES

AMERICAN SPEECH-LANGUAGE-HEARING ASSOCIATION, COUNCIL ON PROFESSIONAL STANDARDS IN SPEECH-LANGUAGE PATHOLOGY AND AUDIOLOGY. (1997). Certification standards for audiology. Rockville, MD: The Association.

BUTLER, K.G. (Ed.). (1986). *Prospering in private practice: A handbook for speech-language pathology and audiology.* Rockville, MD: Aspen Publications.

GARDNER, H.J., & STONE, M.T. (1998). To save time and labor, consider these audiological report checklists. *The Hearing Journal, 51*(10);86–89.

HEARING INSTRUMENT MANUFACTURERS' SOFTWARE ASSOCIATION (HIMSA). (1993). *NOAH: One standard for all.*www.himsa.com.

HOSFORD-DUNN, H., DUNN, D.R., & HARFORD, E. (1995). *Audiology business and practice management.* San Diego: Singular Publishing Group, Inc.

ISKOWITZ, M. (1998). Report writing. *Advance,* February 23, (p. 25.) JACOBSON, J.T., & NORTHERN, J.L. (Eds.). (1991). *Diagnostic audiology.* Austin, TX: Pro-Ed.

JOINT COMMISSION ON ACCREDITATION OF HEALTHCARE ORGANIZATIONS. (1996). *Comprehensive accreditation manual for hospitals: The official handbook.* Oakbrook Terrace, IL: The Commission.

KAY, S., & PURVES, I.N. (1996). Medical records and other stories: A narratological framework. *Methods of Information in medicine, 35*;72–87.

McCOLLOM, H.F., JR., & MYNDERS, J.M. (1984). *Hearing aid dispensing practice: Planning-starting-operating.* Danville, IL: Interstate Printers & Publishers.

MILLER, R.M., & GROHER, M.E. (1990). *Medical speech pathology.* Rockville, MD: Aspen Publishing.

NORTHERN, J.L., & ENGLISH, G.M. (1991). Otological evaluation. In: J.T. Jacobson, & J.L. Northern (Eds.), *Diagnostic audiology.* Austin, TX: Pro-Ed.

RIZZO, S.R., & TRUDEAU, M.D. (Eds.). (1994). *Clinical administration in audiology an speech-language pathology.* San Diego: Singular Publishing Group, Inc.

ROESER, R.J. (1996). *Roeser's audiology desk reference.* New York: Thieme Medical Publishers, Inc.

STACH, B. (1997). *Comprehensive dictionary of audiology: Illustrated.* Baltimore: Williams & Wilkins.

STACH, B. (1998). *Clinical Audiology: An introduction.* San Diego: Singular Publishing Group, Inc.

WOOD, M.L. (1991). *Private practice in communication disorders.* San Diego: Singular Publishing Group, Inc.

Chapter 11

Infection Control

Robert J. Kemp and Aukse E. Bankaitis

Outline

Infection control is an important healthcare issue that significantly affects many aspects of clinical practice. The nature of the audiology profession inherently exposes both clinician and patient to numerous potentially infectious microbes. Surprisingly, infection control receives limited, if any, attention in the form of didactic course work at undergraduate or graduate levels of training. Ideally, basic concepts from the field of biology, microbiology, virology, and immunology should be understood to appreciate infection control because what audiologists do in the clinic and how procedures are performed influence not only hearing healthcare outcomes and patient satisfaction but also the overall health of clinicians and patients. All too often, infection control is a process taken for granted until an old or new infectious disease emerges. Although a comprehensive summary of biological factors is beyond the scope of this review, the primary goal of this chapter is to provide essential information on basic infection control protocols. Specifically, this chapter will provide audiologists with (1) a history of epidemics and infection control, (2) a review of regulatory agencies governing and monitoring various aspects of infection control, (3) background information on infection and modes/routes of transmission, and (4) guidelines involved in efficient infection control in the clinic.

HISTORICAL PERSPECTIVE OF EPIDEMICS

Throughout our existence, humans have always been susceptible to infectious diseases. From ancient times, the smallpox and measles epidemics slowly spread throughout Roman and Asian civilizations in which one third of the population died. During the thirteenth and fourteenth centuries, the Mongolian army unknowingly carried fleas infected with the bacterium *Yersinia pestis* across Asia, resulting in the infamous Black Death or Bubonic Plague (Krause, 1992). The discovery of the New World by Christopher Columbus resulted in trans-Atlantic travel to foreign lands, thereby providing an extended route for disease transmission. As the world became more industrialized, the tuberculosis (TB) epidemic prevailed in the eighteenth and nineteenth centuries. Advances in aviation elevated mass air travel as the predominant route for the transmission of infectious diseases, reducing the current time window of global exposure to a highly infectious disease to a couple of weeks (Krause, 1992).

Despite such susceptibility, progress in biomedical technology throughout the early and mid 1970s generated a misleading assumption that the spread of all infectious diseases was under complete control in the industrialized world. By that time, the number of smallpox, TB, polio, and other major infectious disease cases significantly declined. With the advent of antibiotics, immunization, and improved sanitation, it was believed that most major infectious diseases were, or would soon be, completely eradicated (Burnet, 1963; Levins et al, 1994). In fact, the scientific interest and allocation of grant support from the National Institutes of Health (NIH) to the field of infectious disease significantly declined with the research impetus redirected toward heart disease and cancer (Krause, 1992).

In the midst of such optimism, however, the threat of infectious diseases seemed to emerge from obscurity in the later end of the 1970s. Legionnaire's disease, toxic shock syndrome, and Lyme disease unexpectedly developed throughout the

Audiology: Practice Management. Edited by Hosford-Dunn, Roeser, and Valente. Thieme Medical Publishers, Inc., New York © 2000

United States. The number of TB cases in the United States suddenly increased. Other continents were similarly experiencing unanticipated disease outbreaks. For example, the deadly Ebola virus spread throughout the African continent, killing 50% of those who became infected (Krause, 1992). Although unheard of in the United States, cholera and typhoid fever were killing thousands in impoverished countries.

Of greatest significance in reaffirming human's susceptibility to infectious diseases was the emergence of acquired immunodeficiency syndrome (AIDS). During the early 1980s anecdotal observations of a rare group of disease manifestations, namely *pneumocystis carinii* pneumonia (PCP) and Kaposi's sarcoma (KS), in a handful of young, previously healthy homosexual men were reported to the Centers for Disease Control and Prevention (CDC), the Atlanta-based epidemiological agency governed by the U.S. Department of Health and Human Services. The first official documentation of what only later became known as AIDS appeared in the CDC's *Morbidity and Mortality Weekly Report* on June 1, 1981 (CDC, 1981). Originally thought of as a "gay" disease, AIDS was quickly affecting individuals from every race, gender, and age group.

As new infectious diseases emerged, infection control became a pertinent issue in healthcare settings; however, the concept of infection control was not new. References to infection control may be found in the Bible regarding leprosy. Ancient forms of infection control involved isolation of people afflicted with leprosy from the general population, which led to the development of leper colonies. In addition to community segregation, clothing and dwellings of those infected were burned. At that time, limited knowledge in current mainstream fields such as microbiology, virology, and infectious diseases resulted in fear and intuition as the driving force of disease containment.

Although such measures of infection control may seem old-fashioned or Medieval, HIV/AIDS generated somewhat of a hysteria in the United States during the 1980s, particularly regarding concerns of the potential risk of infection to healthcare workers providing services to HIV-positive patients. Conversely, patients receiving care from HIV-infected healthcare providers rapidly developed. The emergence of HIV/AIDS and subsequent concerns of transmission served as a catalyst for change in the area of infection control (Kemp & Roeser, 1998). In response to concerns regarding HIV, several regulatory bodies, particularly the Occupational Safety and Health Administration (OSHA), outlined and enacted strict infection control regulations and provided healthcare employers and workers with guidelines for reducing risk of exposure to contagious diseases. Although HIV/AIDS prompted developments in infection control policies, infection control does not encompass an isolated virus or a single disease; rather, infection control is an all-encompassing concept designed to reduce transmission and exposure to all infectious diseases.

REGULATORY AGENCIES CONCERNED WITH INFECTION CONTROL

Several federal and state agencies are responsibile for developing guidelines for the purpose of saving lives and

CONTROVERSIAL POINT

During the initial emergence of HIV, considerable debate regarding universal screening for HIV of healthcare workers developed. Some employers may argue that employing HIV-infected healthcare workers would pose a potential threat to patients and instill fear in patients seeking or requiring services. Individuals against universal screening contend that universal screenings to determine an employee's or potential employee's HIV status exploits the medical right to privacy of healthcare workers. In the past few years several laws passed by federal and state governments retain the rights to privacy for healthcare workers in the workplace and mandatory HIV testing is typically illegal. Although mandatory HIV testing of employees is usually not allowed, courts have upheld mandatory HIV testing policies (Johnsen, 1998).

TABLE 11–1   Regulatory agencies

• OSHA:	Regulates workplace to ensure safe and healthful work conditions
• JCAHO:	Independent, nonprofit standards and accrediting body for healthcare organizations
• CARF:	Standard-setting commission for organizations providing services to persons with disabilities
• EPA:	Protects human health and safeguards natural environment
• FDA:	Consumer protection agency responsible for ensuring safety of foods, cosmetics, medicines, medical devices, fee/drugs for pets and farm animals, and radiation-emitting consumer products

preventing injury or illness in the workplace (Table 11–1). The mission of reducing disease transmission in the healthcare setting also falls within the scope of these agencies. Many different agencies are involved in overseeing infection control according to regulations set forth by OSHA. For example, each state may develop and enforce unique infection control guidelines and regulations; however, each state must minimally enforce federal standards dictated by OSHA regulations. On discretion of the state, OSHA regulations are often expanded to varying degrees, and it is important for audiologists to become familiar with specific guidelines of the state(s) that licenses them because infection control guidelines may significantly differ from state to state. Although it is beyond the scope of this chapter to cover each state's specific regulations, knowledge of OSHA regulations will provide a solid foundation for creating an infection control program.

Occupational Safety and Health Administration (OSHA)

The Occupational Safety and Health Administration (OSHA) is a federal agency governed by the U.S. Department of Labor. Outlined in the Occupational Safety and Health Act of 1970, the mission of OSHA is to regulate the workplace to ensure safe and healthful working conditions by authorizing enforcement of the standards developed under the Act of 1970, assisting states in establishing and enforcing safe and healthful working conditions. This would include training, information and education, and conducting research in the area of occupational safety and health (OSHA, 1998). To accomplish this mission, OSHA relies on the collaborative efforts of both federal and state governments to work in partnership with the more than 100 million individuals throughout the United States who are covered by the Occupational Safety and Health Act of 1970. In conjunction with state affiliates, OSHA establishes and enforces occupational protective standards in an effort to prevent injury and protect the health of American workers. To enforce its standards OSHA conducts unannounced inspections of worksites. Priority inspections are reserved for life-threatening situations or accidents involving deaths of three or more workers injured severely enough to require hospitalization, followed by inspections of high-hazard industries and worksites with previous records of injuries and illnesses (OHSA, 1997).

In response to the concerns regarding potential exposure of HIV in the workplace, in August of 1987, OSHA announced the intent to develop guidelines for protecting healthcare workers from cross-infection of the bloodborne diseases. In addition, OSHA proposed to extend the scope of their mission by monitoring worker safety of healthcare treatment personnel. In the past, monitoring of cross-infection pertained to many groups of workers; however, such precautions were not specifically developed with healthcare personnel in mind. On the basis of the recommended universal precautions issued by the CDC, OSHA submitted a program that was outlined in the *Federal Register* on May 30, 1989. By 1991, the final standard was published. Through the power of federal law, OSHA mandates, oversees, and enforces infection control programs. Field inspectors randomly visit and inspect healthcare settings to ensure that such settings are in compliance with current regulations. Failure of an institution to comply with regulations results in citations and fines.

Joint Commission for the Accreditation of Healthcare Organizations (JCAHO)

The Joint Commission for the Accreditation of Healthcare Organizations (JCAHO) is an independent, nonprofit organization representing the nation's predominant standards-setting and accrediting body in healthcare. The mission of the Joint Commission, as it is often called, is to improve the quality of healthcare provided to the public and accreditation and related services that support performance improvement in

health (JCAHO, 1998). This agency establishes standards and conducts voluntary accreditation programs for hospitals, psychiatric facilities, substance abuse treatment and rehabilitation programs, community mental health centers, organizations providing services for the mentally retarded and developmentally disabled, long-term care facilities, ambulatory healthcare facilities, and home healthcare organizations. JCAHO accreditation is recognized nationwide as a symbol of quality reflecting that an organization meets specific performance standards; to earn and maintain such accreditation, an organization must undergo an on-site survey by the JCAHO every 3 years. Although JCAHO endorsement is voluntary, many healthcare organizations seek accreditation because it assists centers in improving quality care; enhances community confidence and medical staff recruitment; expedites third-party payment, including Medicare and Medicaid eligibility; and favorably influences liability insurance premiums (JCAHO, 1998). The Joint Commission's standards address the level of performance standards in key areas, including patient rights and the anticipated patient outcomes on the basis of what a facility has to offer and the efficacy in which the facility provides services. Participants in this commission include the American Dental Association, American College of Physicians, American College of Surgeons, American Hospital Association, American Medical Association, and the public.

In regard to infection control the Joint Commission sets general guidelines on the basis of OSHA standards that may vary depending on the facility. The facility then creates specific protocols for each department. Each department is usually delegated the responsibility of creating specific programs and protocols on the basis of the general guidelines. It is important for hospitals or audiologists based in healthcare facilities to learn how the general Joint Commission guidelines affect the audiology department. Many institutions now have an infection control coordinator who can be of great assistance.

Commission on Accreditation of Rehabilitative Facilities

The Commission on Accreditation of Rehabilitation Facilities (CARF) is sponsored by 31 rehabilitation/habilitation organizations. This commission sets standards for organizations providing services to persons with disabilities such as spinal cord injuries, chronic pain, and emotional disorders. Like JCAHO, CARF issues general standards based on universal precautions that are then customized by each department in a facility. Membership in the Tuscon, Arizona-based organization is voluntary.

Environmental Protection Agency

The mission of the United States Environmental Protection Agency (EPA) is to protect human health and to safeguard the natural environment. Specifically, the foundation of EPA's development was to ensure (1) that all Americans are protected from significant risks to human health from the environment where they live and work, (2) the implementation of national efforts for the reduction of environmental risk to man and the ecosystem on the basis of the best available scientific information, and (3) fair and effective enforcement of federal laws that protect human health and environment (EPA, 1998a).

Based on the agency's mission, through the Office of Pesticide Programs (OPP), the EPA is responsible for protecting public health and the environment from the risks posed by pesticides and to promote safer means of pest control (EPA, 1998b). This mission remains challenging because pesticide products are found in most homes, businesses, healthcare settings, schools, parks, and other areas. In addition, the EPA's OPP must determine the risk/benefit ratio of pesticides. By their nature, pesticides remain a potential risk to human health and the environment because these biologically active products are specifically designed to kill unwanted living organisms (EPA, 1998b). As such, the EPA directs, executes, and oversees the Federal Insecticide, Fungicide, and Rodenticide Act (FIFRA). Enacted in 1947, FIFRA originally dealt with the use of insecticides and pesticides, some of which, until the adoption of this act, had been misused by the farming industry and community. FIFRA was subsequently amended and expanded in 1962 to include a number of noninsecticide chemicals, such as healthcare chemical disinfectants and sterilants. Recently, FIFRA was substantially revised with stricter guidelines in August of 1996 (EPA, 1998c).

Under FIFRA, the EPA registers all chemical disinfectants and sterilants intended for use on inanimate objects or environmental surfaces. The registration procedures are exacting and, particularly in the case of sterilants, extremely demanding. For a sterilant to earn registration rights, a substance's sporicidal activity must be proven by demonstrating 100% kill of a large quantity of resistant spores that have been carefully applied and dried on the surfaces of 360 replicates. Repeat testing must be conducted a second time with a 100% kill recorded for the second time, otherwise the product is not granted approval. In other words if 1 spore survives the sterilization process on only 1 of the 720 replicates, the product does not meet the criteria of a sterilant and will not be assigned a registration number. Without a registration number displayed on a product's label, sale of that product in the United States is illegal and strictly prohibited (EPA, 1979). Although a product may meet the criteria of a sterilant, the EPA also has the responsibility of reviewing toxicological and hazards data, product literature, and other company information to determine the benefit/risk ratio of a qualified product. For example, even if a sterilant meets the criteria of a sterilant, if a product poses a significant risk to human health and environment, the EPA has the right to deny registration of such a product. As such, successful registration of a potential sterilant or disinfectant involves many months of testing and investigation and costs tens of thousands of dollars. These procedures are necessary to ensure that the products meet EPA standards.

Food and Drug Administration

The Food and Drug Administration (FDA) is a consumer protection agency governed by the U.S. Department of Health and Human Services. The FDA is responsible for ensuring the safety of foods, cosmetics, medicines, medical devices, feed and drugs for pets and farm animals, and radiation-emitting consumer products such as microwaves (FDA, 1998a). The FDA also ensures that product labels are accurate and specific enough so that the contents may be used properly. This agency has been authorized by Congress to enforce several public health laws, including the Federal Food, Drug, and Cosmetic Act, and monitors the manufacturing, importation, transportation, storage, and sale of over $1 trillion worth of goods annually (FDA, 1998b).

In addition, this public health agency operates the National Center for Toxicological Research, which researches and documents the biological effects of chemicals, including sterilants and disinfectants (FDA, 1998b). This responsibility overlaps with the jurisdiction of the EPA, and oftentimes both agencies operate jointly and exchange information. Depending on the type of the product, notification of the FDA without extensive testing may be all that is necessary for marketing. However, as in the case of disinfectants or sterilants, an evaluation process similar to that used by the EPA is required by the FDA. In general, the EPA remains the lead agency in most registrations affecting chemical disinfecting and sterilizing products.

IMPORTANCE OF INFECTION CONTROL TO AUDIOLOGY

Audiologists must be diligent in their efforts for controlling the spread of infectious disease within the context of the clinical setting for several reasons. The hearing healthcare professional's work setting creates an environment where various objects come in direct or indirect contact with multiple patients. From the initial handshake with the patient to the administration of tests, patient care may require the use of headphones, immittance or otoacoustic emissions probe tips, speculae, or probe tubes for real-ear measurement. Although most of these supplies are available in disposable form, disposability does not preclude the spread of infection because these items must be removed from the patient's ears, handled, and disposed of appropriately. In addition, the audiologist may handle several different earmolds or hearing aids throughout the day that have been removed either directly by the audiologist or handed to the audiologist by the patient. From this standpoint alone, the importance of infection control must not be overlooked.

The scope of practice in audiology has significantly changed since the 1960s, and as such, infection control has become a more important issue. Beyond advancements in hearing aid techonology, immittance procedures, or the discovery of otoacoustic emissions that necessitate the use of probe tubes or tips in multiple patients, many audiologists are involved with procedures that may potentially result in exposure to bodily fluids. For example, intraoperative monitoring not only requires the presence of the audiologist in the operating room, but the handling, insertion, and removal of several pairs of needle electrodes. Many clinicians may be involved in the administration of a battery of balance tests that, on occasion, cause patients to become nauseous and sick. Because audiometric procedures require the presence of unoccluded external auditory canals, the scope of clinical practice has expanded to include cerumen management. As more and more of these types of procedures are performed by audiologists, the incidence of exposure to blood and other bodily fluids and subsequent risk of exposure to bloodborne pathogens (i.e., HIV or hepatitis) substantially increases.

Hearing healthcare services are sought by a wide range of patients who vary across several factors such as age, underlying disease, nutritional status, and exposure to past and current pharmacological interventions, and socioeconomic status. These factors indirectly and directly influence the efficacy of the immune system and, as such, audiologists are involved in providing services, both knowingly and unknowingly, to individuals with compromised immune systems. Audiologists often encounter patients who are quite old with underlying diseases such as diabetes, or very young patients with immature immune systems. Furthermore, the recent literature has focused on the effects of compromised immunities on the auditory system. For example, patients with varying degrees of HIV infection, who are at considerable risk for hearing loss developing, are living longer and will most likely seek rehabilitative interventions to improve quality of life (Bankaitis, 1996, 1998a,b). Because diseases like HIV/AIDS, diabetes, and rheumatoid arthritis, or factors such as age influence the efficacy of natural and acquired immunities, great care must be taken to protect patients from contracting opportunistic infections.

INFECTION

Humans are continually challenged by infectious agents from the environment as viruses, bacteria, and other parasites vigorously pursue resources for growth and reproduction. Virtually all cells in the body are vulnerable to infection by intracellular parasites, which include all viruses and several bacterial species, and by extracellular pathogens that include most bacteria, fungi, and parasites. Some of these pathogens are nothing more than mere aggravations, such as the various types of microbes that cause the common cold. Other microbes are opportunistic; opportunistic infections originate from commonplace, ubiquitous organisms that do not produce infection in individuals with intact immune systems but take the opportunity to infect a body with a disabled immune system (Bankaitis, 1996). These agents remain harmless as long as the immune system is intact. When a compromise in immunity is recognized, these same, harmless microbes take advantage of the situation by invading the cells of a weakened system, thereby causing severe infections. Likewise, other pathogens are inherently deadly, including those that cause hepatitis B, TB, or AIDS.

Regardless of the type of microorganism that attempts to infect a body, generally only two attributes are required for a microorganism to produce disease. First, the microbe must be able to metabolize and multiply in or on the infected cell, also referred to as the host. Second, when all conditions are suitable for metabolism and multiplication, the pathogen must be able to sufficiently resist the defenses of the host and the immune system to be able to replicate to the higher numbers required to produce overt disease. Consequently, evolution has provided humans with a complex immune system

to protect and defend the body from infection and to contain these agents when the body is infected.

DISEASE TRANSMISSION

For microbes to infect a body, access to the human body is necessary. As such, microbial transmission represents a two-stage process requiring a mode and a route. For transmission to occur, a vehicle or mode of transmission must be available for the microbe to migrate from one place to another. In other words the germ must find a means to travel from its temporary resting place to the actual host. Activities that increase contact between people promote the transmission of microbes from person to person, thereby increasing the opportunity for cross-infection. For example, particles expelled from the respiratory tract of one person by way of a cough or sneeze may be potentially inhaled by another person. Individuals consistently make contact with their own skin, mouth, and nose only to inadvertently touch another person or a surface or object that will be eventually touched by another person. Microbes may also spread in more indirect means. Disease transmission may occur in humans as a result of exposure to infected animals or from other infected humans by arthropod vectors, such as mosquitoes, mites, flies, and ticks. Other infections may be spread through the ingestion of undercooked food, including *Salmonella* bacterium, or by food handled or prepared by an intestinal carrier of hepatitis A. Water also serves as a mode of disease transmission. During the Midwest floods of 1992, drinking water in many communities became undrinkable as waste treatment plants backed up into water supplies.

Although the manner in which a disease may be transmitted appears endless, four principle modes of transmission exist: contact, vehicle, airborne, and vectorborne. Contact transmission represents the most frequent means of disease transmission in the healthcare setting and may be further subdivided into direct contact, indirect contact, and droplet contact. Direct contact involves the direct physical transfer of organisms between a susceptible host and an infected or colonized person. In the context of audiology direct contact transmission would occur when the audiologist touches the patient's ear with an unwashed (colonized) hand. Organisms on the audiologist's hand would quickly be transferred to the patient's (host) ear. Indirect contact refers to personal contact of the susceptible host with a contaminated intermediate object including instruments, specula, hearing aid ear molds, probe tips, probe mic tubes, or surfaces. Droplet contact occurs when droplets of moisture are expelled from the respiratory tract during talking, breathing, coughing, or sneezing. These droplets carry microorganisms that may be transferred to the mucous membrane linings of the susceptible host by way of the eyelids, nose, and mouth. Droplet transmission is particularly problematic in audiology practice because the nature of audiological services often requires the clinician to remain very close to the patient (i.e., during otoscopic examination, placing earphones on the ears, immittance testing).

Vehicle transmission occurs when a vehicle, such as food, carries the microorganism from person to person. Vehicle transmission applies to diseases transmitted by contaminated items including food (i.e., salmonellosis), water (i.e., legionellosis), and blood or body substances (i.e., hepatitis B or HIV). In contrast, airborne transmission refers to the dissemination of infectious agents by air in the form of either droplet nuclei (residue of evaporated droplets that may remain suspended in the air for long periods of time) or dust particles. These infectious organisms can be widely dispersed by air currents before being inhaled by or deposited on the susceptible host. Airborne contamination is constantly showering surfaces and uncovered objects and is a primary source of indirect contact transmission. Lastly, vectorborne transmission occurs when an animal or insect carries the pathogen and infects the susceptible host. Examples of vectorborne transmission include ticks transmitting Lyme disease or mosquitoes transmitting malaria.

Once a microbe approaches its host by one of the four modes of transmission, the second critical principle of disease transmission involves a portal of entry. Microbes require a means to enter the body. Natural orifices of the body serve as common routes of transmission, including the nose, eyes, ears, mouth, and anus. Because the ears are connected to the respiratory tract by way of the eustachian tubes, a missing or perforated tympanic membrane provides a passage for infectious organisms to invade the respiratory tract and cause systemic infection. Although the human body's skin, mucosa, and other resistive coverings and linings provide nonspecific defenses against microbial invasion, cuts, scrapes, nicks, scratches, and chapped and cracked hands are common routes for microorganisms to enter the body.

Protective Mechanisms Against Disease Transmission

Natural and Adaptive Immunities

Although greatly oversimplified, to protect the body from infection, the immune system generates both nonspecific and specific immune responses. Nonspecific immune responses serve as the initial line of defense against infection, providing humans with what is commonly referred to as natural immunity (Abbas et al, 1994; Clark, 1991; Staines et al, 1993). The natural immune system is represented by a variety of physical barriers, cells, and soluble factors with broad-spectrum antimicrobial activity that react to all foreign agents similarly, without regard to structural or chemical properties of the infectious agent (Weinhold, 1993). For example, the skin serves as a preliminary barrier to infection as do the mucous membranes of the mouth, nose, and throat. Perhaps of greatest importance in natural immunity are the phagocytic cells (Clark, 1991). These cells are found throughout the body and include tissue macrophages and blood neutrophils that are capable of recognizing a broad spectrum of bacteria. Through a process called phagocytosis, these cells bind and internalize bacteria in contained vesicles to kill the bacteria with dozens of cytotoxic compounds.

Relatively effective, nonspecific lines of defense provided by the natural immune system are not foolproof. Nearly all microorganisms have evolved mechanisms, such that natural immunity can provide protection for only a few days (Shountz & Bankaitis, 1998). As a result, the body relies on the adaptive immune system to generate specific immune responses to protect and defend against infection. Adaptive immunity involves the recognition of antigen and the generation of specific immune responses by organs and several immune subsystems. This system is sensitive in detecting the presence of by-products produced by infectious microorganisms called antigens and calls on certain immune cells to defend and protect the body from foreign particles. The adaptive immune system responds to these foreign agents by tagging infected cells in such a way that specialized white blood cells called lymphocytes are able to recognize and destroy infected cells. In addition, phagocytes carry antigen to regional lymph nodes and present the antigen to other lymphocytes.

Natural and adaptive immunity mechanisms are paramount for the maintenance of health. However, more virulent diseases are sometimes too strong to be resisted, especially in the elderly, the infirm, and the immunocompromised person. The course of the infectious process depends on the virulence and titer of microbes and the resistance of the host. Virulence refers to the inherent ability of the germ to break down the host defenses, whereas titer refers to the number of microbes. Little can be done to alter the virulence of the microbes or the resistance of the host. The variable most easily affected is the number of microbes available for transmission. Audiologists must strive to reduce, to an absolute minimum, the number of microbes in the clinical environment on materials, personnel, equipment, instruments, and other areas of patient or personnel contact.

Infection Control

Infection control may be defined as the "…organized effort to manipulate and manage the environment in order to eliminate or minimize exposure to pathogenic microorganisms that may make clinicians or their patients sick" (Kemp et al, 1995, p. 2). A variety of microbes may potentially lead to disease, including bloodborne pathogens such as HIV and hepatitis B virus (HBV) or airborne pathogens such as TB and influenza. Bodily substances may carry micro-organisms and must be guarded against as well. Blood, saliva, mucus (ear drainage), sputum, pus, urine, feces, saliva, semen, and spinal fluid are all potentially infectious materials. Table 11–2 provides a comprehensive overview of diseases and potential sources of these diseases most likely to impact audiology.

SPECIAL CONSIDERATION

Cerumen is not considered an infectious substance unless it is contaminated with blood or mucus. Because complete and appropriate visualization may only be achieved with its complete removal, cerumen should be treated like an infectious substance because of the high likelihood of it containing blood or mucus. Special consideration must be taken when handling hearing aids or ear molds removed from patients' ears that may contain contaminated cerumen.

TABLE 11–2   Infectious diseases important to audiology

Disease	Agent	Potential Transmission Danger	Incubation Period	Potential Outcome
Acquired immuno-deficiency syndrome (AIDS)	Virus	Blood-to-blood contact, blood enters via something as simple as chapped hands.	Average 10 y	Death
Chickenpox	Virus	Blood, saliva, or mucus (ear drainage); provide therapy for infected, subclinical child.	10–21 d	Conjunctivitis, shingles, encephalitis
Common cold	Virus	Blood, saliva, mucus; infected patient sneezes on counter. Receptionist touches counter, touches nose, then breathes on others in the office.	48–72 h	Temporary disability
Cytomegalovirus	Virus	Blood, saliva, mucus; handling toys that infected child put in mouth.	2–8 w	Birth defects, death
Hepatitis A	Virus	Oral, fecal; failure to wash hands after using restroom.	2–7 w	Disability, liver damage
Hepatitis B	Virus	Blood, saliva, mucus; microparticles of cerumen containing dried blood land in eyes or are inhaled while cleaning hearing aid.	6 w–6 m	Chronic carrier, chronic disability, death
Herpes simplex-1	Virus	Blood, saliva, mucus, exudate from sores; touch cold sore while performing otoscopic examination.	2–12 d	Temporary discomfort, herpetic conjunctivitis, herpetic whitlow
Herpes zoster (shingles)	Virus	Blood, saliva, mucus; make contact with vesicle (blister).	6–10 w	Disability
Infectious mononucleosis	Virus	Blood, saliva, mucus; contact with infected saliva or ear drainage	4–7 w	Temporary disability
Infectious meningitis	Virus or bacteria	Blood, saliva, mucus; contact with infected saliva, or ear drainage.	2–10 d	Temporary disability
Influenza	Virus	Saliva, mucus, respiratory droplets (moisture particles from the lungs); provide service for infected patient.	1–3 d	Temporary disability, death
Legionellosis	Bacteria	Respiratory droplets; otoscopic examination requires that practitioner's face comes close to patient's face.	2–10 d	Temporary disability, death
Measles (German) Measles (rubeola)	Virus	Saliva, mucus; contact saliva or drainage of infected lesions.	9–11 d	Congenital defects, temporary disability, encephalitis
Mumps	Virus	Respiratory droplets.	14–25 d	Temporary disability sterility (men)
Otitis externa	Bacteria or fungus	Saliva, mucus, blood, contact with microbes; handle ITEs with bare hands, transferring fungus or bacteria from one patient to the next		Itching, pain, swelling
Pediculosis (head lice)	Lice	Lice transported from scalp by combs and hats; headphones could potentially transfer lice from child to child	Eggs hatch in 7–10 d	Temporary discomfort, itching and scratching
Pneumonia	Virus bacteria	Blood, respiratory droplets.	Varies with organism	Temporary disability, death
Staphylococcus infection	Bacteria	Saliva, mucus, contact with staphylococci colony; audiologist handles ear mold or speculum before disinfecting.	4–10 d	Skin lesions, death
Streptococcus infection	Bacteria	Saliva, blood, mucus, respiratory droplets; same as above.	1–3 d	Heart and kidney problems, death
Tuberculosis	Bacteria	Respiratory droplets, saliva.	Up to 6 m	Disability, death

Adapted from Kemp et al (1995).

TABLE 11-3   Centers for Disease Control and Prevention—universal precautions

1. All healthcare workers should routinely use appropriate barriers precautions to prevent skin and mucous-membrane exposure when contact with blood or other body fluids of any patient is anticipated. Gloves should be worn for touching blood and body fluids, mucous membranes, or non-intact skin of all patients, for handling items or surfaces soiled with blood or body fluids, and for performing venipuncture and other vascular access procedures. Gloves should be changed after contact with each patient. masks and protective eyewear or face shields should be worn during procedures that are likely to generate droplets of blood or other body fluids to prevent exposure of mucous membranes of the mouth, nose, and eyes. Gowns or aprons should be worn during procedures that are likely to generate splashes of blood or other body fluids.

2. Hands and other skin surfaces should be washed immediately and thoroughly if contaminated with blood or other body fluids. Hands should be washed immediately after gloves are removed.

3. All healthcare workers should take precautions to prevent injuries caused by needles, scalpels, and other sharp instruments or devices during procedures; when cleaning used insturments; during disposal of used needles; and when handling sharp instruments after procedures. To prevent needlestick injuries, needles should not be recapped, purposely bent or broke by hand, removed from disposable syringes or otherwise manipulated by hand. After they are used, disposable syringes and needles, scalpel blades, and other sharp items should be planed in puncture-resistant containers for disposal; the puncture-resistant containers should be located as close as practical to the use area. Large-bore reusable needles should be placed in a puncture-resistant container for transport to the reprocessing area.

4. Although saliva has not been implicated in HIV transmission, to minimize the need for emergency mouth-to-mouth resuscitation, mouth-pieces, resuscitation bags, or other ventilation devices should be available for use in areas in which the need to resuscitation is predictable.

5. Healthcare workers who have exudative lesions or weeping dermatitis should refrain from all direct patient care and from handling patient-care equipment until the condition resolves.

6. Pregnant healthcare workers are not known to be at greater risk of contracting HIV infection than healthcare workers who are not pregnant; however, if a healthcare worker develops HIV infection during pregnancy, the infant is at risk of infection resulting from perinatal transmission. Because of this risk, pregnant healthcare workers should be especially familiar with and strictly adhere to precautions to minimize the risk of HIV transmission.

From CDC (1987).

Infection Control Protocols

Regardless of whether the organism is a bacteria, fungus, or virus, the goal of infection control remains the same: reduce or eliminate opportunities for direct or indirect transmission of micro-organisms from person to person. Infection control not only involves controlling exposure between people, but the process is also designed to control exposure between people and the work environment. To optimally achieve infection control, occupational settings providing healthcare–related services rely on infection control programs that outline specific procedures that, when followed, reduce the number of pathogens in the working environment, thereby eliminating cross-contamination and cross-infection.

The development of an infection control program is a necessary and important process for all healthcare settings. Effective infection control programs should incorporate guidelines set forth by the CDC's universal blood and body fluid precautions. Originally outlined in 1987 by the CDC as the Universal Blood and Body Fluid Precautions (Table 11–3), these guidelines are interchangeably referred to as "universal blood and body-fluid precautions," "universal body substance precautions," or "universal precautions." The CDC's universal precautions refer to a set of recommendations regarding the use of protective barriers and appropriate handling of potentially infectious agents designed to prevent transmission of HIV, HBV, and other bloodborne pathogens in healthcare settings. Universal precautions apply to blood, semen, vaginal secretions, and other body fluids containing visible blood (CDC, 1988). Universal precautions also apply to cerebrospinal, synovial, pleural, peritoneal, pericardial, and amniotic fluids; however, these precautions do not apply to feces, nasal secretions, sputum, sweat, tears, urine, and vomitus unless these substances contain visible blood (CDC, 1989). In addition, the CDC's precautions do not apply to saliva except when visibly contaminated with blood or in the dental/orthodontic setting where contamination of saliva with blood occurs (CDC, 1989). Compliance with the universal precautions by treating all bodily fluids as potentially infectious, regardless of the absence of blood contamination, and all patients as potential carriers of an infectious disease, is a strategic mindset for healthcare workers to develop.

ENGINEERING AND WORK PRACTICE CONTROLS

OSHA requires that the practitioner develop "engineering and work practice controls" that will minimize the potential for exposure incidents to occur. For example, a physician may require that nurses never try to place a cap on a used needle, but rather place all used needles in a sharps container. The physician may also require that the container be placed in the area where the needle is used to prevent the nurse from walking around with the needle looking for a container. In this example the physician has put in place work practice control, never recap a used needle, and has engineered out the risk associated with a nurse carrying a needle by placing sharps containers in the proximity of their use. Both actions reduce the risk of an exposure incident in that office. An audiologist may designate one portion of the office as hazardous, where the cleaning and sterilization of instruments takes place. All soiled instruments are taken to this place to minimize the chances of someone accidentally using a soiled instrument before it is cleaned and sterilized. An audiologist may decide to select office space that has a sink rather than one that does not. These are examples of how the practitioner consciously manipulates the work environment to reduce the risks of encountering potential infectious materials and reducing the risks of exposure incidents.

Written Infection Control Plan

OSHA also requires that each facility have a written infection control plan. This plan is to be made available to all workers and it is to provide protocols to be used in the office for infection control. The written plan is the cornerstone of all infection control programs. The following requirements are included in the plan:

1. Exposure classification: Each employee is classified on the basis of potential exposure to blood and other infectious substances.

2. Hepatitis B vaccination plan and records of vaccination: Employees who have the potential for encountering blood or other infectious substances are to be offered the opportunity to receive a hepatitis B vaccination.

3. Plan for annual training and records of training: Each office is to conduct annual training in infection control and is to document the completion of the training.

4. Implementation protocols: These are the actual steps that will be taken in your office to observe universal precautions.

5. Postexposure plan and records: If medically treatable exposure occurs, the office must document the treatment that has taken place and the outcome.

Infection Control Procedures for Audiology

Infection control in any setting revolves around controlling exposure between people and between people and the environment in which they work. The following are specific recommendations that can be incorporated into an infection

control plan. Keep in mind that although no one infection control plan is correct, the presented procedures may serve as guidelines for audiologists to develop their own plans. The recommended guidelines and corresponding protocols are divided into two groups:

1. Those steps that are designed to control exposure from the environment and general housekeeping practices

2. Those steps that are designed to protect the practitioner and patient from human sources of infection

Environmental Infection Control and General Housekeeping Practices

Environmental infection control requires cleaning, disinfecting, and sometimes sterilizing items or surfaces that are reused. These terms are not arbitrarily selected to describe products or procedures. Each has a very specific legal meaning as defined by the EPA. For example, a product that only cleans cannot be called a disinfectant; and a disinfectant cannot be called a sterilant unless it has been demonstrated to meet the requirements of a sterilant. It is important to understand the differences between these terms.

Cleaning

Cleaning means that gross contamination is removed but germs are not necessarily killed. Cleaning is an important precursor to disinfecting or sterilizing because gross contamination must first be removed before these procedures will be effective.

Disinfection

Disinfection means killing germs. Various levels of disinfection depend on how many and which germs are killed. For example, household disinfectants kill a very limited number of germs and hospital grade disinfectants kill a wide variety of microbes. In healthcare settings, it is recommended that hospital grade disinfectants be used (Rutala, 1990).

Sterilization

Sterilization means killing 100% of the vegetative microorganisms and their endospores 100% of the time. Many microbes, when challenged, will revert to a spore form of life that is much more resistant than the vegetative form. If the spore is not killed, it may become vegetative again and cause disease. The preferred sterilization technique is heat under pressure in an autoclave. Unfortunately, most implements used by audiologists would melt in these sterilizers. Also, these chambers are quite expensive to buy and maintain. Consequently, "cold sterilization" with chemicals may work best for audiologists. This is accomplished by soaking instruments in 2% glutaraldehyde for 10 hours; glutaraldehyde in a concentration of 2% or higher is currently the only chemical approved by EPA for sterilization. Glutaraldehyde solutions are effective for use and reuse for 14 or 28 days, depending on the solution. It is extremely important that the scope and ability of chemical disinfectants be investigated before using sprays and disinfectants. For example, contrary to popular belief, bleach is a disinfectant, not a sterilant.

PROTOCOL 11–1

Surface Disinfection

Surface disinfection is a two-step process. *First clean, then disinfect, the contaminated surface.* Cleaning removes the gross contamination, disinfection kills the germs. Many products contain a cleaning agent compounded with a disinfectant and, as a result, these products may be used for both cleaning and disinfecting. A fast and efficacious program of surface disinfection incorporates the following steps:

1. Select a hospital-grade, EPA-registered, disinfectant/cleaner, spray, or towelette. Disinfectant towelettes are helpful for objects that may be damaged by a spray, such as headphones or hearing aids.

2. Spray surface or wipe with towelette. Wipe away all gross contamination with a paper towel, towelette, or coarse brush if necessary.

3. Spray or wipe the surface again, this time leaving it wet for the time specified on the label, then wipe dry. It is during this *dwell time* that the germs are killed.

Adapted from Kemp et al (1995).

When to Disinfect

Disinfection is acceptable on "noncritical" items, those items that do not touch blood or other infectious substances. The operating principle is to clean first, then disinfect. Noncritical items in an audiology setting might include earmolds, in-the-ear (ITE) hearing aids, headphones, specula or any object or surface that is not contaminated with blood, ear drainage, or cerumen that contains such bodily fluids. All these items should be disinfected before handling or reuse, but sterilization

PITFALL

Alcohol and bleach should be avoided as disinfectants in the hearing healthcare field because these agents destroy plastic, rubber, and silicone materials so often used to make headphones, hearing aids, and earmolds.

PITFALL

Objects touched by patients are often contaminated with the bacteria *Staphylococcus*. In one study of physicians' stethoscopes, 26 of 29 stethoscopes were contaminated with the organism (Breathnach et al, 1992).

is not required (Protocol 11–1). For example, an ITE aid or ear mold should not be handled with bare hands until the item has been disinfected. The audiologist may need to ask patients to place appliances on a tissue or into a container until it can be cleaned and disinfected (Fig. 11–1). Gloves should be worn while disinfecting the appliance or a disinfectant towelette should be used to hold, clean, and disinfect the appliance (Protocol 11–2).

PEARL

Disinfectant towelettes can be very helpful for disinfecting objects that cannot be submerged, such as hearing instruments and headphones.

PROTOCOL 11–2

Handling ITEs and Earmolds

How many times does a patient simply hand his or her ITE/CIC instruments or earmold directly from the ear to someone's bare hand? This is a practice that must be controlled because the danger of spreading fungal and bacterial infections is very high, not to mention that the appliance may have blood or ear drainage on it. Some type of plan should be implemented to ensure that the hearing instrument is disinfected before handling it. One solution is to wear gloves to receive the aid, but if this seems impractical these simple alternatives should be tried:

1. Receive the hearing aid or earmold in a disinfectant wipe. Once in the wipe, wipe the aid or earmold all over, disinfecting it.

2. Have the patient place the appliance in a bowl or a dish, then disinfect it with a wipe.

3. Ask the patient to place the earmold in the ultrasonic cleaner containing a disinfectant solution.

Other things to consider about handling earmolds and ITE instruments include the following.

1. Always wear gloves when cleaning aids on the repair bench. The chance of encountering dried blood or mucus within cerumen found in the sound ports or on the aid is very high.

2. Sterilize the picks and probes used to clean the aid when encountering blood, drainage, or cerumen that contains either. Disinfect these tools when blood, drainage, or cerumen containing either is not found.

3. Never use the diagnostic stethoscope on an aid that has not been disinfected properly. Always disinfect the stethoscope using a disinfectant towelette before attaching it to another aid.

Adapted from Kemp et al (1995).

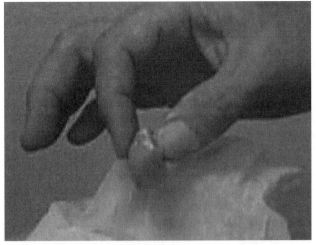

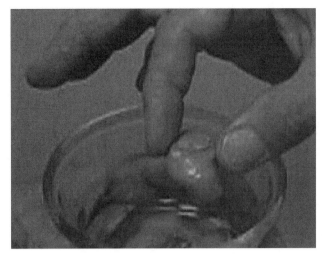

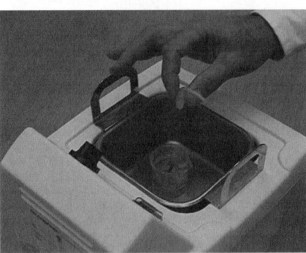

A

B

C

Figure 11–1 When receiving earmolds or ITE/CIC instruments, have the patient place the object in a disinfectant wipe **(A)**, place the object in a bowl or dish before picking it up with a disinfectant wipe **(B)**, or place the object into an ultrasonic cleaner **(C)**.

Surfaces in work areas should also be disinfected regularly. Routine disinfection should be performed on repair benches where earmolds and hearing aids are cleaned, patient "touch" surfaces such as examination chair arm rests, and the reception counter.

Waiting room toys and motivation devices must be disinfected frequently. Toys should be nonporous and easily disinfected. Plastic materials are easier to maintain than painted wood or metal surfaces. Because children invariably place toys in their mouths, great care should be taken when handling objects covered with saliva. Hands should always be thoroughly washed after contact with a potentially infectious item (Protocol 11–3).

When to Sterilize

Critical items, those that may contact blood or mucus, require sterilization. Cerumen is not an infectious substance per se but often contains dried blood or mucus. If visible blood is in or on cerumen, then that cerumen specimen is a potentially infectious substance and the instruments contacting it must be precleaned and then sterilized. One difficulty is that the nature of cerumen, its color and viscosity,

PROTOCOL 11–3

Waiting Room and Motivational Toys

Office toys almost always end up in children's mouths and are common vectors for passing disease. The following information can be used to help control this problem and ensure a safe environment for children:

1. Always use nonporous, easily cleaned toys, preferably those that can get wet. This will allow the use of a spray disinfectant, or a disinfectant towelette.

2. Disinfect these toys daily or on a routine basis. It is highly probable that the toy was placed in a child's mouth.

3. Be careful when handling these toys and be sure to wash your hands thoroughly using an antibacterial soap after touching them. Wearing gloves to pick the toys up would be advisable.

4. Replace old, broken, or worn out toys. Avoid placing stuffed animals, small toys, and nonwashable items in environments frequented by young children.

Adapted from Kemp et al (1995).

PROTOCOL 11–4

Sterilization

Instruments that contact blood, ear drainage, or cerumen containing either are *critical* instruments and *must* be sterilized before reuse. Remember, gross contamination must be cleaned away first. If using heat sterilization, follow the manufacturer's guidelines. If using chemical sterilization with 2% glutaraldehyde, the following steps are recommended:

1. Prepare the solution in a covered, plastic tray that is approved for use with glutaraldehyde. Wear gloves when handling the solution. Do not use glutaraldehyde in an ultrasonic cleaner because this will create fumes.

2. Clean the instruments then submerge them. Ten minutes for high-level disinfection, 10 hours for sterilization.

3. Remove instruments and rinse with sterile water or wipe with a disinfectant towelette to remove the residual glutaraldehyde. Allow to air dry.

4. Change the solution at least every 28 days as instructed on the label or sooner if the solution becomes visibly soiled or viscous.

Glutaraldehyde fumes may irritate the eyes and nose and can cause respiratory problems. Persons who handle the chemical should wear rubber gloves and safety goggles. Good ventilation is necessary in cabinets and rooms where it is stored and where instruments cleaned with it are stored. Be sure to store it in a covered tray.

Adapted from Kemp et al (1995).

make it very difficult for the clinician to determine whether blood, particularly dried blood, is present. For this reason, instruments like curettes used in cerumen removal, impedance probe tips, and otoscopic specula should be sterilized after use when visibly contaminated with cerumen, ear drainage, or blood. The process requires cleaning first with an ultrasonic cleaner, disinfectant towelette, or cleaning brush, then sterilizing the instruments in an autoclave or 2% glutaraldehyde (Protocol 11–4).

SPECIAL CONSIDERATION

Glutaraldehyde, although an effective sterilant and disinfectant, must be handled very carefully. This chemical should never come in contact with skin or clothing. Persons who handle it should wear gloves and safety glasses. Glutaraldehyde fumes may irritate the eyes and nose and can cause respiratory problems. Good ventilation is necessary in rooms and cabinets where the soaking tray is stored. Soaking trays should have a lid that should be kept closed when not accessing the tray. Never use glutaraldehyde in an ultrasonic cleaner because the cavitation created by the machine spreads the glutaraldehyde fumes.

CONTROLLING THE HUMAN SOURCE OF INFECTION

Medical Case History

If feasible, a full medical history of a patient can assist in reducing potential exposure. For example, identifying a case of shingles (herpes zoster) while taking a medical history would alert the clinician to question an unusual looking sore. Identifying a patient taking an anticoagulant (blood thinner; one brand is Coumadin, the generic name is warfarin) would warn the practitioner of a greater potential for excessive bleeding. It may be impractical to ascertain case histories in a group setting like schools or industry. Still, when possible, a medical case history should be taken.

Hand Washing

As previously mentioned, hand washing is critical to any infection control program (see Figure 11–2 and Protocol 11–5). Ideally, hands should be washed before and after each patient. This is often a challenge for audiologists because access to a sink and running water is often inconvenient or impossible. An antimicrobial "no rinse" hand degermer may effectively be used. Most of these products have an alcohol base, which dissipates quickly with no need for drying with a towel. Alcohol is an example of a germicide that is used both as a disinfectant for skin and inanimate objects. However, other germicides may not serve this dual purpose. It is important to be aware of a germicide's ingredients and properties and whether it is suitable for use on human skin.

When hand washing facilities are used, the skin must be washed by rubbing vigorously to clean hands, wrists, and

SPECIAL CONSIDERATION

A good infection control program requires frequent hand washing, which can lead to chapping. Unfortunately, chapping is a problem in infection control because it allows organisms into the body. Care must be taken to use medical grade lotion soap, which helps to protect hands with emollient-rich formulas. Hand lotion may be used to further care for hands, but care should be taken to avoid petroleum-based lotion that renders latex gloves ineffective.

lower forearms. The use of a medical grade liquid antibacterial soap that contains emollients to protect hands from drying is recommended. Medical grade antibacterial soap is gentler than household antibacterial soaps because it is designed for people who wash their hands more frequently than the average person. Bar soap is a great breeding ground for germs and should be avoided.

Gloves

All audiometric procedures, including hearing and immittance screenings performed by audiologists, should begin

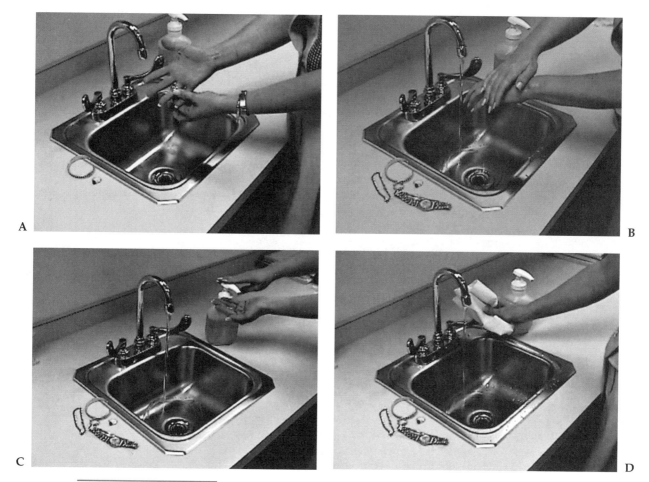

Figure 11–2 Proper hand washing includes removing jewelry (rings, watches, and bracelets) **(A)**; starting the water and applying antibacterial soap **(B)**; washing hands thoroughly, making sure to scrub palms, back of hands up to wrists and forearms **(C)**; and rinsing under water and drying with paper towel. When finished, the water is turned off using the paper towel **(D)**.

with a thorough inspection of the ear, surrounding facial area, and scalp. An otoscopic inspection of the circumaural region and earcanal should be conducted, confirming that the skin is intact and that no blood or ear drainage is present. After completing this inspection, a determination of the necessity of gloves can be made. Gloves should be worn whenever the patient has a draining ear, when blood is present, when sores or lesions are evident on the ear or scalp, or when a medical history indicates an infectious disease.

Gloves should be worn prophylactically when the risk of encountering infectious substances is high. In audiology practice, using gloves should be considered during cerumen management, for real-ear measurements, and while handling ear-mold impressions. Furthermore, gloves should be worn by audiologists providing intraoperative monitoring services in the operating room for several reasons. Monitoring involves insertion of needle electrodes, and gloves should also be worn while handling, inserting, and disposing of needle electrodes to reduce the risk of exposure to bodily fluids.

During closing procedures, when monitoring is no longer used, the audiologist may choose to disconnect the electrode

---

PEARL

It is often difficult for an audiologist to find a sink for hand washing, particularly in private practice where the only sink is often in the bathroom. Waterless hand degermers are an excellent way to clean and disinfect hands in the absence of soap and water.

---

leads from the patient interface and retrieve intraoperative monitoring cables. Because the floor directly below the patient may be soiled with blood products, gloves should be worn during clean up. Gloves should also be worn when cleaning up spills of infectious waste and while disinfecting a contaminated area. After use, gloves should be properly discarded and hands should be washed immediately after removing gloves. Unless grossly contaminated with blood or other bodily fluids, gloves should be discarded in the regular trash (see "Waste Management," which follows) (Protocol 11–6).

PROTOCOL 11–5

Hand Washing

The single, most important activity that limits the spread of infectious disease in the office is washing hands regularly and thoroughly. It is important to always wash hands before and after eating, adjusting contact lenses, handling waiting room toys, performing sterilization procedures, applying cosmetics or lip balm, smoking, or handling undisinfected earmolds or ITE aids. Always wash your hands after removing gloves, contacting any potential or actual contamination, toileting, or completing the day's work. Use of the following guidelines will safeguard against the spread of infectious diseases:

1. Remove all rings and put them in a safe place away from drains. Micro-organisms cannot be eliminated from skin beneath rings and growth is facilitated in warm, moist dark spaces such as exists under rings. Such colonization is a potential risk to the patient and to the employee.

2. Wash hands before and after each patient. When water is not available, use a "no rinse" antibacterial hand degermer. When water is available, use a medical grade antibacterial soap containing emollients to keep your hands from drying out too much.

3. Start the water and apply a liquid antibacterial soap. Lather up the soap, scrubbing your palms, the backs of your hands and up over your wrists onto your forearms for a minimum of 10 seconds. Clean all surfaces, especially under fingernails and between fingers.

4. Thoroughly rinse off the soap under running water.

5. Dry your hands by blotting using a paper towel. Rubbing with the paper towel is chafing to the skin.

6. Turn off the water with the paper towel, not your clean hand.

7. Wash your hands after removing gloves.

8. Wash hands before and after eating, adjusting contact lenses, handling waiting room toys and undisinfected earmolds or ITE aids.

9. Use lotion as needed to keep hands from chapping. Avoid petroleum-based lotions because these negatively affect latex gloves.

Adapted from Kemp et al (1995).

PEARL

Double gloving decreases the risk of inadvertent puncture (Enders, Jones, Jones, and Mornsey, 1990). Studies have demonstrated both a decreased inner glove puncture rate and a decreased cutaneous exposure when double gloves are used (Murr & Lee, 1995).

PITFALL

Various types of electrodes are used in the operating room for intraoperative monitoring, including subdermal needle electrodes and hook wire electrodes. Needles should not be recapped, particularly when hook wire electrodes are used, because this electrode type involves insertion and immediate removal of a hyperdermic needle into tissue. Recapping needles is the single most common cause of needle sticks (Gold & Tami, 1998).

Protective Apparel

Safety glasses and disposable masks are necessary when risk of splash or splatter of potentially infectious material exists, or when the clinician or patient is at risk of airborne contamination. Cerumen removal by irrigation may require safety glasses or masks if the splash of the irrigation is significant. Also, safety glasses and a mask should be worn when working with a grinding or buffing wheel to reduce the chance of microorganisms and particles of plastic from being inhaled or landing in eyes. Also, masks should be worn in the presence of patients with TB or immunocompromised individuals who may be at risk from droplet contact. Disposable headphone covers should be considered to reduce the risk of cross-contamination. These can be particularly important for mass screenings.

Vaccination

One of the most effective forms of controlling infection is through vaccination. Measles, mumps, rubella, tetanus, influenza, tuberculosis, smallpox, polio, pertussis (whooping cough), diphtheria, hepatitis A, and hepatitis B are all preventable through vaccination. Vaccinations should be seriously considered for all healthcare professionals.

PROTOCOL 11–6

Gloves

Follow these guidelines for proper use of gloves:

1. Select latex (or vinyl if you or your patient shows sensitivity to latex) examination gloves making sure that they fit properly. Properly fitted gloves will fit tightly like a second skin. This is important because loose-fitting gloves make for frustration because of a lack of dexterity. This frustration is the main reason people stop wearing gloves.

2. Always change gloves between patients. If a glove becomes torn or perforated, replace it.

3. If questioned about the use of gloves, explain that gloves are worn to protect patients and to provide the best in modern care. Most people expect gloves to be worn. Most other healthcare professionals wear gloves as a precautionary measure.

4. Use the following procedure to safely remove gloves, making sure that the hands do not make contact with potentially infectious material. First, peel off one glove from wrist to fingertip, then grasp it in the gloved hand. Next, using the bared hand, peel off the second glove from the inside tucking the first glove inside the second glove as it is removed. Wash hands thoroughly when completed.

Adapted from Kemp et al (1995).

Waste Management

Waste (gloves, wipes, paper towels, etc.) that is contaminated with blood or ear drainage or cerumen containing blood or ear drainage can be placed in the regular trash unless the amount of blood or mucus is significant. Materials containing significant amounts of blood should be discarded in impermeable bags labeled with the symbol for biohazard. This would include gross amounts of material; that is, biohazard bags are not needed for the regular amount of cerumen removed from a patient's ears. Rather, biohazard bags should be used for large amounts of visible blood and the materials used to clean it up. This waste should be picked up by a waste hauler licensed for medical waste disposal. When placing lesser contaminated waste in the regular trash, an attempt should be made to separate it from the rest of the trash to minimize the chance of clean up personnel making casual contact with it. This can be accomplished by placing such waste in small plastic bags or wrapping it in paper.

Instruments with sharp points or edges, including scalpel blades or needles, must be discarded properly. Approximately 4.4. million healthcare workers in the United States receive an estimated 800,000 needle sticks and other injuries from sharp objects annually (29 CFR Part 1910.1030, 1991).

When disposing of sharp instruments in the operating room, the use of a kidney basin or similar object should be used to transport the sharp instruments from the vicinity of the patient to the sharps container. A sharps container is usually a red-colored, durable plastic container found in every operating room. The container is labeled as a biohazard that must be handled by a licensed waste disposal company.

> **PEARL**
>
> Latex gloves interact with silicone impression material keeping it from setting up properly. Wash hands thoroughly before taking an impression, then wear gloves to remove the impression and for handling it after it is removed from the ear.

> **SPECIAL CONSIDERATION**
>
> In the event of blood or bodily fluid exposure, any exposed skin or wound should be immediately washed with soap and water. The incident should be clearly documented and reported to appropriate hospital personnel. If the patient's HIV status is unknown, informed consent should be obtained to test the patient's HIV status. Baseline HIV testing should be obtained to confirm HIV status of the exposed healthcare worker at the time of exposure. Periodic retesting at 6 weeks, 3 months, and 6 months after exposure is recommended (CDC, 1989). Healthcare workers occupationally exposed to HIV have the option of undergoing postexposure treatment with the antiretroviral zidovudine (AZT) in an effort to protect against seroconversion.

CONCLUSIONS

Infection control is an important aspect of healthcare. Recommended procedures and guidelines are not complex; however, infection control protocols do require diligence and consistency. When taken for granted, insufficiently executed, incorrectly applied, or completely ignored potential consequences often put the health of patients and healthcare workers at a considerable risk of contracting a life-threatening infection or disease. The information covered in this chapter should provide audiologists with a basic appreciation for infection control and the necessary guidelines to develop clinic-specific infection control policies.

REFERENCES

ABBAS, A.K., LICHTMAN, A.H., & POBER, J.S. (1994). *Cellular and molecular immunology* (2nd ed.). Philadelphia: W.B. Saunders.

BANKAITIS, A.E. (1996). Audiological changes attributable to HIV-infection. *Audiology Today, 8*(6);14–16.

BANKAITIS, A.E. (1998a). Preface. *Seminars in hearing, 19*(2); 117–118.

BANKAITIS, A.E. (1998b). An introduction to HIV/AIDS. *Seminars in Hearing, 19*(2);119–130.

BREATHNACH, A.S., JENKINS, D.R., & PEDLER, S.J. (1992). Stethoscopes as possible vectors of infection by staphylococci. *British Medical Journal, 305*;1573.

BURNET, M. (1963). *Natural history of infectious diseases* (3rd ed.). London: Cambridge University Press.

CDC. (1981). *Pneumocystis pneumonia*—Los Angeles. *MMWR, Morbidity and Mortality Weekly Report, 30*;250–252.

CDC. (1988). Update: Universal precaution of transmission of human immunodeficiency virus, hepatitis B virus, and other bloodborne pathogens in health-care settings. *MMWR, Morbidity and Mortality Weekly Report, 37*;377–388.

CDC. (1989). Guidelines for prevention of transmission of human immunodevidiency virus and hepatitis B to healthcare and public-safety workers. *MMWR, Morbidity and Mortality Weekly Report, 38.*

CLARK, W.R. (1991). *The experimental foundations of modern immunology.* (ed. 4). New York: John Wiley & Sons.

ENDERS, D., JONES, T.A., & MORRISEY, M.S. (1990). The effectiveness of double gloving in otolaryngology. *Clinical Otolaryngology, 15*;535–536.

EPA. (1998a). EPA's mission. Available: http://www.epa.gov/epahome/epa.html.

EPA. (1998b). Office of pesticide programs. Available: http://www.epa.gov/pesticides/about.htm.

CDC. (1987). Recommendations for prevention of HIV transmission in healthcare settings. *MMWR, Morbidity and Mortality Weekly Report, 36,* (suppl); 2S.

EPA. (1998c). FIFRA, FQPA, and other regulatory and legislative information. Available: http://www.epa.gov/opp00001/regleg.htm.

EPA. (1979). US Government EPA Definitions, DIS/TSS-1.

FDA. (1998a). Frequently asked questions. Available: http://www.fda.gov/opacom/faqs/genfaqs.html.

FDA. (1998b). The food and drug administration: An overview. Available: http://www.fda.gov/opacom/hpview.html.

GOLD, S. & TAMI, T.A. (1998). Otolaryngological manifestations of HIV/AIDS. *Seminars in Hearing, 19*(2);165–176.

JCAHO. (1998). Facts about the Joint Commission on Accreditation of Healthcare Organizations. Available: http://www.jcaho.org/about_jc/jcinfo.htm.

JOHNSEN, B. (1998). Legal support for patients and audiologists with HIV. *Seminars in Hearing, 19*(2);215–226.

KEMP, R.J., ROESER, R.J., PEARSON, D.W., & BALLANCHANDA, B.P. (1995). *Infection control for the professional of audiology and speech language pathology.* Olathe, KS: Iles Publications.

KEMP, R.J. & ROESER, R.J. (1998). Infection control for audiologists. *Seminars in Hearing, 19*(2);195–204.

KRAUSE, R. (1992). The origin of plagues: Old and new. *Science, 217*;1073–1078.

LEVINS, R., AWERBUCH, T., BRINKMANN, U., ECKARDT, I., EPSTEIN, P., MAKHOUL, N., DE POSSAS, C., PUCCIA, C., SPIELMAN, A., & WILSON, M. (1994). The emergence of new diseases. *American Scientist, 82*;52–60.

MURR, A.H. & LEE, K.C. (1995). Universal precautions for the otolaryngologist: Techniques and equipment for minimizing exposure risk. *ENT Journal, 74*;338–346.

OSHA. (1997). *OSHA facts: Common sense at work.* Washington, DC: U.S. Department of Labor.

OSHA. (1998). Introduction. Available: http://www.oshaslc.gov/OshAct_data/OSH_ACT1.html.

RUTALA, W.A. (1990) APIC guideline for selection and use of disinfectants. *American Journal of Infection Control, 17*(52);99–117.

SCOUNTZ, T. & BANKAITIS, A.E. (1998). Basic anatomy and physiology of the immune system. *Seminars in Hearing, 19*(2);131–142.

STAINES, N., BROSTOFF, J., & JAMES, K. (1993). *Introducing immunology* (2nd ed.). St. Louis: Mosby.

WEINHOLD, K.J. (1993). Basic concepts of the immune response and the immunology of HIV infection. In J. Bartlett (Ed.), *Care and management of patient with HIV-infection.* Research Triangle Park, NC: Glaxo, Inc.

Chapter 12

Cerumen Management

Ross J. Roeser and Phillip L. Wilson

The human earcanal is the primary acoustic pathway to the auditory system. Because of its fundamental role in audition, audiologists are required to have a thorough understanding of all aspects of earcanal anatomy, physiology, and pathophysiology. Audiologists must also be able to examine the earcanal properly and identify normal structures and abnormal conditions. In addition, the practice of performing cerumen management in routine practice is now commonplace in audiological practice.

This chapter covers the topic of cerumen management. The rationale for including cerumen management in audiology practice is discussed. Normal and abnormal aspects of earcanal anatomy and physiology are presented, followed by a thorough description of issues and procedures to carry out cerumen management.

CERUMEN MANAGEMENT IN THE PRACTICE OF AUDIOLOGY

The presence of occluding cerumen in the earcanal is a pathological condition; it can cause conductive hearing loss and tinnitus, vertigo, and skin irritation with accompanying itching and pain. Cerumen removal will result in immediately improved hearing; in fact, if sensorineural sensitivity is normal, cerumen removal will restore hearing sensitivity to normal levels.

Figure 12–1 shows audiometric data from a 58-year-old patient with impacted cerumen. As shown in this figure, a severe hearing loss is present when the earcanal is impacted

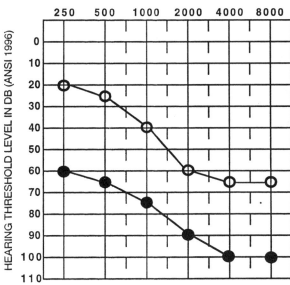

AUDIOGRAM

FREQUENCY IN HERTZ

Figure 12–1 Audiometric data from a 58-year-old man with and without impacted cerumen. Before cerumen removal, results showed a severe hearing loss (*closed symbols*). After cerumen removal, thresholds improved to a moderate loss (*open symbols*).

with cerumen. After cerumen removal, thresholds improve by about 30- to 35-dB to the moderate level. This case study clearly illustrates the effect of impacted cerumen on threshold sensitivity and provides an example of the potential improvement in communication abilities that can result when cerumen is removed.

Beyond the removal of occluding cerumen that results in hearing loss and other possible sequelae, the practice of audiology requires that the earcanal be reasonably clear of cerumen for a number of routine procedures; for others an earcanal completely free from cerumen is required. Included are the following:

- Making earmold impressions for hearing aids
- Probe microphone measures
- Using insert earphones
- Electrocochleography

273

- Electronystagmography
- Immittance measures
- Otoacoustic emissions

The degree to which an earcanal is required to be free of cerumen depends on the audiological procedure to be performed. The introduction into the market and popularity of completely-in-the-canal (CIC) style hearing aids requires taking deep impressions of the earcanal. Because of the sensitivity of the earcanal and the need for an excellent fit for this style of amplification, an earcanal completely free of cerumen is required. Placement of the otoblock near the tympanic membrane may present problems to the patient if some cerumen remains in the earcanal because the otoblock may cause the cerumen to be moved against the tympanic membrane. An inaccurate impression, caused by the presence of cerumen in the earcanal, may cause a hearing aid that is either uncomfortable or likely to create feedback. Cerumen management is typically required before taking impressions for CIC hearing aids.

The necessity for a completely clear canal is not so great when taking impressions for in-the-ear (ITE) and in-the-canal (ITC) style hearing aids or behind-the-ear (BTE) earmolds. However, for any type of hearing aid the more accurate the impression the more likely the hearing aid will fit properly. Cerumen management is a prerequisite when taking ear impressions for a significant number of patients.

Real-ear measures of hearing aid characteristics require the placement of a probe microphone in the earcanal near the tympanic membrane. The small diameters of the probe tubes can easily be clogged with cerumen, which will confound results of the probe microphone measurement. In addition, excessive amounts of cerumen may create unusual resonances in the measurement, not representative of hearing aid performance at the tympanic membrane (Ballachanda, 1995). For these reasons a clean earcanal is essential for accurate and effective probe microphone measurement of hearing aid performance.

The use of insert earphones has several advantages in audiometric testing (see Chapter 11 in *Diagnosis*). As a result, the use of insert earphones is becoming more popular in standard audiology practice, not only for routine threshold audiometry but also in the performance of auditory brainstem response (ABR) and electrocochleography. The presence of significant amounts of cerumen within the earcanal can change the output characteristics of earphones and response characteristics of the earcanal (Ballachanda, 1995; Gerling et al, 1992; 1997). In addition, as with the insertion of an otoblock for taking ear impressions, the insertion of the insert earphone into the earcanal may force cerumen toward the tympanic membrane, increasing earcanal blockage. Excessive or impacted cerumen may even fill the opening of the insert earphone, which would significantly reduce the sound pressure level of the stimuli reaching the tympanic membrane.

Electronystagmography (ENG) relies on the ability of the examiner to direct a flow of air or water directly against the tympanic membrane. The presence of excessive or impacted cerumen may result in inaccurate results, and cerumen management is required before testing when an excessive amount of cerumen is present.

When performing immittance measures and otoacoustic emissions, a probe tip is placed into the external earcanal. If significant amounts of cerumen are present, the probe tip can clog with excessive cerumen and result in invalid findings. For example, with immittance measures test results indicating a flat tympanogram with absent reflexes would result. Earcanals with enough cerumen to clog immittance and otoacoustic emission instrument probe tips must be cleaned for test results to be obtained.

In addition to the need for cerumen management in routine audiological testing, cerumen management is an important part of the hearing–healthcare delivery system. Rather than performing cerumen management as part of audiological practice, if patients are referred for cerumen management, a delay in diagnosis and treatment will occur. In addition, the patient may have questions regarding the audiologist's level of training and skills or even competence. Confusion may be created about the case managers for audiological treatment.

A more pragmatic issue in referring patients with excessive/impacted cerumen to physicians' offices is that it does not ensure effective treatment. Survey data show that cerumen is typically removed in physicians' offices by individuals who have little or no formal training in the anatomy of the earcanal or in the procedures and precautions necessary for safe and effective cerumen removal (Sharp et al, 1990). Mahoney (1993) reports in a study of cerumen impaction among nursing home residents in Massachusetts that it was often difficult to get physicians to respond to requests for cerumen removal. She noted that the physicians responsible for the care of these elderly residents apparently assumed the patients had permanent age-related hearing loss and did not believe that the removal of impacted cerumen was of enough importance to warrant the time involved to clear the impaction. However, more significant from Mahoney's study was the finding that of those individuals who did receive treatment for impacted cerumen, most ears remained impacted after treatment. This information does not necessarily imply that physicians do not have the knowledge and skills necessary to successfully manage excessive cerumen. It does imply that very often physicians believe that cerumen management is a low priority and that the procedure is often relegated to other personnel who may or may not have the necessary skills.

Audiologists have the academic training and requisite skills to perform cerumen management. Over the last several years the American Speech-Language-Hearing Association (ASHA), the American Academy of Audiology (AAA), and the Academy of Dispensing Audiologists (ADA) have included cerumen removal as a part of the scope of practice for audiologists. At the same time, many state licensing laws have been rewritten to include cerumen management as a recognized procedure to be performed by the licensed audiologist. Improved opportunities in graduate training programs and heightened awareness of the need for cerumen management by audiologists has significantly increased the number of audiologists who are practicing cerumen management in routine practice.

Some audiologists choose not to practice cerumen management, which is their prerogative. It appears that uncertainty regarding the appropriate procedures and the fear of liability for a patient being injured are the primary deterring factors (Primus & Skordas, 1996).

The issue of liability is important in this discussion. Like other clinical procedures, audiologists must recognize that cerumen management entails risks, including injury to the earcanal, perforation of the tympanic membrane, exacerbation of chronic middle ear disease, and possible damage to the ossicular chain (Sharp et al, 1990). Primus and Skordas (1996) surveyed 500 audiologists on their cerumen management practices. For those audiologists choosing not to manage cerumen, patient injury and the audiologist's liability for injury were among the main concerns. Every procedure performed in an audiologist's practice potentially can result in a malpractice lawsuit. A successful outcome is not guaranteed when any procedure is performed. An audiologist's protection in the event of litigation is to have demonstrable knowledge, skill, and experience to perform the procedure. Practitioners increase their chances of success in these situations by using their knowledge, skill, and experience to consider all aspects of the procedure, to perform the procedure with care, and to document the procedure accurately.

Whether a specific audiological procedure is covered by an insurance carrier is not always clear, and contacting the carrier will not necessarily clarify procedures or practices that are covered or the extent to which they are covered. A typical response from an insurance carrier when asked whether a specific procedure is covered will be vague and indicate that the procedures are covered if they do not violate existing law and are included as part of normal audiological practice (Manning, 1992). Clinicians are individually responsible to ensure they are practicing according to the standard of care within the scope of their practice.

Audiologists can perform cerumen management safely and effectively by taking a thorough case history, understanding the contraindications for cerumen management, and selecting the method most likely to achieve the desired result. If this general series of actions is taken, the risks in removing cerumen are as minimal as most other procedures audiologists routinely perform.

ANATOMY

Figure 12–2 shows a cross section of the human earcanal. The S-shaped earcanal is a membranocartilaginous structure that begins at the pinna and terminates at the tympanic membrane. The outer one-third to one-half of the earcanal is cartilaginous

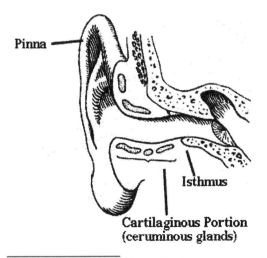

Figure 12–2   Cross section of the human earcanal.

and is covered with relatively thick skin. The remaining portion of the earcanal is bony and is covered with a thin layer of skin that is sensitive to pain. A narrowing of the canal called the isthmus is located at the boundary between the cartilaginous and osseous portions of the earcanal. This narrowing at the isthmus restricts the ability to visualize the tympanic membrane.

PEARL

Practitioners should be particularly careful not to scrape the deep portions of the earcanal when using mechanical removal because it may cause pain for the patient and is more likely to bleed.

Cerumen, the waxy substance found in normal earcanals, is primarily composed of the secretions of two types of glands found in the cartilaginous portion of the earcanal. Sebaceous glands produce a fatty substance called sebum and modified apocrine (ceruminous) glands produce apocrine sweat. Sebum and apocrine sweat combine with desquamated epithelial cells, dust, and other small foreign bodies and shed hair to make up cerumen (Perry, 1957).

The two types of cerumen are the "dry" or "rice-bran" type and the "wet" or "sticky" type. The dry type of cerumen is found in 78 to 87% of the Asian population (Matsunaga, 1962). The Asian population has a tendency for underproducing cerumen, resulting in dryness of the external earcanal (Meyers, 1977; Perry, 1957). This clinical observation suggests a scarcity of sebaceous and apocrine glands for Asians (Perry, 1957). The dry type of cerumen is odorless because of the reduced number of apocrine sweat glands found in the Asian population, apocrine sweat being primarily responsible for the odor of cerumen (Matsunaga, 1962). Presence of an odor accompanying cerumen in the Asian population is of diagnostic significance because it often indicates the presence of an accompanying pathological condition (Matsunaga, 1962).

The "wet" or "sticky" type of cerumen is prevalent in 95 to 98% of Caucasians and Negroid racial types (Petrakis, 1969). Provided no pathological condition is present, the distinction between the two types of cerumen is so clear that distinguishing between them can be made by a simple inspection of the earcanals.

Chromatographic analysis of wet and dry cerumen samples has shown that cerumen type is due to differences in quantity and composition of ear wax lipids. Dry cerumen contains aqualene, triglycerides, free fatty acids, cholesterol, nonlipid substances, steryl esters, and wax esters. However, wet cerumen does not contain the nonlipid substance, steryl esters, and wax esters (Inaba et al, 1987).

Dry cerumen is brittle and appears "ashlike and flaky" and ranges in color from light gray to brownish gray. Because it is exposed over time to air, bacterial activity, oxidation, and dehydration, it changes its color from golden brown to almost black (Matsunaga, 1962). Clinicians must be aware of the normal color variations of cerumen types when examining earcanals and have familiarity with the association between color and consistency of cerumen and race. The decision to remove cerumen from an earcanal must be made on the basis of the conclusion from otoscopic examination that the material in the earcanal is, in fact, cerumen and not some other substance, such as blood or purulent material.

PEARL

Clinicians must be aware of the normal color variations of cerumen and have familiarity with the association between color, consistency, and race.

Cerumen type is inherited as a simple mendelian trait, with the dry type allele (mutational gene group) being recessive to the wet type (Bass & Jackson, 1977). The genetically based polymorphic nature of cerumen has been used to study both genetics and anthropology (Matsunaga, 1962).

PHYSIOLOGY

Although the physiological factors that control the sebaceous glands in the earcanal are not fully known, the function of the apocrine (ceruminous) sweat glands has been well established. Perry (1957) studied cerumen production by direct visualization of the skin of the distal portion of the earcanal in 150 subjects. Production of apocrine sweat increased in the presence of smooth muscle stimulants (pitocin); adrenergic drugs (epinephrine and norepinephine); and the emotional states of anxiety, fear, and pain. Ceruminous glands also increased production when the canal wall was cleaned or rubbed in an action called "mechanical milking." Perry also found in some cases that vigorous chewing caused earcanal distortions that caused the same milking effect.

Cerumen cleans and lubricates the earcanal. Literature reports that the earcanal is protected from bacteria, fungus, and insects by cerumen (Adams et al, 1978; Caruso et al, 1980; Hawke, 1987). The cleaning function is the result of epithelial migration. Cerumen produced in the earcanal migrates toward the earcanal entrance. Dust and other small particles adhere to the cerumen and are cast off as the cerumen is extruded. Alberti (1964) studied this "conveyor belt" process by quantifying the growth, migration, and desquamation of the skin covering the tympanic membrane and deep earcanal in 62 human subjects. Weekly estimates of rate and migration patterns were made from dye spots placed on the eardrumhead for each subject with hand-made sketches and serial photography. Migration was found to be centrifugal from the umbo spreading to all quadrants of the tympanic membrane. Near the umbo the rate of migration was equivalent to the rate of growth of a fingernail. The rate of migration accelerated as the markers moved away from the umbo, with the most rapid migration taking place on the anterior wall of the external earcanal.

Jaw motion also helps to clean the earcanal. Debris attached to the earcanal wall is dislodged during speech and chewing as the jaw rotates vertically and horizontally about the terminal hinge axis of the temporomandibular joint, which makes up the inferior portion of the earcanal (Edwards & Harris, 1990).

The lubricating function of cerumen occurs because of the high lipid concentration of sebum, the substance produced by the sebaceous glands. This high lipid concentration accounts for its hydrophobic properties because it acts as a natural emollient. Harvey (1989) used chromatography to analyze lipid concentrations in wet-type human cerumen and found the major constituents to be cholesterol, squalene, and several series of long-chain fatty acids and alcohols. Bortz et al (1990) made a similar observation.

PEARL

Allowing the patient to visualize the amount of cerumen removed from the earcanal may increase the patient's future efforts to be seen on a timely basis for cerumen management, especially if multiple hearing aid repairs have been needed for the patient.

Cerumen's cleaning and lubricating function is better understood than its antibacterial properties. Some controversy exists because some histological and histochemical studies have failed to support cerumen as a bactericide. Creed and Negus (1926) found that freshly secreted cerumen contained no bacteria, but quickly became contaminated with bacteria. They concluded that cerumen's protective function was to prevent the entrance of dust and insects into the earcanal, acting like a type of "flypaper." Perry and Nichols (1957) supported this finding by observing that cerumen did not inhibit the growth of *Pseudomonas aeruginosa*, when this bacteria was cultured from the earcanals of 45 healthy adult volunteers. After examining the effect of cerumen on the organism's growth, it was determined that no inhibition was present.

Other studies have found that cerumen is effective against certain bacteria. Chai and Chai (1980) showed the viability of *Haemophilus influenzae*, *Escherichia coli* K-12, and *Serratia marcescens* were reduced by more than 99%, and the viability of two *P. aeruginosa* isolates (*E. coli* K-1, *Streptococcus*) and two *Staphylococcus aureus* isolates was reduced by 30 to 80%. Stone and Fulghum (1984) also showed that a suspension of cerumen in a buffered medium inhibited the growth of certain bacteria (*S. aureus*, *Staphylococcus epidermidis*, *Streptococcus pyogenes*, *Streptococcus* sp. L22, *E. coli*, *S. marcescens*, *propionibacterium acnes*, *corynebacterium* spp JOM 125 and 138). On the basis of the more recent studies, it can be concluded that cerumen most likely provides some bacterial protection against some strains of bacteria. The presence of cerumen in the earcanal acts as an oily barrier, preventing the ingress of microorganisms into the skin, and contains antimicrobial substances, including lysozyme, IgA, and fatty acids (Osborne & Baty, 1990).

The warm, dark, moist conditions in the earcanal are conducive to the growth of fungus. Hawke (1994) called the earcanal the "greenhouse of the human body." A study by Megarry et al (1988) documented the antifungal properties of cerumen. It was shown that human cerumen inhibited the growth of *Candida* and *Aspergillus*, two species of fungi commonly encountered in otomycosis. The growth of fungus requires an environment with low acidity, and the presence of fatty acids in cerumen may inhibit fungal growth (Osborne & Baty, 1990).

Although the amount of cerumen in earcanals varies widely, more striking is the variation in the amount of cerumen across certain populations. Table 12–1 provides data

TABLE 12–1 Prevalence of excessive/impacted cerumen in different populations*

	Sample Size	Prevalence (%)
Children		
Roche et al (1978)	224	10
Bricco (1985)	349	10
Adults		
Gleitman et al (1992)	892	5–34[†]
Lebensohn (1943)	794	2.5
Lebensohn (1943)	3258	8
Perry (1957)	111	17
Hopkinson (1981)	500	4
Foltner (1984)	100	9
Cooper (1985)	587	5
Individuals with mental retardation		
Nudo (1965)	494	36
Fulton and Griffin (1967)	191	28
Brister et al (1986)	88	22
Dahle and McCollister (1986)	18	31
Crandell and Roeser (1993)	121	28
Geriatric population		
Mahoney (1987)	133	34–57[‡]
Lewis-Cullinan and Janken (1990)	226	35
Mahoney (1993)	104	25–42[§]

[*] Adapted from Roeser et al (1992).
[†] The prevalence was age dependent, with the older subjects having a higher prevalence.
[‡] Thirty-four percent of the subjects were found to have impacted cerumen and an additional 23% had moderate-to-large amounts of cerumen for a total of 57% with excessive/impacted cerumen.
[§] Twenty-five percent of the subjects were found to have impacted cerumen and an additional 17% had moderate-to-large amounts of cerumen for a total of 42% with excessive/impacted cerumen.

from children and adults and from two special populations: individuals with mental retardation and the geriatric population. In children, two studies found the prevalence of excessive cerumen to be about 10% (Bricco, 1985; Roche et al, 1978). On the basis of clinical experience, the 10% prevalence found in these studies appears to be high and may be due to the low number of subjects in the samples. Clinical experience would suggest that the prevalence of excessive cerumen in normal children is similar to adults and ranges from about 3 to 5%.

As shown in Table 12–1, data from seven studies found the prevalence of excessive cerumen in adults to be from 4 to 34%. Lebensohn (1943) studied the largest sample of adults. In two groups of naval personnel aged 20 to 50, results showed occluding cerumen in 2.5% of 794 reserve midshipmen and in 7.7% of 3258 officers. No hypothesis was given for the sizable difference between the two groups. Methodological differences and sample size may account for some of the variability in prevalence rates shown in Table 12–1. A general tendency exists for the studies with the larger sample sizes to have lower prevalence rates. However, these data also suggest that complex interactions may account for occluding cerumen.

Histochemical studies were performed on cerumen samples from 90 subjects with normal and excessive cerumen to determine whether excessive accumulation resulted from failure of normal migration, physiology, or hyperactivity of the ceruminous glands (Mandour et al, 1974). Enzymatic

histochemical examination on biopsy specimens of earcanal skin strips was performed. Results showed the lumina of the glands was distended in those with excessive cerumen, with the appearance of secretion in the apical parts of the lining of cells, indicating increased secretory activity. This finding suggests that in this study population, excessive cerumen is due primarily to an increase in the activity of the ceruminous glands.

Although Robinson et al (1990) agree that increased cerumen production may account for excessive cerumen in some patients, they argue that cerumen type affects the process. In two studies Robinson et al (1990) analyzed hydrated cerumen plugs taken from cerumen samples of 28 individuals and found that those with wet-type cerumen of the hard variety were more commonly found to have chronic and recurrent cerumen impaction. Hard cerumen plugs also contained more sheets of keratin than soft cerumen plugs. From their results they conclude that patients with chronic and recurrent cerumen impaction have a disorder of keratinocyte separation, resulting in a failure in the breakup or separation of the individual keratinocytes, which normally occurs in the earcanal. This condition reduces the integrity of the outwardly migrating sheets of epithelium (Robinson et al, 1990). Taken together the results of the Mandour and Robinson studies suggest that excessive cerumen is related to a complex interaction of multiple factors.

Several studies suggest no apparent gender difference in the chemical make up or amount of cerumen in the earcanal

(Cipriani et al, 1990; Mandour et al, 1974; Roche et al, 1978; Yassin et al, 1966). Seasonal factors and marked racial differences in the appearance and chemical composition of cerumen have been reported. Cipriani et al (1990) studied cerumen over a 9-month period (November to July) and found decreasing triglyceride production as the seasons progressed from the winter to the summer months. It is suggested in this study that a relationship exists between seasonal diet and triglyceride levels in the earcanal, and a correlation is postulated between earcanal infectious pathological conditions and triglyceride levels.

As shown in Table 12–1, patients with mental retardation and geriatric patients are two populations that clearly have a high prevalence of excessive cerumen. Nudo (1965) was among the first to document that patients with mental retardation are more likely to have excessive cerumen than the general population. He found that 34% of 178 individuals in a residential center for mentally retarded adults had abnormal amounts of cerumen or foreign bodies in their earcanals and that 23% exhibited hearing loss. Fulton and Griffin (1967) reported that 55 of 191 subjects (28%) had impacted cerumen, with 29 of those (54%) having bilateral impaction and 26 (46%) having unilateral impaction. Comparing otoscopic results from 44 mentally retarded adolescents to a typically developing control group matched for age and sex, Brister et al (1986) found a prevalence of excessive cerumen of 34% for the subjects with mental retardation; none of the normal controls were found to have excessive or impacted cerumen.

Crandell and Roeser (1993) studied longitudinal data from 117 adults with mental retardation (20 to 67 years of age) living in a privately owned residential center to document prevalence rates of excessive and impacted cerumen. Retrospective data analysis was performed by examining annual audiological and otoscopic records from a 12-year period. Results from otoscopy were categorized into (a) nonoccluded (less than 50% occluded), (b) excessive cerumen (50 to 80% occluded), and (c) impacted cerumen (greater than 80% occluded). Of the 586 otoscopic examinations performed, 165 (28%) revealed excessive or impacted cerumen. Another significant finding was that recurrence of excessive and impacted cerumen occurred in 54% of those with *excessive* cerumen on the first examination and 66% of those with *impacted* cerumen on the first examination. These findings clearly show that individuals with mental retardation have a propensity to have excessive cerumen on serial examinations. The specific reason for abnormal cerumen accumulation and this propensity for serial problems is unknown. Clearly, regular otoscopy and earcanal management is a necessity for this population, and healthcare professionals working in these settings must be aware of the negative effect of excessive and impacted cerumen on the hearing health of those afflicted.

As individuals age, the secretion of the ceruminous glands decreases, as does the actual number of ceruminous glands. This results in a drier type of cerumen. This fact coupled with an increase in the number and coarseness of hairs in the earcanal, especially in men, causes an increase in the percentage of geriatric patients who have excessive cerumen (Ruby, 1986). Gleitman et al (1992) clearly demonstrated the relationship between age and an increase in excessive and impacted cerumen when they compared the extent of impaction to the chronological age of 892 subjects. A linear relationship was found in data showing that 5% of the youngest age group (26 to 44 years) had excessive cerumen, whereas 34% of the oldest age group (65 to 74 years) had excessive cerumen.

Mahoney (1987) screened 133 elderly subjects and found that 82 (34%) had impacted cerumen and an additional 56 (23%) had "moderate to large" amounts of cerumen. In a follow-up investigation of 104 nursing home residents, 62 to 100 years of age, 25 to 42% were found to have ears with moderate to large amounts or impacted cerumen (Mahoney, 1993).

Lewis-Cullinan and Janken (1990) performed otoscopic examinations on a random sample of 226 individuals 65 years of age or older. In addition, a four-frequency screening was performed at 40 dB HL on all subjects. If excessive cerumen was found during otoscopy, a follow-up rescreen was performed after cerumen removal. Thirty-five percent of the subjects had occluding cerumen. After cerumen management, 75% of the subjects had improved hearing sensitivity on the 40 dB screening. These figures clearly suggest the need for routine management of the earcanals of the geriatric population.

PATHOPHYSIOLOGY

Complications of excessive cerumen in the earcanal include tinnitus, vertigo, itching, pain, external otitis, and hearing loss (Adams et al, 1978; Bricco, 1985; DeWeese et al, 1973). Chronic cough has also been reported (Raman, 1986). The larynx is innervated by the vagus nerve, and the auricular branch of the vagus nerve serves the posterior and inferior wall of the earcanal and concha area of the pinna. Reflex coughing and sneezing sometimes occur when the earcanal is manipulated during procedures such as cerumen removal because of this innervation.

PEARL

Because of vagal nerve innervation of the earcanal and the possibility of cardiac dysrhythmia (syncope), patients should be seated in a chair with surrounding support in the event they lose consciousness.

Vagus nerve connections between the earcanal and tympanic membrane and the cardiac muscle also explain why cardiac depression has been seen during earcanal irrigation (Prasad, 1984). Although cardiac depression is rare, clinicians should take note of the possibility during earcanal manipulation (cerumen management, ear impression taking, ENG testing, etc.) and be aware that loss of consciousness may result when it occurs. Patients must be seated with proper support during earcanal manipulation so that loss of consciousness does not result in head trauma.

Myers et al (1987) report one case of pseudodementia, a deterioration in mental and behavioral functions that simulate dementia, associated with impacted cerumen. Although this is an isolated report, indicating that pseudodementia must be a rare consequence of cerumen impaction, it reinforces the discomfort that occlusion of the earcanal for long periods can cause possible associated behavioral manifestations.

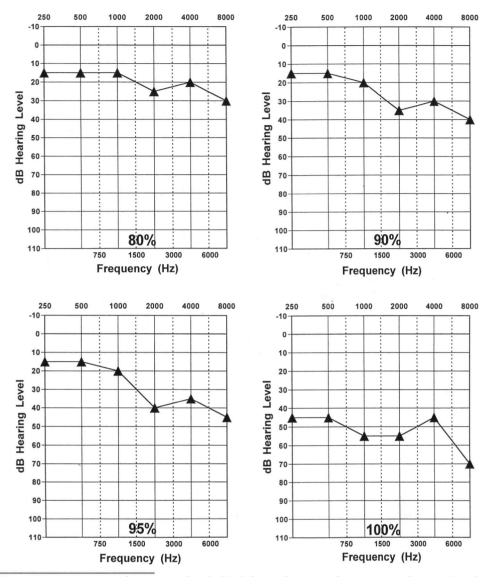

Figure 12–3 Amount of pure tone threshold shift as a function of percentage of earcanal occlusion. (Data are from Chandler [1964]. They were converted from 1951 ASA to 1996 ANSI values.)

Excessive cerumen affects auditory thresholds by gradually decreasing high-frequency sensitivity as the amount of cerumen increases. Figure 12–3 presents data from Chandler (1964), who systematically occluded the earcanals of two subjects from 80 to 95%. As shown, when the earcanal is occluded between 80 and 90%, hearing loss is restricted to the high frequencies, and thresholds decrease only 15- to 20-dB. As occlusion increases to 90 to 95%, high-frequency thresholds decrease by 25- to 35-dB. Only when the earcanal is totally occluded (100%) does threshold sensitivity decrease in the low frequencies, with a pure tone average shift of 40 dB. This sudden loss of low-frequency hearing explains why patients complain of sudden-onset hearing loss when complete occlusion occurs. These patients likely had gradually increasing amounts of high-frequency loss as the occlusion increased, but it was not until the loss affected hearing in the speech frequencies that the behavioral consequence of the loss had its full impact. Of course the threshold shifts found by Chandler

would be added to any pre-existing sensorineural hearing loss, as was shown earlier in this chapter in Figure 12–1.

In contrast to excessive cerumen, *asteatosis* is a condition in which cerumen is underproduced or absent in the earcanal. Because of lack of proper lubrication and accompanying dryness of the earcanal, patients with asteatosis will complain of earcanal itching. Prescriptive and over-the-counter topical ointments are helpful for these patients.

CERUMEN MANAGEMENT

Knowledge and Skills Required

Because a procedure is within the scope of practice of an audiologist does not necessarily mean that the audiologist should perform the procedure. Professional ethical codes stress the competency of the practitioner and the safety of the patient. The Ad Hoc Committee on Advances in Clinical Practice of

ASHA prepared the document, "External Auditory Canal Examination and Cerumen Management" (ASHA, 1992). In this document the committee outlined the education, training, and knowledge and skills necessary to perform cerumen management and the precautions each audiologist should consider before undertaking cerumen management procedures (Table 12–2). As shown in the Table 12–2, ASHA recommends that before cerumen removal audiologists have education and training in otoscopy, medical conditions of the earcanal, cerumen removal, and supervised experience in cerumen removal. Precautions include actions that may protect the audiologist from potentially liability-producing procedural omissions. The ASHA document suggests that audiologists should question regulatory bodies about limitations on their scope of practice, inquire with liability insurance carriers about their position on this procedure, examine specific institutional restrictions at the audiologist's place of employment, follow the Universal Precautions of the Centers for Disease Control Morbidity and Mortality Weekly Report (Centers for Disease Control, 1988), institute an emergency medical assistance plan, and obtain the informed consent of the patient. The knowledge and skills ASHA recommends audiologists to have before performing cerumen management focus on otoscopy, recognizing abnormal conditions of the earcanal and tympanic membrane, and determining whether safe removal can be accomplished or referral is necessary.

Infection Control

PEARL
Hand washing is the most effective procedure to prevent the spread of infection and disease.

Chapter 11 in this volume covers the topic of infection control in detail. As pointed out in this chapter, cerumen is not a medium for infectious diseases, including the AIDS virus (ASHA, 1990). However, because of the possibility of skin lacerations, and the potential for cerumen to contain blood, the universal precautions to prevent the risk of disease from blood-borne pathogens must be followed carefully when managing cerumen (Centers for Disease Control, 1988). Whether gloves should be used routinely for cerumen management as an infection control procedure is an individual clinical decision. Some practitioners will choose to glove, whereas others will not. However, whenever blood is present or when dealing with certain patients, such as those who are immunocompromised, gloves become a necessity.

TABLE 12–2 Education and training, precautions, and knowledge and skills recommended for cerumen management by the ASHA Ad Hoc Committee on Advances in Clinical Practice (ASHA, 1992)

Education and Training

1. Use of pneumatic otoscopy, recognition of the canal and tympanic membrane condition, and removal of cerumen.
2. Knowledge of medical conditions that might have an impact on the safe performance of cerumen management.
3. Supervised experience in these procedures.

Precautions

1. Inform institution and/or regulatory bodies (state licensure boards) that these procedures are within the scope of practice of audiology.
2. Check with appropriate state licensure board(s) to determine whether there are any limitations on the scope of audiology practice that restrict the performance of these procedures.
3. Check professional liability insurance to ensure that there is no exclusion applicable to these procedures.
4. Check medical policy, institutional insurance coverage and delineation of practice privileges for the specific institution to ensure that there are no restrictions applicable to an audiologist performing these procedures.
5. Follow the Universal Precautions, to prevent the risk of disease from blood-borne pathogens (Centers for Disease Control, 1988; ASHA, 1990).
6. Know who to contact in the event of an emergency or if medical assistance is needed.
7. Obtain informed consent by explaining the procedures to the patient, and maintain complete and adequate documentation.

Knowledge and Skills

1. Otoscopy-obstruction/medical conditions.
2. Otoscopy-mobility of eardrum.
3. Otoscopy-status of earcanal and tympanic membrane.
4. Otoscopy-cerumen verification/proceed to remove or refer.
5. Pinna inspection/otoscopy for abnormal conditions.
6. Emergency procedures needed.
7. Cerumen removal methods and need for referral.

Procedures for Cerumen Management

Procedures for safe and effective cerumen management have been well documented (Ballachanda & Peers, 1992; Bradley, 1980; Burgess, 1977; Carne, 1980; Graber, 1986; Larsen, 1976; Manning, 1992; Marshall & Attia, 1983; Mawson, 1974; Salomon, 1967). As pointed out by these reports, when proper techniques are followed, effective cerumen management is a relatively simple and safe procedure. In fact, cerumen management can be performed as a self-management procedure with an over-the-counter ceruminolytic to soften the cerumen and irrigation with a rubber bulb to remove it from the earcanal (Jurish, 1991). The American Academy of Otolaryngology–Head and Neck Surgery even recommends patient use of over-the-counter ceruminolytics and irrigations when it can be established that the tympanic membrane is not perforated (AAO-HNS, 1991).

To ensure minimum risk and maximum efficiency, audiologists who manage cerumen must carefully follow accepted procedures. Accepted procedures require the preliminary steps of taking an appropriate case/medical history and performing an otoscopic examination of the earcanal. Some clinicians also perform premanagement audiological and/or immittance tests and use a ceruminolytic to soften the cerumen. The removal of cerumen is accomplished by any of several or a combination of several procedures, including mechanical removal, irrigating the earcanal with an oral jet irrigator, and suction.

Preliminary Steps

Examine the Earcanal

Visual examination of the earcanal and tympanic membrane (Sullivan, 1997) is an essential preliminary step in all audiological procedures from simple screening to comprehensive diagnostic evaluation. During cerumen management, examination of the earcanal is performed as a preliminary step to ensure that the material in the earcanal is, in fact, cerumen. Historically, otoscopy has moved from direct observation without the aid of special lighting or special instruments, to handheld otoscopes, to the use of video otoscopes. Video otoscopes contain a miniature video camera that places a highly

defined color image of the earcanal and tympanic membrane onto a television monitor (Sullivan, 1997).

Figure 12–4 shows two types of handheld otoscopes. The Welch Allyn Model 25020 is in common use and features a rechargeable battery and disposable specula. The Hotchkiss

otoscope provides for easy insertion of an instrument into the ear for the removal of cerumen without the parallax error common with conventional otoscopes.

The development of fiber optics and miniaturization of videocamera components provided for the development of the video otoscope. The first models were introduced to audiologists in 1983 by Jedmed (Sullivan, 1997). An example is shown in Figure 12–5. The video otoscope facilitates examination of the earcanal, patient education, referral of abnormal conditions to physicians, and treatment of occluding or excessive cerumen. (Sullivan, 1997).

The examination of the earcanal is essential before performing audiological procedures to identify problems in the earcanal that might complicate the procedure or make the procedure useless or unnecessary. The presence of excessive or

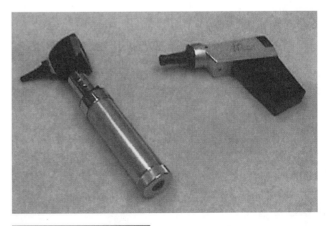

Figure 12–4 Two types of handheld otoscopes: the Welch Allyn on the left and the Hotchkiss on the right.

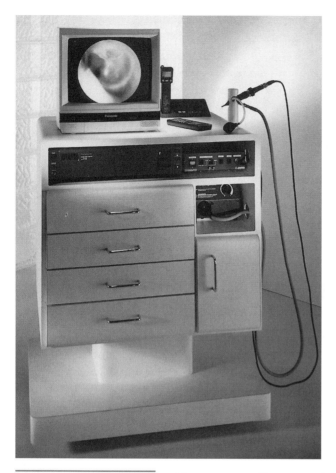

Figure 12–5   Example of a video otoscope. (Courtesy of Starkey Labs, Inc.)

occluding cerumen is such a finding that might necessitate postponing a procedure until cerumen removal has been accomplished. Figure 12–6 shows an example of a normal earcanal and one with a cerumen occlusion that would prevent audiological procedures and ear impression procedures or

hearing aid treatment from occurring without proper management. On otoscopic examination, the earcanal should be visualized to determine whether any unusual conditions require otologic referral. The tympanic membrane should also be examined carefully, and normal landmarks should be noted (Fig. 12–7). If the tympanic membrane does not appear healthy, appropriate referrals should be made. When occluding material obscures the tympanic membrane, the audiologist first must make sure that the material is cerumen. The presence of any matter in the earcanal that might represent purulent drainage, blood, or other foreign bodies should be referred for medical examination. Procedures for removal of the cerumen must then be considered on the basis of its type, consistency, texture, and location. The otoscopic examination also enables the audiologist to view and incorporate the patient's individual earcanal characteristics into any treatment plans. It is important to note the size and shape of the earcanal and determine the relative location of the tympanic membrane, as well as any earcanal turns or bends that deviate from expected patterns. If cerumen management is to be carried out, the otoscopic examination also must be made to locate the blockage precisely to assist in developing a strategy for the removal of the cerumen. On the basis of this thorough visual inspection of the earcanal, the audiologist can proceed with planned audiological procedures, referral for medical examination, or treatment to remove cerumen deemed to interfere with planned procedures.

Take an Appropriate Case/Medical History

Perforation of the tympanic membrane or the presence of myringotomy (polyethylene) tubes are universal contraindications for cerumen management by earcanal irrigation. Good clinical judgment must be used to determine whether patients should be referred to their physicians (or an otolaryngologist) for cerumen management if any of the following are present:

a. Recent earache

b. History of ear surgery

c. Drainage

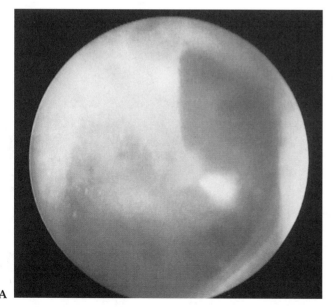

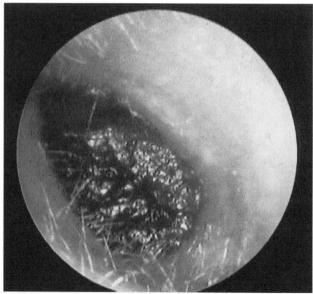

A   B

Figure 12–6   A normal earcanal (**A**) and an earcanal occluded with wet-type cerumen (**B**).

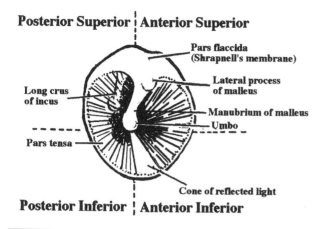

Posterior Superior | **Anterior Superior**

Pars flaccida
(Shrapnell's membrane)

Lateral process
of malleus

Long crus
of incus

Manubrium of malleus

Umbo

Pars tensa

Cone of reflected light

Posterior Inferior | **Anterior Inferior**

Figure 12–7 The landmarks of the normal tympanic membrane.

d. Dizziness

e. Diabetes mellitus

f. Acquired immune deficiency syndrome (ASHA, 1990)

g. Blood thinning medications

h. Any other possible condition that would put the patient at risk

Irrigating the earcanal is contraindicated in the presence of diabetes mellitus and AIDS because of the possible development of malignant external otitis (*Pseudomonas* osteomyelitis), a life-threatening disease precipitated by external otitis. Trauma to the earcanal that is possible from irrigation may result in an innocuous infection of the squamous epithelium of the earcanal. This infection can progress to the underlying soft tissue, cartilage, blood vessels, or bone and eventually lead to cellulitis, chondritis, or osteomyelitis of the temporal bone. If untreated, invasive external otitis may lead to osteomyelitis of the base of the skull, multiple cranial-nerve palsies, meningitis, and even death (Zikk et al, 1991). From the preceding it is clear that the medical history must include questions about diabetes or AIDS; patients having either condition should be referred to their physician for cerumen management. For these patients, earcanal irrigation is contraindicated in favor of mechanical removal or suctioning under direct (microscopic) visualization (Zikk et al, 1991).

Optional Steps

Premanagement Audiometric and Immittance Data
This step is especially important when the tympanic membrane cannot be visualized by otoscopy. Cerumen management with water irrigation is contraindicated when the earcanal is partially occluded (not impacted), obscuring the tympanic membrane, *and* any of the following are present:

1. A conductive component on the audiogram

2. The inability to maintain an hermetic seal when performing immittance measures

3. A flat (type B) tympanogram *and* a high earcanal physical volume

Obviously, any of the preceding findings would suggest tympanic membrane perforation or middle ear pathological conditions.

Cerumenolytic

When hard, dry, occluding cerumen is present, it is best if a softening agent (a ceruminolytic, mineral oil, or another recognized softening agent) is placed into the earcanal before irrigation (see Fig. 12–8). It is best also if the softening agent is used two to three times daily for 3 to 5 days before cerumen extraction. However, if the 3- to 5-day period is not possible, using the softening step for as long as possible (30 to 45 minutes) before the removal process should prove beneficial. Otherwise, cerumen removal may be impossible with irrigation and the earcanal may be left abraded, sore, and possibly bleeding, which would make it difficult or impossible to perform any further audiological testing requiring a clear earcanal.

Table 12–3 is a list of the commercially available ceruminolytics and several other common agents that have been used to soften cerumen. As shown, the composition of the over-the-counter ceruminolytics is identical across the various brands that are available. A new marketing approach is *Audiologists Choice*; this product is distributed only through audiologists. In addition to the ceruminolytics listed in Table 12–3, other prod-

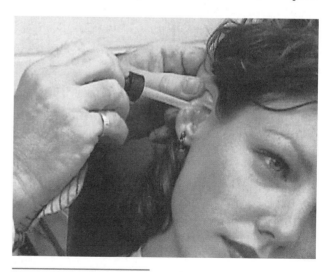

Figure 12–8 Use of a ceruminolytic before cerumen management provides softening of the debris and may facilitate cerumen removal.

TABLE 12–3   Summary of commercially available ceruminolytics and other products used for softening cerumen

Brand Name	Type	Composition
Audiologists Choice[*]	OTC[†]	Carbamide peroxide (6.5%) and glycerine
Auro Ear Drops	OTC	Carbamide peroxide (6.5%) and glycerine
Bausch & Lomb	OTC	Carbamide peroxide (6.5%) and glycerine
Cerumenex Drops	Rx	Triethanolamine Polypeptide Oleatecondensate
Debrox	OTC	Carbamide peroxide (6.5%) and glycerine
Murine Ear Drops	OTC	Carbamide peroxide (6.5%) and glycerine

Other Products for Softening Cerumen

Baby oil
Colace liquid (Docusate Sodium)
Hydrogen peroxide (3%)
Mineral oil
Sodium bicarbonate
Virgin olive oil

[*]Distributed only through audiologists.
[†]OTC, over-the-counter.

ucts shown are baby oil, Colace liquid, hydrogen peroxide, mineral oil, sodium bicarbonate, and virgin olive oil. All these products have been reported to be effective in softening cerumen.

SPECIAL CONSIDERATION

When cerumen is impacted, hard, and dry, removal may be difficult. In such cases, providing the patient with a ceruminolytic and scheduling a second visit in at least 2 to 3 days will avoid possible pain, abrading of the skin of the earcanal, and possible bleeding.

Several studies comparing the efficacy of different ceruminolytics and other agents have been reported in the British literature. Three studies assessed the effectiveness of ceruminolytics by measuring the amount of water needed to irrigate the earcanal successfully after the use of the ceruminolytic. Bailes et al, (1967) found one ceruminolytic (Waxsol) more effective than another (Cerumol). However, Burgess (1966) and Saintonge and Johnstone (1973) failed to note any major differences between the preparations they evaluated. Included were olive oil, Xerumenex, maize oil, and "Dioctylmedo" ear drops (a wetting agent). In-vitro evaluations of Cerumol, olive oil, Waxsol, sodium bicarbonate, Cerumenex, and Dioctyl ear capsules have shown mixed results (Fraser,

1970; Horowitz, 1968). Fraser (1970) concluded that in-vitro studies are inadequate as a means of assessing the efficacy of wax solvents because they do not consider skin irritation and because they do not provide actual information on the process of cerumen removal. Finally, Fahmey and Whitefield (1982) reported data from a multicenter trial comparing Exterol, Cerumol, and glycerol. Although their conclusion was that Exterol is markedly superior to the other ceruminolytics, their data were not compelling.

In a more recent study Robinson & Hawke (1989) found that a 10% solution of sodium bicarbonate was a more effective ceruminolytic than any of several organic liquids including glycerine, olive oil, Cerumenex, Auralgan, and alcohol. The action of sodium bicarbonate disintegrated experimental 250-mg blocks of actual human cerumen in a matter of minutes compared with several days for some of the organic liquids. The authors indicated that cerumen underwent significant swelling after treatment with the solution of sodium bicarbonate. It was also noted that the ceruminolytic used would depend on the type of removal procedure that was contemplated.

Overall, results from the preceding studies do not appear to support using one ceruminolytic over another, although ceruminolytics containing sodium bicarbonate appear to have some disintegrating advantage. The choice of whether to use a ceruminolytic or not will be made by individual clinicians. Reports on the clinical application of ceruminolytics have shown that when ears have hard, dry, impacted cerumen, the process of removal is significantly facilitated by administering a ceruminolytic for 2 to 3 days before removal (Roeser et al, 1991, 1992).

Informed Consent

Before cerumen management, after the patient is seated comfortably in a chair, the procedure to be used should be explained to the patient carefully and permission to proceed should be obtained. Explaining the procedure and potential risks will provide the necessary information to the patient for "informed consent." For patients with hearing impairment it is advisable to have printed materials describing the procedure and the risks.

Cerumen Removal Protocols

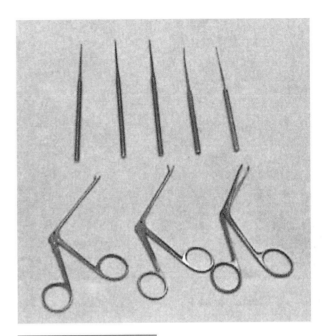

Figure 12–9 Various-sized cerumen currettes or spoons (Mandour et al, 1974) and alligator forceps (*below*) used for mechanical removal of cerumen.

PEARL
During cerumen management illuminating the earcanal with a head mirror, head lamp, or otoscope is very important.

Cerumen management can be accomplished with mechanical removal, suction, or water irrigation. The following describes the procedures used for each technique separately. However, it should be pointed out that in routine practice it is not unusual to use a combination of these approaches routinely.

Mechanical Removal

Mechanical removal is, by far, the most commonly used procedure for removing cerumen when the earcanal is partially occluded and the material is not adhering to the skin of the earcanal.

PEARL
When inserting any instrument into the earcanal, to avoid injury to the patient if sudden movement occurs, the clinician's hand should be braced on the patient's head.

The following instruments, equipment, and supplies shown in Figure 12–9 are needed to carry out the procedure:

- Various sterile instruments, including wire loops, dull ring curettes, forceps, and alligator forceps
- 4 × 4 gauze for cleaning instruments
- Otoscope specula to improve precision of instrument use

A step-by-step procedure for mechanical removal of cerumen is as follows:

1. On the basis of findings from the otoscopic examination, the instrument to be used is selected.
2. The patient's earcanal is straightened with the examiner's free hand by gently pulling the pinna slightly backward and upward. The free hand and forearm are used to steady

and control the patient's head by having him or her press against them.

3. The use of a fiber-optic otoscope as a light source, use of both eyes to achieve depth perception, and insertion of an instrument through the specula to guide the position of the curette and to improve depth judgment (see Figs. 12–10 and 12–11) is recommended.
4. The instrument is inserted into the earcanal against the cerumen, either on the lateral or superior/posterior position, and the cerumen is gently dislodged and removed from the earcanal. When curettes are used, loosening the debris and gently rolling it laterally is the goal in most situations. If a specula is used, removal of the specula and curette simultaneously will prevent the cerumen from "fouling" the specula and blocking the vision of the practitioner.
5. Cerumen that is hard and dry may adhere to the skin lining of the canal. Removal of cerumen in this case may cause patient discomfort, injury to the canal wall, and bleeding. For these cases the use of a ceruminolytic for 30 to 45 minutes to soften the debris may provide a better result.
6. If most of the cerumen has been successfully removed but a cleaner canal is needed for a procedure, such as probe microphone measurements or taking ear impressions, it may be advisable to use suction or irrigation rather than risking injury to the patient by scraping the canal wall.

Suction

Suction equipment is typically available through medical supply companies; an example of a suction system is shown in Figure 12–12. Appropriate sized suction tips must be chosen on the basis of the patient's earcanal shape and size.

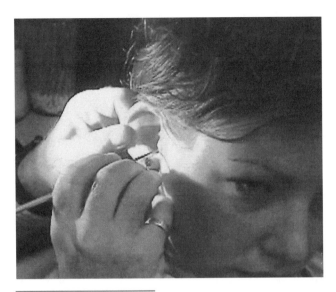

Figure 12–10 Mechanical removal is carried out by bracing the hand holding the instrument against the patient's head and carefully inserting the instrument into the earcanal, while straightening the canal by lifting the pinna with the opposite hand.

PEARL

To be effective, a suction instrument with at least 21 inches/Hg vacuum is needed.

Cerumen extraction using suction is particularly appropriate when the cerumen is very soft or semiliquid and can be found near the entrance to the canal (Ballachanda & Peers, 1992). It is possible that the suction device may become clogged during the procedure. Manning (1992) suggested that a warm cup of water be available to suction through the tip periodically to keep the pathway clear. Large pieces of cerumen should not be suctioned through the apparatus because these are also likely to cause clogging of the line.

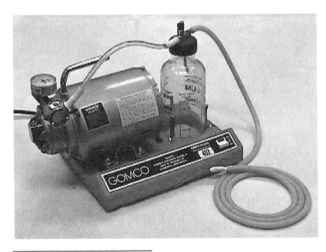

Figure 12–12 Example of a system used for suctioning cerumen.

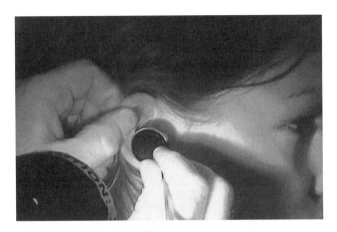

Figure 12–11 Using a speculum during mechanical removal can be useful in straightening the earcanal and keeping it open while the instrument is used to remove debris.

Some indication exists that the sound created by the suction device may create temporary threshold shifts. Young children are often frightened by the loudness of suctioning; for this reason suction may not be as well tolerated for this population.

The step-by-step procedure for earcanal suctioning is as follows (Manning, 1992):

1. Before the procedure begins, the patient should be instructed about the sound of the suction in the earcanal to prevent surprised discomfort.

2. A 4 × 4 gauze pad and cup of water should be available in a convenient location to clean the internal and external portion of the suction tip and tubing when necessary.

3. Using the knowledge gained from a thorough otoscopic examination, identify the location of the cerumen in the earcanal and insert the suction tip through a specula, held in place by the hand braced against the head, onto the surface of the cerumen.

4. Increased suction pressure can be achieved by use of the thumb to cover the suction hole on the suction tip.

5. Vacuum the cerumen from the earcanal by gently moving the suction tip into the cerumen.

6. Sometimes a piece of cerumen may attach itself to the suction tip without being vacuumed through the system. If this happens, remove the suction tip and the specula simultaneously and clean the tip with the 4 × 4 gauze pad.

7. Large or hard cerumen that is not suctioned from the earcanal may need to be extracted with either mechanical removal or irrigation.

Irrigation

Irrigation is commonly used with more complete occlusions and when the cerumen is hard and dry. Irrigation typically results in a cleaner canal, but water may be present and must be removed before carrying out many audiological procedures.

The following instruments shown in Figure 12–13 are needed to carry out the irrigation procedure:

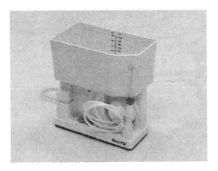
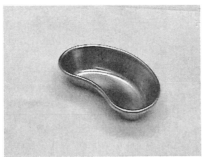
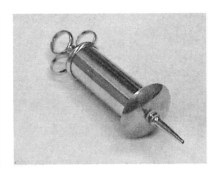
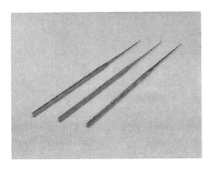
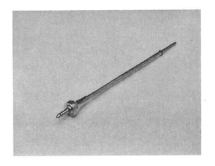

Figure 12–13 Irrigation of the earcanal is accomplished with an oral jet irrigator (*top left*), kidney-shaped bowl (*top center*), and cerumen currettes or spoons (*lower left*). Also shown (*lower right*) is an alternate attachment for the oral jet irrigator. The alternate attachment specifically directs the water flow away from the tympanic membrane. An aural bulb or an aural syringe (*top right*) can also be used.

- An oral jet irrigator (*must be used at low setting*)
- A kidney-shaped basin to catch the water
- A plastic sheet to cover patients and prevent water from spilling on them
- Towels to wipe up excess water
- Ear curettes
- Cotton swabs

An oral jet irrigator may be chosen for this protocol over an ear syringe because it has the advantage of providing a constant, controlled pulsating pressure stream, whereas the pressure produced by an ear syringe is highly variable. Although the use of an oral jet irrigator for managing cerumen has been recommended by some (Roeser & Roland, 1992; Seiler, 1980), it is clear that damage to the ear can result unless low pressure settings are used. Bailey (1983) stated that external otitis and perforation of the tympanic membrane with a secondary purulent otitis media can result from using an oral-jet irrigator in the earcanal. In addition, he speculated that frequent use could result in cochlear damage. However, he later acknowledged that oral jet irrigators can be used without complications if patients have strong, healthy tympanic membranes (Bailey, 1984).

The most compelling data on the potential hazards of the use of oral jet irrigators for cerumen management are from Dinsdale et al (1991). Case studies were presented on three patients who had otologic insult from the use of an oral-jet irrigator for cerumen management. All three patients had perforations of the tympanic membrane with associated hearing loss. Moreover, vertigo, ataxia, nausea, and vomiting were present in two of the patients. In addition to these case studies, Dinsdale et al (1991) reported data from irrigating

CONTROVERSIAL POINT

The use of an oral jet irrigator to manage cerumen has been deemed unacceptable by some practitioners because high pressures will cause damage to the tympanic membrane. However, when used at proper pressure settings, oral jet irrigation of the earcanal is safe and highly effective.

the earcanals of "fresh" cadavers with an oral jet irrigator at full power and at one-third power. Tympanic membrane perforations were created in three (6%) of the 50 ears, two at one-third power and one at full power.

PEARL

Never turn the oral jet irrigator on while the irrigator tip is aimed into the earcanal. Always physically feel the water stream from the irrigator tip for pressure and temperature before inserting it into the earcanal.

It is clear that potential hazards exist from using an oral jet irrigator for cerumen management. However, if used properly for this purpose, oral jet irrigators are safe and effective. It is *very important* to use a *low pressure setting* with the oral jet irrigator, no more than one fourth of the maximum; higher settings can cause damage to the ear. All precautions necessary should be taken to prevent setting the pressure adjustment at higher levels.

The step-by-step procedure for earcanal irrigation is as follows:

1. A plastic sheet is used to keep the patient dry during the irrigation procedure.

2. The oral jet irrigator is filled with lukewarm water. A thermometer can be used to ensure that the temperature of the water is at body temperature (37°C; 98°F). Cold or hot water cannot be used because the vestibular reflex may be triggered, causing dizziness and possible vomiting.

3. The patient is asked to hold the kidney-shaped basin firmly against the side of the face immediately below the ear, with the head tilted slightly downward (see Fig. 12–14).

4. The patient's earcanal is straightened with the examiner's free hand by gently pulling the pinna slightly backward and upward. The free hand and forearm are used to steady and control the patient's head by having him or her press against them.

5. The oral jet irrigator is turned on and the tip is placed into the kidney-shaped basin. Once it is established that the pressure from the irrigator is not too high, the tip is inserted into the earcanal.

6. The stream of water from the oral jet irrigator is directed against the wall of the earcanal not obscured by the occluding cerumen, usually it will be the superior wall. If the earcanal is completely occluded, the stream is directed at the superior wall of the earcanal at the edge of the cerumen plug. This procedure will build up a slight pressure behind the cerumen plug, fragment it, and force it out. Directing the stream at or against the cerumen plug should be avoided, as this may force the cerumen deeper into the earcanal.

7. Care is taken to ensure that the tip of the instrument is inserted just at the entrance of the earcanal so that space is present to allow drainage of the irrigating fluid. If the entrance is blocked, fluid can not drain, a pressure buildup will occur, and damage to the ear is possible. Also, care is taken so that the tip of the instrument is not inserted too deeply because the inner half of the earcanal is sensitive.

8. The earcanal is irrigated for 20 to 30 seconds. After each irrigation, the ear is checked with an otoscope to determine progress in removing the cerumen. Irrigation continues until the tympanic membrane is sufficiently visible for examination. If the cerumen does not dislodge after several attempts at irrigation, clinical judgment should be used to determine whether further softening for 3 to 5 days will be required before additional irrigation is attempted or possibly the ear presents with a difficult condition that will require medical referral. If medical referral is chosen, the continued use of a softening agent will make the removal process easier during the office visit. It is not advisable to use the softening agent for more than 3 to 5 days.

9. A blunt ear curette or a wire curette (cerumen spoon) is used to remove cerumen that is dislodged through irrigation but remains in, and partially occludes, the earcanal. When using the curette, adequate lighting is ensured with a head mirror or head lamp. The procedure used is to place both hands on the patient's head to stabilize the head and neck. With the curette between the thumb and forefinger, the curette tip is slowly inserted into the earcanal just beyond the dislodged cerumen plug. The cerumen is gently spooned or rolled out. Extreme care is taken not to put undue pressure on the skin of the earcanal.

10. Once the cerumen is removed, the earcanal is examined with an otoscope to ensure that the canal is cerumen free and no bleeding occurs. The earcanal and possibly the tympanic membrane may be slightly reddened.

11. If the earcanal is clear and there is no bleeding, it is dried by insertion of several drops of 70% alcohol solution (at body temperature) into the canal. After using the solution the patient's head is inclined for 15 to 25 seconds to allow any liquid to drain away.

12. The pinna and outer portion of the earcanal are dried with a towel.

13. As a final step, the earcanal is checked with an otoscope to make sure that all of the fluid is drained from it and no blood is present. Bleeding is rare, but should it occur a cotton swab is used to absorb small amounts of blood. If the bleeding is excessive, referral to a physician is needed.

14. The activity is documented in the patient's chart, including a description of the otoscopic examination both pre-management and postmanagement, as well as follow-up audiometric findings.

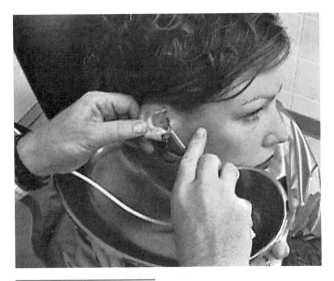

Figure 12–14 While the patient is holding the kidney-shaped bowl, the tip of the oral jet irrigator is inserted into the earcanal allowing space for the water to exit. The water jet should be directed toward the superior margin of the debris, which will allow water to fill the backspace and force the debris from the canal.

CONCLUSIONS

This chapter reviews the physiology and pathophysiology of cerumen and describes issues and procedures for cerumen management. Cerumen is the product of two types of glands in the earcanal: sebaceous glands and modified apocrine glands. Two types of cerumen can be found in the earcanal (dry type and wet type), which is genetically determined. Its function is to cleanse and lubricate the earcanal, and it has some protective properties. Although cerumen normally builds up and falls from the earcanal, in some individuals it does not and becomes excessive or impacted, a finding that is more common for individuals with mental retardation and the elderly. Cerumen management has risks associated with it that can be minimized through proper extraction techniques. The procedures for cerumen management include mechanical removal, suction, and irrigation.

REFERENCES

AAO-HNS. (1991). *Earwax, what to do about it.* Washington, DC: AAO-HNS.

ADAMS, G., BOIES, L., & PAPPARELLA, M. (1978). *Fundamentals of otolaryngology.* Philadelphia: WB Saunders.

ALBERTI, P.W.R.M. (1964). Epithelial migration on the tympanic membrane. *Journal of Laryngology and Otology, 78;*808–830.

ASHA. (1990). Report update: AIDS/HIV implications for speech-language pathologists and audiologists. *ASHA, 32;* 46–48.

ASHA. (1992). External auditory canal examination and cerumen mangement. *ASHA, 34*(Suppl 7);22–24.

BAILES, I.H., BAIRD, J.W., BARI, M.A., BELLETTY, D.R., BILL, C.E.S., BOND, B., CARTER, J., McKENDRICK, J., WELLS, F.D., & WILLIAMS, D.T.A. (1967). Wax softening with a new preparation. *Practitioner, 199;*359–362.

BAILEY, B.J. (1983). Impacted ear wax and a water-pick instrument. *JAMA, 250;*1456

BAILEY, B.J. (1984). Editorial reply to "Removal of cerumen." *JAMA, 250*(11);1456

BALLACHANDA, B.B. (1995). *The human earcanal.* San Diego: Singular Publishing Group.

BALLACHANDA, B.B., & PEERS, C.J. (1992). Cerumen management: Instruments and procedures. *ASHA.*

BASS, E.J., & JACKSON, J.F. (1977). Cerumen types in Eskimos. *American Journal of Physical Anthropology, 47;*209–210.

BORTZ, J.T., WERTZ, P.W., & DOWNING, D.T. (1990). Composition of cerumen lipids. *Journal of Laryngology and Otology, 23;*845–849.

BRADLEY, M.E. (1980). Appliance: A new aid for ear syringing. *Journal of Laryngology and Otology, 94;*457–459.

BRICCO, E. (1985). Impacted cerumen as a reason for failure in hearing conservation programs. *Journal of School Health, 55;*240–241.

BRISTER, F., FULLWOOD, H.L., RIPP, T., & BLODGETT, C. (1986). Incidence of occlusion due to impacted cerumen among mentally retarded adolescents. *American Journal of Mental Deficiency, 91;*302–304.

BURGESS, E.H. (1966). A wetting agent to facilitate ear syringing. *Practitioner, 197;*811–812.

BURGESS, E.H. (1977). Earwax and the right way to use an ear syringe. *Nursing Times, 73* (40);1564–1565.

CARNE, S. (1980). Ear syringing. *BMJ, 280;*374–376.

CARUSO, V.G., & MEYERHOFF, W.L. (1980). Trauma and infections of the external ear. In: M. Papparella & D. Shumrick (Eds.), *Otolaryngology (volume II): The ear* (pp. 1345–1356). Philadelphia: WB Saunders.

CENTERS FOR DISEASE CONTROL. (1988). *Morbidity and mortality weekly report: Perspectives in disease prevention and health promotion* (p. 37). CDC: Anonymous.

CHAI, T., & CHAI, T.C. (1980). Bactericidal activity of cerumen. *Antimicrobial Agents and Chemotherapy, 18;*638–641.

CHANDLER, J.R. (1964). Partial occlusion of the external auditory meatus: Its effect on air and bone conduction hearing acuity. *Laryngoscope, 22;*22–36.

CIPRIANI, C., TABORELLI, G., GADDIA, G., MELAGRANA, A., & REBORA, A. (1990). Production rate and composition of cerumen: Influence of sex and season. *Laryngoscope, 100;*275–276.

COOPER, S.J. (1985, May). *Relationships of hearing protector type and prevalence of external auditory canal pathology.* Paper presented at The American Industrial Hygiene Conference. Las Vegas, NV.

CRANDELL, C.C., & ROESER, R.J. (1993). Incidence of excessive/impacted cerumen in mentally retarded individuals. *American Journal of Mental Retardation, 97;*568–574.

CREED, E., & NEGUS, V.E. (1926). Investigations regarding the function of aural cerumen. *Journal of Laryngology and Otology, 41;*223–230.

DAHLE, A.J., & McCOLLISTER, F.P. (1986). Hearing and otologic disorders in children with Down syndrome. *American Journal of Mental Deficiency, 90;*636–642.

DeWEESE, D., & SAUNDERS, W. (1973). *Otolaryngology* (ed. 4). St. Louis: Mosby.

DINSDALE, R.C., ROLAND, P.S., MANNING, S.C., & MEYERHOFF, W.L. (1991). Catastrophic otologic injury from oral jet irrigation of the external auditory canal. *Laryngoscope, 101;*75–78.

EDWARDS, J., & HARRIS, K.S. (1990). Rotation and translation of the jaw during speech. *Journal of Speech and Hearing Research; 33;*550–562.

FAHMEY, S., & WHITEFIELD, M. (1982). Multicentre clinical trial of Exerol as a ceruminolytic. *The British Journal of Clinical Practice, 36;*197–204.

FOLTNER, K.A. (1984). The case for otoscopic screenings in industrial hearing conservation. *Hearing Journal, 37*(6);27–30.

FRASER, J.G. (1970). The efficacy of wax solvents: In vitro studies and a clinical trial. *Journal of Laryngology and Otology, 84;*1055–1064.

FULTON, R.T., & GRIFFIN, C.S. (1967). Audiological-otological considerations with the mentally retarded. *Mental Retardation, 51*(3);26–31.

GERLING, I.J., BOESTER, K., & YU, J.H. (1997). *The transient effect of cerumen on the external ear resonance.* Paper presented at the annual conference of the American Academy of Audiology. Ft. Lauderdale, FL: Anonymous.

GERLING, I.J., & GOEBEL, J.J. (1992). *Interaural variability in external ear resonance: the effect of debris.* Paper presented at the American Speech-Language-Hearing Association annual convention. San Antonio, TX: Anonymous.

GLEITMAN, R.M., BALLACHANDA, B.B., & GOLDSTEIN, D.P. (1992). Incidence of cerumen impaction in general adult population. *Hearing Journal, 45;*28–32.

GRABER, R.F. (1986). Removing impacted cerumen. *Patient Care, 20*;151–153.

HARVEY, D.J. (1989). Identification of long-chain fatty acids and alcohols from human cerumen by the use of picolinyl and nicotinate esters. *Biomedical Environmental Mass Spectometry, 18*;719–723.

HAWKE, M. (1987). *Clinical pocket guide to ear disease.* New York: Gower Medical Publications.

HOPKINSON, N. (1981). *Prevalence of middle ear disorders in coal miners.* Cincinnati, OH: U.S. Department of Health and Human Services.

HOROWITZ, J.I. (1968). Solvents for ear wax. *BMJ, 4*;583.

INABA, M., CHUNG, T.H., KIM, J.C., CHOI, Y.C., & KIM, J.H. (1987). Lipid composition of ear wax in hircismus. *Yonsei Medical Journal, 28*;49–51.

JURISH, A. (1991). Hearing trouble? Maybe it's earwax. *Prevention, 43*(10);113–117.

LARSEN, G. (1976). Removing cerumen with a water-pick. *American Journal of Nursing, 76*(2);264–265.

LEBENSOHN, J.E. (1943). Impacted cerumen: Incidence and management. *US Naval Medical Bulletin, 41*;1071–1075.

LEWIS-CULLINAN, C., & JANKEN, J.K. (1990). Effect of cerumen removal on the hearing ability of geriatric patients. *Journal of Advanced Nursing, 15*;594–600.

MAHONEY, D.F. (1987). One simple solution to hearing impairment. *Geriatric Nursing, 8*(5);242–245.

MAHONEY, D.F. (1993). Cerumen impaction. Prevalence and detection in nursing homes. *Journal of Gerontological Nursing, 19*;23–30.

MANDOUR, M.A., EL-GHAZZAWI, E.F., TOPPOZADA, H.H., & MALATY, H.A. (1974). Histological and histochemical study of the activity of ceruminous glands in normal and excessive wax accumulation. *Journal of Laryngology and Otology, 11*;1075–1085.

MANNING, R. (1992). *Cerumen management.* Lexington, KY: Eastern Kentucky Speech and Hearing Clinic.

MARSHALL, K.G., & ATTIA, E.L. (1983). *Disorders of the ear.* Boston: John Wright-PSG.

MATSUNAGA, E. (1962). The dimorphism in human normal cerumen. *Annals of Human Genetics, 25*;273–286.

MAWSON, S.R. (1974). *Diseases of the ear* (ed. 3). Baltimore: Williams & Wilkins.

MEGARRY, S., PETT, A., SCARLETT, A., TEH, W., ZEIGLER, E., & CANTER, R.J. (1988). The activity against yeasts of human cerumen. *Journal of Laryngology and Otology, 102*;671–672.

MEYERS, A.D. (1977). Practical ENT: Managing cerumen impaction. *Postgraduate Medicine, 62*;207–209.

MYERS, B.A., SIEGFRIED, M., & PUESCHEL, S.M. (1987). Pseudodementia in the mentally retarded. A case report and review. *Clinical Pediatrics, 26*;275–277.

NUDO, L. (1965). Comparison by age of audiological and otological finding in a state residential institution for the mentally retarded: A preliminary report. In: L. Lloyd & R. Frisina (Eds.), *Audiological assessment of the mentally retarded: Proceedings of a national conference* (pp. 137–277). Parsons, KS: Parsons State Hospital and Training Center.

OSBORNE, J.E., & BATY, J.D. (1990). Do patients with otitis externa produce biochemically different cerumen? *Clinical Otolaryngology, 15*;59–61.

PERRY, E.J., & NICHOLS, A.C. (1957). Studies on the growth of bacteria in the human earcanal. *Journal of Investigative Dermatology, 27*;165–170.

PERRY, E.T. (1957). *The human earcanal.* Springfield, IL: Charles C. Thomas.

PETRAKIS, N.L. (1969). Dry cerumen: A prevalent genetic trait among American Indians. *Nature, 222*;1080–1081.

PRASAD, K.S. (1984). Cardiac depression on syringing the ear: A case report. *Journal of Laryngology and Otology, 98*;1013.

PRIMUS, M.A., & SKORDAS, J.D. Cerumen management in audiological practice. (1996). Poster session presented at the annual meeting of the American Academy of Audiology. Salt Lake City, UT.

RAMAN, R. (1986). Impacted ear wax: A cause for unexplained cough? *Archives of Otolaryngology, Head and Neck Surgery, 112*;679.

ROBINSON, A.C., & HAWKE, M. (1989). The efficacy of ceruminolytics: Everything old is new again. *Journal of Otolaryngology, 18*;263–267.

ROBINSON, A.C., HAWKE, M., & NAIBERG, J. (1990). Impacted cerumen: A disorder of keratinocyte separation in the superficial external earcanal? *Journal of Otolaryngology, 19*;86–90.

ROCHE, A.F., SIERVOGEL, R.M., & HIMES, J.H. (1978). Longitudinal study of hearing in children: baseline data concerning auditory thresholds, noise exposure, and biological factors. *Journal of the Acoustical Society of America, 64*;1593–1601.

ROESER, R.J., ADAMS, R.M., ROLAND, P.S., & WILSON, P.L. (1992). A safe and effective procedure for cerumen management. *Audiology Today, 3*(3);20–21.

ROESER, R.J., ADAMS, R.M., & WATKINS, S. (1991). Cerumen management in hearing conservation: The Dallas (Texas) Independent School District Program. *Journal of School Health, 61*(1);47–49.

ROESER, R.J., & ROLAND, R. (1992). What audiologists must know about cerumen and cerumen management. *American Journal of Audiology, 1*(5);27–35.

RUBY, R. (1986). Conductive hearing loss in the elderly. *Journal of Otolaryngology, 15*;245–247.

SAINTONGE, D.M., & JOHNSTONE, C.I. (1973). A clinical comparison of triethanolamine polypeptide oleate-condensate ear drops with olive oil for the removal of impacted wax. *The British Journal of Clinical Practice, 27*(12);454–455.

SALOMON, J.L. (1967). New technique for rapid ear irrigation. *Journal of Occupational Medicine, 9*(11);576–577.

SEILER, E.R. (1980). Ear syringing. *BMJ, 280*,1273.

SHARP, J.F., WILSON, J.A., ROSS, L., & BARR-HAMILTON, R.M. (1990). Ear wax removal: A survey of current practice. *BMJ, 301*;1251–1253.

STONE, M., & FULGHUM, R.S. (1984). Bactericidal activity of wet cerumen. *Annals of Otology, Rhinology and Laryngology, 93*;183–186.

SULLIVAN, R.F. (1997). Video otoscopy in audiologic practice. *Journal of the American Academy of Audiology, 8*(6);447–467.

YASSIN, A., MOSTAFA, M.A., & MOAWAD, M.K. (1966). Cerumen and its microchemical analysis. *Journal of Laryngology and Otology, 80*;933–938.

ZIKK, D., RAPOPORT, Y., & HIMELFARB, M.Z. (1991). Invasive external otitis after removal of impacted cerumen by irrigation. *The New England Journal of Medicine, 325*(13);969–970.

Chapter 13

Designing an Audiology Practice

Ian M. Windmill, David R. Cunningham, and Karen C. Johnson

THE CHALLENGE OF DESIGNING A PRACTICE

An audiologist's home-away-from-home is the audiology clinic, be it a hospital-based facility, an educational setting, a community clinic, or a private practice. As with any home, comfortable surroundings make for comfortable living and therefore the design and aesthetics of the facility can have a significant impact on job satisfaction and, more importantly, on the quality of the service provided to patients. Ultimately this translates to the economic success of the facility and for this reason the location, layout, and design of the audiology facility in which one practices can be critically important.

Designing a new audiological office or clinic requires careful and deliberate planning. More importantly, it requires the ability to conceptualize and visualize the daily operations that are likely to occur within the physical boundaries of the space. It requires farsightedness and anticipation of the changes that may occur in the practice over the next year, 5 years, 10 years, and beyond. The rewards of working in a facility that has been well designed are significant, not just in terms of financial gains but also for employee, staff, and patient satisfaction. A poorly designed facility will impose limits on service provision that ultimately will work against the mission of the practice and undermine the morale and efficiency of the staff.

A real challenge awaits the individual confronted with the task of designing an audiological office or clinic. "Confronted" is an appropriate word because the task can be daunting, particularly if one has little background in space planning, commercial real estate, or interior design. Few persons in health professions, including audiologists, have training in these areas. Conversely, few space planners, real estate agents, or interior designers have backgrounds in audiology, so the necessity of working with persons who have expertise or experience in each of these areas is an important part of the design and development process. Although one may believe that the cost and "hassle" associated with locating and retaining these experts are prohibitive, the long-term and short-term advantages of this expert advice far outweigh the cost involved. One of the first steps in planning a new clinic or office, therefore, is to recognize the importance of seeking expertise in those areas unfamiliar to the audiologist and to seek out experts in architecture, commercial real estate, space planning, and/or interior design.

PEARL

Seek expert advice to aid in the planning, development, construction, and decorating of an audiological clinic. Although cost may be involved, the expertise can be invaluable.

In many cases, however, the expertise in these areas may be readily available. For example, most hospitals employ or contract with space planners, architects, and interior designers and therefore little time or energy may need to be expended in identifying the consultants. Many professional office building or retail locations may also contract with design professionals or at the very least be able to recommend consultants. Also remember that many regulatory issues may need to be addressed in the design and construction of a medically related facility, particularly if that facility is within a hospital. Persons with expertise in healthcare design and construction can help you avoid mistakes that result in cost overruns or unnecessary delays.

The focus of this chapter will be on the design and planning of an independent audiological practice, but special consideration will be made of hospital-based practices. Most of the concepts are universal and apply not only to the variety of audiological practice settings but also to any professional practice. One factor that will not be discussed is the specific costs associated with the design of an audiological practice. Given that each facility will have unique characteristics, will be located in different economic areas, and will have different budgetary constraints, combined with factors such as regional

291

differences in costs and inflationary trends, discussion of specific costs becomes difficult at best and at worst meaningless. It will be assumed, however, that the budget for any design project is an important consideration, if not the single most significant constraint, in the design and construction of a new facility. Readers are cautioned to apply the information contained in this chapter in light of any financial or budgetary boundaries that may uniquely apply to their situations.

THE DESIGN PROCESS

The process of moving from the *idea* of a new facility through planning, construction, and finally, occupation and use consists of several steps, each intertwined yet each requiring specific considerations (Table 13–1).

Initially, the "idea" is formulated, out of either need or desire, for a new practice facility. The next step is the planning stage in which the basic operational plans are developed. This is then followed by the search for an appropriate location. The layout stage, in which the actual floorplans and construction blueprints are developed, follows with the interior design stage completing the process (Saphier, 1992). Although the order may seem obvious and logical, the stages are not mutually exclusive, and continuous consideration of each stage is necessary to complete the project. For example, the location of the facility must be chosen before a floor plan can be developed because the specific dimensions of the space will significantly influence both the size and location of each room and its associated functions. Conversely, the choice of location is based on the specific services one is likely to provide (e.g., hearing aid dispensing vs. diagnostic procedures) and on the square footage requirements necessary to perform these services.

The adage of "haste makes waste" applies to the design of an audiology facility. Rushing the process can result, at the least, in unnecessary delays or frustrations and, at the most, in years of frustration from rushing a facility to completion that was inadequate, poorly planned, or aesthetically displeasing. It is better to take the necessary time to ensure a facility meets all one's requirements and needs. Too much time, energy, and money goes into the planning and development of an audiological practice, and extending the search for a location, builder, decorator, or appropriate floorplan is a small price to pay for literally years of pleasure in a well-planned practice or clinic.

Getting the Idea

At some point, the *idea* of establishing a new audiology clinical facility comes to mind. Generally, the reason for considering this idea can be attributed to factors such as the need for more space, the need for a different location, the need to expand services, or the need to strike out on one's own. For example, an existing full-service audiology practice located in a medical complex with poor parking and access may wish to reduce the burden and inconvenience to patients returning for hearing aid follow-ups and therefore desire to establish a satellite location closer to the patient base. A hospital-based clinic may be required to find a new location because of expansion of adjacent departments or its own services. Or perhaps the desire exists to start an independent freestanding practice.

The time when the idea becomes more than a passing thought and when serious consideration and discussion begin is the time to begin gathering information and exploring the options available. The reason the idea for a new facility first

TABLE 13–1 Steps in the design of an audiological clinic or practice

Step	Stage	Components
I	Idea	Occurs as a result of an immediate need. Consider all present and future possibilities for the facility.
II	Planning	Generate a list of audiological, business, and miscellaneous services and procedures that are *likely* to occur in the facility. Assign procedures to "rooms." Determine approximate square footage required for the facility.
III	Location	Decide city and state for practice location. Evaluate locations within city. Use SWOT technique to make informed decision about practice location. Choose specific site and enter into lease/buy agreement.
IV	Layout	Sketch potential floorplans. Evaluate patient, staff, and employee movements. Meet with architect. Finalize floor plan.
V	Construction	Evaluate and review construction progress for any changes.
VI	Interior design	Decide on image of practice. Meet with interior designer to develop ideas. Complete design.

occurred probably is indicative of the general type of services that will be provided. But where is the best location? How much will it cost? Who will finance the project? Who will design the facility? Begin to gather information on patient demographics, locations, real estate companies, and banking/ financing requirements. Take to your car and drive through prospective practice areas, taking notes about building or space for rent, noting traffic patterns and accessibility. When you see "For Rent" signs, call the real estate agent for a tour or information. Gather data on pricing, construction, and leasing. Visit other audiological practices for ideas. Contact the local business development offices for information on future commercial or residential developments in prospective areas.

Now is also the time to consider the future possibilities for the practice and the needs and growth patterns that may occur over a more extended time. In addition to meeting an immediate need, one also should consider other questions. Will the practice continue to expand? Will more staff be added? Will more services be added? Will other locations be considered in the future? At this stage in the process all possibilities should be considered. No commitments have been made; no contracts signed; no construction or consulting bills are outstanding, so the attitude can be pie-in-the-sky. Consider all the potential possibilities for the facility rather than restrict thinking to a single need. Although some services can be added after construction is completed, much less opportunity may exist to add space. Realistically consider every possibility, particularly in light of the business plan, then accept or reject each idea as part of the developing plan. Modifications are easy to make at this stage in the process. Realistic modifications will continue to occur throughout the process, particularly when factors such as available square footage or costs are considered.

Plan, Plan, and Plan Again

The primary goal of the planning stage is to develop a firm outline of the daily operations that are likely to occur in the practice, along with a general idea of the square footage requirements. In addition, the planning stage should include the development of a list of any special requirements, such as "at the door parking" or "first floor location." The daily operations, square footage, and special requirements are necessary before beginning the actual search for a location.

Begin by listing all the audiological services and procedures that will or are likely to occur in the site. The list should detail both the type of service and the instrumentation and space requirements for each. For instance, a "pediatric audiological evaluation" is an example of an audiological service that includes a variety of procedures. Sound-field and visual reinforcement audiometry require the use of a sound booth with specific dimensions that will have an obvious influence on space planning. In addition to the audiological procedures, generate a list of all other "business" operations that will also occur in the facility. In freestanding practices it is likely that the business operations will include such things as coding and billing, accounting, or transcription. In a hospital-based clinic, there are likely to be far fewer business operations directly within the facility than might be necessary in a freestanding practice. Finally, generate a list of miscellaneous

functions or spaces that do not fall under the business or audiological operations list. These include storage space, kitchens, and bathrooms. Do not forget to include the waiting room. It is easy to overlook these nonaudiological aspects of a practice or to not give them sufficient attention, but each can be very important to the ensuring efficient operation of the practice. Although it is true that these operations are not revenue producing, lack of attention to the business needs of the facility can result in reduced efficiency and lost productivity. Table 13–2 lists many operations that may be considered within both the audiological and business sides of a facility.

After the itemization of the services and procedures that are likely to occur within the practice, the operational requirements for space can be discerned. The focus at this time is to develop a general idea as to the type and size of the rooms necessary to accommodate all aspects of the practice. Generate a list of "rooms" assigning all audiological, business, and miscellaneous functions previously identified to each room. When making room assignments, consider the ways in which different services interface with each other. Patients should be easily accommodated within the facility, including any interactions with the business aspects of the practice, and there should be little if any space conflicts for a patient. For example, if the immittance instrument is placed within a sound booth, it can never be used while another patient occupies the sound booth. If the practice is designed only to accommodate a single audiologist and patient at a time, this may not be an issue. However, if multiple patients or staff are scheduled at overlapping times and access to an immittance unit may be necessary at times, then the location of the immittance instrument must be considered in light of these potential conflicts. Perhaps an immittance instrument should be located in a separate room or perhaps more than one immittance unit is required. Consider the number of patients, audiologists, and support staff on-site at any given time, especially during peak business hours. How many persons will be on-site and what simultaneous operations will occur? On the business side, how much room will be necessary for files or storage, not just in the next year but over the next 5 years? Does the secretary/receptionist need access to a copy machine or fax machine, and how much space is needed for each piece of equipment? How much storage space is needed for audiological supplies, such as forms, brochures, and hearing aids?

PEARL
Do not forget to include the other members of the staff, particularly the support staff, in the space planning discussions. The receptionist or billing clerk may have entirely different perspectives on patient, staff, or information flow and be able to identify and offer solutions to problems not considered before.

At this stage in the design process, each "room" is merely a conceptual designation for space-planning purposes.

TABLE 13-2 Operations that may be included in an audiological practice

Audiologic operations	Business Operations
Audiologic evaluation	Coding
Audiometry, tones, and speech	Filing
Immittance audiometry	Billing and collections
Otoacoustic emissions	Computer services
Visual reinforcement audiometry	Reception
Play audiometry	Accounting
Electrophysiologic procedures	Administrative operations
Evoked potentials	Waiting room
Electronystagmography	
Vestibular procedures	Miscellaneous operations
Rotational testing	Kitchen
Posturography	Break room
Vestibular rehabilitation	Bathroom
Central auditory processing evaluations	Storage—audiological supplies
Amplification procedures	Clothes closets
Hearing aid evaluations	Storage—cleaning supplies
Selection and fitting amplification	
Assistive listening devices	

Whether these spaces are actually divided by walls or not will be decided at a later time. For example, evoked potentials and electronystagmography (ENG) may be both initially assigned to a "room" for electrophysiological procedures. Equipment that uses the same computer for both auditory brain stem response (ABR) and ENG would necessitate these procedures occur within the same space. On the other hand, trends and referral patterns may suggest a much greater use for each procedure in the future, necessitating that each be given a separate "room." The process of designating rooms should not be done quickly. After an initial list is made, share it with others who may be involved in the daily operations and get their feedback. Remember at this time no floor plans and no space restrictions exist, so adding or subtracting "rooms" can be easily accomplished (Table 13–3).

When the operations are sufficiently divided among the "rooms," an estimate of the square footage required for each room can be generated. This is not quite as easy as it sounds. For example, the dimensions and square footage associated with a sound room can be determined easily from the specifications supplied by the manufacturer or distributor. However the operations that occur *around* the soundroom contribute to the overall space requirements. These operations include space for the doors to open, the placement and type of audiological testing instruments (audiometer, compact disc player, visual reinforcement audiometry equipment), movement patterns of the audiologist and patient around the sound room, and the air-conditioning and ventilation requirements of the booths. A room with ENG must accommodate the ENG instrument, including the light bar, the patient table, movement of the audiologist around the patient, and access to water and supplies. The "footprint" of each piece of equipment, each movement, and each accessory must be identified. In addition, items such as a sink or casework, cabinets or counters, cleaning accessories, printers and cabling, must all be taken into account. Despite your best efforts, it will be impossible to plan for every operation, dimension, or square foot within a facility. Although a perfect space plan can be developed conceptually, the reality is that things change over time. External influences, growth, or changes of equipment and services are examples of changes that cannot be realistically anticipated. Therefore it is a good idea to add about 20% more square footage onto each room estimate to account for these changes, to accommodate instruments or procedures not considered, or for procedures that might be added in the future.

<table>
<tr><td>PEARL</td></tr>
<tr><td>Do not forget to plan ahead for space to counsel patients and their families. This is particularly true in sites in which rooms or equipment is shared by more than one audiologist. Nothing is more disruptive to the counseling process than having to move from room to room while going over test results or having other staff members walking in and out of a room while delicate counseling is going on.</td></tr>
</table>

Using this approach often results in a total square footage estimate much greater than originally contemplated during the idea stage of the planning process. The figures can be scary when considered in terms of the cost per square foot to renovate, or more commonly, for monthly rent. Remember that the estimates for room size generally do not account for "dead" space such as closets, hallways, and restrooms. After totaling the square footage requirements for each room, it is reasonable to add an additional 20 to 25% square footage to account for the dead space. This process provides a reasonable *estimate*

TABLE 13–3 "Room" assignments*

Room Number/Title	Functions Included	Square Footage
1. Waiting	Seating for 10 persons	150
	End tables	
	Coffee service	4
	Literature/magazine stand	3
	Approximate total	$160 \times 1.2 = 192$
2. Reception/Secretary	Desk/work area—corner unit	60
	Filing rack—wall mounted	10
	Fax	5
	Copy machine	5
	Supplies	20
	Approximate total	$100 \times 1.2 = 120$
3. Audiometry I	Sound booth + control room	150
	Room for door swing	60
	Hall space	40
	Approximate total	$250 \times 1.2 = 300$
4. Audiometry II	Immittance	100
	Otoacoustic emissions	
	Video otoscopy	
	Approximate total	$100 \times 1.2 = 120$
5. Evoked Potentials	Auditory brain stem response	120
	Electronystagmography	
	Approximate total	$120 \times 1.2 = 144$
6. Hearing Aid	Selection, fitting, dispensing	150
	Probe microphone unit	
	Computer with NOAH	
	Earmold supplies	
	Hearing aid supplies	
	Chairs for family	
	Approximate total	$150 \times 1.2 = 180$
7. Business Office	Billing	150
	Collections	
	Coding	
	Administrator	100
	Approximate total	$250 \times 1.2 = 300$
8. Storage	Miscellaneous supplies	40
	Approximate total	$40 \times 1.2 = 48$
9. Break Room	Small kitchen	100
	Approximate total	$100 \times 1.2 = 120$
10. Bathroom	Bathroom	20
	Approximate total	$20 \times 1.2 = 24$
	Subtotal	**1548**
	Dead space (20%)	**$\times$ 1.2**
	Total Estimated Square Footage	**1857.6**

*In the example, operations that are likely to occur within the practice have been assigned to rooms. Each "room" is evaluated for the total square footage required should those operations be assigned. Each room's total is inflated by 20% and then the grand total is also inflated by 20% to account for dead space. The final estimate provides a guideline for space required when searching for a practice location.

of the needed square footage for a new audiological practice. This estimate can then be used as a guide when embarking on the process of identifying a location for the practice.

If the square footage requirements are out of line with the budget or space available, meet with a space planner to determine where cuts can be made or where special considerations, such as a waiting room shared with other tenants in a building, can be integrated into the plan. The space planner can give better estimates of the space needs associated with the type of facility you are planning. Special requirements may be needed for medically related facilities or as required by statues such as the Americans with Disabilities Act, which must also be considered.

SPECIAL CONSIDERATION

If planning space in a hospital, do not forget to check current accreditation standards by the Joint Commission on Accreditation of Healthcare Organizations, particularly those pertaining to patient confidentiality, access, safety, and transportation. Failure to take current requirements into consideration during the planning stage may result in the need to make costly modifications after the plans or construction has been completed.

Armed with the general knowledge of the types of services and their associated space and facility requirements, it is now time to begin looking for the appropriate location. For hospital-based clinics, the choice of location is typically limited, if any choice exists, because it is rare for a hospital to have multiple spaces available at any one time. Furthermore, audiology facilities have certain construction or dimensional constraints, such as the size and weight of the sound booths, that may prohibit the use of certain space. Space within hospitals is often at a premium and typically the choice is to take what is available, even if the dimensions or square footages do not match the need, or to wait, perhaps an extended time period, until "other" space becomes available.

Maximum flexibility in design is afforded the freestanding practice located in a separate building designed specifically to house the audiology practice. Dimensions and layout can be designed to meet the specific and exact needs of the facility. Perhaps the most common location for a practice is in a professional building or shared occupancy space such as retail or commercial space. The professional building commonly includes other medical professionals and therefore has probably been designed to accommodate the construction, equipment, and space requirements for an audiological practice. Although exact square footage requirements cannot always be met, many choices are often available in a variety of locations with similar space dimensions that meet the target needs.

Location, Location, Location

This section of the chapter will consider factors pertaining to selecting a location for a freestanding audiology practice.

"Freestanding" refers to practices that are physically located outside of a hospital, multispecialty outpatient clinic, or rehabilitation agency. A freestanding practice might, of course, have administrative or contractual relationships with other types of facilities. The general term *location* implies at least three subsets: the macrolocation or geographical region of the country; the microlocation (town, city, community) within a region; and site or specific building that houses the practice. Each of these will be discussed separately despite the fact that several overlapping issues pertain to all these considerations. Before undertaking these presentations, however, the reader should be reminded that getting expert advice from consultants who specialize in demographics, relocations, business statistics, and real estate (leasing and purchasing) is generally in one's best interest. Some of the information required to make an informed decision about practice location can be obtained at little or no cost from chambers of commerce, service and business organizations, government agencies, leasing agents, libraries, and the like. Gathering data of this type is a vital first step. It is a good idea to arm oneself with as much of this information as possible *before* formulating specific questions for paid consultants like accountants, lawyers, public/relation marketing firms, and demographers.

PITFALL

Never consult with paid experts until you have done your own homework. Whether the issue is marketing, demographics, or zoning, learn enough about the subject to formulate specific questions for consultants. This will save you time and money.

Macrolocation

If one is in a situation that allows movement to any part of the country desired, how will one decide which region is best suited to personal and professional needs and goals? Some would argue that choosing a macrolocation should be done dispassionately, that is "rationally." They would advise one to put aside personal preferences regarding climate, recreational resources, and access to extended family members or friends and advise selecting a location based solely on hard factual data relating to "regional economic trends," "population shifts," "business climate," and so forth. Although no one would dispute the importance of these factors, launching a business venture like an audiology practice in an area of the country that is fundamentally disagreeable with one and one's family is foolhardy. It is our belief that overseeing a successful practice in a geographical region that is unsatisfying personally will ultimately lead to problems that money cannot solve. If one dislikes snow, one should not locate in the north; if one needs the seashore, one should not move to the Midwest. If being close to one's aging parents is important, make plans accordingly. Of course, the whole of society is fluid and in a constant state of flux: family and friends relocate, businesses close, regional economies expand and contract, opportunities change to liabilities, and so forth. Nevertheless, a clinician's fundamental "happiness" depends as much on his or her personal environment as it does on financial rewards. One should make these decisions as much for the "long haul" by considering the totality of one's satisfaction quotient. One not only practices audiology, one lives in the location that selected.

Having said these things, however, we are reminded of a quotation from Hosford-Dunn et al (1995) . . . "personal preferences have an immediacy that tends to obscure other more objective considerations. Little if any research is needed to know where you would *like* to practice, but a great deal of marketing research is needed to learn where you would do *best* to practice." With this counterbalancing admonition, the factors that will help us "zero in" on a location will be discussed.

Because choosing a "macrolocation" involves a comparison of broad geographical areas, the factors that aid in deciding these matters are also necessarily broad. The use of a comparison chart, such as the one shown in Table 13–4, will be useful in making a final determination. Information of this type can be obtained from sources such as the U.S. Bureau of the Census, national business magazines and journals, economic development councils, state governments, business bureaus, major newspapers in the region, chambers of commerce, universities, the U.S. Bureau of Labor Statistics, public libraries, or from the Service Corps of Retired Executives.

Microlocation

"Microlocation" refers to a town or city within a broad geographical region. Some of the information gathered to decide on the macrolocation would help answer questions about the community in which one wishes to locate. In comparing two or more cities, however, one needs to ask more specific questions. To help answer these questions, charts such as seen in Tables 13–5 and 13–6 (Baxter, 1994) are helpful.

The following important questions that pertain to selecting not only a specific microlocation but also an area within the community should be answered. This list is adapted from Hosford-Dunn et al (1995).

- Is the city expanding geographically?
- Is the city growing economically?
- Are businesses/industries opening/closing?
- What are the population demographics (age, educational level, income, occupational types, marital status, and number of dependents)?
- How is the real estate market (average home costs, property values, length of time to sell, age of homes)?
- Is the population stable, transient, or seasonal?

TABLE 13–4   Choosing a macrolocation

	Region A	Region B	Region C
Audiologist/population ratio			
Overall economy			
Main industries			
Unemployment rate			
Health insurance trends			
Healthcare trends			
Climate/weather			
Cost of living			
Cultural amenities			
Cultural/ethnic mix			
School systems			
Higher education			
Transportation			
Overall demographics			
Population trends			
Population age			
Housing costs			
Taxes			
Shopping/entertainment			
Economic potential			
Per capita income			
Disposable income			
Proximity to family/friends			
Places of worship			
Recreational opportunities			
Licensure laws			
Competition			
Other (_____)			
TOTALS			

Give 3 points for more favorable, 2 points for neutral, and 1 point for less favorable; identify the *five* most important factors to you and *double* the point value for these.

TABLE 13–5 Evaluating communities, resources, and potential

Professional Considerations	Community A	Community B	Community C
1. I can meet requirements for obtaining a state license. (Audiology and hearing aid dispensing.)			
2. Desirable office space is available and affordable.			
3. Laboratories (in town or reached by shipment) do good work and costs are reasonable.			
4. Trained or trainable auxiliary personnel are available at reasonable cost.			
5. The local hospitals and managed care organizations recognize audiologists as providers of covered services.			
6. State and/or regional associations are active. Continuing education is available at a reasonable cost.			
7. Educational facilities for postgraduate work are accessible.			
8. Supplementary salaried work is available.			
9. Other audiologists are cordial. Collaboration is available.			
10. Referrals and consultations can be obtained.			
11. The community is sympathetic to a modern concept of audiology.			
12. I can create a competitive and viable "niche."			
13. SWOT analysis is mostly positive.			
14. Referrals are likely to materialize.			
15. I sense a suitable level of professionalism.			
TOTAL			

Family Living	Community A	Community B	Community C
1. The town has an attractive residential area.			
2. Houses are available to rent or buy at a price within the budget.			
3. Property taxes are reasonable.			
4. Schools are modern; teachers seem enthusiastic; level of education appears high.			
5. Park and playground facilities are adequate.			
6. Favorite recreation is within driving distance.			
7. Cultural activities are suitable.			
8. Shopping facilities are good.			
9. The community is progressive and well managed.			
10. The family likes the area and will feel at home.			
11. Climate is good.			
12. Proximity to extended family/friends is acceptable.			
13. Spouse has appropriate work/educational opportunities.			
14. Place of worship is available.			
15. We have contacts in the community.			
TOTAL			

Each community under consideration may be rated on the following charts. A "yes" answer receives a 5, a "maybe" 3, and a "no" 1. Columns for each community in each category can be added and the results compared.

TABLE 13–5   (continued) Evaluating communities, resources, and potential

Economic Potential	Community A	Community B	Community C
1. Population increase compares favorably with state and national increases.			
2. Audiologist/population ratio is lower than state average.			
3. Income level is high.			
4. Retail sales show healthy growth.			
5. Industry is stable and growing.			
6. Wages are high.			
7. Consumer credit and collection records are good.			
8. Fee schedules reflect rise in cost of living.			
9. Average gross profits of audiologists in area compare favorably with state and national averages.			
10. Professional and business people questioned say the town can use another audiologist.			
11. I have business/professional contacts.			
12. The penetration of managed care contracting is appropriate for my practice goals.			
13. I can gain access to HMO, PPO, and POS contracts.			
14. My "patient mix" (proportion of private pay, third-party payors, etc.) is likely to be favorable.			
15. Unemployment rate is low.			
TOTAL			

	Community A	Community B	Community C
Family living			
Professional considerations			
Economic potential			
TOTAL			

Adapted from Baxter (1994).

- Will recreational and cultural amenities meet our needs? How about places of worship?
- What are the transportation modes? Are they convenient for my patients?
- What is the quality of the schools? Colleges and universities?
- Will I feel comfortable in the cultural/ethnic mix?
- What are the traffic patterns within the city? Are there areas to be avoided?
- What are the zoning restrictions in the area of interest in the city?
- What is the tax structure (real estate, business, personal property, occupational, sales, income, etc.)?
- Is there evidence of civic pride and cooperation? Does the government seem effective?

- Who are the main employers? Are these industries/businesses stable?
- What kinds of health insurance are residents likely to have (HMO, PPO, Indemnity, Medicaid, Medicare)?
- What are the characteristics of the workforce (blue collar, union, white collar, industrial, managerial, farming, professional)?
- What is the socioeconomic and educational level of the population?
- Is one area of the city growing more rapidly than others?
- Will residents be likely to need/use and afford these services?
- Who are the competitors? What is the nature of their practice (specialty clinic, hospital-based, physicians, and retailers)?

TABLE 13–6   Checklist for characterizing practice locations

City or town

Economic considerations

1. Source of income
   - ❏ Farming
   - ❏ Manufacturing
   - ❏ Wholesale/retail
   - ❏ Professional/managerial

2. Trend
   - ❏ Highly satisfactory
   - ❏ Growing
   - ❏ Stationary/stagnant
   - ❏ Declining

3. Permanency
   - ❏ Old and well established
   - ❏ Old and reviving
   - ❏ New and promising
   - ❏ Recent and uncertain
   - ❏ High turnover

4. Diversification
   - ❏ Many and varied income sources
   - ❏ Many of the same income sources
   - ❏ Few income sources
   - ❏ Dependent on one industry

5. Stability
   - ❏ Constant
   - ❏ Satisfactory
   - ❏ Subject to wide fluctuations

6. Seasonality
   - ❏ Little or no seasonal change
   - ❏ Mild seasonal change
   - ❏ Periodical—every few years
   - ❏ Highly seasonal in nature
   - ❏ Tourist-dependent

7. Business climate
   - ❏ Attracting several new investments
   - ❏ Some new commercial projects
   - ❏ Corporate headquarters stable
   - ❏ Corporate holdings volatile

8. Future
   - ❏ Most promising
   - ❏ Satisfactory
   - ❏ Uncertain
   - ❏ Poor outlook

Population

1. Income distribution
   - ❏ Mostly wealthy
   - ❏ Well distributed
   - ❏ Mostly middle income
   - ❏ Poor

2. Trend
   - ❏ Growing
   - ❏ Large and stable
   - ❏ Small and stable
   - ❏ Declining

3. Living status
   - ❏ Own homes
   - ❏ Pay substantial rent
   - ❏ Pay moderate rent
   - ❏ Pay low rent

Competition

1. Number of competing services
   - ❏ Few
   - ❏ Average
   - ❏ Many
   - ❏ Too many

2. Nature of competing services
   - ❏ Relatively low-tech; large service gaps
   - ❏ Average level of competence
   - ❏ Organized network/full service
   - ❏ Sophisticated delivery systems/ leading edge

3. Type of competing service
   - ❏ Unattractive
   - ❏ Average
   - ❏ Old and well established

The town as a place to live

1. Character of the city
   - ❏ Homes neat and clean
   - ❏ Lawns, parks, streets, etc., neat, modern, attractive
   - ❏ Banking facilities adequate
   - ❏ Transportation facilities adequate
   - ❏ Professional services adequate
   - ❏ Utilities facilities adequate

2. Facilities and climate
   - ❏ Schools
   - ❏ Churches
   - ❏ Amusement centers
   - ❏ Medical and dental services

TABLE 13–6 Checklist for characterizing practice locations *(continued)*

The Actual Site

1. The number of other providers of services of the same kind as yours _____

2. Traffic flow
   Sex of pedestrians _____
   Age of pedestrians _____
   Destination of pedestrians _____

3. Transportation
   Transfer points _____
   Highway _____
   Kind (bus, streetcar, auto, railway)_____

4. Parking facilities
   ❏ Large and convenient
   ❏ Large enough but not convenient
   ❏ Convenient but too small
   ❏ Completely inadequate

5. Unfavorable characteristics
   ❏ Fire hazards
   ❏ Industry
   ❏ Vacant lot—no parking possibilities
   ❏ Garages
   ❏ Smoke, dust, odors
   ❏ Poor sidewalks and pavement
   ❏ Unsightly neighborhood building

6. Professionals on the block
   ❏ Physicians
   ❏ Psychologists
   ❏ Lawyers
   ❏ Others

7. History of the site

   _____
   _____
   _____
   _____

8. The premises
   ❏ Away from noise sources
   ❏ Handicap accessible
   ❏ Office easy to find
   ❏ Hard to get around within building

Adapted from Baxter (1994).

- Which ZIP codes contain more of the population that I'm most likely to serve?
- Is office space available at a reasonable cost in these areas?
- Are these areas on public transportation routes?
- Are these areas easy to reach by automobile (traffic patterns, congestion, safety, etc)? Would access be convenient?
- Are these areas considered "safe" (low crime rates, negotiable traffic flow, less intimidating to younger and older persons)?
- What is the general attitude toward healthcare providers? Audiologists?
- What is the travel time from home to practice site? From patients' homes to practice? Can this city support the practice? Does a need exist for services here?
- What healthcare facilities exist (hospitals, rehabilitation agencies, nursing homes, clinics, etc)?
- How do residents usually pay for healthcare (private pay, third-party, etc.)?
- Are there any gaps or niches that my practice can fill?
- What is the reputation of competing professionals, clinics, retail offices, physicians and hospitals?

- Do I have "connections" in this community (family, friends, colleagues, bankers, business and government leaders, civic organization members, etc.)?
- Can I afford to practice in this city? Community? (housing costs, rental/leasing costs, taxes, transportation utilities, etc.)?

PEARL

Location, location, location: it is a lot easier to upgrade equipment and furnishings than it is to change practice sites. Choose the very best site you can afford now.

In addition to studying the information sources just mentioned, take advantage of the marketing departments of some of the major hearing instrument and equipment manufacturers. It is obviously in the manufacturers' best interests to help select a location that increases the probability that the practice will be profitable now and in the long run. In essence, one is "partnering" with the manufacturer in this venture.

Chances are good that the manufacturer has more experience (and resources) in making business decisions. Their expertise should be used to your mutual advantage. Several of the larger manufacturers offer free or low-cost market survey and demographic data to assist in selecting a suitable location. If some cost is involved in gathering these data, it can often be paid back by agreeing to purchase "x" number of hearing aids from a particular manufacturer within a specified period of time. Although some discounts on the single unit price of the hearing instruments purchased from that source may be given up, "co-oping" with the manufacturer may be a relatively simple way of securing the funds necessary for carrying out a thorough market survey and demographic analysis of a particular region/city. When contemplating establishing a new practice or a satellite location in the same region, it is often helpful to contact hearing instrument manufacturers who have been good business partners as an early step in the process. They might be able to save a considerable amount of time and money. Although their data can be extremely useful, one should corroborate their findings with independent research. If their report and your data are in essential agreement, perhaps the right location has been found.

The SWOT Technique

Another "tool" for making informed decisions about locating a practice is a technique known as SWOT: *s*trengths, *w*eaknesses, *o*pportunities, and *t*hreats (Cunningham & Erekson, 1994). SWOT analysis requires you to list strengths, weaknesses, opportunities, and threats that you and your advisors believe to pertain to planting your practice in one or another location. An example of SWOT analysis is shown in Table 13–7. The same analysis should be applied to other potential locations as a means of comparison.

Another important consideration related to choosing a viable practice location is the probability of garnering referrals from agencies, other professionals, schools, clinics, industries, and the like. This sort of analysis goes well beyond merely identifying potential referral sources. It is also more critical than locating a practice in the proximity of potential referrers. It is *strongly* recommended that one estimate the actual number of referrals expected on a monthly basis from each source. These data, although they are only best estimates, will be useful in deciding between and among various locations within the community. These data are also invaluable in preparing a business plan, especially the proforma profit and loss statement section. In this regard, it behooves one to do a thorough projection of the number of referrals, by source, that one is likely to receive in a specified period of time. To achieve this, potential referral sources must be visited on an appointment basis. This opportunity should be used to introduce yourself and to describe your credentials, experience, and range of services. Ask the facility director to characterize his or her population's general need for your services and to estimate the number of patients he or she is likely to refer to you each month. Quite often the response will be given as a range (i.e., "you might expect to get two to four referrals each month from our agency." Accept this estimate at face value, do not press for more precise data, and under no circumstances make the director feel that he or she is being pressured for any sort of commitment. Take the midpoint of this range and enter it into

TABLE 13–7 Illustration of the SWOT technique as applied to choosing a practice location

Strengths
- This part of the city is expanding.
- Most of the population is older than 40.
- The socioeconomic level is high.
- My office will be close to my home.
- Referral sources are close by.

Weaknesses
- I have no personal contacts here.
- Public transportation routes are not convenient.
- Rush hour traffic is congested.
- Three competitors are close by.
- Many retirees in this community are on a fixed income.

Opportunities
- Plenty of prime office space is available here.
- Leasing rates are reasonable.
- Other healthcare facilities are locating here.
- A major competitor is retiring soon.
- Two new retirement villages are under construction here.

Threats
- The large ACME manufacturing plant closes next year.
- The ENT practice may begin dispensing soon.
- Zoning restrictions are under review.
- The new expressway might divert traffic elsewhere.
- Managed care insurance options are popular with residents here.

the chart shown in Table 13–8. Tally the estimates and use these figures as a means of comparing two or more potential microlocations. Do not underestimate the value of this exercise. The magnitude of the differences among various locations may be surprising. A partial list of potential referral sources is given in Table 13–9 as an aid to stimulating the search. This list is adapted from Loavenbruck and Madell (1981).

Once this list of potential referral sources has been studied and those most likely to recommend your services have been identified, use their referral estimates to complete a chart such as the one given in Table 13–8.

PEARL

The SWOT technique can be used for helping to make nearly any decision that involves complex or conflicting considerations in any aspect of your business or personal life.

Choosing a Specific Site

Now that decisions have been made regarding the macrolocations and microlocations, it is time to focus on choosing a specific site (building) to house the practice. One of the first

TABLE 13–8 Monthly referral estimates for location # _____

Source	Referral Probability			Total/ Month
	Low	Likely	High	
Steven Smith, M.D.		3		3
Jones Nursing Home	2			2
ACME Manufacturing Co.	3			3
Pediatric Associates, P.S.C.			8	8
East End Medical Associates, P.S.C.		2		2
Boone County School District		4		4
S.H.H.H.			2	2
Schriner's Children's Hospital			7	7
Easter Seal Speech & Hearing Clinic		4		4
All-Care Rehab Agency	2			2
James Dawson, M.D.		2		2
E.N.T. Associates, P.S.C.			6	6
Cumberland Community Hospital			6	6
Tri-County Nursing Home		2		2
Mid-South Medical Specialists		4		4
H.M.O. Contracts		6		6
GRAND TOTALS	7	27	29	63

Adapted from Loavenbruck and Madell (1981).

considerations is the match between the "practice model" and the sites that are under consideration. The practice model has two components: (1) the actual way in which the practice will be structured (private "medical model" vs. public "retail" setting; "walk-in" dependent vs. referral-based "appointment only," etc.); and (2) the "image" that one hopes to convey (e.g., mall "retailer" vs. "doctoring" professional; "premier" products and services vs. discount oriented, etc.). These decisions need to be given serious thought. These judgments will be influenced significantly by a number of correlative factors. The following are examples:

- *Likely referral sources:* Will other professionals who refer to you be comfortable with the site (and style) of your practice? For example, will physicians perceive the site as on par with their own offices, image, and service quality? Is it reasonably close to the most likely referral sources? Is it easy to find?

- *Congruence with the population base:* Does the site "fit" the lifestyles, attitudes, and consumer habits of the population under consideration (i.e., price-driven vs. quality-oriented)? What expectations will the patients bring to the office? Will they expect valet parking or are they willing to park on the 7th floor of the parking garage? How will they react to the other offices and businesses

around the practice? What is the overall impression the site creates? Would patients like the "feel" of the site? Would an "upscale" site be intimidating to the typical patient? Would a strip mall site surrounded by a discount store, a large grocery, and a fast food restaurant be seen as convenient or crass? Do you know your population base well enough to characterize their likely response to these questions?

- *Topographical considerations:* Will the site be within the "topography" of other service-oriented enterprises (i.e., are "like-minded" businesses clustered in the proximity of the site)? Is the topography or "cluster" a professional office building? A medical center? A senior-services (nutrition, health information center, etc.) complex? A health-oriented complex (e.g., a site that includes an optician; a pharmacy; a health food store; a physician, dentist, or chiropractor)? Is the location of the site associated with related, high-quality services? Does the proximity of other health professionals increase the likelihood of mutual cooperation and referrals (e.g., might the neighboring optometrist or podiatrist refer patients because they are in the same complex? Would the site attract walk-in consumers who notice the office while using the services of other professionals? Would those who are waiting for

TABLE 13–9   Possible referral sources

• Construction companies	• Heavy equipment operators
• Rehabilitation agencies	• Hospitals
• Clinics	• Industrial/manufacturers
• Insurance companies	• Lawyers
• Learning disability specialists	• Nursing homes
• Public school	• Private and parochial schools
• Preschools and kindergartens	• Otolaryngologists
• G.P./family medicine	• Neurologists
• Internists	• Geriatrics/gerontologists
• Oncologists	• Neurosurgeons
• Neonatologists	• Others (opticians, dentists, etc.)
• Retirement villages	• Intermediate care facilities
• Parent-teacher associations	• Psychologists
• Social workers	• Senior citizens clubs
• Musicians	• Theaters/movies (ALDS)
• Places of worship (ALDS)	• Hunting/shooting clubs
• Fire and police organizations	• Speech-language pathologists
• Railroads	• Service clubs (Elks, Lions, etc.)
• School nurses	• Self Help for the Hard of Hearing (SHHH)
• HMOs	• Consumer groups
• Skilled nursing facilities	• Special Olympics
• Women's service clubs	• Other audiologists
• Labor unions	• Colleges and universities
• American Cancer Society	• Plant safety engineers (OSHA)
• Deaf community organizations	• Social service agencies
• Pilots' association	
• Retired personnel groups (SCORE, AARP, etc.)	
• Organizations for the handicapped	

Adapted from Loavenbruck and Madell (1981).

family members to see another professional be likely to "drop in" to ask about your products or services? Would the topography of an enclosed shopping mall or a strip mall induce consumers to "drift" into the site while marketing, banking, visiting the post office, or bookstore?

• *"Gut-Reaction" to the Site:* When you drive or walk by the site and observe its full "ambiance," what do you see and how does it feel? Commercial? Professional? Confusing? Inviting? Busy? Imposing? Impressive? Congested? Modern? Dated? Clean? Progressive? Can you find a single adjective to describe the site? Do you like the description? Would you send your own family member there? Do you see your own image in the site? Does it feel comfortable to you?

Perception matters, but so does substance. The choice of an office space depends on a number of concrete and practical considerations. In addition to the obvious size and square footage requirements, some of the most basic attributes include the following:

• *Affordability:* Check the budget section of your business plan carefully. Know what can be afforded, but also know that you cannot afford to make a gross error in site selection. Within reason, it might make sense to stretch the budget to get the best site possible. Remember, it is not difficult to move up to more expensive clinical equipment

or better office furniture later, but it is much more difficult (and costly) to upgrade your site.

• *Configuration:* Is it possible to function in the space? Are the number of rooms appropriate? Are the rooms of appropriate size? Will the space require extensive architectural modifications? Who will pay for them? Are utilities, power sources, sinks, lavatories, and the like well placed? Are the plumbing, heating/air conditioning, lighting and window placement adequate? Does the site lend itself to easy reconfiguration? Will the floor support the weight of sound booths?

• *Site within the site:* Is the office off the main lobby? Near the entrance? Easily found within the building? Visible by pedestrian traffic in the corridors? Too near noise sources? Opposite the elevator bank? At street level? Clustered near similar services? Near a busy pharmacy or clinic? Would

---

PEARL

Bankers and lenders are also partners in your venture. Their expertise and advice about suitable practice sites in the community can be extremely valuable.

finding the office be confusing for elderly patients walking from the parking garage?

- *Related costs:* Does the lease include utilities? If not, what are the estimated utility charges? Are utilities separately metered? For what taxes is the tenant responsible? Who pays (tenant or landlord) if taxes are raised during the term of the lease? What is the tenant's share of "common use fees" (i.e., the cost of services like snow removal, exterior building and parking lot lighting, building maintenance and security, housekeeping, lawn maintenance, and the like)?

- *Parking and access:* Is parking adequate near the site? (At-the-door "surface" parking is preferable to high-rise parking towers.) Is valet parking a possibility? Will the practice's patients have to pay for parking? If so, what is the cost? Can the tenant validate parking tickets? If so, what's the cost to the tenant? What are the costs associated with personnel parking? Are "reserved " spaces available? What distance will patients have to walk to reach the office? Is the entire distance free of barriers to those in wheelchairs? Is the "route" to and from the parking area and the office easy to find and follow? Are curb cuts, ramps, elevators, handrails, and the like easily negotiated by handicapped individuals?

- *Purchasing a stand-alone structure:* Would the purchase of an existing stand-alone building be an advantage? (Consider factors such as tax advantages, long-term real estate investment opportunities, owner equity accumulation, etc.) Might part of the space be subleased to related businesses to improve walk-in traffic and visibility? Would rental income help offset mortgage installments? Would renovation costs be affordable? What is the potential resale value of the property? Consider zoning restrictions and real estate tax rates. Additional costs may be incurred in bringing an older facility into compliance with current fire, building, safety, and Americans with Disabilities Act regulations.

- *Constructing a new facility:* Is a suitable building site available in the part of town you are interested in? Can you afford it? This gives you the opportunity to custom design the facility to meet your specific requirements. The use of a qualified architect and contractors is a must. Regular planning sessions and construction site visits are essential to monitor progress. A construction time frame and a performance contingency must be included in construction contracts. It is important to use only insured and bonded contractors and obtain copies of paid bills or quit claims as work progresses. This is because subcontractors and suppliers can put a lien on your property if the general contractor fails to pay bills in full and on time.

Leasing/Renting an Office

Most private practice owners generally begin by leasing (or renting) an office site. Leasing should not be undertaken without competent legal counsel. Lease agreements (contracts) offered by the landlord are prepared by the attorney. They are written in such a way as to protect the landlord and his or her property. They are not necessarily written to afford the protection and options that the practice might require. Indeed, the landlord's "standard" contract is often presented to the tenant as if it were cast in stone and essentially nonnegotiable. The document often looks so "official" as to have the effect of intimidating the potential tenant. *Never assume that a lease contract is immutable. All* of the covenants and language are subject to negotiation and revision by the tenants and their lawyers. Your counsel will review the document very carefully with you and recommend changes and additions that are in your best interest. A complete description of a suitable lease contract is beyond the scope of this chapter. However, some of the key issues that must be considered follow:

- An accurate description of the "demised premises" (site), including location, size (square footage), condition, and the like.

- The names and addresses of the landlord and tenant.

- The date that the lease actually begins ("commencement date").

- The "term" (length) of the lease (e.g., 1 year, with a 3-year option, etc.) along with specifics regarding renewal.

- What "leasehold improvements" (build-outs, renovations) will be done; who will pay for them (tenant or landlord)? (NOTE: be certain to include detailed architectural drawings of these improvements as an appendix to the contract.)

- The monthly rental rate, utilities cost, "common area fees" (janitorial, security, etc.), insurance, and security agreements. The dates that rent is due and any provisions for late charges.

- Clear descriptions of circumstances and causes under which the lease can be broken before the termination date; an enumeration of penalties, fees, forfeiture of deposits, and the like must be included.

- A description of how the office can be legally used, along with a list of prohibited uses (e.g., noisy manufacturing processes, unapproved use of toxic chemicals).

- A covenant restricting the use of the other offices in the building by competing businesses and professionals. (NOTE: this may be more difficult to negotiate than other points in the contract.)

- Options for the tenant to "sublease" the premises in whole or in part and the conditions of rental payment in this circumstance. Size, location, and type of signage to be used on the exterior and interior of the building.

- Parking availability and restrictions; parking fees (if applicable).

Other Factors in Site Selection

Research has demonstrated that consumers exhibit "spatial choice behaviors" when selecting their destinations. These choices are often based on subjective rather than objective or physical realities (Cadwallader, 1981). Consumers appear to use "cognitive mapping" (Parfit 1984) as an important variable in deciding which locations or destinations are most suitable. "Convenience" is more than merely choosing a designation that is closest to their home or place of business. Convenience also relates to selecting sites that are within their cognitive map. For example, consumers will visualize your site in relation to other "anchor points" that they are already familiar with.

An anchor point is a site that has some significance to the consumer. It might be a major shopping mall, a notable city landmark, a school building, a fire station, or the like. It would behoove one to locate (and describe the location in marketing materials) with the typical client's cognitive map in mind. A site that is "one block of east of town hall," "across the street from Mid Town Mall," or "beside the grocery store" is easier to find (and identify with) than merely a street address.

Hosford-Dunn et al (1995) offer the material in Table 13–10 as an aid in selecting a specific practice site. Use it to make careful comparisons between and among the places that are under consideration.

From Floorplan to Construction

Choosing the location for a practice is a significant accomplishment, but after that the real work begins. Now the space must be configured within the location to meet the operational needs of the practice. Configuring the space leads to a formalized drawing from which construction will proceed. A floorplan is a drawing that in its final version details the location of every construction-related aspect of the facility, including the walls, doors, electrical outlets, plumbing fixtures, casework, lighting, computer cabling, and sound booth location. An architect will be responsible for producing a final version of the floorplan with all the details, but at this time the concern should be primarily with the location of the walls and rooms.

The location chosen for the practice, in part, influences the energy and effort that are required to configure or layout the space. One may have chosen a particular location because its space is already configured in an acceptable manner for the practice. Little or no construction is required and existing rooms can be readily adapted to the audiological and business needs of the practice. More commonly, space needs reconfiguring, in part or in whole, to meet the practice needs

of the new occupant. The thought of tearing down existing walls and constructing new ones; of putting in new carpeting, ceiling tiles, and casework; and of adding lights, electrical outlets, and acoustic barriers evokes thoughts of a significant financial investment. Typically, however, contracts for renting space in commercial professional buildings will include a building allowance that is applied toward the cost of the renovation, particularly for major construction costs. If this is the case, the floorplan can be developed from a blueprint of the walls that define the boundaries of the space. In other words, the layout of space should be done as if the space were completely void of any existing walls. It should be noted, however, that the building allowance can be limited and that items such as sinks in all rooms can cause the allowance to be easily exceeded. This will result in an additional up-front cost or an increase in rent if the allowance is amortized over the length of the lease. For persons constructing a new building for a practice, the floorplan can take whatever shape or configuration desired, probably only limited by the size and shape of the land on which the building is to be built. Obviously, it is easier to design a facility without restrictions than it is to design a facility that must be "fit" into existing space, but constructing a new building adds significantly to the overall effort necessary to see the facility to completion.

PEARL

If possible, go to the location chosen with a roll of masking tape and "layout" the locations of the walls, doors, and the like. Scaled to actual size, the taped walls helps visualize the movements of patients, staff, and operations, making impractical layouts obvious.

Using the lists of rooms and operations previously developed, the next step is to begin sketching possible configurations of the space. As a starting point, use fixed points within the boundaries. For example, if the entrance door cannot be moved, it is logical to assume the waiting room will be located near that fixed point. As a sketch develops, consider patient and staff traffic patterns. Consider the movement of persons within the space from the time they enter the practice until the time they leave. The location of the sign-in window, the size and shape of the waiting area, the movements of patients through the facility, and the location for paying bills or for consulting with the business manager should be considered. The goal is to create a plan that minimizes confusion and congestion and maximizes use of space. How does patient traffic flow if the appointments are for audiological evaluations versus hearing aid evaluations? How do patients flow if they "walk-in" for a hearing aid repair or for batteries? How does staff enter and exit the building? How do movements of staff during office hours influence the location of rooms? Remember that the "rooms" contain certain operations that may have special requirements and therefore may not be very flexible in size or location.

Most often, persons contemplating the layout of a new facility have an idea about how the various audiological and

TABLE 13–10   Comparative features and cost analysis of office sites

Factors	Location 1	Location 2	Location 3
*Site features**			
Location			
Parking			
Accessibility			
Physical suitability			
Room for expansion			
Safety/security			
Image			
Estimated value in 10 y			
Zoning			
Competition			
Community			
Distance from referral sources			
Distance from my home			
Vehicular traffic patterns			
Pedestrian traffic flow within building			
Visibility to patients			
Convenience			
Relation to "anchor" points			
Noise levels			
TOTAL POINTS:			
Cost variables[†]			
Rent or depreciation			
Heating			
Electricity			
Other utilities			
Wages			
Insurance			
Advertising rates			
Personnel costs (salaries and benefits)			
Remodeling/construction costs			
Common use fees (snow removal, etc.)			
Security			
Parking fees			
Signage requirements			
Consultant fees			
Travel (To and from home)			
TAXES[‡]			
Property			
Personal property			
Income			
Sales			
Payroll			
City/county/state			
TOTAL $$:			

*Rate as "good" (10 points), "average" (5 points), or "poor" (1 point).
[†]List costs in dollars.
[‡]Use estimated or exact cost per year in dollars.
Adapted from Hosford-Dunn et al (1995).

> ## PEARL
>
> Be sure to plan ahead for enough electrical outlets in your sound booths and treatment rooms. This is especially important if you plan on bringing equipment like portable audiometers, otoacoustic emissions systems, or immittance units into the booth.

> ## PEARL
>
> Do not settle for any floorplan that does not meet either your immediate need or fit with the long-term possibilities. Continue to manipulate the drawings until an acceptable floorplan is developed.

business operations interface with each other. If not, insight into these interactions can be gained by examining the strengths and weaknesses of the current facility or by visiting other audiological facilities and practices. Carefully examine the working and space relationships between staff, services, and patients to identify the reason things work well or the reasons they do not. Evaluate space and patient flow. Evaluate the spatial relationship between various departments (professional staff, bookkeeping, billing, receptionist, waiting room, testing or treatment rooms) and the ways these interactions enhance or detract from efficient operations. Could operations be improved by locating specific services closer or farther apart? Do patients move easily through the facility or do logjams occur at certain times during the day? Is it important for the business aspects of the practice and the audiological aspects be within contiguous space? Are walk-in patients easily accommodated? Insight into the operational aspects of other practices provides guidance for the floorplan of your new facility.

For an audiological facility, the location of the sound booths is perhaps the most important first consideration in space planning, particularly if the booths are the large double-room, double-wall types. Typically these booths will remain wherever they are first installed, and all future changes in space will work around the booths. Smaller booths, such as a seven by seven (7×7) single-room, single-wall booth, can be moved, although not easily, if future changes so dictate. Background noise factors have to be considered in developing the space layout. When planning the location of the sound booths also remember accessibility factors, particularly with regard to getting patients in and out. Accessibility in this regard relates to three factors: (1) the height of the doorsill, (2) the ability to maneuver patients in front of the booth, and (3)

whether the door swings in or out. In hospitals, sufficient space must be left near the doors of the booth to allow stretchers and wheelchairs to be maneuvered into the booth. Although it is unlikely that stretchers would be of concern in a freestanding private practice, patients in wheelchairs would not be uncommon. Allowance for floor space to accommodate an elevated surface or a ramp should be included in the plans. A new facility can be planned to incorporate a dropped floor where the booths would be located, thus lowering the doorsill to ground height. Although this improves accessibility, it also virtually eliminates any possibility of moving the booths in the future.

It is important to work with both the manufacturers of the sound booths and the installation company during the planning stage. Understanding the exact dimensions of the booth, the air handling systems, and the space required for the doors to open is necessary when planning around the booth. The location and dimensions associated with the sound booths will dictate initial aspects of the space plan.

> ## PEARL
>
> Many buildings are constructed with the walls extended just into the ceiling area but not joining the floor above. This allows sound energy to pass easily from one room to another. Insist that walls extend fully to the floor above, and that all openings between rooms be sealed. Include the use of acoustic barriers; usually sound batting, in the walls and ceilings of sound-sensitive rooms.

> ## SPECIAL CONSIDERATION
>
> If one plans to carry out auditory-evoked potential tests, medical grade wiring with isolated grounding in the rooms in which you plan to perform the procedures may be included. Although line interference from other electrical sources is typically associated with hospital settings, it can also be an issue in office settings in which multiple pieces of equipment (e.g., computers, printers) share a common ground.

Sound booths today also present a unique planning problem in relation to fire control systems within buildings. Many building codes require all rooms to contain sprinkler systems or other forms of fire control. Installing sprinkler systems in sound rooms compromises the acoustic integrity of the booths. A special waiver may be required to avoid this problem. Schedule a meeting with the fire inspector to discuss this matter before installation.

Patient confidentiality has always been important, but the need to ensure patient confidence is even more critical in today's litigious society. Space and room configurations should be planned in a manner to ensure confidentially. Conversations about patients, whether in direct counseling, in conversations among the professional staff, or in phone conversations, need to be protected. The best place to begin consideration of this matter is during the layout stage. A popular concept in space planning has been an "open" design, whereby many of the barriers between the waiting room and the office are removed, thus allowing patients to "see and hear" many of the operations that take place. Although this may create a sense of intimacy and connectedness between the patient and the office, it also allows confidential conversations to become public knowledge, potentially compromising the patient-audiologist relationship.

Take your time when sketching possible floorplans. Develop several different layouts using entirely different combinations of space. In addition to the walls and sound booths, preliminary consideration of items such as access to water, electrical connections, lighting, heating and ventilation, and computer locations should be made. This is particularly true if these things will directly influence the floorplan. Preliminary sketches should include items such as casework, cabinets, sinks, and file racks.

After generating a series of preliminary sketches, it is time to visit an architect. The architect can provide a more realistic draft that will include any or all building restrictions or codes. Remember that an architect, even one with expertise in medical facilities, is not an audiologist and therefore does not know details regarding the operations within the practice, therefore communication throughout the design and detail process is critical. Before meeting with the architect, make sure the sketches are realistic and readable but also include a list of each individual room and the functions therein. Note any special restrictions, such as the need for acoustic barriers, that may be necessary in any given space. In addition, make sure the architect has an idea of any budgetary constraints that might influence the design.

Finally, one must convey a sense of the type of atmosphere one would like to create in the space because the final drawings will need to detail any specialized construction that contributes to the image and look of the practice. The final "look" of the practice is composed of a combination of the furnishings and the layout. Lighting, wall location, carpeting, and ceilings contribute to both form and function. A contemporary office design may incorporate curved glass walls, which influence both floor space available for use and the types of functions that occur on either side. Those construction components that help to create the look will need to be incorporated into the floorplan.

Details of construction are added after a finalized floorplan is developed. The location of electrical outlets, sinks, casework and cupboards and the use of acoustic barriers in the walls, electrically shielded outlets, and carpeting or tiled floors is added to the plans. One should participate in all decisions in this regard and carefully review all plans before construction. Only when fully satisfied that the plans meet the practice's needs and fall within acceptable budgetary constraints should one proceed to the construction phase.

During the actual construction, pay close attention to the details, comparing the plans to the evolving product. If deviations are noted, bring it to the attention of the construction crews immediately. If substantial changes are necessary, get with the construction foreman and architect immediately because it is much easier and less costly to make changes before the construction proceeds farther. Attention to the details at this point is imperative to ensure the facility is designed according to your needs. Visit the facility daily and examine every aspect of the construction. Remember, haste makes waste. Do not rush the construction to completion. The days and productivity lost because of the need to reconstruct space after the facility is completed will be substantially more than that lost during the initial construction phase caused by changes.

Decorating and Interior Design: The Final Touches

As the saying goes, you never get a second chance to make a first impression. The first thing any new patient "sees" at your office is the waiting room, and the design of the waiting room can speak volumes about your practice. Even before the patient sees the audiologist, attitudes about your practice, professionalism, and care to be rendered are being formed in the patient's mind, based solely on the impression created by the look of your office. This impression being formed by the patient actually began as he or she responded to a referral, an ad, or a recommendation. It continued its formation through scheduling of an appointment and was further entrenched by the location and look of the building in which the practice was established. The look of the waiting area can go a long way to either solidify that reputation or to counter the impression. It is hoped that the impressions up to the point the patient walks in the door are positive and the look of the waiting room does nothing but solidify the impression. If, however, the interactions have been negative, the look of the waiting room can have a positive influence and cause the patient to change his or her impression. In the worst case scenario, the waiting room creates a highly negative impression, detracting from any or all the good efforts in patient care supplied by the staff. The goal during the interior design phase is to use decorating, color schemes, and furnishings that create an environment that evokes trust, confidence and professionalism from the moment patients enter until they leave.

The image created in the waiting room is a combination of size, color, furniture, lighting, and accessories. This image can play a significant role in the long-term viability of the practice, and its importance cannot be overstated. Remember that the image created in the waiting room needs to be carried forward throughout the practice. This can be as simple as adding a wallpaper border around the ceiling of the examination rooms that matches the wallpaper in the waiting room. Also remember that the staff will occupy the practice on a daily basis, and their work environment should be decorated in a manner that evokes trust, faith, and a willingness to put forth a good effort. It is very easy to minimize the budget for staff amenities and create a situation in which the staff does not feel as though they are an important part of the practice. Consult with the staff to gain an insight as to their preferences for furniture and color schemes. Involve them in the process from the beginning. If they feel like they have contributed to the selection of the decorating, they will feel vested in the practice and are more interested in seeing the practice succeed.

No hard and fast rules exist as to the color scheme, types of furniture, and accessories used in completing the process of designing your practice. The final image created is a combination of a variety of factors, including (a) personal and staff preferences, (b) the predominant type of patient served, (c) the image of other tenants and the surrounding community, (d) the type of services rendered, and (e) the budget. You and your staff must be present in the practice on a daily basis so the preferences of the staff and yourself are very important and should not be sacrificed solely to please patients. If the predominant patient population is geriatric, as may be typical with a dispensing practice located near a large retirement area, the interior design should reflect values and styles consistent with this population. Try to achieve a suitable balance between a style that is pleasing to your patients and your staff. The image of the surrounding community will also influence the interior design. If the building in which you are located is "upscale," your interior design should also reflect this attitude. Patients expecting an upscale practice will be disappointed if they enter a facility with a "cheap" design. A patient's first impression should not be one of disappointment. Finally, the budget is typically the most important issue when preparing to decorate and furnish a practice. When progressing through the design and development process, it is easy to underestimate the budget for interior design. For example, the number of chairs used in a modest size practice is impressive. Waiting room chairs, examination chairs, chairs for the booths, chairs for family members, and chairs for staff add to a significant expense. Combined with tables for the waiting room, table lights, pictures for the walls, framed diplomas, workstations for hearing aid repair, worktables for equipment, desks, file cabinets, storage cabinets, wallpaper, borders, plants, pots for the plants, bookshelves, books and magazines for the waiting room, holiday decorations, literature racks, and display cases, the expense for interior design can be great. If first impressions are truly that important, however, be liberal in budgeting for furniture and decorating.

Hosford-Dunn et al (1995) describes four types of interior design typically seen in the patient waiting areas of professional offices:

- *"Gracious Living"*: A quiet and subdued mood prevails. Furnishings are conservative and comfortable. Amenities such as coffee service are obvious and attractive. Informative magazines are present, as are professional cards, brochures, and newsletters. Chairs, not couches, are used as seating. The nature of the practice layout makes the staff activities apparent but discreet.
- *"Modern and Efficient"*: The furnishings are contemporary with designer fabrics, colors, and lighting. No food amenities but informative current magazines are present and an informational display containing brochures and informational literature is obvious. Ample seating is present. Staff activities occur out of sight of the waiting area.
- *"Spare and Basic"*: The mood is relaxed and although the furnishings are nondescript they are adequate. Fluorescent lighting is used. New magazines are present but older magazines have not been removed. Educational or professional brochures are not adequately refreshed. Seating may or may not be adequate. Staff activities are audible but not discriminable from the back rooms.
- *"Cold and Untouchable"*: The mood is distant but clinical. Furnishings are angular and metal and color is lacking. Glossy magazines are present but no informational or professional literature is present. Seating is adequate and staff activities occur out of sight of the patient.

Obviously the goal is to avoid cold and untouchable. The other design styles can be adequate depending on the image desired and the size of the practice (Hosford-Dunn et al, 1995, p. 158.) Remember that the image may be created with the paying customer in mind, but the employees and staff will need to live with that look every day. Employees spend a significant amount of time in the practice environment and therefore their comfort should also be factored into the design, particularly with regard to work areas, chairs, and work space utility. Patients, however, pay the bills, and therefore their impressions may be the more important of the two.

Consulting with an interior design specialist can help ensure the appropriate look is created. In addition to the yellow pages, interior designers can be also be found through the builder or property manager, through many commercial furniture outlets, or through the recommendations of friends and colleagues. We have found that the designers recommended through the property manager or through commercial furniture stores are very helpful in this regard. Most interior designers will work hard to not only understand the type of look you are trying to create but to achieve it even on a limited budget.

Interior design specialists, particularly those who have expertise in commercial or professional design, have access to a wide variety of manufacturers, fabric styles, accessories, furniture, carpeting, and color schemes and have the ability to make parts of the design work collectively to create the image you desire. Although it may seem easy to visit the local discount office supply store to get office furniture, the furniture selection is typically limited and is not tailored to the health professional's needs. Furthermore, the selection of wall coverings, wall hangings, lighting, and accessories is even more limited, if available at all. The interior designer can pull together all these things from many sources. Although the use of an interior designer may seem expensive, many of these specialists derive their income through the sale of the merchandise rather than the consultation service itself. More importantly, the time and energy spent seeking everything from carpeting to wall pictures can more than exceed the cost of a designer. In many ways a designer may be less expensive in the long run.

Whether engaging the services of an interior designer or coordinating the interior design yourself, consider the following points in your deliberations:

- When selecting colors, remember to choose them on the basis of long-term satisfaction rather than the popular colors of the time. Like clothes and fashion, popular colors change quickly and can leave the office looking dated.
- Bright or primary colors appeal to children, whereas adults prefer softer colors.
- Dark colors can be depressing, whereas brighter colors stimulate. Greens and blues can be soothing (Hosford-Dunn et al, 1995, p. 155).
- When selecting furniture, consider the predominant population. Do not select fine antiques for a pediatric setting.
- If the practice will serve persons with ambulatory difficulties, ensure waiting room and examination chairs have arms to assist with standing. Do not forget the chairs in the sound booths. Avoid use of chairs with casters or rollers as a safety precaution.
- Be sure to include child-friendly furniture, sized to fit and treated to last.

- If children are likely to be in the waiting area, either as patients, siblings, or offspring, reserve a play area that includes a sufficient number of toys. Keep this area separate from the main waiting area. Both parents and other adults will appreciate the thoughtfulness.
- Consider adding visually stimulating entertainment such as a television or aquarium. Use a VCR to play popular children's movies. Cable the system so the VCR and movies remain out of reach of children.
- Ensure the clinical environment is well lit without being sterile. Remember many patients have visual deficits.
- Ensure areas of interest such as educational or brochure displays are well lit and easily accessible.
- Lighting in the waiting areas can be more subdued yet bright enough to allow patients and their families to read.
- Consider adding a display case in the waiting room. This case can be used to display products for sale such as hearing aid batteries and cleaning supplies, as an educational exhibit (e.g., hearing aids through time), or to display personal professional mementos such as awards and accomplishments.
- Be sure to include a location for magazines and reading material. Do not forget to constantly rotate the reading material.
- Make sure the patients can clearly determine their course of action when they enter the practice for the first time. Use appropriate signage for check-in.
- A phone or coffee service area in the waiting room adds an air of concern that the patient's time is as valuable as yours.

- Use diplomas or other professional material as decorations within the practice, either in the waiting rooms, on hallways, or in examination rooms.
- Use of live plants enhances the appearance of a practice but significantly detracts if the plants are not cared for appropriately. Use of artificial plants is an adequate substitute, but be sure to dust them frequently.

CONCLUSIONS

Designing an audiological practice is a significant undertaking but can yield tremendous personal and professional satisfaction. This satisfaction is felt at several distinct steps in the process. The first sense of accomplishment occurs when the decision is made to act on the *idea*. The second important satisfaction marker occurs when a firm *concept and plan for* the facility and its services has been developed. Searching and choosing a *location* gives the project tangible evidence of the progress. The finalization of a floorplan detailing the *layout* of your practice adds a personal component to the project. The *construction phase* yields two important events: the start of construction provides further tangible evidence of the progress toward an independent practice; and the end of construction signals that the practice will soon be ready to occupy. The addition of the sound booths and audiological instrumentation signals the professional nature of the space. Last but not least is the addition of furniture, decorations, accessories, and other amenities that complete the *interior design* and provide an image for you and your practice.

It's time to unlock the doors and see patients.

REFERENCES

AMERICANS WITH DISABILITIES ACT OF 1990. (1991). Public Law 101-336, 42, U.S.C. 12101 et seq. U.S. Statutes at Large, 104, 327–378.

BAXTER, J. (1994). Locating and equipping an audiology practice (Appendices E and F). In: H. Hosford-Dunn, J.H. Baxter, E. Cherow, A.I. Desmond, G. Jacobson, J.L. Johnson, P.F. Martin, D.L. Eger, & C. Cooper (Eds.), *Development and management of audiology practices* (pp. 15–23). Rockville, MD: American Speech-Language-Hearing Association.

CADWALLADER, M. (1981). Towards a cognitive gravity model: The case of consumer spatial behavior. *Regional Studies, 15* (4);275–284.

CUNNINGHAM, D.R., & EREKSON, N.R. (1994). Financial management. In: S.R. Rizzo, & M.D. Trudeau (Eds.), *Clinical administration in audiology and speech-language pathology* (pp. 213–246). San Diego: Singular Publishing Group, Inc.

HOSFORD-DUNN, H., DUNN, D.R., & HARFORD, E.R. (1995). *Audiology business and practice management.* San Diego: Singular Publishing Group, Inc.

LOAVENBRUCK, A.M., & MADELL, J.R. (1981) Planning the dispensing program. In: A.M. Loavenbruck, & J.R. Madell. *Hearing aid dispensing for audiologists: A guide for clinical service* (pp. 13–30). New York: Grune & Stratton, Inc.

PARFIT, M. (1984, May). *Mapmaker who charts our hidden mental demands* (pp. 123–131). Washington, DC: Smithsonian Institution.

SAPHIER, M. (1992). *Office planning and design.* New York: McGraw-Hill.

Chapter 14

The Business Plan and Practice Accounting

Gyl A. Kasewurm

Outline

When I established my private practice, I did not bother to write a business plan. The business did not require a large investment, and some of my spouse's "banker buddies" were willing to extend him a loan with few questions asked. However, the bankers were reluctant to finance my business because I had failed to prove that an audiological private practice could be a profitable venture. Sure, I had years of education and a burning desire to succeed, but those characteristics do not guarantee a successful business. Fifteen years later, I realize why I needed a business plan and how many problems could have been avoided if I had written one.

Business planning is the process of creating a model or picture of the owner's goals and expectations for the business. That model, the business plan, provides essential information to outline what the organization will look like. A business plan can serve as a priceless tool in evaluating success throughout the life of the business. The plan describes the who, what, when, where, why, and how of a good adventure story. In my private practice much of my business style reflects my personality. Although a business plan must present the facts, it should also stress the uniqueness of the business and what impact that will have on potential customers. In other words a business plan should inspire an interested reader.

This business blueprint encompasses the development of strategic and operational plans. The strategic portion of the plan should cover in detail the first 12 months of the business and explain the next 2 to 5 years in lesser detail (McKeever, 1994). The process begins by identifying the aims of the organization, known as the vision or mission statement, and takes the reader through an analysis of the concept. This phase investigates the business environment, the organization's capabilities, the competitive advantage, and its basis for growth. The action steps involve setting objectives and developing strategies for key areas of the business, followed by an implementation process.

The business plan is a multipurpose tool, containing several different sections, which assist the writer in planning and operating a business. Although the business plans of major corporations can stretch to several hundred pages, many entrepreneurs plans may be as short as 10 pages. The length of each section should be tailored to the particular needs of the individual business owner. Detailed planning forces the naive businessperson to examine every aspect of the business before money is invested. The owner can easily change strategies, markets, or the nature of the business on paper without losing any hard-earned cash. These decisions will determine the course of the business for years to come.

If the goal of the business plan is to obtain financing, the writer must remember that the financier may read hundreds of plans. For maximum efficiency, the plan should be short, concise, and easy to read.

PITFALL

The business that fails to plan, plans to fail.

One of the principal reasons for business failure is lack of planning. According to the Small Business Administration, approximately 1 million new businesses are established in America each year. Of these, approximately 200,000 will survive the first 5 years. When pondering the concept of business planning, one critical fact seems to emerge: all businesses need a business plan. Federal Express, one of the largest venture capital investments ever with more than $70 million in sales, still prepares an annual business plan.

A well-written business plan will serve as a guide throughout the life of the business, and lenders are not likely to grant

Audiology: Practice Management. Edited by Hosford-Dunn, Roeser, and Valente. Thieme Medical Publishers, Inc., New York © 2000

a capital request without detailed information that will lead them to believe the business will succeed. The essential directive is to provide sufficient information to support the objectives, strategies, and tactics being developed without making the document so lengthy as to bore the reader. Detailed information that is of interest, but not essential to the arguments supporting the document, should be included in the appendices. Many sources recommend that initial preparation of the business plan begin 6 months before the need to use it, allowing time to evaluate and critique the business venture (Pinson & Jinnett, 1996). This painful but necessary exercise will demonstrate that careful consideration has been given to the business's development and show that the entrepreneur has done his or her homework. A well-written business plan will clarify the focus of the business and provide a logical framework from which the business can develop and grow during the subsequent 3 to 5 years (Hosford-Dunn et al, 1995).

In addition to probing existing strengths and weaknesses, the plan should paint a realistic view of the expectations and long-term objectives of the business. It is better to abandon an idea in its infancy than invest a lot of time and money before learning that the idea will not work. The annual *Hearing Instrument* or *Hearing Journal* surveys can serve as excellent resources, projecting the average business the private practitioner may expect in the first few years. Obviously, these figures will vary according to the location of the business, target market, and the degree of commitment of the business owner.

PEARL

A well-written business plan provides a road map for years to come.

BEFORE YOU START WRITING

Although I am the perpetual cheerleader for private practice, not everyone possesses the drive or desire to start a business. Certain characteristics are helpful in maintaining a private practice. Being an entrepreneur generally means several years of long hours, hard work, and financial sacrifice with no guarantees of success. People who go into business focused solely on the trappings of success are likely to fail. A potential business owner should be motivated by love of their work, the joy of helping others, and the desire to be independent and autonomous (see Chapter 8 in this volume for a discussion of this topic).

McKeever (1994) identified a number of characteristics that create successful entrepreneurs. Before making the decision to start a private practice, the entrepreneur should ask the following questions:

- Are you a self-starter? A small business owner must possess drive and initiative. Responsibility for getting the job done rests on the shoulders of the owner.
- Do you like and get along with people? Nearly all small businesses succeed through people, primarily customers and employees. Individuals who dislike interpersonal contact on a regular basis are at distinct disadvantage in a private practice.

- Has your career exposed you to the workings of a small business? The most valuable experience for opening your own business is working in someone else's. The small business environment is something that must be experienced to be appreciated.
- What is the main reason for opening your own private practice? The most pervasive characteristic of entrepreneurs is that they do not enjoy working for someone else. These individuals enjoy making their own decisions and will do whatever it takes to get the job done.
- Are you prepared to work 60 or more hours a week for an indefinite period of time? Small business owners often describe their work load as 16 hours a day, 7 days a week. Experience indicates that successful private practitioners work long hours for many years before they have a chance to relax.
- Do you like to win? Private practice in audiology can be a very competitive business. The best entrepreneurs focus on winning and outselling the competition.
- Do you have excellent organizational abilities? The ability to organize people and tasks is essential for a small business owner. A disorganized person is generally busy losing patients and money.
- How is your health and energy? If you have not gotten the idea by now, owning a private practice can be exhausting and stressful. An entrepreneur needs physical stamina and emotional strength to endure the first few years.

Operating a business is a very demanding endeavor that can take a great deal of time and energy. Before making the decision for self-employment, sit down and write strengths and weaknesses and then analyze whether those will blend into a successful business opportunity. The owner must remember that a road may be long and bumpy, but if the destination meets the expectations, it will be worth the journey.

CONTENTS OF THE PLAN

The Cover Sheet

The *cover sheet* of the business plan is like the cover of a book. The image should be attractive and should contain the following information:

- Company name
- Company address
- Company phone number (including area code)
- Logo, if you have one
- Names, titles, addresses, and phone numbers of the owners or corporate officers
- Month and year in which the plan is issued
- Number of the copy
- Name of the preparer

The preceding information need not be presented in an elaborate fashion. However, if the plan is used to obtain financing, a new cover sheet should be used for each proposal. Figure 14–1 gives examples of cover sheets.

```
┌─────────────────────────────────┐
│          COVER  SHEET           │
│                                 │
│                                 │
│           EARS TO YOU           │
│         234 RINGY CIRCLE        │
│       ANYWHERE, USA 49000       │
│          (555) 555-1212         │
│                                 │
│                                 │
│      John Cerumen, President    │
│          555 Tinnitus Row       │
│         Jamestown, NY 12345     │
│           (616) 429-9999        │
│                                 │
│                                 │
│    Mary Peters, Vice-President  │
│          345 Tragus Lane        │
│         Jamestown, NY 12345     │
│           (616) 429-8876        │
│                                 │
│                                 │
│    William Weird, Secretary     │
│          177 Concha Blvd.       │
│          Quatro, NY 12678       │
│           (616) 429-0065        │
│                                 │
│                                 │
│    Vonda Jane Ast, Treasurer    │
│          678 Tragus Point       │
│          Gylville, NY 12906     │
│           (616) 429-2288        │
│                                 │
│                                 │
│    Plan prepared June, 1998     │
│    by the Corporate Officers    │
└─────────────────────────────────┘
```

A

```
┌─────────────────────────────────┐
│      Financing Proposal         │
│              for                │
│          Ears to You            │
│                                 │
│                                 │
│                                 │
│                                 │
│      To be Submitted to         │
│   Pinnacle Bank and Trust Co.   │
│                                 │
│                   Suzy Radishio │
│                     John Tames  │
│                    Ears to You  │
│                234 Ringy Circle │
│              Anywhere, USA 49000│
│                 (555)555-1212   │
└─────────────────────────────────┘
```

B

Figure 14–1 (A,B) Sample cover sheets.

The Executive Summary

The executive summary, also known as the statement of purpose, addresses and explains key elements of the business. The business objectives should be stated on the first page of the business plan. The executive summary illustrates how the proprietor intends to use the plan once it has been developed and explains the current state of the company, what products or services it will offer, its market, its competition, and its

finances. This is a quick overview of all aspects of the business in an attempt to introduce the company to the readers. If someone were to read only the executive summary, he or she would learn the name and nature of the business, its legal structure, the amount of the loan request, and a repayment schedule. If the plan is being used for internal use only and not for the purpose of obtaining a loan, the statement would be a summary of the business and its goals for the future. Because this section introduces and summarizes the essence of the business plan, the writer must determine what he or she most wants the reader to know about the business idea. These ideas must be condensed into a few paragraphs that can be read and absorbed quickly and easily.

The executive summary presents an opportunity to convince the reader that the plan is worth reading and yet leave enough unsaid to require a deeper look. In this section the writer emphasizes the positive aspects of the business idea and minimizes the negative aspects. For instance, if a unique market niche has been discovered, the entrepreneur should include this in the executive summary but eliminate the fact that no prior experience operating a business exists. Individuals who read the business plan are busy and probably have many specific questions that need to be addressed in the remainder of the plan. The reader will form an immediate impression of the prospective company from this section, and first impressions are lasting ones.

SPECIAL CONSIDERATION

The executive summary may determine whether the reader will review the entire plan.

The following key words are helpful in formulating the executive summary (Pinson & Jinnett, 1996):

What is	the business name?
	the legal structure?
	the product or service to be provided?
	the loan needed for?
	to be used for collateral?
Where	is the business located?
How	much money is needed?
	will the loan be repaid?
When	was the business established?
	is the loan needed?
	can repayment begin?

The short and businesslike summary will usually be no longer than one page but can be longer if necessary. A sample of an executive summary is found in Figure 14–2.

Table of Contents

A table of contents follows the executive summary, which is expanded and supported in the remainder of the business plan. The table of contents helps a prospective lender understand the road map of the plan. As with any professional document, its appearance affects how others react to it. A

Ears to You Corporation

Ears to You Corporation, an S Corporation established in 1996, is a private practice providing audiological services and hearing aids to hearing-impaired consumers. The business, located at 234 Ringy Circle, Anywhere, USA, is seeking capital in the amount of $75,000 for the purpose of opening a second facility at 345 Presbycusic Way in Anywhere, USA. Funding is needed in time for the office to be opened on January 1, 2000.

The increased incidence of hearing loss and the growth of the over-80 population have created a growing clientele base, which in turn has led to a 20% rise in revenue for each of the past two years. This increase in clientele has necessitated the addition of a new facility to better serve our patients. Repayment of the loan and interest can begin promptly within 30 days of the receipt of funds. The loan can further be secured by company owned real estate that has a 1999 assessed value of $156,000.

Figure 14–2 Sample executive summary.

professional look and feel further increase the chances of the plan being well received. Do not put a page number on the beginning of each section, so that individual segments may be updated at any time. Every business plan should include the following three main ideas:

- The business
- Financial data
- Supporting documents

Because a business plan may be a lengthy document, the table of contents will guide the reader to sections of particular interest. The executive summary states the intended journey of the business and the table of contents makes it easy to locate stops on the tour. When seeking a loan from a financial institution, the plan should be specific as to the use of the lender's money, and these uses must be supported in the remainder of the document.

Although the statement of purpose appears at the beginning of the document, it may be drafted after completion of most of the business plan. It is only after the entire plan has

been thoroughly investigated that one is able to effectively and concisely complete the statement of purpose. Entrepreneurs who attempt to write the statement of purpose first often end up with a vague and shallow communication. Although the statement of purpose need not border on the dramatic, it must succeed in generating immediate interest. Ending the summary on a personal note allows an opportunity to convey an assessment of the business' history to date (if there is one) and feelings about its future. For example: "The founders of Ears-R-Us are greatly encouraged by the need for audiological services among the 28 million hearing-impaired persons in the country and we believe that…"

Description of the Business

The description of the business comprises the heart of the business plan by summarizing the organizational structure of the business. This section should address questions such as: What exactly is the business? How will it be run? Why will the business succeed? When describing the business operations, the writer should include appealing aspects of the business and any unique factors that may influence the success of the business (Pinson, 1996) (see Fig. 14–3).

Determining the central focus of the business and goals for the business 5 years ahead is one of most important decisions a business owner will make. A private practice can take many directions, and it is wise to decide the projected focus long before the doors open. If it is impossible to describe an idea clearly, the writer will want to take more time to forge a road map. Throughout the business plan, it is important to inform the reader of all major factors, positive and negative, that may have an impact on organizational aspects of the operation. This section should provide the reader with the concept of how the business will work and why it will survive in a competitive marketplace.

Before writing the description of business section, the writer should ask the following questions:

- What business will I be in?
- What is the status of the business? Is it a startup or an expansion of an existing business? A takeover or buyout?
- What is the business' form? Sole proprietorship, corporation, partnership?
- What are the economic trends and how will they contribute to the success of the business?

- Are there any local economic factors that will influence the business (e.g., Does the location present a concentration of Seniors?)? Have any major industries in the vicinity closed?
- Will the business contract with physicians, HMOs, hospitals, clinics, other dispensers or industries that will contribute to the success of the business?
- What kind of experience do I have in this type of business?
- How will the business be unique? What procedures will be used in an attempt to outshine the competition?
- Will the business have any special relationships with suppliers that may contribute to the success of the business?

By examining the central focus of the business, the writer can estimate possible sources of revenue. Once goals for revenue are determined, the owner can begin planning how to generate the needed revenue to operate profitably. Financial goals and projected revenues should be incorporated into the description of business.

Products or Services

In this section of the business plan the writer must devote attention to the products and services that the business will provide. It is necessary to describe the products and services that the business will offer and qualifications needed to provide the services. Once again, the writer should seize every

---

Professional Hearing Services, Ltd. is a full-service clinic specializing in helping hearing – impaired consumers to hear better. This clinic provides services to patients of all ages, including those who are handicapped or physically limited. During the coming year, Professional plans to concentrate more heavily on patients with vertigo, which affects millions of Americans. Several local physicians have expressed a need for such services, and revenue is projected to increase by 25% from the vestibular evaluations.

Professional Hearing Services, Ltd. concentrates on providing excellent customer service by providing walk-in hours for patients who need repairs or adjustments. Professional, which has been in business since May 1984, is currently open Monday through Friday from 8am until 5pm with additional hours by appointment. Professional specializes in fitting programmable hearing aid technology. The business, which presently serves 4000 patients, is open year round and located at 458 Bubby Blvd. in St. Joseph, Michigan.

Figure 14–3 Sample description of business.

Amplification systems, when properly fit and maintained, can provide significant benefit to persons with hearing loss. Improvements in hearing aid technology render a multitude of fitting options and flexibility.

Miniaturization of hearing aid circuitry and the ability to interface hearing aids with computer based programs provides the user with the opportunity to use state of the art technology and offers a cosmetically acceptable alternative to the larger behind-the-ear instruments. Improvements in fitting procedures have increased the accuracy of fitting frequency specific gain and compression characteristics. Automatic signal processing, digital processing, and directional processing have the potential to increase user satisfaction by reducing the effects of background noise on the primary speech signal of speech.

In addition to prescribing and fitting hearing aid technology, Ears R Us will offer comprehensive hearing aid fitting services. Patient satisfaction surveys will be used pre-and post-fitting to assess the benefits of amplification in conjunction with target gain validation through the use of real ear measurements.

Ears R Us will offer comprehensive hearing, middle ear and vestibular assessments for patients of all ages. Treatment for vestibular disorders will be based upon test results and will be provided through the use of a modified Epley maneuver. Studies have cited that 79-100% of patients with Benign Paroxysmal Positional Vertigo experience relief of their dizziness following therapy employing the Epley maneuver.

Figure 14–4 Sample products and services.

opportunity to discuss the uniqueness of the business and how it will differ from the competition (see example in Fig. 14–4).

Entrepreneurs are more familiar with their profession than the readers are. Therefore it is important that characteristics of the products and services be explained in a clear and concise fashion. State what stage of development the business is in and include any products or services that the business plans to offer in the future. Share information on extended warranty programs or unique service programs that the business will offer. The writer may want to consider including case studies to support these claims.

A detailed description of the core products the business will sell should be highlighted in this section of the business plan (Brandt, 1997). The writer need not include each product that will be sold, but rather the type of products that the business will offer, such as linear, programmable, and digital hearing aids. The next step is to explain the services the business will sell and how those services will benefit the target market. For example, when a private practitioner dispenses a hearing aid, peripheral services include the delivery, fitting, routine servicing, repairing, and annual evaluations of the unit.

Because the average life of a hearing aid is 3 to 5 years, the products and services section of the business plan should explain how this life cycle will have an impact on the profitability of the business. Hearing aid technologies continue to evolve, and this evolution will have an impact on hearing-impaired consumers and the future growth and profitability of the business. The plan should project peak sales months and when capital may be needed for key equipment purchases. Audiology is a unique profession. The anticipated increase in the incidence of hearing impairment and the fact that 75% of consumers fail to use amplification could have an impact on patient flow and business profitability. Although it may be the writer's belief that audiological products and services are special, this perception is not necessarily shared by the reader.

One of the most important aspects of management is giving the target market a reason to consume the products and/or services. The plan must explain why the projected business will be better equipped to satisfy the needs of the public and why the services offered will surpass those of the competition. Potential customers have needs, and a variety of ways exist to meet those needs. Audiologists sell products and provide services that work hand in hand to benefit hearing-impaired consumers. Essentially, the business must present the products and services in such a way that the consumer believes their communication needs can be satisfied. In addition, it is important to mention suppliers and why they were chosen from the wealth of resources.

SPECIAL CONSIDERATION

Audiologists should specialize in the products and services that best meet the needs of their target markets.

Management and Personnel

This section of the business plan will characterize the qualifications of the business owner and the individuals who will play key roles in operating the proposed business. The management team will be responsible for the success or failure of the business venture. According to *Business Digest*, more than 50% of small businesses fail within the first 2 years and fewer than 10% exist after 10 years. Although these figures may not accurately describe audiological private practices because no industry statistics exist for our profession at present, Dunn and Bradstreet has compiled a number of reasons for the failure of small businesses.

- Poor choice of business type
- Owner not suited to small business
- Lack of knowledge of attracting customers
- Insufficient planning and investigation
- Failure to get proper professional advice
- Poor choice of legal form
- Insufficient capital
- Poor pricing practices
- Owner living beyond income of the business
- Lack of knowledge of finances and record keeping
- Poor credit granting practices
- Poor inventory management
- Inadequate borrowing practices

PITFALL

Most business failures result from poor business management and not from a lack of knowledge of the profession.

The primary objective of a business plan is to sell the target audience on the business idea, and a large part of the sales job is convincing the reader that the entrepreneur is competent, talented, and has what it takes to run a successful business. Therefore this section of the business plan should include who will be responsible for specific duties and why the individuals are qualified to perform those duties. The writer should report the following attributes of the persons who will be involved in the business (adapted from Lasher, 1994):

- *Personal background and status:* A bank wants to lend money to people, not companies.
- *Employment history:* Investors want to know what types of responsibilities the prospective business owners have had.
- *Experience in the industry:* Lenders want to make certain the owner is qualified to run the business.
- *Experience in small business:* Exposure to the workings of a small business will be an asset.
- *Management experience:* Any business owner spends a great deal of time supervising employees. College training does not usually provide experience in this area.
- *Education and training:* Six to 8 years of college will show your lender that you are knowledgeable and capable of providing the proposed products and services.
- *Motivation:* It is beneficial to give your investor some idea of why you are going into business. Starting a private practice requires commitment and dedication.
- *Health and energy:* Lenders need to be assured that the entrepreneur is capable of the long hours required to start a business.

The writer should organize all the preceding information into a short and concise statement in half a page or less to avoid boring the reader or appearing egotistical. In many private practices the audiologist will carry the major responsibility for most of the jobs. However, an organization with a formal structure is better able to achieve its goals. It is important to realize that an audiologist who is a business owner will be unable to be responsible for everything. A wise entrepreneur uses legal, financial, computer, insurance, and marketing experts to share in the duties of the business. Most importantly, the audiologist/owner should focus efforts on what he or she is trained to do as an audiologist and ask for assistance in areas in which he or she is unqualified or uninterested. The plan should include the names of outside experts that will be used in managing segments of the business plan. No need exists to discuss every employee in equal depth. However, it is essential to describe the preceding characteristics in the primary participants in the business. It is helpful to chart the organizational structure of the business. An example of such a chart is found in Figure 14–5.

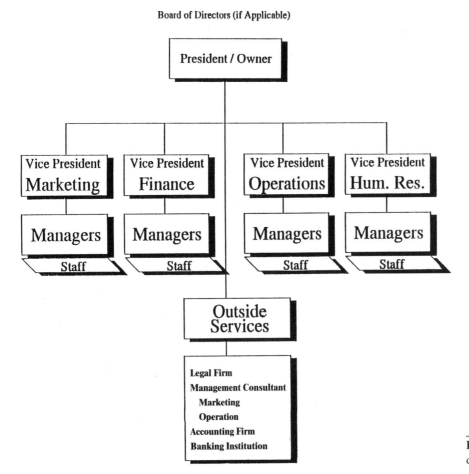

Figure 14–5   Sample organizational chart.

Profile of the Target Market

The target market of the business can be defined as, "That group of customers with a set of common characteristics that distinguishes them from other customers" (Pinson, 1996). It is the job of the management team to identify the target market and to delineate the customer groups to which the business expects to sell. The plan's emphasis should be in the area that the audience sees as most critical, and the plan must offer to meet the measurable goals and objectives valued most by the target market. By focusing on exact customer groups with particular characteristics, business planners often discover new opportunities. A service business should define exactly how wide a geographical area it plans to cover. For most businesses, the area is dictated by a reasonable driving time for the customer to travel to the office or for the professional to travel to the customer. The business planner must then decide whether enough customers are within the geographical area to support the business.

In the target market section of the business plan, the writer must state the potential consumers of products and services, the geographical size of the marketplace, and the anticipated growth potential of the target market. Once the demographic information is processed, the writer may want to add services or products that will cater to the needs of the target market. For instance, if the business is located next to a gun club,

management may want to concentrate a segment of the business on fabricating custom molded earplugs.

An established practice should begin by focusing on existing customers. Who are they and what do they have in common? A new business should ask, "Who will be our customers and how will their needs best be met?" To survive, any business requires a steady stream of customers that desire the products and services the business offers. The reader will take the business plan more seriously once he or she realizes that the entrepreneur has identified the profile of his or her average customer.

PITFALL

The only business that will survive will be one that meets the needs of the consumers in the target market.

The following are helpful questions in completing the target market section of the business plan (adapted from Pinson and Jinnett, 1996):

- What are the geographical markets? For instance, what counties or ZIP codes in the state will the business serve?

- What are the economic markets? Is the business targeting white-collar, blue-collar, retired with $40,000 or more income a year, and so forth?

- What is the age range of the target market? What group will the private practice specialize in?

- What is the size of the target market?

- Will the market grow or shrink? As in most targeted market areas, persons with hearing loss are increasing dramatically, but is the competition increasing as well?

- What are the social activities of the target market? Is the population active or retired? Will any of the activities contribute to the business?

- What barriers must the business overcome to open the market? For example, might the business wage a campaign against a large dispensing chain office across the street?

- What product prices will the target market bear?

- For an established business, how much of the target market is composed of existing patients.

Understanding the Competition

Before initiating a business, the entrepreneur must formulate a business strategy. A business is unable to be strategic without knowing its competition. *Direct competition* is a business offering the same products or services to the same market, and *indirect competition* is a business offering the same products or services to a *different* target market (Couthard et al, 1996). The distinction between direct and indirect competition is most often determined by the method of delivering the service. For instance, audiologists who provide services to nursing home patients are indirect competition to audiologists in school systems. Every business must evaluate the competition and try to determine an untapped market for the practice. In addition, the competition can provide a valuable source of information: What do they do well? What could you do better? How do they satisfy their customers? What type of pricing structure do they maintain? Where and how do they advertise? Hearing aid manufacturers have insights into the habits of your competitors and are able to provide information and understanding into the market share that the business can expect. The business plan should compile competitive information that can give the practice the edge to survive in an aggressive marketplace.

The flow of competition will largely depend on barriers to entry into the marketplace, such as large capital requirements or slow and restrained growth of the market. Quite often, the eventual performance of a prospective business is influenced by external factors over which the business has little or no control. In addition to expanding current markets and perhaps creating new markets, the owner of a new business will be forced to take customers away from the competition and plan a strategy to keep those customers. Analyzing the competition will reveal who the competition is, where they are located, what products or services they offer, and how the new business can provide a unique and needed service to consumers. Technological change remains a force that drives the marketplace. However, state-of-the-art technology is not always the answer to securing a major portion of the marketplace. Often, just ensuring that the business offers a variety of levels of technology will be enough to carve out a section of the market. Defining the competition will enable the business to establish a battle plan for capturing its share of the target market.

SPECIAL CONSIDERATION

Business owners must know their competition, be familiar with what they do, and focus on what their businesses do better.

Marketing

In the marketing section of the business plan the author needs to convince the audience that a real opportunity exists and that the proposed business can capitalize on it. This section identifies what methods will be used to reach potential customers and how customers will be informed of the products and services that the business will offer. A marketing strategy should explain how the business will organize and implement its plans to achieve desired sales performance. Although meticulous detail is not necessary, the reviewer must gain understanding of how the business intends to market its products and services.

The Michigan Small Business Planning Guide (1989) suggests investing 10% of gross revenues into a marketing budget. Although many private practitioners believe that hearing-impaired consumers will seek out audiologists for their education and professional qualifications, practical experience proves that consumers will obtain services from someone they have heard or read about. Pinson and Jinnett's *Anatomy of a Business Plan* (1996) suggests that targeted promotions are often the safest and most economical way of reaching the potential market and are an excellent way of stretching advertising dollars. When composing the marketing section of the business plan, the entrepreneur must consider what will cause customers and prospects to remember the business when they have need of services.

Although it is important to ask customers for referrals, "word of mouth" advertising alone will fail to grow a business. Happy customers will tell 0.7 other people, whereas unhappy customers tell 7 to 11 other people (Pinson, 1996). On the basis of these figures, this means of advertising will not spread a message to the masses of hearing-impaired consumers.

An advertising budget needs to include monies for signage, brochures, business cards, stationery, and everything that gives the public an image of the business. It is a good idea to hire a professional to establish a marketing campaign that will meet the needs of the prospective target market. Portraying the wrong image to consumers could be the hole that sinks the company ship. Everyone has seen businesses with superior locations and unique products go broke and close their doors. In most cases the fatal problem can be attributed to poor marketing and promotion.

Many business owners ignore the potential for effective advertising of their service or product. The market is there:

the 1997 annual *Hearing Instrument* survey indicated that 75% of hearing-impaired consumers fail to solicit the services of an audiologist or a hearing instrument specialist, and this number is growing daily with the increase in the incidence of hearing loss and the growth of the aging population. As audiologists, it is our duty to educate the public on the benefits of amplification and the need to have services provided by the most qualified professionals.

Many methods are available to reach the market segment, including direct mail, television, radio, newspaper ads, and others (see Chapter 7 in this volume). The cost varies by type and the targeted market. Virtually every manufacturing company has a marketing department that can assist private practitioners. A business can take advantage of advertising slicks and programs already developed by manufacturers and professional organizations.

Direct mail has proven to be an effective way to deliver the sales message into the hands of prospective customers. In direct mail a business sends information about products or services to names on a mailing list. Where does one obtain these names? Either a business compiles the list from previous customers or the names can be rented or purchased from brokers or manufacturers. An inexpensive flyer sent to a specific geographical region may be an appropriate piece to use until the private practitioner can compile his or her own customer list.

Display ads are large, often colorful, quarter, half-page, or full-page ads that can be placed in newspapers, magazines, or trade journals. These ads often include a photo or illustration in the promotional material in an attempt to attract a large readership. Evoking a mood with the ad may emotionally motivate consumers to pursue the products or services offered by the business. The marketing program must stress the benefits of the products and services in an effort to motivate the reader to call the office for an appointment. Because people are inundated with advertisements, the display ad should stand by using type styles, pictures, formats, and layouts that are different from the competition. The ad must ask consumers in some forceful way to open their wallets. The cost of display advertising varies according to size of the ad, number of colors, circulation of the publication, and type of readership.

Special events, such as open houses, are often excellent ways of promoting a response to an ad. These events are usually held over 1 to 2 days and feature the demonstration of some product or service. The business may have special pricing or additional services offered to any customer who purchases amplification during the event. Direct mail or display advertising may be used in conjunction with the promotion of a special event. In addition, open houses are often more successful when accompanied by a visit from a manufacturer's representative.

Another form of advertising that reaches a large number of potential customers is radio advertising. Unfortunately, so many ads compete for the attention of the consumer that the message may be lost if it fails to grab the listener's attention. Radio listeners cannot see the product, and *The Perfect Business Plan* by Lasher (1994) suggests that the retention of audio messages is much less than visual messages. The radio ad should be simple and straightforward, repeating the name of the company many times throughout the commercial. To target a specific market, the business owner should contact the radio station and determine the best time to reach the targeted consumer. Before producing a radio commercial, the entrepreneur should note which radio ads catch his or her attention.

Television can also serve as a forceful advertising medium, and local cable TV stations often provide a cost-effective medium for a private practice in audiology. Television commercials can create excellent name and face recognition. Lasher suggests that television advertising provides a visual, audio, and written message. If the private practitioner decides to pursue this medium, it is usually best to interview and hire a professional to produce a professional ad that will portray an appropriate message about the business.

Publicity is "free" media coverage such as press releases that can provide credibility for a business. When a business pays for an advertisement, the practice is telling the customer that their product or service is good. When a member of the media or someone else outside the organization gives the business' products or services a boost, consumers may perceive it as impartial judgment, and the publicity may be worth several paid advertisements.

Business and community involvement through participation in civic events and membership in business organizations is another means of promotion. Most civic organizations have weekly programs and are looking for educated and interesting speakers. Although it may be difficult to find time to devote to public speaking, the effort can provide dividends for years to come.

In summary, the business planner should report how promotional dollars will be spent, why those avenues were selected, how the message will reach the target market, when the promotional campaign will begin, how much the marketing plan will cost, and what format the advertising will take. Timing is important. The marketing plan will require contacting promotional resources well in advance to determine publication schedules. For example, if a business is to open in July and the telephone directories are published in September, it may need to place the telephone ad in April.

Pricing

The pricing structure of the business is critical to success and is determined through market research and analysis of financial considerations. (NOTE: For a more advanced resource on pricing, consult Hosford-Dunn et al [1995].) Basic marketing strategy is to price within the range of price ceiling and price floor. The price ceiling is the highest price a consumer will pay for a product or service on the basis of a perceived value. The price floor is the lowest amount at which the business is able to offer a product or service, meet all costs, and still make a desired profit. Reason would suggest it is wise to know what the competition is charging. However, the pricing structure of a business should be made on the basis of profitability and not on what the competition is charging.

A business owner must decide early what payment policies will be used and how the policies will be enforced. The owner must not be routinely seduced into creating special payment options for patients. Although excuses abound for not making immediate payment, most patients will make arrangements for payment if the office does not waver on the payment structure. If a patient cannot pay cash for the purchase, credit card or finance options should be available.

The business will need to consider the nature of the demand for the products and services being offered and the image the business is attempting to project. In addition to meeting all the costs of operating a business, the business must generate a profit. A viable business operates between the price ceiling and the price floor. The difference allows for discounts, bad debts, and returns.

It is important to establish the relationship between price and cost. A common planning error involves establishing a retail price that provides an adequate margin over cost only to discover that most hearing aids are sold during an "open house," which provides for a discount on each unit. This can result in a lack of revenue to cover overhead expenses. Price and cost assumptions must be explicit in the plan and must be used as input to the financial projections.

Pricing may be a marketing concern because price, quality, service, and profitability are tied together. Although no mechanical formulas exist for making price decisions, the following are a few guidelines to follow (Hill & Jones, 1992):

- The price of goods and services should reflect the product or service itself and also an intangible image factor. Positioning or predetermining the perceived value in the eyes of the consumer can be accomplished through promotional activities. To be successful, the owner must decide what the business offers that the competitor does not. This unique benefit or service should be promoted to the consumers.

- Identify the business objectives. Is the business attempting to buy market share with low prices? Maximize profits? Remain competitive? Build up a new product line? Pricing is inherently strategic, so the business objectives must be clear.

When determining the price of a product, one immediate objective is to determine the sales volume necessary to reach the break-even point (see the discussion of break-even analysis later in this chapter).

Financial Information

The first sections of the business plan described the physical setup of business and shared plans for finding and reaching potential customers. The financial section is the quantitative interpretation of everything stated in the text portion of the plan. Well-executed financial statements provide the means to look at the profitability of the business. The financial documents included in the plan are not just for the purpose of satisfying a potential lender or investor, they are streets on the road map designed to serve as a guide during the life of the business. To be effective, the financial section must be current and up to date (Covello & Hazelgren, 1995). This means examining the financial statements periodically and measuring the actual performance against projections.

A business's financial statements are numerical representations of what the business is doing physically. The idea beyond these statements is to portray a picture of what is happening within the company and between the company and the rest of the world. Because lenders and financial backers focus on dollars and cents, it is important to prepare competent, professional financial projections for the business. In the revenue area the business plan should begin with a forecast of how many of each particular product will be sold at what prices. When approaching a financial forecast, the business planner should project every product the business expects to sell and how much it expects to charge for those products. Annual reports published by *Hearing Instruments* and *Hearing Journal* may be helpful in determining what the average private practice produces in a month. Financial projections should be broken down into monthly forecasts for years 1 through 5.

The business plan should include the following: Profit and Loss Statement (see Figs. 14–6 and 14–7), Balance Sheet (Fig. 14–8), and the Cash Flow Worksheet (Fig. 14–9).

Profit and Loss Statement (Also Known as an Income Statement)

This document will be used to project revenues over time. The most important element in all the projections is the anticipated sales volume. The credibility of this forecast is so important that an entire section of the marketing plan may be devoted to supporting this projection. The owner must calculate the costs of goods and/or services, as well as the anticipated fixed overhead costs. The net difference of total revenue less total costs will determine the profit and loss of the business. This statement shows how much money a company will earn during an accounting period. Although no set of projections will be 100% correct, experience and practice tend to make the predictions more accurate. Even if the projections are inaccurate, they will provide a benchmark against which to measure short-term goals. Most income statements have a general form similar to that shown in Figure 14–6 and a specific form like the one shown in Figure 14–7.

Small businesses should make 5-year projections for both planning purposes and income projections, whereas an existing business should include financial statements for 2 immediately preceding years. In addition, the business plan for an established business should include copies of the past three tax returns to substantiate the projected financial claims.

The Balance Sheet

In simple terms the balance sheet lists everything a company owns and everything it owes at a moment in time. The firm's

Profit and Loss Statement

Sales	$100,000
Cost of Goods Sold	30,000
Gross Margin	70,000
Expenses	35,000
Earnings Before Interest and Taxes	35,000
Interest Expense	1,000
Earnings Before Tax	34,000
Tax	7,000
Net Income	$ 27,000

Figure 14–6   Sample profit and loss worksheet.

money comes from people who have lent or extended credit in one form or another. These actions create a liability on the part of the firm to pay the money back. Funds may also come from owners who have invested their own money into the company. Such investments of owners are called equity. A balance sheet has two sides. One side lists all the company's assets, whereas the other side lists all the company's liabilities. The balance sheet is really an equation: Assets = Liabilities + Equity. Balance sheets are designed to show how the assets, liabilities, and net worth of a company are distributed at any given time. In general, all companies, large or small, use the same categories arranged in the same order when composing a balance sheet. An example of a balance sheet can be found in Figure 14–8.

The balance sheet gives a profile of the worth of the company's assets: cash, accounts receivable, inventory, equipment, property, and all the company's liabilities, such as accounts payable, notes payable, taxes and interest payable, and salaries. The differences between assets and liabilities constitute the company's net worth. If the business has a track record when the business plan is developed, the business sheet show considerable equity. If this is a new venture, the balance sheet may show little or negative equity.

Cash Flow Statement

The cash flow statement shows the reader where the firm's money came from and what it was spent on during a specified period. Cash flow statements involve the inflow and outflow of cash. Inflows are usually represented by positive numbers, whereas outflows are negative numbers. It is common practice to use parentheses to indicate negativity rather than a minus sign. A cash flow worksheet can be found in

Profit and Loss
May 1998

	May '98
Ordinary Income/Expense	
Income	
Income	99,306.75
Income-Ind.	2,419.00
Total Income	101,725.75
Expense	
Acct Fees	75.00
Advertising	3,333.43
Auto Loan	1,626.86
Bank Chrg	90.88
Charity	300.00
Cleaning	340.00
Dues	50.00
Earmolds	30.25
Education	1,440.66
Entertain	450.00
Equipment	149.99
Equipment - Main	2,358.17
FICA - employer	1,710.77
Gifts	179.67
Hearing Aids	43,563.66
Insurance Health	289.07
Insurance-Disab	427.92
MedWH - emp	400.09
Office Maint.	150.00
Office Util	296.03
Outside service	1,873.81
Payroll	
Gross	27,593.00
Total Payroll	27,593.00
Postage	116.00
Postage Lease	175.14
Rent	2,114.21
Returns	381.38
Supplies	1,158.91
Telephone	1,645.11
Travel-Bus	4,215.89
Total Expense	96,535.90
Net Ordinary Income	5,189.85
Net Income	5,189.85

Figure 14–7   Sample profit and loss statement.

Figure 14–9, or a completed cash flow statement can be found in the Appendix.

Cash and profitability are not synonymous terms. It is possible to have cash and yet be operating at a loss. Conversely, it is possible to be operating profitably, yet have no cash. The question that must be addressed is, "How much cash is needed to be operating profitably?" The first step in cash flow forecasting is to estimate how much the business is expected to sell or receive in income for a given period of time. If the business is dealing in products, the plan should forecast the number of units the office expects to sell and multiply this number by the cost per unit and then translate these figures into the expected dollar volume of sales.

BALANCE SHEET			
ASSETS		**LIABILITIES**	
Cash	$10,000	Accounts Payable	$10,000
Accounts Receivable	14,000	Taxes Payable	2,000
Inventory	12,000	Notes Payable Short term	12,000
Total Current Assets	36,000	Current Liabilities	24,000
		Long Term Debt	18,000
		Total Liabilities	42,000
Fixed Assets			
Equipment	50,000		
Accum Depreciation	(10,000)	Total Capital/Equity	34,000
Total Fixed Assets	40,000		
		Total Liabilities	
Total Assets	$76,000	and Equity	$76,000

Figure 14–8   Sample balance sheet.

If a business receives only cash for products, operating cash inflow will be identical to total sales. Cash-flow in a business that sells products on credit will depend on the collection of accounts receivable. Cash-flow projection is an estimate of cash the business expects to receive, not the value of the invoices. Payments are recognized in the cash-flow forecast in the period they are received, not when the debt is incurred. To determine the net effect, summarize the amount of cash inflows and subtract the total of the cash outflows.

The plotting of expected revenues, expenses, assets, liabilities, and equity forecasts the level of cash flow. Cash-flow totals are a critical index of how successful the business will be, and this forecasting estimates the timing of cash flowing into the business and out of it. To assess the feasibility of a venture, the owner must assess how much cash is necessary to acquire the capital resources necessary to establish the business. This is known as *fixed capital*. The amount of cash needed to support the trading of the business until the proceeds of sales are received is known as *working capital*.

The cash-flow forecast considers cash received into the business from all sources, including sales, capital funds, and loan funds. In addition, this forecast should include cash paid out by the business, including operating expenses, expenditures on capital items, and loan repayments. Obviously, it is essential that the amount of money flowing into the business exceeds the amount flowing out. If outflows exceed inflows, sooner or later the business will fail. Small businesses are especially vulnerable to cash-flow problems because they tend to operate with inadequate cash reserves.

Break-Even Analysis

A break-even analysis provides a sales objective, expressed in either dollar or unit sales, at which the business will be breaking even. That is, neither making a profit or losing money. Once the break-even point is known, the business will have an objective target to aim for. Increased sales do not necessarily mean increased profit. For instance, doing a high volume of Medicaid work may mean a lot of "work" but very low profit margins and, consequently, very little profit.

Fixed costs are those costs that remain constant no matter what the sales volume may be. These include rent, salaries, benefits, and taxes. *Variable costs* are those costs associated with sales, including cost of goods, variable labor costs, and sales commission. The net operating profit of an enterprise is represented by the gross revenue for the period less the total fixed costs for that period. The break-even point for a business is the point at which all of the variable and fixed costs are met, but no operating profit is achieved.

The Lake Michigan College Business Planning Workbook (1997) suggests the following formula for computing the break-even point:

$$\text{Break-even point in sales} = \frac{\text{Fixed expenses}}{\text{Gross profit per unit}}$$

Cash Flow for the Period of _____ *to* _____

1) **Beginning Cash Balance** _____
2) **Cash Receipts**
   a) **Cash Sales** _____
   b) **Accounts Receivable collected** _____
   c) **Loans and Other Cash Income** _____
3) **Total Cash Available (1+2a+2b+2c)** _____

4) **Business Expenditures**
   a) **Products** _____
   b) **Advertising** _____
   c) **Insurance** _____
   d) **Interest** _____
   e) **Office Supplies** _____
   f) **Rent** _____
   g) **Salaries** _____
   h) **Telephone** _____
   i) **Dues** _____
   j) **Other Expenses**_____ _____
   k) _____ _____
   l) _____ _____

5) **Total Expenses (4a thru 4l)** _____

6) **Loan Principal Repayments** _____

7) **Other Cash Paid-Outs** _____

8) **Total Cash Paid-Outs (5 + 6 + 7)** _____

9) **Ending Cash Balance (3 – 8)** _____

Figure 14–9 Sample cash flow worksheet.

This break-even formula determines how many units the practice must sell to pay fixed expenses. It subtracts the variable expense per unit from the sales income for each unit and the difference per unit is then applied to fixed expenses. The break-even quantity is the number of units that must be sold to cover those fixed expenses. The following is an example of the break-even concept.

Ears R Us sells hearing aids for $1000 each and the hearing aids cost the business $250 each, which results in a gross profit per unit of $750. The total of the fixed costs is $15,000 per month (rent, utilities, advertising, salaries, supplies, and so on). Using the preceding formula, it can be determined that dividing the monthly fixed cost of $15,000 by the gross profit per unit of $750 gives a break-even point of 20 hearing aid sales per month.

$$\text{Break-even point} = \frac{15,000}{750} = 20 \text{ units}$$

Another pricing technique is to adopt a rule of thumb that the cost of goods does not exceed a certain percentage of gross revenues. *The American Hearing Aid Associates Manual* (1998) suggests that the cost of goods does not exceed 30% of gross revenues. For a more complete description of these and other pricing approaches, consult your accountant or Chapter 7 in this volume.

Financing Proposal

The purpose of this section is to assist the entrepreneur in turning a business plan into a financing proposal that fits the business and capital needs. Most financing deals rarely progress beyond the first screening. Therefore the proposal must be attractive enough to warrant attention and tailored to the needs of the intended audience. Most small business people should turn to their local bankers first. If the business needs more equity than is available from the bank, the entrepreneur may search for a financier who routinely invests in small businesses, or contact parents, grandparents, or the richest living relative.

A bank loan consists of money that will be repaid over a period of time at an additional cost (interest). The money an owner invests in a business is equity, that is, money that will not be repaid unless a portion of the business is sold or a partnership is formed. Debt financing does not lead to sharing ownership of the business, whereas equity financing does. An owner who is unable to obtain financing should consider acquiring a partner who will share ownership of the business. From a banker's standpoint, the higher the debt, the riskier the deal, and short-term loans are generally less risky than long-term loans.

Every lender wants to answer one very basic question before approving a loan for a new business: "Will the borrower be able to repay the loan and interest as planned?" To answer that fundamental question, lenders may ask more detailed questions. When dealing with a local bank, the owner may want to emphasize the reliability of the past credit history and include supporting documents. First impressions are often lasting ones so it is important to dress well and to have the documents available that the lender may request. If the loan request is denied, the entrepreneur may choose another lender in the area who may be more willing to finance the business venture.

Application and Expected Effect of the Loan

One of the reasons an entrepreneur needs a business plan is to generate needed resources from lenders or investors. Once the plan has been polished to perfection, it is ready to be used in the campaign to obtain financing. The plan needs a statement of the total cash needed to expand or begin the business and should summarize the precise financial needs for the venture and identify how the resources will be used. In the case of financing the cash flow projections will reflect how the funds are to be repaid, and in the case of capitalization involving partners the projections will give an indication of the growth of equity and the anticipated timetable for the sharing of profits.

Asking for money can be an intimidating process. However, remember that lenders are in the business of loaning money. It is the writer's job to convince the lender that the loan will be repaid as promised and at a profit to them. When requesting funds, make certain to ask for ample funds to ensure that the business is not undercapitalized. It is vital to have enough money on hand to buy equipment, pay salaries, and cover unexpected costs. *The Business Planning Guide* (Michigan Small Business Development Center, 1989) recommends that a new business have enough working capital to carry the business through a full 3 months of operation. This section of the plan should contain responses to the following questions:

- How is the loan or investment to be spent?
- What items will be purchased?

- Who are the suppliers?
- What are the pricing structures?
- What specific models of equipment will be purchased?
- How much will be paid in sales tax, installation charges, freight, or delivery fees?

A banker may be interested in using equipment or property as collateral for the loan, or alternately the owner may consider the possibility of leasing the necessary equipment or getting the equipment from a hearing aid manufacturer. If a shortage of cash is projected, a lease arrangement may enable the business to purchase the essential equipment over time. The business owner should keep in mind that leasing forces the owner to pay more because of the additional interest that will be paid.

SPECIAL CONSIDERATION

The reasons a lender will not finance a business will sometimes be more valuable than the money.

Risks

The business owner faces a number of risks in starting a business. The following questions should be addressed in the plan:

- What happens if the owner becomes incapacitated or dies?
- What if the business is destroyed by fire?
- What if a former employee establishes a similar business in your target market?
- What if a patient sues over a faulty product or negligent service?

Obviously, it is impossible to anticipate everything a new business may encounter. However, it is a good idea to provide a section that illustrates the planner has thought about the unexpected and has ideas on what to do if things do not go as planned. This is called a contingency plan. The written business plan need not present the contingency plan in great detail. Rather, this detail must be in the mind of the business owner when the idea is presented to potential financial backers.

A good contingency plan has two parts. First, it spells out warning signals that may indicate the business is off course and, second, it explains the actions needed to correct the problem. The problem with most new businesses is that the owner does not anticipate having difficulties until the business is already in trouble. This is especially true in small businesses where running out of cash is often a problem.

Good business planning establishes a system to monitor operations so the discovery time for problems is as short as possible. This process involves monitoring financial results and carefully analyzing the implications of any changes. A contingency plan should address the need to implement an action plan quickly and decisively. For example, if the financial forecast projected selling 10 aids in the first 6 months and the business sold only 4, how would the business meet its debt and payroll obligations? A system should be devised to establish when the business is beginning to slide into trouble. For example, management may establish a policy that states if revenue is down X% for 2 consecutive months, adjustments will be made to compensate for the losses.

Some business plans do not include a section explicitly dealing with contingency planning but rather the issue is dealt with in the financial section. The main purpose of the risk section is to convince the reading audience that time was spent considering problems that the business may face, and options are provided in case problems occur.

Conclusion

The conclusion section of the business plan summarizes the key elements of the plan and demonstrates the consistency between the overall corporate aims, the present position analysis, and the proposed business strategies. The elements of a well-constructed conclusion to a business plan may comprise the following (adapted from Lasher, 1994):

- Aims of the business venture.
- Key success factors required to meet those aims.
- To what extent the enterprise can satisfy the requirements of the key success factors.

- Major challenges the business may face in meeting the requirements of the key success factors and thus achieving its objectives.

A sample of a conclusion is found in Figure 14–10.

MAPPING THE FUTURE

By this point in the business plan, the writer has done a lot of work. The owner knows what products will be sold, to whom they will be sold, who the competition is, how the product will be marketed, what the risks are, and what kind of finances will be involved in the business venture.

The next step is to create a time line for the business plan that will establish the occurrence of specific events. This section of the business plan determines the time frame of the operations and assists in planning special events, such as the purchase of equipment, hiring of additional employees, seasonal highs and lows, and vacations. When starting a business, the owner is faced with a monumental set of tasks that can be organized and predicted through the completion of a time line of events necessary to open the business by a certain date.

Gordon Hearing Aids is an audiological private practice that aims to provide quality services and superior products to the more than one hundred thousand consumers in Berry County, Michigan. Marketing objectives include introduction of at least two new high technology products per year, direct mail advertising sent twice yearly to all residents of Berry County and expansion of services into Vanna County, Michigan.

The business seeks to provide wealth for its owners through an annual net profit of 25%, which will allow reinvestment in the company to continually upgrade facilities and equipment. A human resource objective is to expand the skill base of company employees which will lead to an increase in personal productivity. The firm's key success factors have been identified as economic efficiency, maintenance of high standards of quality, increase of target market coverage and customer satisfaction.

Gordon Hearing Aids is recognized as an industry leader. With very little marketing effort, it has maintained sales close to its capacity and at its current level of personal productivity. The business is financially sound and exemplifies exceptional customer service and high standards of quality in the market it currently serves.

Figure 14–10 Sample conclusion.

If the writer has created a well-thought-out business plan, he or she now has a check in hand and is ready to begin the business journey. Suddenly faced with a large sum of money, the business owner may spend the money carelessly until reality hits and the owner realizes that he or she has squandered the cash that the business needs to survive the first year. Instead, the owner needs to prioritize and schedule purchases to ensure the business follows the path that the plan has paved. Success does not begin when the checks start rolling in. Success begins long before, as the owner attacks and meets all necessary goals to get the business on the road to profitability. Although nothing is easy, a private practice in audiology can be a lucrative and thrilling ride for the person who is willing to devote the time and energy needed to succeed.

PEARL
Good planning and persistence breed success and nothing feels as good as success.

Appendix
Sample Business Plan

The following example of a business plan was used by an audiologist who recently went into private practice. Note that it contains most, but not all, of the business plan components discussed in this chapter.

AUDIOLOGICAL ASSESSMENTS, INC.

January 1999

Karen Jolly
President

488 E. Joiner Lane
Grand Fork, Michigan 49987
(616) 997-6549

MISSION STATEMENT FOR AUDIOLOGICAL ASSESSMENTS, INC.

Audiological Assessments, Inc., (AA) was established to provide quality comprehensive audiometric services, including diagnostic audiometric assessments, vestibular assessments, vestibular rehabilitation for benign paroxysmal positional vertigo, hearing aid sales, and service to a diverse patient population. AA is a nondiscriminatory practice.

STATEMENT OF PURPOSE

AA is seeking $45,000 for the purpose of equipment and supplies, property rental located at 488 E. Joiner Lane in Grand Fork, Michigan, renovations and furnishings for the office space, and maintenance of sufficient cash reserves to operate an audiology practice offering diagnostic audiometric evaluations, hearing aid sales, vestibular assessments, and vestibular rehabilitation for benign paroxysmal positional vertigo. This sum, along with the $10,000 cash equity and $50,000 offered as collateral, will be sufficient to finance this company through the start-up phase so the business can operate at a profit.

DESCRIPTION OF BUSINESS

AA is an audiology practice specializing in diagnostic audiological assessment, hearing aid sales, including conventional and programmable technology, vestibular assessment, and rehabilitation for benign paroxysmal positional vertigo (BPPV).

According to the National Institutes of Health 1991–1993, the prevalence of chronic impairment as a result of dizziness affects more than 2 million people in the United States alone. Vertigo or dizziness is the most common reason for seeking medical care in the population older than 75. It is estimated that 15 to 23% of individuals older than 65 who experience falls do so as a result of vertigo. The most common balance disorder is BPPV.

BPPV is particularly amenable to therapy. Several treatment regimens have been suggested in the literature. AA will use a modified Epley maneuver to remove debris from the semicircular canals. Studies have cited efficacy rates of 79 to 100% successful after one treatment.

AA will provide the diagnostic testing for vestibular disorders on the referral from a physician. Treatment by means of a modified Epley maneuver will be suggested for those patients with BPPV (the most common cause of dizziness in adults younger than 50).

A key component in identifying balance disorders, communication disabilities, and pathological conditions of the ear is through a thorough diagnostic audiometric evaluation. Audiometric assessment can help determine the need for medical treatment or amplification.

The fastest growing population in the United States is that of persons older than 85. This group will show an increase by 91% between the years of 1976 and 2000. Approximately 60% of these people will report a significant hearing *loss*. An even greater number will report associated problems including tinnitus and vertigo.

Amplification systems, when properly fit and maintained, can provide the hearing-impaired person with significant benefit. Improvements in hearing aid technology have opened up a multitude of fitting options and flexibility.

Miniaturization of hearing aid circuitry and the ability to interface hearing aids with computer-based programs not only provides the user with the opportunity to use state-of-the-art technology, it also offers a cosmetically acceptable alternative to the larger behind-the-ear aids fit in the 1970s. Improvements in fitting procedures have increased the accuracy of fitting frequency-specific gain and compression. Automatic signal processing and digital processing capabilities have increased user satisfaction by reducing the effects of background noise on the primary signal of speech.

PERSONNEL

Vestibular Assessment and Rehabilitative Audiologist—This position must be held by a certified audiologist. Past experience with electronystagmography (ENG) testing or special course completion for hands-on testing and assessment is necessary.

Karen Jolly will be the primary service provider for vestibular services. She has 10+ years of experience with ENG testing. Karen has completed two educational courses on assessment and treatment of BPPV offered by Dr. Susan Bauer and Dr. Marian Girardi.

Testing and rehabilitative services will also be provided by Darlene Lewis, MA, CCC/A, audiologist. Ms. Lewis has experience providing rehabilitation services for BPPV. She will be working part-time at AA.

Dispensing Audiologist—Duties will be to sell hearing aids, provide hearing aid rehabilitation and consultation, provide hearing aid repair, and remake services. This position must be filled by a licensed dispensing audiologist or an audiologist with a hearing aid trainees license. A minimum of 2 years experience with hearing aid selections and fittings is preferred. Candidates must hold current certification CCC/A and proof of license.

Administration—Duties will include patient scheduling, billing insurance companies, assisting with patient establishment, document payments and receivables, filing, assisting with correspondence, and contacting patients for new and follow-up appointments. This candidate needs to have a clean and professional appearance. He or she must be able to interact with patients and other professionals with a courteous, friendly attitude. Knowledge of computer-based billing, word processing, and file management is preferred but not necessary if the candidate shows a willingness and ability to learn.

AA will offer comprehensive hearing aid fitting services. AA will use the latest fitting procedures such as DSL[i/o], IHAAF, and FIG 6 and the latest technology available for real-ear measurements and target gain assessments. This ensures that our patients get the professional services needed and the maximum benefits from amplification. Prefitting and postfitting patient satisfaction surveys will be used to quantify hearing aid fitting success in conjunction with target gain validation through the use of real-ear measures.

MARKETING PLAN

AA will target Northern Gent, Montuyday, and Megarstar counties. Services will be promoted to physicians and clients in these areas. Marketing highlights should advertise that AA employs the only full-time audiologist in Northern Gent county. The closest full-time audiologist and sound booth is in the town of Lincoln. AA provides vestibular assessment, vestibular rehabilitation for BPPV, audiometric services, and hearing aid sales in one location. AA will participate with BCBS, Medicare, Medicaid, PPOM, Priority Health, and Blue Care Network. Physicians will be attracted by our insurance participation, ease in scheduling, comprehensive services, and Ms. Jolly's reputation as an exceptional diagnostic audiologist. Customers will be attracted by our location, word of mouth reputation, insurance participation, services, and competitive prices. Information will be disseminated through advertisements in local newspapers, brochures sent to physicians, and flyers sent to previous hearing aid clients.

COMPETITION

Grand Fork currently has 11 hearing aid dispensing audiologists and 4 hearing aid dealerships offering hearing aid services. These companies are located in 19 different main offices and satellite locations. Most of the hearing aid dispensers are located in the southeast and southwest Grand Fork areas. In the northeast, competition will come from a Miracle Ear satellite office and Rapp Solartone, both located on Prainer Avenue. These locations do not employ an audiologist and are unable to provide comprehensive audiological services, hence, no physician referrals. Neither of these locations provides vestibular assessment or rehabilitation services.

Three locations provide vestibular assessment at this time. St. John's Hospital, Drs. Harry and Byrns, and West Fork Ear Nose and Throat. None of these locations provide rehabilitation for BPPV. A physical therapy group is located at St. Mary's Hospital that provides vestibular rehabilitation, but they do not provide audiometric or vestibular assessments.

FINANCIAL OVERVIEW

AA is an audiology private practice offering diagnostic audiometric evaluations, hearing aid sales, vestibular assessment, and vestibular rehabilitation for BPPV. On the basis of data from similar businesses in the Grand Fork area, it will take up to 8 months for AA to become a profitable corporation. The start-up costs for these first 8 months is projected to be $71,000, which includes an investment of approximately $45,000 in equipment.

A personal investment from David and Karen Jolly in the amount of $40,000 and an approved line of credit for $40,000 will be sufficient to finance this company through the start-up phase and into the second year when the company will be profitable. In addition, David will continue with his current employment as a petroleum transfer engineer. A detailed budget estimate of the initial 2 years of operation included projected expenses and revenues is included.

Profit and Loss
(Projected Income) Statement For Period Ended _____

Company Name _____

	Mo 1	Mo 2	Mo 3	Mo 4	Mo 5	Mo 6	Mo 7	Mo 8	Mo 9	Mo 10	Mo 11	Mo 12	Total	Ratio
Revenue														
1) Gross Sales (Total Revenue)														
2) Less Sales, returns & allowances														
3) Net Sales (1-2)														
Cost of Goods Sold														
4) Beginning Inventory														
5) Plus: Purchases														
6) Total Goods Available (4+5)														
7) Less: Ending Inventory														
8) Total Cost of Goods Sold (6-7)														
9) Gross Profit (Gross Margin) (3-8)														
Operating Expenses														
10) Advertising														
11) Automobile														
12) Depreciation														
13) Dues/Subscriptions/Licenses														
14) Insurance														
15) Interest														
16) Legal and Professional														
17) Office Supplies														
18) Payroll Expenses (Taxes)														
19) Rent														
20) Salaries														
21) Taxes-Sales, etc.														
22) Telephone														
23) Travel & Entertainment														
24) Utilities														
25) Wages - Employees														
26) Other Expenses: _____														
27) _____														
28) _____														
29) _____														
30) TOTAL OPERATING EXPENSES (10+29)														
Profit Before Taxes (9-30)														
Taxes - Federal _____														
Taxes - State _____														
Taxes - Local _____														
Profit After Taxes _____														

Figure 14–A1 Sample profit and loss worksheet.

Cash Flow Projection by Quarter, Year Two

	A	B	C	D	E	F
		1st Qtr.	2nd Qtr.	3rd Qtr.	4th Qtr.	Total
1						
2	Cash Receipts					
3	Receivables	$3,200				$3,200
4	Wholesale	$38,900	$54,800	$76,500	$94,800	$265,000
5	Retail	$41,000	$37,400	$48,600	$53,000	$180,000
6	Other Sources			$12,000	$15,000	$27,000
7	Total Cash Receipts:	$83,100	$92,200	$137,100	$162,800	$475,200
8	Cash Disbursements					
9	Cost of Goods	$57,528	$66,384	$90,072	$106,416	$320,400
10	Variable Labor			$604	$2,196	$2,800
11	Advertising	$2,000	$2,305	$3,125	$3,695	$11,125
12	Insurance	$950	$950	$950	$950	$3,800
13	Legal and Accounting	$500	$500	$500	$500	$2,000
14	Delivery Expenses	$1,600	$1,844	$2,500	$2,956	$8,900
15	*Fixed Cash Disbursements	$12,630	$12,640	$12,640	$12,640	$50,550
16	Mortgage (rent)	$2,628	$2,628	$2,628	$2,628	$10,512
17	Term Loan	$1,602	$1,602	$1,602	$1,602	$6,408
18	Line of Credit			$12,140	$15,360	$27,500
19	Other (see notes)					
20	Total Cash Disbursements:	$79,438	$88,853	$126,761	$148,943	$443,995
21						
22	Net Cash Flow:	$3,662	$3,347	$10,339	$13,857	$31,205
23						
24	Cumulative Cash Flow:	$2,424	$5,771	$16,110	$29,967	$54,272
25						
26	*Fixed Cash Disbursement					
27	(FCD)	Year Two				
28	Utilities	$2,640				
29	Salaries	$39,000				
30	Payroll Taxes and Benefits	$4,875				
31	Office Supplies	$360				
32	Maintenance and Cleaning	$360				
33	Licenses	$115				
34	Boxes, Paper, etc.	$800				
35	Telephone	$1,800				
36	Miscellaneous	$600				
37	Total: FCD/yr	$50,550				
38	FCD/qtr	$12,638				

This spreadsheet was prepared using the Excel spreadsheet program from Microsoft. ®

Figure 14–A2 Sample cash flow projection year two.

Capital Budget

Product Description	Current Est.	Month 1	Month 2	Month 3	Month 4	Month 5	Month 6	Month 7	Month 8	Month 9	Month 10	Month 11	Month 12	Total
Audiometer	$ -												$0	$ -
Sound Booth	$ 3,700.00	$ 3,700.00												
Tympanometer	$ 1,700.00	$ 1,700.00												
Currents and Headlight	$ 300.00	$ 300.00	$0	$0	$0	$0	$0	$0	$0	$0	$0	$0	$0	300.00
Otoscope	$ 200.00	$ 200.00	$0	$0	$0	$0	$0	$0	$0	$0	$0	$0	$0	200.00
Procedure Table	$ 1,000.00	$ 1,000.00	$0	$0	$0	$0	$0	$0	$0	$0	$0	$0	$0	1,000.00
Vestibular Testing Unit	$ 20,000.00	$20,000	$0	$0	$0	$0	$0	$0	$0	$0	$0	$0	$0	20,000.00
Phonics Box w/ Real Ear	$ 2,500.00	$ 2,500.00	$0	$0	$0	$0	$0	$0	$0	$0	$0	$0	$0	2,500.00
Grinding Wheel w/ Attachment	$0	$0	$0	$0	$0	$0	$0	$0	$0	$0	$0	$0	$0	-
NOAH Software	$ 1,000.00	$ 1,000.00	$0	$0	$0	$0	$0	$0	$0	$0	$0	$0	$0	1,000.00
Fax Machine	$ 300.00	$ 300.00	$0	$0	$0	$0	$0	$0	$0	$0	$0	$0	$0	300.00
Copy Machine	$ 600.00	$ 600.00	$0	$0	$0	$0	$0	$0	$0	$0	$0	$0	$0	600.00
Computer (2)	$ 5,000.00	$ 5,000.00	$0	$0	$0	$0	$0	$0	$0	$0	$0	$0	$0	5,000.00
Printers (2)	$ 500.00	$ 500.00	$0	$0	$0	$0	$0	$0	$0	$0	$0	$0	$0	500.00
Phone System	$ 2,000.00	$ 2,000.00	$0	$0	$0	$0	$0	$0	$0	$0	$0	$0	$0	2,000.00
Furniture	$ 5,000.00	$ 5,000.00	$0	$0	$0	$0	$0	$0	$1,000	$0	$0	$0	$0	5,000.00
Misc.	$ 2,000.00	$ 1,000.00	$0	$0	$0	$0	$0	$0	$0	$0	$0	$0	$0	2,000.00
Total Capital Expenditures	**$ 44,800.00**	**$ 44,800.00**	**$0**	**$0**	**$0**	**$0**	**$0**	**$0**	**$1,000**	**$0**	**$0**	**$0**	**$0**	**$ 44,800.00**

Operating Expenses

Product Description	Per Year Estimate	Monthly Estimate	Month 1	Month 2	Month 3	Month 4	Month 5	Month 6	Month 7	Month 8	Month 9	Month 10	Month 11	Month 12	Total
ASHA, AAA, MAA Dues	$ 370.00	$ 30.83	$ -	$ -	$ -	$ -	$ -	$ -	$ -	$ -	$ -	$ -	$ -	$ -	
Dealers Exam	$ 740.00	$ 61.67	$ 400.00	$ -	$ -	$ -	$ -	$ -	$ -	$ -	$ -	$ 340.00	$ -	$ -	740.00
Corporate Publications	$ 3,000.00	$ 250.00	$ 1,500.00	$ -	$ -	$ -	$ -	$ -	$ 1,000.00	$ 1,000.00	$ -	$ 500.00	$ -	$ -	3,000.00
Advertisements	$ 6,500.00	$ 541.67	$ 200.00	$ 2,500.00	$ 200.00	$ 200.00	$ 200.00	$ 200.00	$ 200.00	$ 2,000.00	$ 200.00	$ 200.00	$ 200.00	$ 200.00	6,500.00
Liability Insurance	$ 600.00	$ 50.00	$ 50.00	$ 50.00	$ 50.00	$ 50.00	$ 50.00	$ 50.00	$ 50.00	$ 50.00	$ 50.00	$ 50.00	$ 50.00	$ 50.00	600.00
Employment Insurance	$ 1,200.00	$ 100.00	$ 100.00	$ 100.00	$ 100.00	$ 100.00	$ 100.00	$ 100.00	$ 100.00	$ 100.00	$ 100.00	$ 100.00	$ 100.00	$ 100.00	1,200.00
Wages/FICA	$ 31,377.08	$ 2,368.08	$ 2,368.08	$ 2,368.08	$ 2,368.08	$ 2,368.08	$ 2,368.08	$ 2,368.08	$ 2,368.08	$ 2,368.08	$ 3,108.11	$ 3,108.11	$ 3,108.11	$ 3,108.11	31,377.08
Lease w/ remodel	$ 21,000.00	$ 1,750.00	$ 1,750.00	$ 1,750.00	$ 1,750.00	$ 1,750.00	$ 1,750.00	$ 1,750.00	$ 1,750.00	$ 1,750.00	$ 1,750.00	$ 1,750.00	$ 1,750.00	$ 1,750.00	21,000.00
Construction Cost															
Utilities	$ 2,400.00	$ 200.00	$ 200.00	$ 200.00	$ 200.00	$ 200.00	$ 200.00	$ 200.00	$ 200.00	$ 200.00	$ 200.00	$ 200.00	$ 200.00	$ 200.00	2,400.00
Phone	$ 2,400.00	$ 200.00	$ 200.00	$ 200.00	$ 200.00	$ 200.00	$ 200.00	$ 200.00	$ 200.00	$ 200.00	$ 200.00	$ 200.00	$ 200.00	$ 200.00	2,400.00
Supplies	$ 2,400.00	$ 200.00	$ 200.00	$ 200.00	$ 200.00	$ 200.00	$ 200.00	$ 200.00	$ 200.00	$ 200.00	$ 200.00	$ 200.00	$ 200.00	$ 200.00	2,400.00
Maintenance/Cleaning	$ 1,200.00	$ 100.00	$ 100.00	$ 100.00	$ 100.00	$ 100.00	$ 100.00	$ 100.00	$ 100.00	$ 100.00	$ 100.00	$ 100.00	$ 100.00	$ 100.00	1,200.00
Training/Education	$ 2,400.00	$ 200.00	$ -	$ -	$ -	$ -	$ -	$ 500.00	$ 800.00	$ 200.00	$ 200.00	$ 200.00	$ 200.00	$ 200.00	2,400.00
Travel/Entertainment Exp.	$ 2,400.00	$ 200.00	$ 200.00	$ 200.00	$ 200.00	$ 200.00	$ 200.00	$ 200.00	$ 200.00	$ 200.00	$ 200.00	$ 200.00	$ 200.00	$ 200.00	2,400.00
Lawyer Fees	$ 2,100.00	$ 175.00	$ 100.00	$ 100.00	$ 100.00	$ 100.00	$ 100.00	$ 100.00	$ 1,000.00	$ 100.00	$ 100.00	$ 100.00	$ 100.00	$ 100.00	2,100.00
Corporate Fees/License	$ 500.00	$ 41.67	$ -	$ -	$ -	$ -	$ -	$ -	$ 500.00	$ -	$ -	$ -	$ -	$ -	500.00
Accountant Fees	$ 2,000.00	$ 166.67	$ 500.00	$ 100.00	$ 100.00	$ 100.00	$ 100.00	$ 100.00	$ 500.00	$ 100.00	$ 100.00	$ 100.00	$ 100.00	$ 100.00	2,000.00
Misc.	$ 2,400.00	$ 200.00	$ 200.00	$ 200.00	$ 200.00	$ 200.00	$ 200.00	$ 200.00	$ 200.00	$ 200.00	$ 200.00	$ 200.00	$ 200.00	$ 200.00	2,400.00
Total Expenses	**$ 84,987.08**	**$ 6,836.88**	**$ 8,068.08**	**$ 8,068.08**	**$ 6,768.08**	**$ 6,768.08**	**$ 6,768.08**	**$ 6,368.08**	**$ 8,358.08**	**$ 8,768.08**	**$ 6,708.11**	**$ 7,548.11**	**$ 6,708.11**	**$ 6,708.11**	**$ 84,617.08**

Projected Revenue

Service/Sales	$ per test	Month 1	Month 2	Month 3	Month 4	Month 5	Month 6	Month 7	Month 8	Month 9	Month 10	Month 11	Month 12	Total
Vestibular Testing	$ 250.00	0	0	1	2	3	3	4	4	6	6	8	10	47
Vestibular Treatment	$ 120.00	0	0	0	2	1	1	1	2	2	2	3	3	15
Hearing Test	$ 70.00	0	8	12	16	20	20	20	25	25	25	30	30	231
Hearing Aid Sales	$ 500.00	0	4	4	6	8	10	10	14	14	16	20	20	126
Total Revenue		$ -	$ 2,560.00	$ 3,090.00	$ 4,620.00	$ 6,270.00	$ 7,270.00	$ 7,620.00	$ 9,990.00	$ 10,490.00	$ 11,490.00	$ 14,460.00	$ 14,960.00	$ 92,720.00

Figure 14–A3 Sample business portfolio.

Business Portfolio

Net Income Projections	Month 1	Month 2	Month 3	Month 4	Month 5	Month 6	Month 7	Month 8	Month 9	Month 10	Month 11	Month 12	Total
Total Capital Expenditures	$ 44,800.00	$ -	$ -	$ -	$ -	$ -	$ -	$ 1,000.00	$ -	$ -	$ -	$ -	$ 45,800.00
Total Operating Expenses	$ 8,068.08	$ 8,068.08	$ 5,768.08	$ 5,768.08	$ 5,768.08	$ 6,368.08	$ 8,368.08	$ 8,768.08	$ 6,708.11	$ 7,548.11	$ 6,708.11	$ 6,708.11	$ 84,617.08
Total Liability	$ 52,868.08	$ 8,068.08	$ 6,768.08	$ 6,768.08	$ 6,768.08	$ 6,368.08	$ 8,368.08	$ 9,768.08	$ 6,708.11	$ 7,548.11	$ 6,708.11	$ 6,708.11	$ 130,417.08
Total Revenue	$ -	$ 2,960.00	$ 3,090.00	$ 4,620.00	$ 6,270.00	$ 7,270.00	$ 7,520.00	$ 9,990.00	$ 10,490.00	$ 11,490.00	$ 14,460.00	$ 14,960.00	$ 92,720.00
Net Income	$ (52,868.08)	$ (5,408.08)	$ (3,678.08)	$ (1,148.08)	$ 501.92	$ 901.92	$ (848.08)	$ 221.92	$ 3,781.89	$ 3,941.89	$ 7,781.89	$ 8,251.89	$ (37,697.08)

First 8 months cost = $ 102,744.64
First 8 months income = $ 41,320.00
First 8 months net = $ (61,424.64)

Figure 14–A3 *(continued)* Sample business portfolio.

REFERENCES

AMERICAN HEARING AID ASSOCIATES. (1998). *Structure of a business plan*. Published in the AHAA Training Manual.

BRANDT, S. (1997). *Focus your business* (pp. 123–134). Friday Harbor, WA: Archipelago Publishing.

COUTHARD, M., HOWELL, A., & CLARKE, G. (1996). *Business planning: The key to success*. South Melbourne, Australia: Macmillan Educational Australia PTY LTD.

COVELLO, J., & HAZELGRAN, B. (1995). *Your first business plan*. Naperville, IL: Sourcebooks.

HILL, C., & JONES, G. (1992). *Strategic management* (pp. 169–197). Boston, MA: Houghton Mifflin Co.

HOSFORD-DUNN, H., DUNN, D., & HARFORD, E. (1995). The business plan. In: *Audiology business and practice management* (pp. 55–76). San Diego, CA: Singular Publishing Group.

HYYPIA, E. (1992). *Crafting the successful business plan*. Englewood Cliffs, NJ: Prentice Hall.

LAKE MICHIGAN COLLEGE. (1997). *Business planning workbook*. Benton Harbor, MI: Lake Michigan College.

LASHER, W. (1994). *The perfect business plan*. New York: Bantam Doubleday Publishing Group.

McKEEVER, M. (1994). *Hoooow to write a business plan*. Berkeley, CA: Nolo Press.

MICHIGAN SMALL BUSINESS DEVELOPMENT CENTER. (1989). *Business planning guide*. Dover, NH: Upstart Publishing Co.

PINSON, L., & JINNETT, J. (1996). *Anatomy of a business plan*. Chicago, IL: Upstart Publishing Co.

SIEGEL, E., FORD, B., & BORNSTEIN, J. (1993). *The Ernst and Young business plan guide*. New York: John Wiley & Sons.

SMITH, F. (1988). Private practice: Are you ready? *ASHA*, January; 31–33.

Chapter 15

Managerial Accounting for Daily and Long-Term Practice Success

Daniel R. Dunn

This chapter is not intended to turn audiologists into accountants. It is important, however, that audiologists be conversant with common accounting terms and basic concepts to better manage their practices and protect their assets. An accountant is one of the key professionals that every small business and practice needs to survive in today's complex business environment.

At the minimum, an established practice should use an accountant to review the quarterly performance and provide business and overall financial advice on topics such as lines of credit, retirement planning, profit sharing, and investments. An accountant should also be used for tax planning and preparation. These services can provide relatively inexpensive protection against some catastrophic financial events.

At the other end of the scale, startup practices need an accountant to set up the accounts; do the bookkeeping on a weekly or monthly basis; handle payroll and prepare all the monthly, quarterly, and annual taxes. Hands-on accounting and bookkeeping services represent substantial but necessary expenses to the fledgling practice. Accounting and bookkeeping errors and omissions can produce financially devastating effects on a practice. An accountant is a necessary but expensive insurance policy for the fledgling practice.

The sooner a practice assumes its own bookkeeping, the sooner it can reduce a significant expense. Fortunately, in today's business environment, several excellent accounting software packages offer effective and inexpensive solutions to simple bookkeeping and accounting needs (e.g., QuickBooks and QuickBooks Pro from Intuit, Money from Microsoft, Peachtree Office Accounting from Peachtree Software). These simple-to-use, Windows-based packages use double-entry bookkeeping systems that grow with the practice and can be copied onto diskettes to provide the latest updates to the practice's accountant.

Managerial accounting strives to provide current and future-oriented information for the business owner or manager (Engler, 1990). In this chapter the focus is on information that is generated internally and used internally to run the business. In addition to internal accounting, this chapter addresses some practical issues that are often obscure to new business owners. It covers day-to-day bookkeeping, registration with government entities, proper tax forms, and meeting filing dates. Chapters 14 and 16 in this volume discuss financial accounting, business plans, and ratio analysis.

ACCOUNTING

How does an audiologist answer the questions of how the practice is doing or if it is meeting plans or budgets? The questions cannot be answered by just looking at the checking account, which only indicates the cash balance at a specific point in time. A checking account does not reflect the obligations that place a demand on cash assets of the practice, demands that may exceed the balance in the account. What is needed is a system to identify, define, measure, report, and analyze the sources of income, as well as the various elements of direct and indirect costs associated with providing and marketing the services of the practice. The practice does this by establishing an *accounting system*.

> ### PEARL
>
> **It should never cost more to obtain information than the information is worth.**

The proper coding of revenues and expenses is vital. The audiologist needs an accounting system that is designed and

Audiology: Practice Management. Edited by Hosford-Dunn, Roeser, and Valente. Thieme Medical Publishers, Inc., New York © 2000

customized to provide a framework for accurate and usable information. The value of information is measured in its usefulness to the end user and the cost-effectiveness of acquiring and providing that information. A well-designed accounting system is simple and logical. It provides information to both internal and external users. Internally, the information must be meaningful, flexible, and current to be a useful tool for the practice. Externally, it must convey the health of the business and, when used on a pro-forma basis, predict future expectations.* For small, privately held businesses, like most audiology practices, the external users are generally creditors. Loans and lines of credit limits reflect a balance between the financial needs of the practice and the risk tolerance of the creditor. The lower the risk or the more financially viable the practice, the more credit the creditor is willing to extend.

The popular bookkeeping and accounting software packages currently on the market not only do financial record keeping but also provide the quality of reporting that is necessary for internal use and for building pro-forma reports. The practice's accountant should be familiar enough with these packages to help the audiologist configure the applications so that they generate meaningful and customized reports. Selecting an accountant is discussed later in this chapter.

Chart of Accounts

The first step in setting up an accounting system is to establish a *chart of accounts*. Table 15–1 shows the framework for a chart of accounts. It is generic and can be applied to any business endeavor. This chart, referred to as the *ledger* by accountants, provides ranges of account numbers for recording all transactions of the business. Each revenue source and each expense category requires a separate account. In practice, it is not enough to know that revenues totaled $100,000.00 for the month. Effective management and planning dictates that the gross revenue be broken down into measurable and meaningful subsets (e.g., revenue from services, revenue from hearing aids sales, and revenue from supplies and batteries). These gross revenue categories enable further subdivision and extraction of more detailed information, such as revenues or hearing aid sales generated by each audiologist (see Fig. 15–1). They also allow development of rolling trends of revenue distribution, such as hearing aid sales according to manufacturer generated by a each audiologist. Effective account design measures employee contributions and tracks shifts in product sales, shedding light on whether shifts are due to technology changes, changes in contracts, or training and performance.

TABLE 15–1 **Generic framework for chart of accounts**

ACCOUNT NUMBER	DESCRIPTION
101–199	Asset accounts
201–299	Liability accounts
301–399	Owner' Equity
401–499	Revenues
501–699	Operating expenses

*See Chapter 14 for discussion and examples of pro-forma accounting.

The logic of account number selection provides a quick guide to which accounting reports are affected by entries into the ledger accounts. This information is valuable for reviewing periodic reports or working on tax reporting. Looking at the first row in Table 15–1, accounts numbered 100 to 199 are *Asset* accounts. As examples, account 110 may be the practice checking account, account 115 the savings or Money Market account, and account 120 assigned to depreciable equipment (e.g., computers and other office machines). Accounts numbered in the 130s can represent depreciable furniture and fixtures. By using this simple, logical convention, the audiologist recognizes that an account with a 100 number represents an asset of the practice.

Row 2 in Table 15–1 indicates that accounts 200 to 299 are *Liability* accounts. Accounts 210, 211, 212, and so forth may represent accounts payable to various vendors; accounts in the 220s may indicate longer term obligations, such as mortgages or loans. Again, the audiologist can quickly recognize that accounts numbered 200 represent obligations of the practice.

Accounts 300 to 399 represent *Owners' Equity*. These accounts represent the mathematical difference between the assets of the practice and the liabilities of the practice. It is unlikely that more than a few of the 300 accounts will ever be used because these accounts represent the residual investment of the owner offset by any profits or losses.

PEARL

Owners' Equity Accounts represent the mathematical difference between the assets of the practice and the liabilities of the practice.

Financial Statements
Balance Sheet

The first digit of the accounts reveals not only what type of account it is but also whether the account is a *balance sheet* or an *income statement* account. The balance sheet is represented by the first three rows in Table 15–1, as exemplified by the following equation:

Assets = Liabilities + Owners' Equity

Therefore first digits of 1, 2, and 3 indicate that the accounts are balance sheet accounts. It is important to understand that the balance sheet is a snapshot of the practice, taken on a specific date. A balance sheet is always headed with the date, as follows:

Happy Audiology, Inc.
Balance Sheet
December 31, 199X

Examples of the two basic formats for a balance sheet for a small audiology practice are shown in Tables 15–2A and 15–2B. As the name implies, the balance sheet must balance. That is, no matter which format is used, the total of the assets is equal to the total liabilities and owners' equity.

Hearing Aids Sold, Less Returns

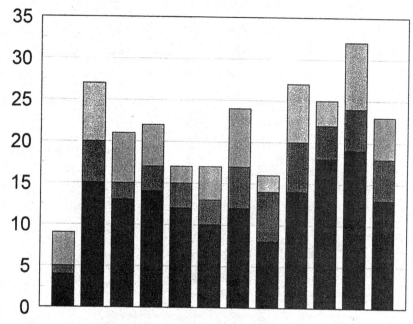

Sales per Audiologist		J	F	M	A	M	J	J	A	S	O	N	D
Audiologist #1		4	15	13	14	12	10	12	8	14	18	19	13
Audiologist #2		1	5	2	3	3	3	5	6	6	4	5	5
Audiologist #3		4	7	6	5	2	4	7	2	7	3	8	5

Figure 15–1   Example of trend analysis derived from accounting data, showing monthly hearing aid sales and returns for three audiologists for a 1-year period.

For non-accountants, especially entrepreneurial audiologists, this balancing may seem counterintuitive at first. If a practice becomes more successful by generating more income than expenses, how does the equation stay in balance? The answer goes back to the accounting equation, which forms the backbone of the balance sheet. The equation can be restated as follows:

Owners' Equity = Assets − Liabilities

In other words, whatever monies are left over after liabilities are accounted for goes to the owners. Net income from the income statement (see next section) goes straight to the equity section of the balance sheet. If the owners do not elect to take the monies out of the business as a distribution, the monies stay in the business as part of the owners' equity. In startup practices, owners' equity on the balance sheet typically represents the amount the audiologist loaned the business as seed money.

Income Statement

The remaining rows (4, 5, and 6) of the chart of accounts shown in Table 15–1 are income statement accounts. They are also commonly known as *profit and loss (P&L)* statement accounts. Accounts 400 to 499 are *revenue* accounts, with numbers assigned for all categories of income (e.g., battery sales, hearing aids, repairs, diagnostics, ear molds, supplies,

TABLE 15–2A   Report form balance sheet

Happy Audiology, Inc.
Balance Sheet
January 31, 199X

Assets

Cash . . . .$ 8,230
Accounts Receivable . . . .$ 1,600
Equipment. $25,000
Less Accumulated Depreciation. . . . . (5,000) 20,000

Total Assets $29,830

Liabilities

Accounts Payable. . . . .$ 4,830
Total Liabilities . . . .$ 4,830

Owner's Equity

Capital Stock. 20,000
Retained Earnings 5,000

Total Liabilities and Owner's Equity $29,830

TABLE 15–2B   Account form balance sheet

Happy Audiology, Inc. Balance Sheet January 31, 199X	
Assets	
Cash	$ 8,230
Accounts Receivable	1,600
Equipment	$25,000
Less Depreciation	5,000
Total Assets	$29,830
Liabilities	
Accounts Payable	$ 4,830
Owner's Equity	
Capital Stock	20,000
Retained Earnings	5,000
Total Liabilities and Owner's Equity	$29,830

refunds, discounts, write offs). It is important to understand that refunds, discounts, and write offs are income. They are *not* expenses, because they appear as negative numbers and their net effect is to reduce revenue.

Accounts numbered 500 to 699 are *expense* accounts. Twice as many expense account numbers are available as revenue numbers because most businesses have more sources of expense than of revenue. For example, a startup practice may assign a single account for insurance expenses. But, as the practice grows, it may need to assign new account numbers for various types of insurance (e.g., comprehensive, malpractice, disability, medical, workers' comprehensive, key employee or officer's life). The same scenario applies to advertising. As the practice grows, it needs separate accounts to track Yellow Pages, print media, broadcast media, and so forth. As always, the objective is to create accounts that generate usable information.

Because entries in the 400, 500, and 600 accounts reflect revenues and expenses of the practice, they directly affect the bottom line (in contrast to accounts 100 to 300). The income statement (or P & L) reports on the performance of the practice for a *period* of time that is indicated in the report heading. The period can be annual, quarterly, monthly or even daily, but it must be indicated in the heading to have value to the user. Table 15–3 is an example of a monthly P & L statement.

The income portion of the P & L is composed of the 400 accounts. Total income, also called revenues, is the sum of all 400 numbered accounts. In Table 15–3, the income of the hypothetical practice for the month of January was derived solely from battery and warranty sales, which yielded a total income of $116.00.

Gross profit, also called net revenues, is the balance remaining after cost of goods is subtracted from total income. In Table 15–3, cost of goods is $500.00, which exceeds total income. The result is a negative gross profit or loss of ($384.00).*

The bottom half of the P & L itemizes expenses by summarizing activity of all 500 and 600 accounts for the accounting period. Total expenses is the sum of that activity. In Table 15–3, expenses for rent, phone, advertising, and office needs totaled $1600.00.

Net income, also popularly known as the "bottom line," is the money left over when total expense is subtracted from gross profit. The practice had a gross loss (negative gross profit) and substantial monthly expenses, yielding a negative net income, or a net loss, of ($1984.00).

TABLE 15–3   Profit and loss statement

Happy Audiology, Inc. Profit and Loss January 199X	
Income	
Battery	16
Warranty	100
Total Income	116
Cost of Goods Sold	
Battery	500
Total COGS	500
Gross Profit	(384)
Expense	
Rent	600
Telephone	400
Advertising	275
Office expense	325
Total Expense	1600
Net Income	(1984)

Bookkeeping and Accounting Terms

It is often difficult for people outside the field of accounting to distinguish between bookkeeping and accounting. Bookkeeping is the record keeping phase of accounting that posts transactions to the ledger. Accounting includes bookkeeping, but it also involves designing the accounting system, preparing the reports and statements, developing budgets, analyzing costs, income tax work, and interpreting the accounting information for making business decisions. The first accounting skills the audiologist needs to acquire are those of bookkeeping. Accurate posting of information by means of good bookkeeping skills is very important to the practice. It is the foundation on which all other accounting activities rest.

Accounting equation: Assets = Liabilities + Owners' Equity

---

*Common accounting convention indicates negative values by enclosing the numbers in parentheses.

As already discussed, this equation forms the basis for all accounting information and is therefore known as the *accounting equation* or the *balance sheet equation*. The importance of the equation is that all transactions should leave the equation in balance. This means that every sale and purchase is reflected in the equation through the use of *double-entry* (debit and credit) bookkeeping so that the equation is always in balance. Out-of-balance conditions indicate that there are bookkeeping errors.

PITFALL

Out-of-balance conditions indicate bookkeeping errors.

Debits and Credits

A confusing concept for those outside the accounting profession is the use of the terms *debit* and *credit*. The simplest way to consider these terms is to think of them as corresponding to left and right, where debit is left and credit is right. Asset accounts, which comprise the left side of the accounting equation, normally have a debit (left side) balance.* For instance, cash in the business checking account has a debit or left side balance. Conversely, liability or equity accounts are on the right side of the accounting equation and therefore have a credit (right side) balance. This is often demonstrated in textbooks by using a *T account* model as shown in Table 15–4. Notice the account *cash* is shown with a left side or debit balance. As an asset account, it has a natural debit balance; additions to the account are recorded by debit and reductions by credit. If an account has a natural credit balance, increases in the account balance are recorded by credit and reductions by debit. Always remember: debit is left side and credit is right side.

For example, if the practice purchases a stock hearing aid from a manufacturer for inventory, it has increased its inventory (asset) account by the cost of the instrument plus shipping or other costs incurred to bring the instrument to a ready-for-sale condition. For bookkeeping purposes, this increase is accomplished by debiting the inventory account (a left side account) for the proper amount. To keep the accounting equation in balance, the accounts payable account for the manufacturer, which is a liability (right side) account, is credited for the same amount. Conversely, when the vendor's statement is paid at a later date, the left side asset account (checking or cash) is credited or reduced. If everything stops here, the accounting equation is out of balance because the practice has reduced a liability account (accounts payable) by paying the statement. To complete the transaction and bring the accounting equation back into balance, double-entry bookkeeping posts a debit to the accounts payable for an equal amount. Thus it is demonstrated that *not only does the accounting equation have a right and left side but each account has a right and left side.*

---

*The exception is an overdrawn asset account, which would have a credit or right side balance until the overdraw is corrected. If the practice writes a check for more than the balance in the checking account, the account will have a credit balance.

TABLE 15–4 Example of T account for an asset account

Cash	
Beginning $2500.00	

Manual and PC Accounting

The previous discussion focused on the bookkeeping aspect of accounting. Accurate posting of the books provides the practice with real-time data to make informed decisions and improve the overall efficiency of the practice. This bookkeeping activity can be done manually at the end of the day or concurrently using previously referenced personal computer applications. By using an accounting software package, the audiologist or front office person can accomplish much of the bookkeeping function automatically while creating the patient's invoice. As part of entering transactions, accounts are updated and the accounting equation is kept in balance. If the application is properly coded in the software during setup, the applications will collect the information necessary for report generation and income tax preparation. Selecting the proper Internal Revenue Service (IRS) schedule or form during initial account setup is best facilitated by using an accountant. The advantage of automatically posting transactions to the correct schedules and forms throughout and at year end is increased bookkeeping accuracy and efficiency.

DAY-TO-DAY DATA COLLECTION FOR BOOKKEEPING

The following scenario of a simple transaction is one way to expand the discussion of the financial complexities that practices handle every business day. Discussion points and simple tracking forms will be developed from the scenario to cover the many business and accounting facets of such a simple event and to help the audiologist envision the interactions.

Tracking Patients and Transactions
Sign-In Sheet

The scenario should begin with a sign-in sheet. The sign-in is a simple form headed with the name of the practice. It has columns for signature, printed name, reason of visit, and so on. The form is like the one shown in Table 15–5. It is simple to design and print, using a personal computer and word processing software. It can be changed or printed as the needs of the practice dictate.

This simple record holds much useful information for the practice. It provides a patient name for each encounter and a count of the total patient encounters for the day. The names are a source for building the patient database. The sign-in sheets provide a hardcopy record of patient contacts that are useful for bookkeeping, audit, or legal requirements. The encounter counts are used to develop trend data that characterize growth patterns, seasonal trends, and even

SCENARIO

It is 9 AM Monday morning, day one of the practice, and the first patient comes through the door and stops at the front desk. He asks the price on 13A batteries. He orders two packs, pays the price, and leaves. The practice has just had its first encounter. How will the practice handle this event? The business questions to be answered by the budding entrepreneur after such a simple exchange are complex and staggering. Rare does the novice audiologist have enough awareness to understand how many separate events just occurred. Questions include what happens to the money collected? Is something written down or recorded? Who was this patient? Was any demographic information gathered? Where did the batteries come from? How much did they cost? How was the price determined?

PEARL

Make sure before the start of business every day that a new sheet and a functioning pen are available. It demonstrates a level of professionalism to make sure the sign-in sheet is current and a working pen is available throughout the day.

Trending from the Sign-In Sheet

A simple example of trending from the sign-in sheet is to total the number of patient encounters each day on a separate data collection sheet. At the end of the week, the practice has a count for each day of the week and a weekly total. By continuing the process week after week, the practice develops trend data that provide an average count of encounters per day of the week, per week, or per month. Graphing such information reveals business trends and provides a graphical representation of practice growth, as shown in Figures 15–2A and B. Trend data can stimulate productive inquiries on the whys of slow months or missed pro-forma estimates. Comparing this information to pro-forma estimates of practice growth allows revision of estimates as needed.

Establishing and Tracking the Cost of Goods

Open Accounts

Scenario questions addressed in this discussion relate to cost and pricing. How was the price determined? Where did the batteries come from? How much did they cost? A logical sequence begins with where the batteries came from. Once the source is identified, the cost can be determined and the appropriate patient price set. Pricing is addressed in Chapters 7 and 14.

Tangible products and accessories that a practice sells to its patients are purchased from third-party vendors. These include batteries, hearing aids, assistive listening devices, and

identifies busy days of the week. This information helps plan for staffing, training, advertising, and scheduling.

The sign-in sheet is also useful as a daily check of cash receipts. It provides a check of reasonableness. If the practice has 20 encounters on a particular day, is it reasonable to have cash receipts for one pack of batteries? Perhaps it is. It could also be a flag of employee dishonesty or poor protocols and procedures. A high number of encounters matched with a low volume of battery and supply sales may indicate noncompetitive pricing or inattention to customer needs. Letting a patient out the door without making sure they have enough batteries or other supplies is a disservice to the patient and to the bottom line of the practice. Seeing to the battery and supply needs of the patients enhances the quality of service and can develop a source of revenue.

TABLE 15–5   Example of sign-in sheet

PLEASE SIGN IN

DATE: _12/11/99_

NAME	SIGNATURE	PURPOSE OF VISIT
Earl Lobe	Earl Lobe	Batteries
Lotta Cerumen	Lotta Cerumen	Test
Earline Drum	Earline Drum	hearing aid

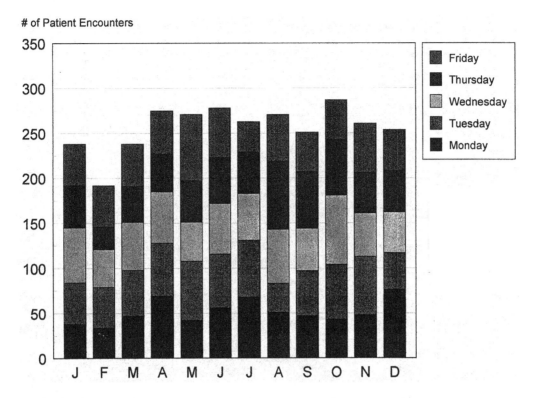

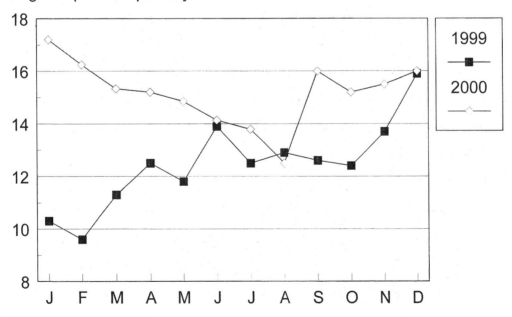

Figure 15–2 Two examples of trending analysis using data from the sign-in sheet. **(A)** Average number of patients per day of the week, shown monthly for a 1-year period. **(B)** Comparison of the average number of patients seen per month in 1999 and 2000.

any number of supplies. To obtain these items, a practice must establish business relationships by opening accounts with selected manufacturers and suppliers. The alternative is to order items and pay with a credit card or cash on delivery (COD). An open account has the advantage of providing "ship to" and "billing" addresses. It establishes the practice as a retailer, which leads to wholesale pricing and perhaps other price incentives for volume purchases or timely payment. Lower costs for the practice mean lower expenses, leaving more room for larger profit margins or competitive pricing in the marketplace. Activity through the account develops a track record and a business relationship with the vendor.

Opening an account is similar to opening a personal credit account, except that the audiologist selects vendors and not vice versa. Vendor selection is usually based on past experience, recommendations from colleagues and mentors, visiting vendor displays at professional conferences, or studying the advertising in industry and profession publications.

The practice needs sources for items such as batteries, hearing aids, supplies, and assistive devices. With these needs identified, the audiologist contacts selected vendors, completes the credit application, and forwards them to the vendors' credit departments, often by fax for quick turnaround. The vendors then assign account numbers to the practice and send statements of their terms and conditions to the practice. Early on, before the practice has an established track record with a company, an account may function more like a personal account than a business account; the practice may have to pay by credit card or COD for initial orders until a payment relationship is established. As the business relationship develops, the terms and conditions of the account will change to reflect the practice's continued business with the vendor. An added benefit of this business track record is that the practice can use established vendors as credit references when it opens accounts with other vendors

Tracking the Cost of Goods

The practice needs to establish a liability account (account payable) for each vendor with whom it does business. Then, as the products are received, the invoice is used as a source document to enter the cost into the vendor's payable account. When the vendor's statement arrives, the practitioner reconciles the account to the statement. To facilitate this process, it is a good habit to file hardcopy invoices by vendor and attach reconciled invoices to the practice's copy of the statement. It is also good practice to identify each entry in the payable account with the vendor's invoice number. This habit requires a bit more time and effort when posting entries to the account, but greatly reduces reconciliation time at month end. The advantages of entering the invoices as they arrive are that the practice always knows what it owes and the reconciliation is simpler.*

Tracking and Protecting Income

The scenario questions of what happens to the money collected are addressed here. The recording of transactions was covered as part of the discussion on bookkeeping. The rigorous attention to recording events as they occur cannot be stressed too often. Many businesses get into severe financial difficulty with a casual approach to the cash collection aspect of the business. Money is the fuel that makes the engine of the practice go. The practice will soon run out of fuel if the practice fails to collect or if unscrupulous employees or others help themselves to this resource. It is imperative to record encounters as they occur and keep daily cash receipts in a cash draw and out of view. Also, the practice must make regular and frequent deposits. Daily deposits collecting dust in the cash drawer do not fill the practice's asset accounts; they also increase temptation. The impact of the loss of several days deposits can be devastating. If the deposits are in the bank, temptation is reduced, and loss through misappropriation is avoided. Money in the bank can bear interest and bank accounts are protected by FDIC insurance up to $100,000.

Daily Encounter Form

The *daily encounter sheet* shown in Table 15–6 is a useful tool for record keeping. A good daily control is to reconcile the financial transactions of the practice on a daily basis as shown in Table 15–6. This sheet is the source document for calculating the day's deposits. It records the patient's name; the procedure or encounter; the dollar amount of the transaction; and whether it was cash, check, or credit card. The form can be modified to post receivables from previous encounters. This is helpful because all monies, checks, and cash received will be part of the daily deposit.

The encounter form should be updated at the completion of each encounter. Bad habits of not recording encounters as they occur leads to confusion at the end of the day when one is trying to reconstruct the day's events. It is always easier to reconstruct events from good records. The sample form in Table 15–6 provides a cross-check for math errors. In that sample form the total of the *amount* column is the total of receipts for the day. Cash transactions are also entered in the *cash* and *deposit* columns; likewise transactions by check are entered in the *check* and *deposit* columns. These three columns are totaled at the bottom. Comparing these totals with the daily bank deposit, the cash total should equal the cash for deposit, the check column should total the checks for deposit, and the deposit total should equal the cash plus checks. The difference between the amount total and the deposit total should equal the credit card total. If the practice bills insurance or allows payment plans, then another column should be added to reflect balances due from transactions.

---

*A difference occurs when entering invoices into the payable account that depends on whether the practice is accrual or cash basis. If the practice is accrual basis, the invoice amount is immediately posted to the cost of goods. If the practice is cash basis, the cost of goods is not updated and the expense is not recognized until the check is written.

TABLE 15–6 Daily encounter sheet

DATE _12/11/99_

DAILY ENCOUNTER

PATIENT NAME	PROCEDURE	AMT	CASH	CHK	DEP TOTAL	CR CARD	TOTAL
LOBE, E.	13x2	16⁰⁰	16⁰⁰		16⁰⁰		16⁰⁰
CERUMEN, L	HE + 13x3	124⁰⁰		124⁰⁰	124⁰⁰		124⁰⁰
DRUM, E	2x HEARING AID	2500⁰⁰				2500⁰⁰	2500⁰⁰
Daily total:	***********	2640⁰⁰	16⁰⁰	124⁰⁰	140⁰⁰	2500⁰⁰	2640⁰⁰

The encounter sheet, when matched with the sign-in sheet, patient invoices, and appointment schedule, gives the practice a good snapshot of the day's activities and what should appear on the daily deposit. For example, if two patients are scheduled for hearing aid delivery on this day and it is customary to receive payment on delivery, then the encounter sheet should show two large deposits. If not, it serves as a trigger to inquire why money was not collected and when it is due. If four patients are scheduled for annual hearing tests and warranty renewal, the audiologist should expect the encounter sheet to reflect those encounters.

Accounts Receivable

The encounter sheet is easily adapted to grow with the practice and meet the practice's information needs. The encounter sheet can be expanded as the practice grows to record payments received on accounts receivable from patients or from third parties such as insurance companies. These payments should be added to the daily transactions to make up the total daily deposit. The practice also can add columns to the encounter sheet to capture referral source information or reflect discounts and allowances.

Invoices and Receipts

The practice should provide invoices or receipts for every encounter. These become source documents for each line of the encounter form and a hard copy record for the patient. Some practices only do this when asked, but it is prudent to provide invoices with each encounter. At the end of the day it is simple to match invoices to lines on the encounter sheet as a check of completeness.

Receipts or invoices can be produced by hand, using multi-part documents purchased at business supply stores or automatically using accounting software. Computer-generated forms have the following several advantages:

- They automatically merge with patient information in the database and perform mathematical calculations, saving time and reducing errors.
- They print as the transaction closes, saving time for the patient and the audiologist.

In the computer-generated sales receipts shown in Figure 15–3, each receipt is numbered automatically, has the patient's name, a description of the service, the method of payment, and the check number when applicable. These are useful fields for completing the end-of-day reconciliation and characterizing the practice according to sources of income and methods of payment. Receipt copies are stored with the daily encounter form. Some practices put copies in the patients' charts as well, but this is time consuming and creates thick charts. Another easy thing to do with the computer is to run an income statement for that day only to match to the daily encounter form.

Daily Deposit

At the end of the day the *daily deposit* is compiled and cross-checked against the encounter sheet, the sign-in sheet, the individual invoices, and the appointment schedule. All the documents are gathered together along with a front and back copy of the deposit slip as a daily package and filed as part of good record keeping. This daily package is used to make sure bank deposits match. At the end of the month it and the other daily packages for the month are used to reconcile the bank statement.

HAPPY AUDIOLOGY, INC.
1234 PERFECT PLACE
EUPHORIA, AK 99999

Sales Receipt

DATE	SALE NO.
12/11/99	1

SOLD TO: LOBE, EARL

CHECK NO.	PAYMENT METHOD	PROJECT
	Cash	

DESCRIPTION	QTY	RATE	AMOUNT
SIZE 13A BATTERY	2	8.00	16.00

Thank you for your business. Total $16.00

HAPPY AUDIOLOGY, INC.
1234 PERFECT PLACE
EUPHORIA, AK 99999

Sales Receipt

DATE	SALE NO.
12/11/99	2

SOLD TO: CERUMEN, LOTTA

CHECK NO.	PAYMENT METHOD	PROJECT
123	Check	

DESCRIPTION	QTY	RATE	AMOUNT
DIAGNOSTIC SERVICE		100.00	100.00
312 SIZE BATTERY	3	8.00	24.00

We appreciate your prompt payment. Total $124.00

HAPPY AUDIOLOGY, INC.
1234 PERFECT PLACE
EUPHORIA, AK 99999

Sales Receipt

DATE	SALE NO.
12/11/99	3

SOLD TO: DRUM, E.R.

CHECK NO.	PAYMENT METHOD	PROJECT
	Master Card	

DESCRIPTION	QTY	RATE	AMOUNT
BTE INSTRUMENTS	2	1,250.00	2,500.00

We appreciate your prompt payment. Total $2,500.00

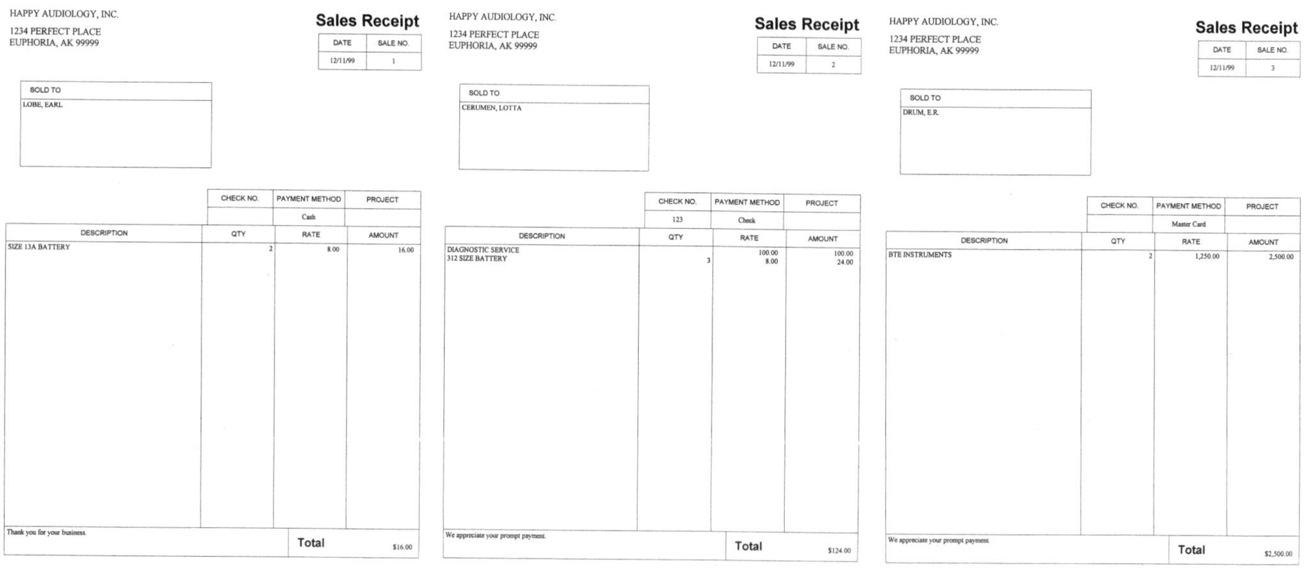

Figure 15–3 Examples of computer-generated sales receipts, sequentially numbered, for different service products, and with different payment methods.

BUSINESS DECISIONS AND BUSINESS EVENTS

Business Form

One of the early decisions a new business must make is selecting the form of business organization.* This is done because, other than a sole proprietorship, the various forms of partnerships and corporations generally require the filing of contracts and other legal agreements. These two forms of business need to file with the Internal Revenue Service and affected states to acquire tax payer identification numbers. These numbers are used to file quarterly reports, tax returns, and make payments for withholding, unemployment, and sales transactions as required. The simplest form of business, the sole proprietorship can operate and file most taxes using the proprietor's social security number. However, if the sole proprietorship hires employees, it must file for a separate tax payer ID number. Thus it is often suggested that even sole proprietorships apply for tax payer ID numbers from the beginning.

Despite the legal differences among the three forms of businesses, only a few differences exist in their respective financial statements. These differences are discussed to clarify what the financial statements represent. In the equity section of the balance sheet a proprietorship lists the capital balance by the owner's name (e.g., Fred Jones capital account). The approach is much the same for partnerships. Corporations do not list the stockholders' names. Instead, the stockholders' equity is divided into *contributed capital* and *retained earnings*. Contributed capital reflects stockholder or owner investment. Retained earnings reflect the corporation's profits.

Different terms are used to describe payments to the owners depending on the legal form of the business. Payments to owners of proprietorships or partnerships are called *withdrawals*. In partnerships each partner has a separate draw account. Just as there is a Fred Jones capital account, there is a Fred Jones draw account to show the withdrawals from the practice. Corporations distribute equity to the owners by payments that are called *dividends*. For small corporations, this is not much more formal than that of a proprietorship or partnership. But, large publicly held corporations must observe a very formal procedure that involves the following three key dates:

- The *date of declaration*, when the board declares the dividend.
- The *date of record*, when owners of stock on that date are paid the dividends.
- The *date of payment*, when the dividend is paid to the stockholders of record.

The biggest difference in the financial statements occurs in the amounts paid to company managers. For corporations, salaries paid to managers are reported as expenses. In contrast, if the owner of a proprietorship or partnership functions as a manager, no salary expense is reflected on the income statement. This distinction has practical importance because most new businesses start out as proprietorships or partnerships, and this difference requires special consideration when analyzing the income statement.

For example, the formula for return on equity (ROE) reflects the net income divided by owners' equity as shown by the following formulas:

$$ROE = NI / BOE$$

where *NI* = net income and *BOE* = beginning owner's equity.

When the value of the owner's managerial efforts is not factored into the P & L as an expense, net income is higher than if the practice is organized as a corporation. This conveys an unrealistic impression of how well the practice is doing. To accurately reflect the performance of the business,

*See Chapter 16 for a more in-depth discussion on this topic.

the fair value of the owner's efforts needs to be represented by modifying the equation as follows:

$$MROE = NI - V / BOE$$

where *NI* = net income, *V* = dollar value of owners efforts, and *BOE* = beginning owners' equity.

The MROE has another practical application for audiologists in sole proprietorships or partnerships. The MROE should be compared with other investment alternatives available to the owner to determine whether the practice is producing an adequate return on the investment of the owner(s)' resources. This means that if the audiologist sets a fair value on his or her work week, the practice's bottom line may not be as impressive as it looks. Perhaps this real return on the audiologist's effort and investment is insufficient compared with other approaches that earn a better return on investment. The audiologist needs to decide whether the MROE from the practice is worth the effort.

Accounting Basis

Some small businesses and professions, such as physicians, accountants, and lawyers, record revenues and expenses on a *cash basis*. This means that revenues are recognized when cash is received and expenses are recognized when cash is paid out. Problems usually surface at year end. For example, services rendered in December 1998, for which the practice receives payment in 1999, would record as 1999 revenues. Similarly, expenses incurred in December 1998 that are not paid until 1999 are 1999 expenses. This is considered improper matching of expenses and revenues. It is the main reason that the cash basis accounting is not considered a "generally accepted accounting procedure" (GAAP).

However, cash basis *can be* considered acceptable when the results approximate those that would be obtained under an *accrual basis* of accounting in which the revenue and expenses are recorded as they occur. Small business and professions generally meet that requirement because payment is usually expected when service is rendered. Exceptions would fall outside the realm of materiality as discussed in the following paragraphs.

Materiality is an important principal of accounting. It is a term that is used or implied throughout this chapter. Materiality is more a concept than a rule because no hard and fast rules exist to define what is material (Larson & Miller, 1995). Decisions as to what is material and what is not are determined by management in consultation with the accountant. The litmus test of materiality is that it is information that is required for an individual of average intelligence and experience to form an informed decision. In the decision to use the cash basis of accounting, the basic idea is that requirements of accounting principals may be ignored if the effect on the financial statements is unimportant to their users. In other words, cash basis may be used if it is unlikely to produce an error large enough to misrepresent the financial statement information.

Another way of looking at materiality is one of scale. In a startup practice an expense of $3000.00 is likely to be material. But that same expense incurred by a multibillion dollar corporation is likely to be lumped together with many other similar expenses before it even shows up on the firm's financial statements. By itself, the $3000.00 would disappear as part of rounding off the numbers to make them usable to the end user.

Reporting

As a business, a practice is required to comply with a certain base level of reporting to the federal government. In most cases the same level of reporting is required for state governments, with additional state and local sales tax reporting. State and local requirements vary and are not described in this chapter. The chapter addresses usual federal requirements and stresses that the reader be aware state requirements may mirror these federal requirements.

EIN

One of the first contacts a practice is likely to have with the IRS is the need to obtain a Employer Identification Number (EIN). This is a nine-digit number issued by the IRS. It is used to identify the tax accounts of the practice. The audiologist can use IRS Publications *1635* and *583* to understand the use of the EIN and how to file returns, respectively. File *Form SS-4* to request the IRS issue an EIN.

Government Forms and Dates

Whenever a practice hires an employee, there are requirements that are mandated by the federal government in the form of IRS and the Immigration and Naturalization Service (INS) Filings. These forms are required regardless of the business form of the practice. An employee must complete a *FORM W4* for the employer to determine withholding requirements for the IRS and the Social Security Administration (SSA). The employer is also required to complete and maintain on file a *FORM I9* for each employee. The best way to obtain the latest versions of these forms is from the Internet as shown in Table 15–7.

When a practice has an EIN, it receives a coupon book for use in meeting many of its reporting and paying requirements. The coupons have multiple uses, which are designated by different markable fields on the form. The practice must submit the form along with deposit to its bank for payment of withholding, social security taxes (FICA), Medicare, and federal unemployment taxes (FUTA). The frequency of these payments is based on the history of payment by the practice; the higher the obligation the more frequent the payment requirements. In the future the IRS plans to arrange for automatic withdrawals from the practice's business bank accounts. Table 15–8 shows the most basic reporting schedule for a small practice.

Monthly filers deposit their FIT and FICA withholdings on the 15th day of the following month using Form 941. In other words, January FIT and FICA withholdings must be deposited by the 15th of February, and so on throughout the year. Failure to meet filing deadlines results in substantial penalties. State requirements often match federal requirements.

Table 15–8 represents a basic obligation of a small business or practice. As the practice grows in income and employees, the requirements for reporting increase dramatically. As stated early in the chapter, it is a good investment for the practice to contract with an accounting professional to

TABLE 15–7   Internet addresses for ordering forms

Forms via the Internet		
Federal Service	Form	Internet Address
INS	I-9	www.ins.usdoj.gov/forms/download
IRS	W-4	www.irs.ustreas.gov
IRS	All other	www.irs.ustreas.gov

TABLE 15–8   Basic reporting schedule

Basic Filing Dates	
Jan 31	W2s to employees, 1099s to contractors, Form 940, deposit FUTA for prior 4th quarter, Form 941 and Form 945 annual return of withheld FIT
Feb 15	Any W4 or W5 updates are to be initiated
Feb 28	Form 1096 along with 1099s, Form W3 along with W2s
Mar 15	File calendar year corporate returns
Apr 15	Individual, partnership returns
Apr 30	1st quarter 941 deposit, 1st quarter 940 FUTA deposit
Jul 31	2nd quarter 941 deposit, 2nd quarter 940 FUTA deposit, Form 5500
Oct 31	3rd quarter 941 deposit, 3rd quarter 940 FUTA deposit

calculate and determine the correct filings and filing dates. It is a prudent use of financial resources and a prudent savings of a professional's time and energy.

ACCOUNTANTS FOR AUDIOLOGY PRACTICES

Licensing

Audiologists need to exercise some care and judgment in selecting an accountant. Not all accountants are alike in their training, just as not all hearing health care providers are alike. Accountants are not all Certified Public Accountants (CPAs). To become a CPA, an individual must meet educational and experience requirements and pass the CPA examination. The steps are much like those required to become a certified audiologist, except that CPAs must also take and pass a course in professional ethics (American Institute of Certified Public Accountants, 1998). Like a certified audiologist, this licensing holds the CPA to a higher standard of professional service to the public than is required by law of an uncertified accountant or bookkeeper. However, a CPA may not be necessary for some of the bookkeeping and accounting needs of the business.

In selecting an accountant for the practice, licensing and experience in the field are important, as are recommendations from respected sources. Familiarity with technology and expertise in the business form of the practice are very important factors to consider, especially if the practice is a Sub Chapter S-Corporation.*

Computer Literacy

Technological sophistication is an important factor that the audiologist must consider when selecting an accountant. Throughout this chapter, it is recommended that an accountant be consulted when setting up accounting software and configuring computer-generated reports and forms. Just as some audiologists choose not to enter the computer age, some accountants are also not computer literate. It makes little sense for a practice that uses personal computer accounting software to rely on the services of an accounting firm that is not fully computerized or capable of handling the practice's account with compatible software. Unfortunately, it is not uncommon for practices to generate computer information but have to print out hardcopy for delivery to their accounting firm, which then manually enters the information in their system. This is incredibly inefficient and expensive for the practice.

PITFALL

Just as some audiologists choose not to enter the computer age, some accountants are not computer literate.

---

*See Chapter 16 for discussion on S-Corporation.

Interview the accountants. Visit their office and see whether their environment resembles that of the practice. If the technology use seems compatible, solicit their input on software applications that will be compatible with their applications and meet the practice's needs. The software should be flexible, user-friendly, offer technical support, and offer opportunities for growth.

CONCLUSIONS

This chapter stressed the importance of adopting and maintaining simple, useful bookkeeping and accounting disciplines for internal and external reporting and analysis. Basic bookkeeping and accounting skills can help the practice operate at maximum efficiency, plan and budget for the future, meet its financial and reporting obligations, secure good terms with its creditors, and harbor some peace of mind through increased knowledge. The accounting system must be flexible enough to handle changes in business size and business form. Always, the system must let the audiologist know how the practice is performing and progressing and yield valid data for calculating return on investment.

Audiologists cannot and should not do all these things themselves. It is advisable in most instances to contract with accounting professionals for assistance in steering the practice through the hazards it will face and keeping the practice poised to take advantage of opportunities. By using personal computer-based accounting applications and gaining knowledge and experience, the audiologist can reduce the need for more basic services and devote more resources to proactive business planning and analysis.

GLOSSARY

Accounts payable Liabilities created by selling goods and services on credit.

Accounts receivable Assets created by selling goods on credit.

Accrual basis accounting Preparing financial statements based on recognizing revenues when they are earned and matching expenses to those revenues.

Asset Economic resources owned or controlled by an entity as a result of past events or transactions.

Balance sheet *Statement of financial position* that lists the types and amounts in dollars of an entity's assets, liabilities, and equity at a specific point in time.

Cash basis accounting Preparing financial statements based on recognizing revenue when cash is received and reporting expenses when cash is paid.

Credit Recorded on the right side of a *T account*. An entry that decreases asset and expense accounts and increases liability, equity, or revenue accounts.

Creditors Entities entitled to receive payments from the practice.

Debit Recorded on the left side of a *T account*. An entry that increases asset and expense accounts and decreases liability, equity, or revenue accounts.

Debtors Entities that owe amounts to the practice.

Direct costs Costs that can be directly related or traced to a single cost objective, for example hearing aid or product costs.

Double entry Recording the effects of transactions with equal debits and credits.

Equity The residual interest in the assets of an entity after deducting liabilities.

Expenses Using up the assets of the practice as a result of performing the central operations of the practice.

FICA Federal Insurance Contributions Act. Social Security and Medicare taxes.

FUTA Federal Unemployment Tax.

GAAP Generally accepted accounting practices.

Income Assets received by the practice.

Income statement A report that shows the results of operations (profit or loss) for a period of time.

Indirect costs Costs that relate to more than one cost objective, for example, administrative costs.

Ledger The collection of all accounts used by a business.

Liability Obligations owed by an entity that represent future sacrifices.

Materiality Information that is required for an individual of average intelligence and experience to form an informed decision.

Posting The process of copying information to the ledger.

Revenues Assets received in exchange for the goods and services of the practice.

T account A simple account form used to illustrate how debits and credits work.

REFERENCES

AMERICAN INSTITUTE OF CERTIFIED PUBLIC ACCOUNTANTS. (1998). *Professional ethics for certified public accountants*. Redwood City, CA: California Certified Public Accounts Education Foundation.

ENGLER, C. (1990). *Managerial accounting*. Homewood, IL: Irwin.

LARSON, K., & MILLER, P. (1995). *Financial accounting* (pp. 19–41). Homewood, IL: Irwin.

Chapter 16

Financial Management of Audiology Practices and Clinics

Barry A. Freeman, Joseph P. Barimo, and Gilbert S. Fox, III

FINANCIAL MANAGEMENT PRACTICES

As audiologists, our training often emphasizes diagnostic and therapeutic interventions to the exclusion of information on financial practices and management. Those of us who find ourselves managing or owning businesses do so without significant preparation for the crucial responsibilities that lie ahead. Our models for best practice, in most instances, come from working for and observing our supervisors and managers. Although it is hoped that our role models are effective and efficient business people, too often just the opposite turns out to be the case.

According to ASHA (1990), poor fiscal management is the most significant single cause of business failure. When asked to respond to the question, "What do you wish you had known, but did not, before becoming a clinical manager?" the most frequent response related to financial management skills. Most clinical managers reported that they had not realized how complicated the job of managing a clinical operation would be. Although many reported possessing superior clinical skills, they found difficulty handling such routine tasks as accounting for revenue and expenses, complying with state and federal regulations, and fiscal considerations involved with staffing.

This is an age of downsizing, right-sizing, leveraged buy-outs, mergers, and managed competition. The practicing clinician must assume the role and responsibilities of a financial manager, including assembling and allocating scarce resources (e.g., funding, physical facility, human resources, information) coupled with establishing goals and objectives. Terms such as staffing mix, budgeting, and fiscal fitness must move from the abstract to the concrete.

This chapter provides the knowledge and skills that have practical application in the professional lives of audiologists. The development of this chapter is driven by the progression of activities faced by practitioners. To begin, practitioners must decide on or understand the requirements of an organizational structure. Considerations include the legal, tax, and liability implications of the practice. Once this is in place, a practice plan can be developed. This includes identifying and articulating personal and professional goals; developing budget projections; recruiting appropriate staff; and responding to the changes in the reimbursement system. The development of this plan precedes the process of seeking capital for the proposed practice. All potential sources of capital should be identified and evaluated on the basis of personal, financial, and professional considerations (see Chapter 14 in this volume for further discussion).

If the practice is operational, a financial analysis must be performed. Financial ratios can be used to assess profitability

Audiology: Practice Management. Edited by Hosford-Dunn, Roeser, and Valente. Thieme Medical Publishers, Inc., New York © 2000

aspects of the practice, inventory control, and collection policies. These are easily applied to an audiology practice and are beneficial in capital maintenance.

Financial management also should include planning for the future. Not only should the audiologist invest for retirement, but he or she must also prepare for the purchase of new equipment or expansion of the practice.

The major goals for the reader of this chapter include the following:

- Become knowledgeable about legal and financial structures as they relate to a professional practice
- Become knowledgeable about fiscal considerations when planning and developing programs
- Devise strategies to assess personal and professional financial goals
- Learn to effectively and efficiently manage changes in the reimbursement system
- Develop strategies to identify and analyze sources of capitalization
- Devise strategies to analyze and improve fiscal performance
- Learn strategies to plan for future practice and personal development

ORGANIZATIONAL STRUCTURES FOR CLINICAL PRACTICE

A legal structure should be the initial step in establishing a practice. This decision will have an impact on the legal, tax, and liability aspects of the practice. Those who operate under an existing system—as an employee of a hospital, university clinic, or private practice—need to know the implications and expectations of the principles to establish appropriate goals and strategies and effectively function within the structure. Although three basic legal forms of business organization exist, most businesses and professional practices are sole proprietorships. This business structure accounts for approximately 75% of all small businesses (Gitman, 1997).

Sole Proprietorships

A sole proprietorship is a business owned by a single person who is responsible for the financial planning and daily management of the practice. The proprietor has unlimited liability and is personally responsible for the debts of the business. Creditors have the right to seek restitution by attaching the personal assets of the owner to satisfy business debt. The strengths and weaknesses of sole proprietorships are summarized in Table 16–1.

Partnerships

Some professional practices are co-owned and a partnership is established. This structure enables more than one person to manage and operate the business. Like the sole proprietorship, partnerships assume full responsibility for the debts of the business and personal assets can be attached to satisfy creditors. Once in a partnership, partners cannot sell or transfer ownership without the consent of the other partners. Because less flexibility occurs in transferring ownership, it may be more difficult to raise funds for practice growth. A partnership legally terminates on the withdrawal, death, or retirement of a principal. Table 16–1 summarizes the strengths and weaknesses of partnerships.

Corporations

The personal liability of practice principals can be limited to the personal investment of the stockholders by forming a corporation. This is a legal entity with the power to own property and enter contracts. Corporations maintain limited exposure to the principals. Also, funds can be raised by selling shares of stock without interfering in the daily operation of the business and without the permission of other stockholders. A corporation retains a long charter to maintain stability if a stockholder dies. The shares go to the heirs. A summary of the benefits and weaknesses of incorporation are found in Table 16–1.

Other Organizational Entities

Limited liability corporations (LLCs), limited liability partnerships (LLPs), and Subchapter S corporations provide alternatives to conventional structures. The S corporation is taxed as a partnership but maintains the limited liability of a corporation. The LLC combines the partnership's tax status while maintaining limited liability. Unlike an S corporation, the LLC can own other corporations, and other corporations, partnerships, and non-U.S. citizens can own LLC shares. This permits joint ventures or projects developed through affiliate companies. The LLP is essentially a partnership but is permitted in less than half the states in the country. The LLP is

---

SPECIAL CONSIDERATION

Key terms
- Sole proprietorship: Business owned by one person who is personally responsible for debts of the business.
- Partnership: Co-owned business in which partners assume full responsibility for debts of the business.
- Corporation: A legal business entity with the power to own property, enter contracts, and maintain limited exposure to the principals.
- S corporation: A tax-reporting entity whose earnings are taxed not as a corporation but as the incomes of its stockholders.
- Limited liability corporation: An entity that combines partnership tax status while maintaining limited liability.

Learning outcomes
- Understand the legal and financial implications of various business structures.
- Identify the legal, tax, and liability implications of business structures.

TABLE 16–1   Strengths and weaknesses of forms of business organizations

	Sole Proprietorship	Partnership	Corporation
Strengths	Owner receives profits and losses	Can raise more funds than sole proprietorship	Owners have limited liability—cannot lose more than invested
	Low organizational costs	Borrowing power enhanced by more owners	Can grow with issuance of more stock
	Income taxed as personal income of owner	More available knowledge and managerial skill	Ownership transferrable
	Independence Secrecy	Income taxed as personal income of partners	Long life of firm because does not dissolve at death of owners
	Ease of dissolution		Receives certain corporate tax advantages
Weaknesses	Owner has unlimited liability because total wealth can be taken to satisfy debts	Owners have unlimited liability and may have to cover debts of partners	Taxes higher because corporate income is taxed and dividends paid to owners are taxed again
	Limited fund-raising power may inhibit growth	When partner dies, partnership dissolved	More expensive to organize
	Owner must do everything	Difficult to liquidate or transfer partnership	Subject to greater government regulations
	Hard to give employees long-term career		
	Lacks continuity when proprietor dies	Difficult to achieve large-scale operation	Lacks secrecy because financial reports public

Modified from Gitman, 1997.

taxed as a partnership, but partners are not personally liable for other partners' malpractice. The advice of a good attorney and an accountant are requirements for any practice.

PEARL

A legal structure should be the initial step in establishing a practice to ensure that effective operating principles, goals, and strategies are developed by the persons operating within the structure.

CONSIDERATIONS FOR DEVELOPING A PRACTICE PLAN AND ESTABLISHING FISCAL FITNESS

It is accepted that most American industry is composed of small businesses. Unfortunately, a mistaken impression by many is that entering an independent professional practice merely requires one to "hang up a shingle" and the patients will flock to the door. Unfortunately, many of these new businesses fail during the first 5 years. In this section, considerations for developing a practice plan and establishing fiscal fitness will be addressed.

Although audiologists have a sound understanding of the professional literature, it is important that they recognize their strengths and weaknesses in practice management. Historically, training programs have not provided the skills to develop a financial practice plan. Student value, for example, has been measured in clock hours rather than in patient billing and collections. Audiologists must apply a dollar value to patient services, including planning time, overhead expenses, and follow-up. It is critical to recognize and place an appropriate value on audiological services.

Moreover, not all audiologists enter the profession with the same professional aspirations. Some choose to be employees in a private physician's office, university clinic, or hospital, whereas others seek independent practice. Regardless of the practice setting, the audiologist must have an understanding of the professional and financial objectives of the employment setting. These include patient and personnel

SPECIAL CONSIDERATION

Key terms
- Balance sheet: Summary statement of the firm's financial position at a given point in time.
- Assets: Properties or economic resources owned by the business.
- Liabilities: Debts to others—probable future sacrifices of economic benefits arising from present obligations.
- Current assets: Cash or other assets expected to be sold, collected, or consumed within 1 year or less.
- Current liabilities: Short-term debt expected to be paid or liquidated within 1 year or less.
- Gross profit margin: Percent of sales dollar remaining after goods are paid for.
- Net profit margin: Percent of each sales dollar remaining after all costs and expenses.
- Return on assets: Overall effectiveness in generating profits with available assets.
- Income statement: Financial summary of operating results.
- Line of credit: Agreement between bank and business specifying the amount of unsecured short-term borrowing bank will make available to business.

Learning outcomes
- Identify and articulate personal and professional goals.
- Identify key components and considerations for the development of an effective business plan.
- Learn the key questions and considerations in developing a budget.
- Understand the financial impact of changes in the reimbursement system.
- Learn to develop income and expense projections.
- Develop strategies to improve staffing and retention.

management, issues in reimbursement, obsolescence of equipment, and other expenses. An audiologist with this knowledge becomes a valuable resource for the employer, thereby ensuring better job secuity and value to the practice. Given this overview, it is now possible to view the specific aspects that must be considered when devising a practice plan and establishing fiscal fitness.

Budgeting

A budget is a financial plan delineating the distribution of resources necessary to carry out activities and meet financial goals for a future period of time. In many organizations the responsibility for preparing the budget is usually assigned to several high-level managers. This group is referred to as the budget committee. The committee calls on managers throughout the company for help in the budgeting process. The budget committee's duties are as follows:

- Formulate budget policies compatible with the organization's goals and objectives
- Review budget estimates submitted by department heads
- Revise budget estimates as necessary
- Approve budget estimates
- Analyze budget reports and recommend changes
- Establish the budget time table

For-Profit Budgeting

The specific budget that is found in most organizations is referred to as the master budget. Five subunits usually comprise the master budget: sales budget, direct labor budget, overhead budget, marketing cost budget, and administrative cost budget.

The preparation of the master budget begins with the sales budget. This is a formal plan that forecasts anticipated sales in quantities and in dollars. A sales forecast is a prediction of the quantities expected to be sold on the basis of such factors as past sales, economic and seasonal conditions, pricing policies, and market analysis.

Once the sales forecast and sales budgets are computed, the next phase is initiated. A direct labor budget is a quantitative calculation and listing of planned expenditures for direct labor costs for the coming budget period. The direct labor budget is on the basis of the required services to be rendered.

Following this step is the determination of the overhead budget. This is a listing of each type of planned cost such as rent, repairs, light and power, telephone, maintenance, supplies, and miscellaneous expenditures.

The next component is the marketing cost budget. This is a list of each planned marketing cost for the coming year, such as advertising, travel, rental space, utilities, and miscellaneous. A significant portion of this budget is dictated by the sales budget. Therefore the two are usually prepared in conjunction with each other.

The final piece is the administrative cost budget. This is a listing of each planned administrative cost for the coming year such as administrative salaries, fringe benefits, rent, utilities, insurance, professional dues, and miscellaneous expenditures.

Not-for-Profit Budgeting

Budgeting in most not-for-profit organizations often is different from that just described. Many of these organizations make use of the incremental approach when preparing budgets. In this process the previous period's budget is accepted as a base, and those figures are either increased or decreased depending on whether the entity wants to increase or decrease output during the period. The major advantage of using this approach is that the preparer begins with an already established document that only requires modifications. As a result, the task is significantly simplified in this approach. The major disadvantage of using this approach is that the previous year's inefficiencies are automatically continued. In addition, it is virtually impossible to identify what has been effective.

Another budgeting scheme frequently found in nonprofit organizations is zero-base budgeting. Unlike incremental budgeting, which begins with the previous period's numbers as a base, zero-base budgeting begins with a zero. Each program or project is submitted for review and ranked according to its importance to the organization. In this system the manager is able to choose or eliminate programs.

Budgeting for Professional Development

In developing an annual budget, many practice owners/employers consider nonsalary benefits for staff. An example is investing in professional development. Some larger practice organizations view this as an investment with the reward of better patient service, and some companies also are identifying professional development courses as revenue producers from outside practitioners who participate in the courses for a fee. Therefore financial managers are being required to develop budgets for professional development.

SPECIAL CONSIDERATION

Five general areas to be addressed when planning professional development courses as revenue producers:

1. Select a topic that will have interest to a wide audience. A community survey of interests or speakers may yield suggestions for topics.
2. Determine the market. Decisions must be made about the target audience, professional employment settings, and clinical populations to be addressed in the workshop.
3. Locate the workshop. Factors to be weighed are accessibility, availability, cost of housing and amenities such as dining and social facilities.
4. Time of the workshop. Consideration must be given to dates to avoid other meeting conflicts and holidays. Also, one should be aware of license expiration dates to ensure that the activity will accommodate practitioners requiring continuing education to maintain their professional license.
5. Determine the price. Attendance, affordability, break-even points, profit objectives, and professional discounts are all factors to be addressed in planning. It is best to be conservative in estimates to make the activity affordable and attractive.

Cash Management and Remaining Liquid

Cash is needed to pay the bills. Sources for this cash include collections from audiological services and the sale of products. Bills can be paid from current revenue or cash reserves established over time. On occasion, however, practices may need to establish a line of credit for funds to meet current expenses. Receivables must be managed to ensure adequate cash flow to pay expenses and hopefully make a profit. Many variables must be factored into the estimate of adequate cash flow. For example, the practice payment policies should be reviewed. Should patients be told they are responsible for payment at the time of service? Should insurance be paid directly to the patient? Should practices accept assignment or bill for payments not covered by third parties? Should payment plans be arranged for the purchase of products or services? How often should bills be mailed? These are some issues that impact cash flow. Proper planning can ensure the liquidity necessary to meet expenses.

Numerous factors can affect cash balances. In some regions of the country business will increase during certain seasons. For example, the influx of "snowbirds" living in the warmer climate during the winter impacts Florida. This might increase business and cash reserves compared with other times of the year. A wholesale price change also affects cash reserves. Assume, for example, that hearing instruments typically cost $500 but a new technology is introduced with a wholesale cost of $700. Being excited about the new hearing instrument, a large marketing campaign is developed to promote the new product. Advertisements will require an investment, and it may take time to generate sales. Also, when patients are fit, a 30-day trial is extended during which time no money or only a portion of the purchase price is collected. A financial shortfall in the revenue may be necessary to advertise and purchase the hearing instruments until payments are received from patients. Both the new product and the advertising campaign are good investments that probably will result in increased sales and revenues. It is the short-term financial management that will ensure the ability to remain solvent and to reap the rewards of the investment.

PEARL

Practice payment and collection policies must be established to ensure adequate cash flow to the practice.

Estimating Revenue and Expenses

Revenue goals often are established to assist the management team in determining the financial success of a practice site or the production of an individual practitioner. Revenue and expense data may prompt the manager to recommend expanding certain sites; provide bonuses or incentives to certain employees; or eliminate selected services, personnel, or satellite offices. It is incumbent on the manager to control revenue and expenses to achieve profitability.

Most revenue for practices will be derived from the productivity of the audiologist. Therefore the following five-step process is recommended for estimating facility or practioner revenue:

1. Project the number of procedures/products sold for the month by each practitioner.
2. Multiply the total number of procedures/products sold by the individual by the average reimbursement per procedure/product to determine the total projected revenue produced by that person.
3. Calculate the actual collection percentage of the charges of each practitioner.
4. Subtract overhead costs for each practice location and individual practitioner to arrive at the profit/loss estimates.
5. Total the information for all employees to determine revenue projections for the month.

In terms of operating expenses, include costs of various components directly related to the daily operations of doing business. Categories include expenses such as labor, communications, supplies, and advertising. The following six-step process is useful for establishing an expense budget:

1. Identify fixed costs. These remain constant regardless of sales volume (e.g., rent, utilities, telephone line charges).
2. Identify trends of variable costs because they will change directly with the amount of production (e.g., advertising, cost of goods, supplies).
3. Project existing percentages into revenue total to determine preliminary profit figures.
4. Establish spending targets in variable cost areas to increase profit margin.
5. Establish spending limits in fixed cost areas to enhance profit margin goals.
6. Finalize operating expense budget.

When examining revenue generation, it is necessary to include productivity and related factors. For example, Barimo and Newman (1996) performed a time study for practitioners supervising students in a university training clinic. The results indicated that many were scheduled beyond the 37.5 hours per week required as a part of their employment contract. However, several were scheduled to work less than 30 hours per week or were engaged in activities that were not revenue generating. To accommodate this loss in revenue, adjunct part-time faculty were hired to teach, supervise students, or see patients. This resulted in reduced morale as full-time staff complained of discrepencies in caseloads, duties, and hours spent on the job. In addition, to pay for this part-time staff cutbacks in clinic materials and travel were needed.

As a result, additional time studies were completed to determine the average time required to perform certain tasks. The staff were then given guidelines for scheduling duties, patients, and classes. Consequently, the need for part-time adjunct faculty declined. This permitted full-time employees to maintain an economically productive schedule and lead to a higher level of morale as more money was allocated and invested in these employees.

Profitability

When many audiologists first came into the profession in the 1960s and 1970s, profit was viewed by some as unethical and immoral. Over time, though, practitioners learned that the objective of having a high rate of return on the business plan and investments can occur concurrently with quality hearing care services. Net sales of products and services determine the return rate, the net operating assets including depreciation on equipment and bad debts, and the net operating income. Generally, the more earned on each dollar of sales and the more sales made for each dollar of operating assets, the greater will be the return on each dollar. This type of analysis is beneficial in assessing the potential return on new products and equipment. For example, should a practice purchase otoacoustic emissions or auditory brain stem response equipment? In addition to professional service considerations, the financial return on the investment should be properly assessed by the practice's financial manager.

It is necessary to review various aspects of the business to understand its financial picture. Many management teams use profitability ratios to develop the financial profile. These are quite useful in many businesses but, unfortunately, no standards for the profession of audiology exist because of variations among individual practices. No audiology standard exists for the percentage of practice revenue generated from diagnostic versus product sales. Each practice is unique. Similarly, no industry standard exists for overhead. Some practices, for example, generate 90% of their revenue from the sale of products. Other practices, though, may generate 60% of their revenue from professional services and only 40% from product sales. Therefore a discussion of ratios allows only intrapractice comparisons until standards evolve. That is, at this time, it is possible to use ratios to evaluate changes in the financial picture from year to year within the same practice, but comparing one practice with the next is difficult.

PITFALL

Management teams use profitability ratios to develop the financial profile. Unfortunately, because of variations among individual audiology practices, standards for the profession do not exist. Consequently, comparing one practice to another is difficult.

The Income Statement and Profitability Ratios

A simplified practice statement for the Audiology Practice of America (APA) in Table 16–2 presents income and expenses as a percent of total revenue. This information is valuable for comparing annual practice performance. For example, the APA statement reveals that 64% of the $700,000 total practice revenue is generated from the sale of products. With the advent of managed care and the changes in reimbursement,

TABLE 16–2 Simplified practice statement of the Audiology Practice of America (APA)

	Revenue
Professional Evaluation Services	$250,000 (36%)
Product Sales	$450,000 (64%)
Total Revenue	$700,000
Expenses	
Rent/Overhead	$ 75,000
Equipment Leases	$ 25,000
Advertising	$ 45,000
Salaries	$ 75,000
Insurance	$ 25,000
Other Professional Expenses	$ 75,000
Equipment	$ 16,000
Cost of Goods Sold	$170,000
Total Expenses	$506,000
Net Before Taxes	$194,000 (27.7%)

practices that traditionally had a high volume of diagnostic evaluations have found an increasing dependence on dispensing hearing aids to generate income. It appears that a greater dependence on product sales will result in a higher overhead because of a greater cost of goods sold. The net before taxes for APA, for example, is 27.7% of the total practice revenue. A cursory survey of many independent practices that mix both diagnostic and dispensing suggests that many practices do, in fact, net between 25 and 30%. Without an industry standard, these numbers are more valuable for annual intrapractice assessments.

As the cost of new hearing technology increases as reflected by a higher cost of goods sold, there should be a comparable increase in retail prices. The *gross profit margin* reveals the percentage of each sales dollar remaining after the practice has paid for the products.

$$\text{Gross profit margin} = \frac{\text{Sales} - \text{Cost of goods sold}}{\text{Sales}}$$
$$= \frac{\text{Gross profits}}{\text{Sales}}$$

The gross profit margin for APA is $530,000 which is 76% of total revenue. Generally, the greater the dependence on amplification to generate revenue, the smaller the gross profit margin. Perhaps a more important measure is the *net profit margin*, which measures the percentage of dollars that remain after all costs and expenses, including interest and taxes, have been deducted.

$$\text{Net profit margin} = \frac{\text{Net profits after taxes}}{\text{Sales}}$$

The net profit is frequently used to measure a practice's success, and the margins appear to vary greatly across the industry. It also is useful to compare the net profits to total assets and derive a measure of *return on total assets*. Each practice maintains equipment requiring a substantial financial investment.

$$\text{Return on total assets} = \frac{\text{Net profits after taxes}}{\text{Total assets}}$$

This ratio measures the effectiveness in generating profits from the equipment used in the practice. Too many assets in relation to income may suggest an inefficient use of equipment. Yet, if investment in assets has not been adequate, revenues and working capital may be restricted, which also places a strain on the practice.

Financial Management and Managed Care

In the eyes of the evolving healthcare industry, what previously were profit generators under traditional fee-for-service insurance contracts are now considered expense centers. Filled hospital beds and comprehensive diagnostic assessments no longer are a sign of success in healthcare. In fact, they are expenses and profit reducers in the world of managed care and capitation. The shift to managed care is not merely a matter of reducing prices, it is a combination of lowering the prices, the number of office visits, patient referrals, and diagnostic and surgical procedures (Smith, 1997). Providers such as audiologists must comply with clinically appropriate protocols and are not rewarded for aggressive management. Participation in prepaid capitated health plans requires different financial management strategies than traditional fee-for-service plans.

Capitation relies on big numbers where practitioners are paid a fixed monthly fee for each contract member (per member per month) (Carter et al, 1995). Under capitation, members do not equal patients but, rather, potential patients. Assume, for example, the audiologist agrees to provide diagnostic services for a company with 5000 employees and beneficiaries. These become the plan members. The managed care organization may agree to pay a set fee of 20 cents to the audiologist for each member. Thus the audiologist will receive a monthly check for approximately $83.00 (5000 members × 0.20/12 months) whether 1 or 5000 members schedule appointments. All costs and revenue come from the monthly payment. Profitable practices ensure that capitation revenues offset the utilization costs and understand that an objective of managed care is to minimize cost while maximizing patient service. This reimbursement structure, however, does facilitate financial planning. A fixed payment will be received monthly regardless of the number of patients served during the month.

CONTROVERSIAL POINT

In managed care environments providers such as audiologists must comply with clinically appropriate protocols and are not rewarded for aggressive management.

Another approach to controlling healthcare costs is to require audiologists to discount fees with the promise of significant increases in patient referrals. Proper financial management requires a careful examination of the discount structure, the anticipated increase in patient volume, and whether the practice can handle the increase in patient load (Freeman, 1990). For example, assume that a managed care organization requests a 30% discount in fees, which would be offset by an increase in patient volume. If true, patient volume would need to increase by approximately 45% to offset the discount and generate the same revenue.

Similarly, as practices find significant reductions in revenue generated from diagnostic evaluations, there is an increasing dependence on income from the sale of products. Of course, as discussed previously, the wholesale cost of high-level technology has led to higher retail prices. Oftentimes, practitioners are concerned about setting a price too high and losing patients. Assume, for example, prices are increased by 20%. The practice could afford to lose 16.7% of the current patients and still make the same profit. If no loss in patients occurs, revenue will obviously increase by 20%. Therefore a small increase in prices can have a significant impact on the bottom line profit.

Calculating and analyzing capitated and discounted contracts provide an economic foundation for financial decision making, comparing aspects of the practice and ensuring financial stability. Proper financial management may be the difference between financial liquidity and insolvency. It is worth the time to properly assess the health of the practice.

For further discussion of practice management in managed care environments, refer to Chapters 17 and 18 in this volume.

Recruitment and Staffing Strategies

As previously stated, the changes in our healthcare system have resulted in lower reimbursement for audiology services. Because salaries account for a high percentage of a typical practice's budget, many employers assume that the best way to control costs and offset the reimbursement cutbacks is to replace high salaries with lower ones.

Some work settings elect to save salary dollars by hiring recent graduates for their clinical experience year despite their lack of clinical experience. Employers often assume that if they can recruit these practitioners, it will be cost-effective to hire them for the 1 year while they are completing their requirements for licensure or certification. The risk is that the position will remain unfilled for an extended period of time. Also, when filled, a significant investment in time and training is required to prepare the new employee for the practice experience.

A review of documentation obtained from a national contract therapy company in 1995 (Barimo, 1998) revealed that the average gross revenue generated by recent graduates in clinics, medical practices, and private practice is approximately $250,000 annually. For every month the position remained unfilled, the business estimated losses of approximately $20,000 In addition, the reported cost of retraining a new employee averaged $5000/mo or ($60,000/y). Not filling a position coupled with the burden of retraining a new employee resulted in morale problems and placed a burden on existing clinical staff. In addition, patients often complained about inconsistent service and abandoned the practice during periods of understaffing and frequent turnover.

Of interest are two studies that suggest that employers may be able to control costs by providing a quality and diverse work experience with lower salaries (Barimo, 1998; Weintraub, 1996). When asked to rank order job factors, first time job applicants in speech-language pathology ranked clean and safe working conditions and varied caseload as the top two reasons for accepting a position. Salary ranked as the fifth most important factor. However, before employers adopt this apparent salary cost saving policy, they should consider the expense of replacing practitioners annually.

CAPITALIZATION

After the development of a realistic business plan, decisions must be made about raising the funds to finance or expand a practice. Sources of investment revenue include the following:

- Personal and family savings: Investing the personal savings of the audiologist or a family member would eliminate the middleman. It does place personal dollars at risk and there is a loss of the potential gain and interest earned from the invested principal.

- Life insurance policy cash value: Many insurance policies have cash values that can be borrowed at low fixed interest rates. Many insurance companies have a flexible pay-back period, and borrowing should not affect the policy benefits.
- Banks: Audiologists with a realistic business plan often can go directly to a bank for a loan. Line of credit can be extended and borrowed on an as-needed basis. Also, banks can provide a sum of money deposited into the business checking account. The banks set a payment schedule on the basis of the amount and duration of the loan.
- Hearing instrument manufacturers: Many manufacturers extend loans to audiologists. Some companies function like a bank, requiring a business plan and establishing a fixed payment schedule. Other companies co-op the purchase of equipment through the purchase of hearing instrument products. Although this may be attractive to many practitioners, other audiologists have raised the issue of a possible ethical dilemma.

Table 16–3 presents an example of Dr. Smith who is comparing two methods of financing her practice. Her analysis suggests that she will have a lower tax burden and higher return on equity by borrowing from a bank. Spending her personal inheritance will give her a higher net profit. This is an example of considerations in capitalizing a practice.

FINANCIAL ANALYSIS RATIOS

The ability to assess the health of a business involves analyzing financial ratios of the business's risk and return. Two approaches to ratio comparisons often are made: cross-sectional and time-series.

Cross-Sectional Analysis

The comparison of the performance of one company to several others during the same time frame provides a cross-sectional analysis. It is a form of *benchmarking*, in which a company's ratios are compared with the benchmarked company. This concept has had increased application to audiology as national corporations are purchasing local practices. Significant deviations from the norm may provide information,

TABLE 16–3   Return on equity consideration for Sally Smith, Au.D.

Sally Smith, Au.D., is considering opening a new practice. After analysis, she determined that a $100,000 initial investment would be necessary. She has two ways to obtain the funds. The first is to not incur debt. She inherited $100,000 and can invest that sum in the practice. The alternative would be to personally invest $50,000 and borrow the remaining $50,000 at 12% annual interest. From her analysis, she expects sales to average $300,000 and expenses to be $180,000.

Dr. Smith yields a higher profit of $21,000 (after staff and personal salaries) from the no-debt plan, but this is a 21% rate of return compared with a return rate of 33.6% from the debt plan. In addition, she has access to $50,000 of her inheritance for other investments. She, then, must weigh the slightly lower annual profit against the benefit of having a higher rate of return and use of her personal funds.

Sally Smith, Au.D.
FINANCIAL STATEMENTS

Assets/liabilities/equity	No Debt Plan		Debt Plan
Total personal (inheritance) assets	$100,000		$100,000
Debt (12% interest)	$ -0-		$ 50,000
Equity from personal inheritance	$100,000		$ 50,000
Total debt and equity	$100,000		$100,000
Income statements			
Sales	$300,000		$300,000
Less: Expenses including salaries	$270,000		$270,000
Operating profits	$ 30,000		$ 30,000
Less: Interest expense	-0-	$0.12 \times \$50,000$	$ 6,000
Net profit before taxes	$ 30,000		$ 24,000
Less: Taxes (30%)	$ 9,000		$ 7,200
Net profit after taxes	$ 21,000		$ 16,800
Return on equity (profit/equity)	$\dfrac{21,000}{\$100,000} = 0.21$		$\dfrac{16,800}{\$50,000} = 33.6$

although not necessarily conclusive evidence, of potential areas of concern or opportunities for future growth.

Time Series Analysis

Company performance is evaluated over time in a time series analysis. It is an internal comparison to determine whether the company is growing and progressing in accordance with the business plan. Because industry average ratios for audiology clinical practice are not available, this analysis of the annual growth of the business may be more informative than the cross-sectional analysis.

For this chapter, four ratio categories will be discussed: liquidity, activity, debt, and profitability. Although profitability ratios measure return as discussed earlier in this chapter, the remaining ratios assess risk. The short-run operation of a practice is best determined from the ratios for liquidity, activity, and profitability. Table 16–4 summarizes some cautions in analyzing ratios.

Liquidity Ratios

A business's liquidity refers to its ability to pay bills as measured by (1) net working capital, (2) current ratio, and (3) the quick (acid test) ratio.

Net working capital measures the practice's overall liquidity.

Net working capital = Current assets – Current liabilities

This is a tool for internal control purposes. Often, loans and other assumed borrowed debt will specify some level of permitted net working capital. It forces the firm to maintain an adequate level of liquidity and protects creditors.

Traditionally, many aspects of financial analysis were on the basis of the *current ratio*. This is an estimate of a practice's ability to meet current debt.

$$\text{Current ratio} = \frac{\text{Current assets}}{\text{Current liabilities}}$$

SPECIAL CONSIDERATION

Key terms

- Net working capital: Difference between current assets and liabilities of the business.
- Current ratio: Measure of practice's ability to meet debt.
- Quick ratio: Measures how liquid the business is by comparing assets to liabilities.
- Average collection period: Time needed to collect money owed to the business.
- Financial leverage: Strength of practice's equity that enables it to borrow money.
- Debt ratio: Measures how dependent the practice is on borrowed money.
- Times interest ratio: Shows the practice's ability to make interest payments.

Learning outcomes

- Learn ratios that can be used to asses the various financial aspects of professional practice.

TABLE 16–4   Ratio analysis cautions

- The best information about a company's health is determined from the comparison and analysis of a group of ratios, not a single ratio.
- Comparisons should be on the basis of performance for the same time period. Comparing June for one company against January for another may not account for seasonal differences and may provide an unfair comparison.
- Comparisons may be distorted by pricing and reimbursement policies. Some regions of the country, for example, receive higher third-party reimbursement and some may charge more for products. Yet, overhead may be higher in these regions.

The higher the current ratio, the stronger the practice's ability to meet its bills. If, however, the current ratio is unusually high, this may suggest inefficient use of funds. Perhaps current accounts receivable are not being collected or there is too much cash on hand. Simply, this is the ratio of current assets to current liabilities. Although no industry standard exists for audiology, this ratio should at least be 1.0 to ensure financial obligations are met. Of course, a practice with a current ratio of 1.0 will have no working capital. Many retail businesses have a current ratio between 1.5 and 2.5. Note that sometimes this ratio can be deceiving. For example, suppose additional personal funds of the sole proprietor or partners are invested in the current assets to present a strong cash position or to pay outstanding bills. This may make the ratio higher, but, in fact, the financial position of the company may

be poorer. These numbers should be interpreted with caution although they may present valuable comparative information over a fixed period.

The most demanding ratio used to measure the liquidity of a practice is the *acid test* or *quick ratio* that measures the extent to which cash will cover the current liabilities.

$$\text{Quick ratio} = \frac{\text{Current assets} - \text{Inventory}}{\text{Current liabilities}}$$

This ratio is similar to the *current ratio* except for the inclusion of inventory. Current assets include those readily converted to cash such as cash on hand, marketable securities, and accounts receivable. Inventory often has low liquidity in an audiology practice. Items such as batteries, earplugs, and stock hearing aids may not be easily sold and converted to cash. Therefore inventory is deducted from the assets because it is the least liquid of the current assets. Again, no standards for audiology exist, but the quick ratio should exceed 1.0 to assure overall liquidity. Note that in these liquidity measures, the higher the ratio, the better the practice's ability to meet financial obligations when they come due.

Activity Ratios

Credit and collection policies also should be assessed to determine a practice's ability to convert accounts receivable to cash.

$$\text{Average collection period} = \frac{\text{Accounts receivable}}{\text{Average sales per day }^*}$$

$$^*\text{Average sales per day} = \frac{\text{Annual sales}}{360 \text{ days}}$$

From the APA income statement (Table 16–2), it is clear that the gross revenue of APA from professional services and products is $700,000. This equates to approximately $1945/day of average sales (700,000/360). Assuming accounts receivable of $70,000, the *average collection period* is 36 days (70,000/1945). However, for analysis purposes, assume accounts receivable for *products* is $40,000. Gross product sales from the income statement were $450,000, making the average daily sales $1250 (450,000/360), and the average collection period for products 32 days (40,000/1250).

The collection period is meaningful in terms of the practice's credit terms and the amount of third-party billing. If, for example, the APA management team insisted that staff collect payments for products at the time of sale, then the 32-day average collection period may indicate poor enforcement of office policy. Generally, for an audiology practice, the average collection period should not exceed 1.3 times the credit terms. A patient expected to pay his or her bill within 30 days should not be permitted more than 39 days (30 × 1.3) without action by the collection's department.

Debt Ratios

Practices often consider investing in new equipment or opening a satellite office. Consideration must be given to financial commitments involved in these investments; that is, taking on more debt. Lenders and other potential creditors must be assured that the practice can satisfy the claims of all creditors. Acquiring more debt can provide more *financial leverage*, "the magnification of risk and return through the use of fixed-cost financing such as debt" (Gitman, 1997).

The analysis of debt assists in assessing the degree of indebtedness of the practice and in determining whether the practice can meet fixed payment schedules such as for leases or loans. The *debt ratio*,

$$\text{Debt ratio} = \frac{\text{Total liabilities}}{\text{Total assets}}$$

measures the assets that are financed by creditors. The higher the ratio, the more dependent the practice is on borrowed money. The changes in healthcare have led to a new trend in audiology, the purchase of practices by publicly traded corporations. Often, these practices bring debt, but the mergers also generate additional cash flow, making it easier to service the debt. The owners of the purchased practices are freed of the debt and investors support the acquisitions of these practices because of their positive effect on debt ratios.

In addition to debt ratios are ratios that assess the ability to service debts. The *times interest ratio*,

$$\text{Times interest earned} = \frac{\text{Earnings before interest and taxes}}{\text{Interest}}$$

measures the practice's ability to make interest payments. The higher the ratio, the better the practice can meet interest obligations. Generally, a ratio between three and five is preferred because it means that earnings are at least three to five times higher than the interest payments. This provides a good margin of safety for the practice.

FINANCIAL PLANNING: PREPARING FOR THE FUTURE

The Need for Financial Planning

Among the challenges confronting audiologists are developing investment plans for acquisition of technology, expanding the practice, and preparing for an unforeseen event. The following section will discuss investment options to prepare

audiologists for anticipated and unanticipated events that will dictate their futures.

Basic Investment Tools

Stocks

The terms *stock* or *share* both refer to a fractional ownership interest in a corporation. As "owners," stockholders vote for the company's board of directors and receive information on the firm's activities and business results. Stockholders may share in current profits through "dividends" declared by the firm's board.

When a corporate business is first organized, investors contribute money to fund the enterprise and in return receive shares of stock representing their ownership in the company. If the business is successful, it will grow and have increasing profits, and the shares generally will become more valuable. If the business is not successful, the value of the shares usually declines.

- *Uses:* Investors typically buy and hold stock for its long-term growth potential. Stocks with a history of regular dividends are often held for both income and growth.
- *Risks:* Because the long-term growth of a company cannot be predicted, the short-term market value of the company's stock will fluctuate. If need or fear causes an investor to sell when the market is "down," a capital loss will result. If the market is "up," the investor will realize a capital gain.

Bonds

Whereas stocks represent ownership in a business, bonds are debt. Issued by institutions such as the federal government, corporations, and state and local governments, a bond is evidence of money borrowed by the bond issuer. In return, bond holders receive interest and at "maturity," the principal amount of the bond.

When first issued, a bond will have a specified rate of return or "yield." For example, a 6.0% bond will pay $60.00/y for each $1000 invested. If a bond is traded on a public exchange, the market price will fluctuate, generally with changes in interest rates. Later investors will receive a yield that may be more or less than 6.0%, depending on the price paid for the bond in the open market.

- *Uses:* Bonds are typically bought to generate current income or for capital growth.
- *Risks:* Like stocks, the market price of bonds will fluctuate up and down. If an investor sells a bond before it matures, a capital gain or loss may result. Unless the issuer defaults, bonds held to maturity will recover the principal amount. Because a bond pays a fixed return, inflation risk can be a problem; over time, the dollars received will buy less and less. Also, the interest income received may be subject to current income taxation.

Savings Accounts

Most investors are familiar with a savings account at a bank, savings and loan, or credit union. For many, the generic term *savings account* includes both the traditional savings account (allowing for deposits and withdrawals of small amounts) and fixed-term certificates of deposit for larger sums. Savings accounts are usually prized by investors for two primary characteristics: safety of principal and liquidity. Such accounts are insured against a failure of the savings institution by agencies of the federal government, such as the Federal Deposit Insurance Corporation or the National Credit Union Administration, for up to $100,000 per account.

- *Uses:* Savings accounts are often used as a reservoir for emergency funds or as a "warehouse" for dollars ultimately earmarked for some other purpose. Banks often permit professional practices to have interest-bearing checking accounts. The interest from these accounts can be used to generate current income.
- *Risks:* Because risk of principal loss is small, savings accounts typically have a lower yield than other investments. One "risk" to such accounts is the potential additional interest income not generated in exchange for safety of principal. The relatively low yield can also be heavily impacted by inflation and current income taxes.

Life Insurance

In the past several decades the life insurance industry has developed a number of products that combine the protection of life insurance death benefits with a significant savings element. Policies such as universal life, variable life, and universal-variable life allow practitioners to purchase a single financial instrument providing both life insurance and long-term accumulation goals. These policies may serve as a form of "forced savings" for those who find it difficult to save on a regular basis but who routinely pay their bills. Also, some partnerships take life insurance policies on the partners as a form of buyout for heirs should one partner pass away.

- *Uses:* Life insurance products often are used for long-term savings. Accumulated cash values may also serve as an "emergency reserve" if needed or a source of loans because life policies frequently include features permitting borrowing against accumulated cash values.
- *Risks:* Fixed contracts rely on the assets of the issuing life insurance company. Inflation may negatively impact a fixed return contract. Variable contracts share the risks of the underlying investments. Loans and withdrawals must be carefully structured to avoid negative income tax results.

CONCLUSIONS

Successful financial management often means the practitioner must be willing to take a risk. Many opportunities for contracts, salary negotiations, equipment, and practice growth will be presented throughout the life of a practitioner. This chapter has presented information geared to the audiology student and practitioner relative to the tools necessary to minimize the risks while maximizing the quality of service provided to our patients and the financial rewards that result. The progression of topics attempted to mirror events as they are encountered in the "real world." The information is intended to provide a template for effective fiscal functioning in a clinical setting and specific tools to facilitate financial tasks.

REFERENCES

AMERICAN SPEECH-LANGUAGE-HEARING ASSOCIATION. (1990). *Planning and initiating a private practice*. Rockville, MD: American Speech-Language-Hearing Association.

BARIMO, J. (1998, May). *Managing in managed care*. Presentation at the 1998 FLASHA Spring Conference, Marco Island, FL.

BARIMO, J., & NEWMAN, W. (1996, June). *Productivity, profitability, and livability in the university clinic*. Presentation at the 1996 ASHA Leadership in Service Delivery Conference, Chicago, IL.

CARTER, M.F., SPILLER, M.S., & MATHER, D. (1995). *Capitation rates and managed care manual*. American Academy of Audiology and the Academy of Dispensing Audiologists.

FREEMAN, B.A. (1990, July/August). Private practice. *Audiology Today, 2*,No. 3,44.

GITMAN, L.J. (1997) *Principles of managerial finance*. Reading, MA: Addison Wesley Longman, Inc.

SMITH, B.C. (1997). *Embracing change: How to survive...and thrive...in managed care*. San Diego, CA: United Benefits for Hearing.

WEINTRAUB, A. (1996). *The key elements that would attract a clinician to a CFY position*. Unpublished. Nova Southeastern University, Fort Lauderdale, FL.

Chapter 17

Managed Care and Reimbursement

Paul M. Pessis and Alan Freint

Outline

The landscape of insurance reimbursement continues to evolve as the marketplace becomes more cost-conscious. Most healthcare today is delivered through organized panels of providers who participate in programs established by insurance companies. The care given is provided according to strict contracts and fee schedules to control escalating costs. The process of grouping providers together into healthcare networks and negotiating reimbursement levels created the system we now know as managed care.

Still in its infancy as a participant in the healthcare arena, managed care continues to evolve and define itself. From day to day, variations of one or another plan enter the scene. The common thread appears to be that all plans seek to become more cost-conscious; the *management* in managed care is an attempt to make each provider more conscious of the intensity of services rendered, the costs incurred, and the number of tests ordered for a given diagnosis. Insurance companies expect to rein in medical costs by restricting the number of providers, limiting the procedures performed, and reducing the levels of reimbursement.

How we providers respond to the challenges of the changing insurance marketplace will shape our role in the coming decade. A crucial need exists to understand the concept of managed care: what it means to you as the provider, what it means to your patients, and how it will affect your practice. For all its strengths and weaknesses, managed care is here to stay; it is inescapable. The more familiar and comfortable audiologists are with managed care insurance and reimbursement, the better the chances are that their practices will thrive and financial consequences will be minimized.

This chapter begins by providing a glossary of terms used in the text followed by the background for understanding how the insurance industry has operated in the past and how it has become transformed into the managed care environment we see today. A review of the choices of insurance plans will familiarize the reader with the basics of different forms of coverage, giving insight into how this has an impact on daily office operations. Issues of reimbursement will be examined, and suggestions will be made for practice improvement. Tidbits of information about daily office problems are reviewed. The chapter concludes with three appendices that provide a special practicum section for survival within the managed care environment, sample billing codes for audiology, and sample ICD-9 diagnosis codes. The topics covered in the chapter will arm the reader with the multifaceted knowledge needed for success in the workplace.

GLOSSARY OF TERMS

Allowed Amount In insurance parlance, that portion of the provider's fee that will be considered for reimbursement.
Any Willing Provider Legislation In some states legislation that permits any provider to join existing insurance plans.
Approved Amount See *allowed amount*.

Audiology: Practice Management. Edited by Hosford-Dunn, Roeser, and Valente. Thieme Medical Publishers, Inc., New York © 2000

Bundled A term that describes the combination of several related procedures into one CPT code.

Capitation An insurance program in which the provider shares financial risk with the insurance company, paying the provider a specific amount of money "per member, per month" regardless of the amount of care a member requires.

Carve-out In capitated plans a procedure, or procedures, excluded from general capitation coverage for which the provider will be reimbursed on a fee-for-service basis.

Closed Panel In an insurance plan describes the provider list as being limited to current members; no further providers are being enrolled.

Coinsurance A percentage of the total bill for services that the patient is required to pay.

Conversion Factor A specific multiplier figured annually by Medicare or an insurance company to use for calculating reimbursement for all procedure codes.

Co-pay A specific payment due from a patient at the time of service as part of the insurance plan.

Covered Benefit or Service In an insurance plan a procedure or item that will be considered for payment.

CPT Code *Current procedural terminology* listing of all procedures performed with applicable numeric codes used to report all services rendered.

Deductible A preset dollar amount that a patient must pay before insurance reimbursement begins.

EOB (explanation of benefits) A formal report from an insurance company enumerating the service(s) being considered for payment and the allocation of payment. It also accompanies any denial on the basis of noncompensability.

ERISA Employee Retirement Income Security Act; a federal plan enacted in 1974 to regulate certain labor benefits.

Geographical Practice Cost Index Factor A component of the RBRVS system that attributes different costs for supplying care to patients on the basis of the region of the country in which treatment is provided.

HMO (health maintenance organization) Health maintenance organizations require members to select a primary care physician (PCP) from a given list of providers to act as a gatekeeper. Members receive care at a fixed, prepaid premium. Specialty care requires a written referral from the gatekeeper.

ICD-9 Codes *International Classification of Diseases, Clinical Modification, Ninth Edition*; a compendium of diagnoses with numeric codes.

In-network Care delivered by a provider who is a member of the insurance company's panel.

Insurance Waiver A document executed at the time of performing a noncovered service making the patient responsible for the fee.

IPA (independent practice association) An independent practice association is a group of providers who have united to supply healthcare under contract to insurance companies and businesses.

Limiting Charge For Medicare, the maximum amount allowed to be charged by a nonparticipating provider.

Limiting Charge Exception Report A violation notice sent to a provider when a Medicare patient has been charged more than the fee schedule allows.

MCO (managed care organization) An entity that supplies insurance coverage by means of contracted plans at negotiated rates of reimbursement.

Nonparticipating Provider For Medicare, a provider who bills the patient directly for services.

Open Panel An insurance company that is accepting new providers.

Out-of-network Care rendered by a provider who is not a member of an insurance company's plan.

Participating Provider For Medicare, a provider who bills Medicare directly for services rendered.

Payer Any third party payer including, but not limited to, an insurance company, health maintenance organization, self-insured employer, multiple employer trust, or union trust that has entered into an agreement with a managed care organization (or provider for the MCO) for the provision of healthcare services.

PCP (primary care provider) In managed care the provider who is responsible for the basic care of a patient and coordinating all other needed specialty care.

PIN (provider identification number) A provider identification number used by Medicare for tracking providers and practices.

PMPM (per member, per month) In capitated insurance plans a term that usually refers to a negotiated per capita rate to be paid periodically, usually monthly, to a healthcare provider.

POS (point of service) The point of service plan blends indemnity features and HMO features into one product. In-network care receives 100% coverage; out-of-network care necessitates a deductible and coinsurance.

PPO (preferred provider organization) A program in which contracts are established with providers of medical care. Providers under contract are referred to as preferred providers.

Primary Insurance A person's main source of insurance coverage.

RBRVS (resource-based relative value scale) The system by which procedures are assigned values according to a comparative scale; used by Medicare and many other insurers as the basis for reimbursement.

RVU (relative value unit) In the RBRVS system the basic component of applying a numeric amount to a procedure compared with all other procedures.

Secondary Insurance A person's supplemental, or additional, insurance plan.

Self-Insured Plan A type of insurance plan run by an employer in which all aspects are governed and maintained independently from an outside insurance company.

TPA (third-party administrator) An independent company that runs an insurance plan on behalf of a business or other company.

Unbundled Services listed individually for billing that normally would be grouped together as a combined procedure or included in the primary procedure.

UPIN (unique physician identification number) A number used by Medicare for tracking physicians.

Withhold In some managed care contracts a percentage of monies retained by the insurance company to cover expenses.

Write-Off The amount of a fee remaining (and so, not billed) after payment has been received from an insurance company and the contractual discount taken.

BACKGROUND

Fee-for-Service Insurance

Traditionally, patients enrolled in indemnity plans that covered services rendered by any provider for virtually any condition. Known as "fee-for-service," quite simply, the provider got paid for what he or she billed. This system was based on individual fees set by providers in response to market forces (charging whatever the market would bear.) The specific levels of reimbursement set by each insurance company developed as every company gathered data on the prices charged by each provider and created fee profiles. Payment for healthcare and diagnostic testing was then based on the "reasonable and customary fee," a sometimes seemingly arbitrary amount calculated differently by each insurer as it collated data from different providers over varying time periods. Although the system appeared to be functioning adequately, its weaknesses derived from the fact that prices charged by providers were arbitrarily established and some providers took advantage of the situation to charge excessively high prices. Patients, overall, were happy because they had "freedom-of-choice" in obtaining healthcare because no restrictions were placed on whom they could see or where the services were provided. It was not unusual, however, for some patients to be dissatisfied with the system because the insured often bore the responsibility for the unreimbursed portion of the fees. Any amount beyond the "reasonable and customary" was billed to the patient. The patient frequently resented the financial burden of the unpaid balance; most assuredly, goodwill among the insurance company, the patient, and the healthcare provider was greatly compromised.

Medicare System

Established in 1965 as part of *The Great Society* program of President Lyndon Johnson, the Medicare system provides a national healthcare plan for Americans age 65 or older or permanently disabled people (Title XVIII, 1965). The program is directed by the Health Care Financing Administration (HCFA), a federal agency of the Department of Health and Human Services. Medicare pays 80% of the allowed amount of covered services after the patient has paid a yearly deductible. Initially, Medicare reimbursements were based on the "reasonable and customary fee" model that worked well for many years. As life expectancy of Americans increased, the Medicare budget mushroomed, putting the system at risk

for bankruptcy. A study commission headed by Dr. William Hsiao, Ph.D., at Harvard University sought to establish a consistent and objective method of setting fees for all procedures as a means of controlling medical expenditures. First published in October 1988 (Hsiao et al, 1988), this panel developed what we now know as the *RBRVS* system.

Components of the RBRVS System

Each procedure performed by a healthcare provider is assigned a code number found in the *Physician's Current Procedural Terminology* (CPT), Fourth Edition (AMA, 1997). Typical CPT codes used by audiologists are shown in Appendix B. The backbone of the RBRVS system is the *relative value unit* (RVU), which assigns a relative weighting factor to each CPT procedure according to three specific components: physician/provider work (including effort and skill, time, judgment), practice overhead expenses (equipment costs, maintenance, payroll, rent), and malpractice liability. Some differences exist in reimbursement levels, depending on the region of the country in which the procedure is performed so each of the three RVUs is then multiplied by a *geographical practice cost index factor* to compensate for regional price variations. The RVUs for each procedure are then added together, resulting in a *total RVU* for each CPT code. Finally, to arrive at the *actual fee*, the total RVU is multiplied by the *conversion factor*, a specific dollar amount that is revised annually and adjusted for inflation (Segal, 1995). This calculated price is what Medicare recognizes as the *approved amount*. Table 17–1 is an example of how to calculate reimbursement for CPT 92585 (evoked response audiometry) using the RBRVS method (HCFA, 1997).

In December of every year Medicare publishes and sends to each provider a revised fee schedule for the appropriate locality, listing the allowed amounts for all of the CPT codes. Some reimbursements increase, others decrease. Different fee schedules are used for providers who accept assignment and for those who do not. It is essential for providers to update their Medicare fee schedule annually because accurate billing of patients is necessary. For providers who do not accept assignment, inadvertent overbilling of a procedure whose reimbursement level has been reduced may lead to receipt of a *limiting charge exception report*, a formal notice that a provider has billed a Medicare patient too much. Continued overbilling of Medicare patients may lead to sanctions. For providers accepting assignment, Medicare will automatically reimburse according to the current fee schedule for the locality.

TABLE 17–1 **Example of RBRVS method for calculating reimbursement**

CPT Code	Work	Practice Expense	Malpractice	Total RVUs
92585	0.50	3.25	0.31	4.06

Calculations:

$$0.50 \quad + \quad 3.25 \quad + \quad 0.31 \quad = \quad 4.06 \text{ RVUs}$$

$$4.06 \text{ RVUs} + \$36.6873^* = \$148.95$$

*$36.6873 is the conversion factor (or multiplier) that was applied to all Medicare claims for 1998.

CURRENT SYSTEMS

Managed Care

The cost of healthcare has skyrocketed in recent years, and insurance companies maintain that traditional fee-for-service billing is no longer economically viable. Controlling healthcare costs has become one of the country's priorities. In the early-to-mid 1980s, the first HMOs developed in several regions of the country. Their goal was to limit access to healthcare and clamp down on spiraling costs. This was the birth of the managed care model. Through successes and failures, the concept of managed care became more focused, while the problems with traditional healthcare increased. President Clinton in 1993 appointed Hillary Rodham Clinton to create and implement a managed care health system that would effectively curb costs but allow patients freedom of choice for all medical services (Clinton, 1993). After nearly 2 years, the committee failed to produce a viable plan. Consequently, the insurance industry took this opportunity to implement its own model of cost-control on a widespread scale. The insurers enlisted a limited number of providers under contract to supply services according to a prearranged and discounted fee schedule. Since then, MCOs of all types have been created to impose price controls on every facet of the industry and redesign the healthcare delivery system.

Individual types of MCOs have certain qualities. Common to all MCOs, though, is a limited group of healthcare providers who have signed agreements to supply services by contract at a predetermined and discounted rate. All MCOs use utilization review to judge whether healthcare services are medically necessary and cost-efficient. MCOs provide incentives to their members to use their panel of providers. As illustrated in the discussion to follow, many types of MCOs exist.

Health Maintenance Organization

As the most restrictive of all the MCOs, HMOs require members to select a PCP from a given list of providers to act as a gatekeeper. Members receive care at a fixed, prepaid premium. The gatekeeper controls all access to healthcare for the patient. The PCP's goal is to treat as much of a person's health needs as comprehensively as possible within the primary care setting. By definition, PCPs include family physicians, pediatricians, general physicians, and often internists and obstetrician/gynecologists. Every month, the gatekeeper receives a payment from the HMO for the care of all his or her patients. Known as *capitation*, the payment to the physician is PMPM. Whether the patient comes into the office for treatment or not, the provider receives a monthly payment. The provider assumes some risk for delivering healthcare in this environment, hoping that the capitation payment will cover the true cost of providing service to the patient. The HMO provides a financial incentive by rewarding the PCP for limiting referrals to specialists. Although this restriction curtails costs, it prevents the patient from receiving specialty care unless the PCP believes a justifiable need exists. Should the patient seek care without a referral, it is considered unauthorized, and the patient cannot be billed for the service unless a waiver is signed before care is given.

Some HMO insurance plans are capitating specialists in the same manner as PCPs. The company pays the PMPM allowance and expects the specialist to assume some of the risk of providing healthcare. In many of the plans a referral from the gatekeeper is still required before seeing the capitated specialist.

Although most plans require a *co-pay* (a small, personal payment due from the patient) at each visit, a significant benefit of the HMO plan is the absence of annual deductibles or other additional medical costs. A yearly physical or other health services such as hearing aid, dental, or eyeglass benefits are occasionally included in the basic package.

Reimbursement to providers is made periodically, usually on a monthly basis. Payment to PCPs (and specialists who have capitated contracts), as described previously, is based on the number of patients enrolled each month. Payment to noncapitated specialists is made according to the contracted rates; however, a percentage of the allowed amount of reimbursement, known as a *withhold*, is often kept in reserve to cover the costs of running the HMO. This offset reduces current payments to the providers, but if the HMO runs efficiently and profitably, a portion of the excess monies remaining at the end of the fiscal year may be refunded to the providers.

Types of HMOs

Staff-Model HMO

A staff-model HMO directly employs its physicians and nonphysician providers, compensating them with set salaries, but paying incentive bonuses on the basis of performance and profitability of the HMO. Some hospital corporations own and operate their own staff-model HMOs, using their own hospitals and health centers to save money. Generally, all ambulatory health services are provided under one roof. The staff-model HMO will contract with nonemployed providers for services not available through its employees.

Group-Model HMO

A group-model HMO contracts with independent groups of providers and physicians but does not employ them directly. These practices may be located within HMO-owned facilities but also are seen independently. The provider may share in utilization savings but does not necessarily provide care exclusively for HMO members.

Independent Practice Association-Model HMO

An IPA is a group of providers who have united to supply healthcare under contract to insurance companies and businesses. In the IPA-model HMO, often organized by a hospital, capitated plans are created within the IPA to offer a less expensive, but more restrictive, option of coverage. The IPA providers maintain their independent identities and separate practices and continue to see their non-HMO patients in addition to the contracted HMO members. Each office is staffed and managed by the independent practice, not by the HMO. Any provider who is a member of the IPA is eligible to join the IPA-model HMO; this is known as an open-panel HMO.

Medicare HMO

Certain areas of the country have seen the establishment of Medicare HMO plans that blend the Medicare structure with HMO benefits. Under this plan, a Medicare patient selects a PCP as gatekeeper and is required to obtain referrals for most specialty and ancillary healthcare covered by the HMO. Enticements to the patient such as a free yearly physical with no co-pay or co-insurance fees exist. In addition, many Medicare HMO plans have negotiated with audiologists to provide discounted hearing services and hearing aids. Optical and dental benefits may also be enticements to join; these serve as excellent marketing tools for the Medicare HMO plans.

Point-of-Service

Although also managed by a gatekeeper physician, the POS plan allows some flexibility for the insured to seek specialty care more easily or outside the restricted network of physicians. Still requiring a referral from the PCP, the patient bears a greater financial burden for the visit and is typically responsible for a higher co-pay or greater percentage of coinsurance. Patients with this plan have reduced benefits if they go "out-of-network" or do not obtain a referral.

Exclusive Provider Organization

Fashioned after the PPO, the EPO further restricts the network panel to an even smaller group of healthcare providers. By sending its insured members to a more limited group of providers, the EPO attempts to hold down the cost of the insurance policies. A deductible and co-payment may apply to office visits. Services rendered by unaffiliated providers are not reimbursed.

Preferred Provider Organization

One of the most popular types of managed care organizations is the PPO. In this model, a limited panel of providers supply medical services at discounted rates. PPOs typically are selected by individuals or employers who want to control medical costs but do not want the restrictions of an HMO plan. Patients receive a financial incentive by using providers on the panel. Unlike the HMO subscriber, the PPO beneficiary can receive medical services outside the PPO network more easily, but a patient who does so is personally liable for a larger co-pay, deductible, or share of coinsurance. Overall, though, the incentive is for the patient to remain in-network.

The PPO plan requires the provider to agree to accept payment from the PPO at a predetermined rate, which is typically less than what would be received from the fee-for-service patient but higher than for an HMO patient. The providers accept the discounted payment structure with the hope that an increase in patient volume will occur.

Independent Practice Association

Under the aegis of a hospital or a specialty organization, an IPA is a group of providers who have banded together to seek contracts with multiple insurance companies and programs. The IPA has the strength to negotiate contracts at a more favorable rate because it represents a large number of providers in a wide geographical area. Some IPAs hold contracts with 10 or more insurance plans. These plans may include HMOs, POSs, PPOs, and EPOs.

As with HMO plans, IPAs may withhold a percentage of reimbursement for its HMO contracts. Certain amounts of money may be returned to the provider at the end of the year if a profit has been generated. Noncapitated POS plans, PPO, and EPO payments are made by the insurance company directly to the provider.

Medicare

Title XVIII of the Social Security Act is the statute better known as Medicare (Title XVIII, 1965). Medicare benefits apply to those 65 years and older and to persons receiving Social Security disability payments for more than 2 years. There are two parts to Title XVIII of the Social Security Act: Parts A and B.

Part A covers inpatient and hospice services as well as home health needs. Part A benefits are applicable for only 90 to 100 days per illness. A coinsurance is due from the patient. Part B covers outpatient services. Part B frequently applies when Part A benefits are no longer available. As with Part A, a coinsurance is also collected after an annual deductible of $100 has been met. For Medicare Part B, the coinsurance is 20% of the allowed amount.

Medicare has contracted with various insurance companies throughout the United States to process claims. They are known as Regional Medicare Carriers, and they are responsible for reimbursing the Medicare providers. All Medicare claims are submitted to the Carriers using a HCFA 1500 form or electronically.

Private Contracting

Effective January 1, 1998, as provided in Section 4507 of the Balanced Budget Act of 1997, *certain providers* can opt out of Medicare for 2 years or longer for all covered services they furnish to Medicare beneficiaries. The provider and the Medicare beneficiary would sign a private contract that stipulates the beneficiary relinquishes all Medicare coverage and payment for services furnished by that provider, while the provider agrees not to bill Medicare.

Private contracting does not apply to audiologists. As in the past, procedures covered by Medicare must be submitted according to the appropriate Medicare fee schedule. Hearing aids and other assistive listening devices that are not covered benefits are not subject to limiting charges. Contact your local Medicare carrier for any questions you may have.

A comparison of insurance plan services is found in Table 17–2.

Traditional Indemnity Insurance

Rapidly disappearing from the marketplace, traditional indemnity insurance is on the basis of a fee-for-service model. In this plan a patient has the freedom to seek care from any provider for any service at any time. A claim is then submitted to the insurance company and payment is made. Levels of reimbursement vary widely, depending on the company and

TABLE 17–2 Comparison of insurance plan services

	Provider Panel	Referral Needed?	Deductible?	Hearing Aid Benefits?	Capitated Audiology Services?
HMO	Limited to network panel	Yes	No	Some plans	Variable
POS	Limited to network panel with option to go out-of-network	Yes, for most plans; reduced benefits without a referral	No, if in-network; usually yes, if out-of-network	Some plans	Variable
PPO	Not limited to network; may usually go out-of-network with increased financial responsibility	No	Yes, in most cases	Typically, none	Does not apply
Medicare	Any provider who sees Medicare patients	No	Yes	No	No, fee-for-service
Medicare HMO	Limited to network providers	Yes	No	Variable	Variable

plan. The patient may be responsible for a deductible and coinsurance of varying amounts. Long considered the "gold standard" of care, few of these plans are now available at rates that the average person can afford.

REIMBURSEMENT AND MANAGED CARE ISSUES

If you are not familiar with how to negotiate a contract or if you sign rapidly without fully analyzing a contract, you could suffer financially. When a contract to provide managed care services is offered, it is often presented under pressure to sign and may pit one provider against another colleague. Contracts are often designed to take advantage of a practice by paying too little for services or by requiring extra services to be included at no additional compensation. When evaluating a contract, the following four basic categories should be examined:

1. Points that require clarification
2. Points that refer to additional documents that have not been provided for review
3. Points that need to be negotiated
4. Provisions that are unacceptable for the practice

Contracting with an HMO

One of the first things to look for in a capitation contract is missing information or open-ended clauses. These may be provisions stating that additional documents may be attached and/or changed at the discretion of the HMO and that the provider will still be held to the terms of the document. It is important that all documents and addenda are obtained and that the wording is thoroughly reviewed, adding a notification period for any changes to it. The notification period should equal the time required to break the contract, so if the changes are not acceptable, it is possible to get out of the contract.

In a capitated contract every covered CPT code should be listed individually and the level of reimbursement stated. One should review the list of services the practice provides and highlight any particularly difficult or unusually lengthy procedures. For these select codes, it may be advantageous to use of *carve-outs*. Carve-outs describe certain procedures that the audiologist or specialist provider has excluded from the capitated rate and therefore has designated as reimbursable on a fee-for-service basis. This protects the provider from the cost of having to provide a more expensive service at a monetary loss under the capitated allowance. When signing a contract, knowing what is covered and what is not covered is essential for the financial health of the practice. (See section on the costs of doing business, later in this chapter.)

Contracting with a PPO

Besides listing the exact amount allowed for each CPT code, it is good practice for the provider agreement to require prompt payment from the PPO to compensate for the discounted service. A PPO provider must accept the PPO reimbursement structure and cannot balance bill the patient. It is not uncommon for the patient to be responsible for paying a deductible and a co-payment at the time of an evaluation and management visit. For diagnostic services, however, a co-payment may not be required.

Medicare Participation

Two types of Medicare providers exist: *participating* and *nonparticipating*. A *participating provider* means the provider will "accept assignment." In this case Medicare is billed and reimbursement is paid directly to the *provider*. The patient is responsible for a 20% coinsurance payment (money paid out of pocket) for all services.

A *nonparticipating provider* does not accept assignment, allowing the healthcare professional to collect full payment for care rendered at the time of service. A HCFA 1500 claim form still must be submitted to Medicare on behalf of the patient, but payment is sent to the *patient*. Nonparticipating reimbursement levels are 5% less than for participating providers. Nonparticipating practitioners, however, can choose to bill at a special *limiting charge* rate, which is 10% higher than the participating provider reimbursement levels. Medicare reimburses the patient for 80% of the *participating* rate, regardless of whether the limiting charge fee schedule has been used or not. A nonparticipating provider occasionally may accept assignment; reimbursement will be 80% of the participating provider fee schedule.

Provider status may be changed annually and applies until December 31. No action on the part of the provider is required if no change in status is desired.

PEARL

You are responsible for processing the HCFA 1500 form or filing electronically for every Medicare patient treated for a "covered service," regardless of whether you are a participating or a nonparticipating provider.

Obtaining a Medicare Provider Number

If your office plans to treat Medicare patients, it is required that you obtain a Medicare provider number for *each* provider. Every provider of Medicare services must complete an application for inclusion in the plan and assignment of a PIN.

All claims submitted must include the PIN or payment will not be processed.

An initiative is under way to simplify the identification process by instituting the National Provider Identifier (NPI), a number that will eventually replace all other identification numbers and will remain unique to a particular person for as long as he or she remains in practice, wherever the location (Health Care Services Corporation, 1997). It is hoped that, eventually, all insurers will also use the NPI number to track each provider.

To obtain an application regarding provider identification numbers, contact your local Medicare carrier.

ERISA

It is not unusual for a company to *self-insure*, meaning the company sets money aside in a reserve account to pay for healthcare benefits for its employees. This practice is becoming more and more common as insurance premiums escalate. Self-insured plans are often used by unions, local governments, and school districts. What marks these policies as different from plans issued directly by insurance companies is the fact that the state insurance commission does not have jurisdiction over disputes that may arise with the administrator. Instead, these plans are regulated by the United States Department of Labor under the *Employee Retirement Income Security Act of 1974 (ERISA)*. ERISA is a federal law that governs the funding, vesting, and administration of pension and employee benefit plans. Plans regulated by ERISA cannot be sued by patients for more than the cost of the service for untoward healthcare decisions. These self-insured companies contract for clerical services with a TPA, often an existing large insurance company, that processes and pays claims.

PITFALL

When a TPA is responsible for issuing payment, check the explanation of benefits form to make sure the reimbursement levels are what you contracted for. Sometimes the TPA will pay from a lower fee schedule than is used for other providers or plans, resulting in a decrease in payments. When this occurs, request that the claim be re-evaluated and paid outside the terms of the contract.

Antitrust Issues

In many states, and even on a national level, audiologists have organized into groups to establish and operate Audiology IPAs. Usually, these IPAs are limited exclusively to audiologists and sometimes hearing aid dispensers. As the number of enrolled audiologists increases, issues of antitrust infractions must be considered. Antitrust laws forbid any contract or conspiracy among businesses in restraint of trade (Federal Trade Commission Act, 1994). The law prohibits any person or business from monopolizing, or attempting to monopolize, any market and it prohibits agreement among business firms to fix the price of products or services sold or to boycott to achieve their goals. Specific to healthcare, no consistent opinion exists as to what percentage of providers in a given specialty in a given area constitutes a monopoly. In the past no more than 20% of providers in a limited geographical area were allowed to belong to the same IPA. In some instances, however, 30% or more of providers may be permitted to practice together without violating the Antitrust Act if the network or plan is nonexclusive. Individual situations must be evaluated for conformity with the law. When organizing IPAs, consultation with a healthcare attorney is recommended.

Coding

All third-party payers, whether private insurance companies or governmental agencies, use a numeric coding system for identifying procedures performed by a healthcare provider (see Appendix B). These codes are organized in the *Physicians' Current Procedural Terminology*, Fourth Edition (AMA, 1997) manual. The American Medical Association (AMA) pioneered and instituted the use of this coding system, now recognized as the "gold standard." Diseases also have a standardized numeric coding system known as ICD-9-CM codes, which are published in the *International Classification of Diseases*, Ninth Revision, Clinical Modification Manual (World Health Organization, 1977). Appendix C contains some sample ICD-9-CM disease codes used in audiology practices.

PEARL

Audiologists should know the codes that fall within their purview and work proactively with the AMA and third-party payers to keep the codes relevant as newer procedures and more refined diagnoses become available. For example, several new CPT codes for otoacoustic emissions were recently incorporated into the audiology procedures section after vigorous lobbying by audiologists.

Insurance companies base acceptance or denial of a claim on the pairing of the CPT and ICD-9 codes. Some insurance companies will make payment only if certain, very specific ICD-9 codes are linked to a procedure. Using the "incorrect code" may lead to nonpayment. For example, basic comprehensive audiology (CPT 92557) may be paid when paired with acoustic neuroma (ICD-9 225.1) but may be denied with sensorineural hearing loss (ICD-9 389.10). The audiologist should review rejected or poorly reimbursed claims, noting which diagnoses are linked with denials. Often, a nonspecific code will be rejected, but a more specific code will be accepted.

PEARL

When selecting an ICD-9 category, code to the highest level of specificity for the disease. Insurance companies require that the selected code represent the actual diagnosis and not an ICD-9 code that is being "ruled out."

SPECIAL CONSIDERATION

Use ICD-9 codes that describe symptoms when trying to avoid using a "rule-out" diagnosis, for example, otalgia, dysequilibrium, hyperacusis, and so forth.

Certain conditions may require the administration of multiple procedures before a definitive diagnosis can be identified. When several tests or procedures are performed, a *bundled* code may be available. A bundled code is a single code representing multiple related procedures. The bundled code may carry a lesser reimbursement than if each code were billed separately or *unbundled*. For example, CPT 92557 (Basic audiometry: air/bone/speech) *cannot be unbundled* and billed separately as CPT 92552 (Pure tone audiometry [threshold]; air only), CPT 92553 (Pure tone audiometry: air and bone), and CPT 92555 (Speech audiometry; threshold only). Unbundling is not allowed when billing any third-party payer, and unbundling a Medicare claim can lead to fines, sanctions, and even exclusion as a Medicare provider.

All insurance policies have both *covered* and *noncovered services*. "Covered services" mean that the insurance company will reimburse for a procedure, whereas a "noncovered service" will be denied. When a procedure is a "noncovered service," the procedure still can be administered, but payment is the responsibility of the patient and not the third-party payer.

PEARL

It is important to ascertain before rendering care whether a patient's policy will recognize a test or procedure as a payable service.

Goodwill exists in knowing which benefits are covered and which ones are not; however, this is not always possible. To ensure that the patient acknowledges financial responsibility for benefits that are not covered, patients can be required to sign an *insurance waiver* before providing the service and required to make payment at the time of the visit. An insurance waiver should list the procedural codes in question, the applicable fees, the date of service, and the patient's signature. A waiver should be executed for each new date of service and the patient should always be provided with a copy (Table 17–3).

Billing

Primary Insurance

The patient's major insurance coverage is known as *primary*. The primary insurance company is billed first for all services. The claim, listing all dates of care, CPT codes, ICD-9 codes, and fees, needs to be submitted on the appropriate form (or electronically) in a timely fashion. The insurance company will process the claim and respond with payment, if forthcoming, and an EOB statement (see Table 17–4).

TABLE 17–3   Example of an insurance waiver

_____

Patient Name

_____

Responsible Party (if applicable)

I understand that services provided to me on this date may not be a covered benefit as defined by my insurance company.

I also understand that a referral form, authorization, or precertification has not been obtained from my insurance company before today's evaluation and treatment.

I agree to be personally responsible, and to pay today, for the services rendered to me by (company name).

CPT code and fee

_____

Signature

_____

Date

TABLE 17–4   Sample EOB

XYZ Insurance Company

PPO Name:	ABC Company
Claim Number:	31690994-52
Employee Name:	John Doe
Employee ID:	252-52-5252
Patient Name:	Jane Doe
Relationship:	Spouse
Plan Number:	46657364-52
Patient Acct. No.:	752952052
Date:	August 15, 1999

Service Rendered	Date of Service	Charges	Ineligible or Discount	See Rmk Code	Co-pay	Approved Charges	Deductible	Coins. Amt.	Benefit Paid
92557	7/30/99	$ 65.00	$ 1.00	D1		$64.00	$ 64.00		$0.00
92567	7/30/99	$ 47.00	$18.00	D1		$29.00	$ 29.00		$0.00
92568	7/30/99	$ 22.00	$ 2.00	D1		$20.00	$ 20.00		$0.00
92599	7/30/99	$ 40.00	$40.00	D2		$ 0.00	$ 0.00		$0.00
	Totals	$174.00	$61.00			$113.00	$113.00		$0.00

Remark Code (Rmk Code)
 D1 Discount applied; patient not responsible for discount amount.
 D2 Service(s) not covered.

Benefit Summary

Total Benefit Payable $0.00
Paid by Other Insurance $0.00
Total Benefit Payable $0.00

Deductible (Year-to-Date) $113.00

Secondary Insurance

Some patients are enrolled in two insurance programs, often through a spouse. *Secondary* insurance describes a *supplemental* policy, a policy that is extra, or held by the spouse of the patient and is meant to provide reimbursement for unpaid primary insurance balances. Claims for secondary insurance cannot be submitted until a response has been received from the primary insurance company. The EOB statement from the primary insurer must accompany the claim to the secondary insurance company. In the case of Medicare, payment of secondary claims may be automatic if the patient has "cross-over" or "Medigap" coverage for the secondary insurance company.

PITFALL

Whenever Medicare insurance applies, whether as primary or secondary coverage, the patient must be charged Medicare fees. Failure to comply with the Medicare fee schedule will result in issuance of a limiting charge exception report and possibly fines, sanctions, or both.

Explanation of Benefits

The *EOB* is a formal statement by the third-party payer that lists basic insurance information and delineates how reimbursement is allocated. A sample EOB is shown in Table 17–4. Typical information on an EOB includes some, or all, of the following:

- The date of service: Lists when each service was provided.

- The services rendered: Lists which CPT codes were performed.

- The fees charged: Lists the fees the provider billed for the services.

- The fees allowed: Lists the amount the insurance company will consider for each procedure.

- The noncovered amount: Lists the amount the insurance company will *not* consider for reimbursement. (The patient may still be liable for this amount.)

- The co-pay, if applicable: Lists the patient's per-visit financial responsibility.

- The provider discount: Lists the write-off (adjustment) for the services as contained in the provider's contract.

- The patient's responsible portion: Lists the amount of the total bill that the patient is required to pay.

- The amount applied to the patient's deductible, if applicable: Lists the dollar amount that goes toward satisfying the patient's annual financial responsibility; the patient is also required to pay this amount.

- The amount of reimbursement: Lists the payment from the insurance company to the provider for services rendered.

- The reasons for denial, if applicable: Lists specific reasons for exclusion from coverage.

The EOB is sent to the patient and to the provider. As the provider, it is essential to review the statement carefully and to bill the patient for the following:

- The co-pay: The per-visit payment from the patient as required by the insurance policy, if applicable.

- The coinsurance: An additional amount due from the patient, often a percentage of the allowed amount, if applicable.

- The deductible: A given amount per calendar year that is due from the patient for healthcare, if applicable.

- Noncovered benefits: Specific services that are nonreimbursable by the insurance company, but are billable to the patient.

PITFALL

A patient cannot be billed for any managed care discounts that the provider is required to take under the contract.

Discussion of Explanation of Benefits Statement

Although the insurance company does not provide any reimbursement for Jane Doe, the patient needs to be billed for the amount applied to the deductible ($113.00) and for the $40.00 procedure that was a noncovered benefit under the insurance plan. The eligible services total $134.00 ($65.00 + $47.00 + $22.00). A provider discount or writeoff of $21.00 must be taken against the eligible charges; the patient is not responsible for the discounted amount. Therefore the total due from the patient is $153.00 ($134.00 − $21.00 + $40.00)

SPECIAL CONSIDERATION

Examining and scrutinizing each EOB is essential for every provider so that maximal reimbursement is obtained from both the patient and the insurance company. Discounts taken by the insurance company should be compared against negotiated contracts to verify the accuracy of the writeoffs.

DOING BUSINESS

Determining Levels of Reimbursement

In managed care environments an increased need exists to monitor one's levels of reimbursement relative to the cost of providing the service. No practice can survive without covering the costs of the services rendered. Every provider should calculate the *cost-per-unit*, which describes the actual cost associated with providing the service. It includes the "hidden costs" of overhead, equipment, salaries, insurance, and so forth. Good fiscal management dictates that your billing adequately covers the cost of providing the service. *Cost-to-collection* relates the actual cost of supplying the care to the actual level of reimbursement. By knowing these ratios, the provider will better understand the costs of providing professional services. Using this information, more efficient office practice management may be instituted to achieve higher profit margins.

Annually, each office should calculate the total *allowed amounts* received for each CPT code. The allowed amount signifies the actual reimbursement received under managed care contracts after discounts to your fees have been taken. These figures should then be divided by the total number of each CPT procedure performed as shown.

$$\frac{\text{Total allowed amounts per CPT code}}{\text{Number of procedures performed per CPT code}}$$

$$= \text{Average reimbursement per CPT code}$$

The resulting amount represents the average level of reimbursement received from all insurance plans for each CPT code. By comparing the *average reimbursement* to the *actual cost* of providing the service (as discussed above), the provider will understand whether it is profitable to perform a particular CPT code.

This exercise should be repeated for each insurance plan so that the provider will know whether any insurance plans are paying at such a low level as to not be worth retaining. For some plans, however, continuing to accept relatively low payments for some CPT codes may be tolerable if the revenue from other noncovered services offsets the dollar loss or if the volume of patients referred by the insurance company compensates for the lower reimbursement.

Evaluating the value of certain insurance plans requires a close look at the *net revenues*, not just the cost/collection ratios for each CPT code. The net revenues represent the total monies collected by a practice for services provided and goods sold after withholds and discounts have been subtracted. A well-run, economically efficient practice may be able to absorb the financial loss of providing some services at, or slightly below, the actual cost of the procedures.

Practice Costs

Practitioners should tabulate the *total professional practice costs* annually to make appropriate business decisions. Practice costs include, but are not limited to the following:

- Office equipment, rent, utilities, telephone, maintenance, and others.
- Test equipment: audiometers, impedance bridges, real-ear, sound booths, and others.

- Salaries: professionals, receptionists, office maintenance, and others.
- License fees, professional dues, subscriptions, and others.
- Advertising, promotional literature, and others.
- Legal, accounting, other business costs.

By adding up the costs of all these professional services and dividing the total by the number of procedures performed in your practice, you may arrive at a *per procedure* cost of doing business. Adding this amount to the *actual reimbursement* of each CPT code will provide the practitioner with an absolute value of the *total true cost* of performing each procedure.

Surviving in the Managed Care Environment

Coping with the changes imposed on every practice requires flexibility, ingenuity, and hard work. Several important issues should be addressed.

1. *Marketing the primary care providers:* As an ancillary provider, the audiologist will want to establish and maintain strong ties with primary care providers in the community who are members of the same managed care insurance programs. Many PCPs are not familiar with the audiologist's scope of practice and therefore require education and reminders about who we are and what we do. Preparing referral pads and informational pamphlets for the PCP will simplify the referral process. Intermittent reminders, phone calls, and thank-you letters for referrals will keep the audiologist's name in the PCP's mind.

2. *Cost containment:* Because reimbursement levels for managed care contracts are constantly being ratcheted down, it is essential to control costs within the office. For example, good business practice necessitates evaluating the prices charged by your suppliers and periodically requires renegotiating costs of products and services.

3. *Insurance and benefit verification:* Because patients change jobs frequently and because companies change insurance plans equally as often, it is imperative that your office verify the insurance coverage every time procedures are provided, especially when funded benefits apply. It is beneficial to photocopy the front and back of the patient's insurance card. The card provides the group number, policy number, address for submitting claims, and a phone number for benefit verification. Never assume that the insurance is in force and valid; it is not uncommon to find that a plan has been terminated or the patient was delinquent in paying the premiums.

4. *Increasing patient volume:* Because reimbursement levels have decreased, increasing the number of patients seen may compensate for lost revenue. Direct marketing and advertising will secure increased patient volume, however, it is necessary to have adequate staffing to accommodate the patients. Sending a newsletter to existing patients and the community will remind them of your services. Keeping

your existing patients happy will lead to personal referrals to friends and family. (See Chapter 7 in this volume.)

OUTCOME MEASURES

No question exists that managed healthcare is here to stay. What is still evolving is how comprehensive the list of paid benefits will be for the insured. For example, hearing aids historically were not a covered benefit, even with executive indemnity plans. Now, some HMO plans are offering hearing aid benefits. This is welcome news for the insured but raises reimbursement issues for the provider. Some typical hearing aid plan models include discounting from usual and customary charges, dispensing at a predetermined amount established by the insurance company, or receiving a partial allowance from the insurance company toward the purchase of an amplification system. It is apparent that many insurance companies now recognize that a hearing aid benefit is an excellent marketing tool for promoting a plan, especially when the target market is senior citizens. Because the insurance industry may pay for hearing aids in part or in whole, it needs objective measures for justifying reimbursement. In addition, third-party payers need substantiation of the benefits of the hearing aid when the audiologist recommends programmable digital amplification rather than a standard linear circuit.

The need for such outcome measures is not unique to audiology. The National Committee for Quality Assurance (NCQA) requests this type of information as part of a national emphasis for quality measures. As a profession, audiology can benefit from outcome measures. The implementation of outcome measures creates professionwide standards of care, helps to effectively negotiate with third-party payers for better technology, and serves as a powerful tool when working with patients and when securing other managed care contracts.

Audiologists traditionally have not been consistent in their habits of notekeeping or with standardizing the tests or procedures that should constitute a hearing diagnostic examination or a hearing aid selection and fitting. Documentation and consistency will give a practice an advantage over time with third-party payers and with patients. Performing outcome measures needs to become office protocol.

A significant step in achieving standardized care can be accomplished by standardizing testing. For example, an initial hearing evaluation may be only air thresholds in one facility but may include air conduction, bone conduction, speech audiometry, tympanogram, acoustic reflex, and reflex decay testing at another office. Consistency among practices will make it easier to define what constitutes a diagnostic examination. Once care is more standardized, the insurance companies will be able to optimize reimbursement to the provider.

Measuring satisfaction and benefit from hearing aids is also a priority. Many objective measures are available. As with diagnostic testing, protocols need to be established. Prefitting measures could include diagnostic procedures such as loudness growth tests, desired sensation level (DSL), or independent hearing aid fitting forum (IHAFF). During the fitting process, probe microphone measurements or functional gain responses could be recorded. At postfitting follow-up visits, patients could complete subjective scales such as the Abbreviated Profile of Hearing Aid Benefit (APHAB) or the Client-Oriented Scale of Improvement (COSI), repeated at two weeks, and at 2 months, after dispensing. Establishing standardized care helps the patient, the audiologist, and the third-party payer. The patient and the audiologist will have a concrete representation that the hearing aid system is of benefit, and the insurance company will have substantiation that the amplification is providing good performance especially when the cost of the hearing aids exceeds the basic benefit amount.

The information obtained from outcome measures is sorely needed by the insurance companies. Unfortunately, some MCOs have *nonaudiologists* collecting and interpreting outcome measure results. Audiologists must become proactive and begin to provide third-party payers with accurate and timely information. Our state and national audiology IPAs will be excellent resources for collecting and interpreting these data for the insurance companies. We, as a profession, cannot avoid outcome measures. The findings are invaluable when negotiating new contracts and benefits and should be routine office protocol within every successful practice.

IMPORTANT TIDBITS

Certain protocols must be followed to receive maximum benefit from the third-party payer. The following suggestions are important when trying to maximize reimbursement. Managed care tidbits will be separated into categories: general, Medicare, and HMO/PPO.

General Information

- Know the best linking of ICD-9 codes with CPT codes. For example, some insurance carriers will deny coverage for sensorineural hearing loss but may pay for tinnitus. It is prudent to monitor reimbursement patterns for each managed care contract so optimum coding may be submitted.
- Insurance companies are continually monitoring what practices are charging for individual procedure codes. "Profiles" are kept for each provider and then the data are analyzed. These figures may be used to substantiate reduced reimbursement levels if a provider bills less than the insurance company would normally pay. In simple terms the insurance company will always pay the least amount it can possibly pay.
- Carefully examine and photocopy the patient's insurance card for information regarding co-pays and claims submission. Sending an insurance claim to a wrong (or outdated) address may delay processing. If the claim is returned to you for resubmission to the correct address, it still must be filed within the allowed time frame. If the claim is filed too late and is rejected by the insurance company, the patient cannot be billed for the unpaid service(s).
- Waivers should be used routinely. A medical waiver requires the patient or patient guardian to be responsible for any charges not covered by the insurance company.

The waiver should include the date of service, the procedural codes performed, and the cost of the procedures (Table 17–3).

Medicare

- Claims must be filed within 1 year from the date of service.
- Regardless of whether Medicare is the primary or secondary insurance, the provider is required to bill Medicare fees. Medicare automatically reimburses a *participating provider* according to the correct fee schedule. If a *nonparticipating provider* charges a patient fees higher than allowed by Medicare, the provider can be cited with a limiting charge exception report that states that an overcharge has occurred. The law requires the provider to refund the excess amount back to the patient and to prove to Medicare that a refund has been made.
- A participating provider accepts assignment. Payment from Medicare goes directly to the provider.
- A nonparticipating provider does not accept assignment. Reimbursement payments from Medicare go directly to the patient.

- Medicare requires that 20% of every Medicare bill *must* be collected whether the practice accepts assignment or not. This 20% can never be written off.
- The provider is required by law to file all Medicare claims for the patient. Even if full payment is collected at the time of service (from a nonparticipating provider), Medicare must receive a claim form from the provider documenting the transaction.

- To be eligible for Medicare reimbursement, audiology services must be ordered by a physician. A note in the chart must document this referral, but some regional Medicare directors also require a written referral with appropriate ICD-9 diagnoses.
- If Medicare deems a procedure to be a noncovered benefit, the patient can be billed for the cost of the procedure only if the patient were informed of this fact before testing. A waiver of insurance coverage form (Table 17–3) should be executed and filed in the patient's chart.

HMO/PPO Plans

- HMO and some POS patients need a referral *before* they can be seen for covered services. Seeing these patients without a referral absolves the insurance company from financial responsibility for the claim.
- If a patient does not have a referral, the patient should sign a waiver of insurance (Table 17–3), which stipulates that the patient is responsible for the charges.
- Evaluating and billing the patient needs to be timely. Many referrals have a time limit (often 45 to 60 days) and become null and void if not used within the designated time frame. Also, some insurance carriers will not pay a claim if it is submitted after a specified time period, typically 45 to 60 days.

UTILIZATION REVIEW

In the managed care environment, greater emphasis is placed on the accountability of the practitioner as far as the choice of tests performed and the frequency with which they are ordered. The process of utilization review focuses on carefully evaluating the overall use of medical services and examines the ICD-9 diagnosis linkage to the CPT codes performed. Data are collated, charted, and analyzed for multiple factors, including the following:

1. Appropriateness of performing a specific test for a specific diagnosis
2. Overuse of test procedures to arrive at a specific diagnosis with consideration given to variance between geographical locations
3. Excessive testing of an individual patient

The intent of the utilization review report is to "educate" the provider about his or her practice protocols relative to other practitioners. By restricting the frequency and type of

> ### PITFALL
>
> **Insurance companies routinely disallow certain procedures from reimbursement by citing reasons such as: "This procedure is unnecessary for the medical condition or diagnosis." HMOs and IPAs may review each practice annually and issue a report detailing the use of procedures that are deemed "too frequently performed."**

testing done to arrive at a diagnosis, the insurance company can save large sums of money. Providers who order excessive numbers of tests are known as "outliers" (i.e., they lie at the extremes of the bell curve for numbers of procedures performed). If these providers do not conform to the utilization review parameters, the insurance company may terminate their contracts.

> ### PEARL
>
> **If an insurance company has a practice performance requirement that conflicts with audiology standards of care, the audiologist makes a formal, written protest to the insurance company for review of its policy.**

PATIENT'S BILL OF RIGHTS

Because of the increasing power of healthcare plans to dictate which services are covered and which are not, when care may be rendered or denied, or when patient's confidential information may be disclosed, national legislation to protect Americans' healthcare rights is currently being considered in Congress. Individual insurance companies are also considering their own versions of the Patient's Bill of Rights.

According to the American Medical Association (American Medical News, 1998), to be beneficial to both patients and physicians, the following five important factors should be included:

1. Full disclosure of insurance plan details
2. Elimination of the "gag clause" from insurance plans, restricting physicians from discussing specifics of a patient's insurance plan
3. An independent process for patients to appeal health plan decisions
4. Reasonable access to emergency services
5. Accountability of health plans for their decisions (i.e., when appropriate, allowing patients to sue their health plans, not permitted under ERISA laws at present.)

Because the concept of a Patient's Bill of Rights is in its infancy, multiple revisions will be drafted before becoming law. Insurance company versions of the Bill of Rights will be enacted first because of public pressure. The era of the patient resting power from the insurance company has just begun.

CONCLUSIONS

The evolution of the managed healthcare environment requires that every practitioner learn all he or she can to adapt to the changes of the marketplace. Educating oneself about insurance plans and reimbursement arms the provider with information that is indispensable. The practitioner need not fear managed care; a good understanding of the basics will enable the audiologist to maximize the opportunities for growing his or her practice. Surviving in today's healthcare environment is a continual challenge, but it is not insurmountable. Managed care is a change from the past, yet those who greet it with a positive attitude will be rewarded with success.

Appendix A
Practicum Section
Mini-Primer for Entering the Managed Care Environment

A provider would follow several basic steps in securing managed care relationships. The following list will highlight the most important points:

1. Know the companies providing insurance to patients in your practice. Create a list as patients register, noting specific plans, such as HMO, POS, and PPO types.

2. Are you a provider for the particular plan listed on the patient's insurance card?

3. When patients request that their records be transferred to another practice, ascertain if it is because you are *not* a provider for their insurance plan. Ask the patient to send a letter on your behalf requesting you be included in the provider panel and sent an application.

4. Call provider/member relations explaining that you have patients who are beneficiaries of the insurance company who want *you* to provide ongoing healthcare and also that *you* want to be able to provide care to your patients (and to their other insureds.) Follow-up with a letter including the patient's name and identification data, your name, geographical locations of offices, the number of audiologists and employees, and the services you provide. Show the insurance company how and why you would be a benefit to their provider panel.

5. Make follow-up calls to the insurance company every month or two to check on the status of your application. Try to maintain contact with a specific person in the provider relations department who will be your advocate. Find out whether new providers are welcomed at certain times of the year. Is there a time for annual review of providers when your application might be better received?

6. Negotiating tips
   - *Don't "give up" billing for diagnostic testing.* This is important in your role as a professional. Do not include any diagnostic audiology testing as a benefit included with hearing aid dispensing. Audiological testing should be coded and billed as separate services *apart from* hearing aid services.
   - Ascertain how each insurance company's fee schedule is developed. Is it on the basis of the Medicare RBRVS model, the McGraw-Hill model (a long-standing, independent reimbursement system, once the most prevalent means of valuing procedures), or another method? Are your services to be capitated? If so, apply *carve-outs* to the costliest and most difficult procedure(s) in your

practice so you will be reimbursed on a fee-for-service basis for these specific codes.
   - Know what you need to earn to make a profit. Understand your costs of providing service and be sure you can afford a contract for discounted reimbursement. Obtain a fee schedule that includes payment levels for each code you perform.
   - If you are considering entering into a capitated contract, know what population is covered so you can predict the intensity of need for supplying services to this group. Calculate how many lives must be included to make the contract financially feasible.

PEARL

For example, if a capitated contract provides diagnostic hearing services and the member population is predominantly composed of senior citizens, it is likely that there will be high use of your services.

   - If you are trying to negotiate with an insurance company that represents a broad geographical area, it may be advantageous to include other audiology practices in your vicinity by creating an audiology IPA within your region or state.
   - Have a managed healthcare attorney review all contracts, paying special attention to the following.
     ▼ What is the life of the contract?
     ▼ Terminating a contract by either party.
     ▼ When fees are reviewed and adjusted.
     ▼ Are there withholds?
     ▼ How promptly are payments made?
     ▼ Who is the administrator of the plan (the company itself or a third-party administrator)?

HOW TO STREAMLINE PATIENT INTAKE

- Have patient check in with receptionist.
- Obtain the patient's insurance card and make a photocopy of the front and back to keep on file. Check to see if patient also has a secondary insurance plan.

- Have patient complete an information form, custom-tailored to fit your practice. Include the full legal name, address, phone (home and work), date of birth, social security number, emergency contact, and so forth. Include a statement regarding release of medical information for insurance purposes, a statement regarding the assignment of medical benefits (important if you are filing insurance claims for payment), and some practices may wish to include a statement regarding a waiver of coverage acknowledging that certain procedures may not be covered benefits under the insurance plan. The patient should sign the form, agreeing to the above terms. Also, include a space for the patient's physician's name and who referred the patient to you (if different from the physician).

- It would be expeditious to have a prepared history form for the patient to complete before the evaluation. Ask for a brief description of the reason for the office visit, followed by a short paragraph detailing the problem. Include a checklist of related questions, making it simple for the patient to understand and complete. An example for a single subject heading might be as follows:

Tinnitus:	☐ Right Ear	☐ Left Ear	☐ Both
	☐ Constant	☐ Intermittent	☐ Pulsatile
	☐ High-pitched	☐ Low-pitched	
	☐ Ringing	☐ Buzzing	☐ Hissing

Repeat this format for each area of questioning. Finally, obtain a list of allergies, medications, major illnesses, and a family history of hearing-related disorders.

- Prepare a routing slip/superbill that includes common procedural codes (CPT) and diagnosis codes (ICD-9) specific to your practice to use as a checklist for billing the patient and filing insurance. This should remain with the patient during the office visit and be given to the discharge clerk at the end of the visit to simplify the checkout process.

PROVIDER ENROLLMENT IN MANAGED CARE

For audiologists to become providers in a managed care plan, they must apply to, and be accepted by, the credentialing board of the insurance company. This is not always possible because the panel of providers may already be full (a *closed panel*) or audiologists may not be recognized as providers under the plan. In the case of a closed panel the audiologist may enlist the help of a beneficiary of the insurance company

to write a letter to the provider relations department requesting inclusion with their existing panel of providers. Success with this approach depends on the responsiveness of the company to its insured members.

Some states have enacted *any willing provider* legislation that requires an insurance company to offer to any provider in the state inclusion in the managed care plan, subject to the contracted rates. Insurance companies in states without this law are free to limit provider participation as they see fit.

HOW TO SET UP BILLINGS AND ACCOUNTS PAYABLE TO TRACK SERVICES AND REIMBURSEMENTS

Choosing a computer software system appropriate to your practice is a difficult and time-consuming task. To optimize the benefits of the system, several key points are included.

1. Be sure the software is designed as a medical model, specifically created to list the following.

   - The date of service

   - The procedure

   - The fee

   - The diagnosis code(s)

   - The co-pay (if applicable)

   - The contract discount or write-off

   - Payments received (and the source, i.e., the patient or the insurance company)

   - The balance due from the patient

2. Be sure the software is logical and able to be followed by office staff. Is the screen format user-friendly?

3. Select a system that is data based in orientation.

4. Verify how easy (or difficult) it is to create data reports.

5. Visit an office that has been using the software for a reasonable length of time and sit down with the receptionists, billing clerks, and office manager to find the strengths and weaknesses of the system.

Appendix B
Audiology CPT Codes
Sample of Basic Audiology Procedures

CPT CODE   *DESCRIPTION*

Hearing Evaluation

92552	Pure tone audiometry (threshold); air only;
92553	air and bone
92555	Speech audiometry threshold;
92556	with speech recognition
92557	Comprehensive audiometry threshold evaluation and speech recognition (92553 and 92556 combined)
92565	Stenger test, pure tone
92567	Tympanometry (impedance audiometry)
92568	Acoustic reflex testing
92569	Acoustic reflex decay test
92582	Conditioning play audiometry
92584	Electrocochleography
92585	Auditory brain stem–evoked response recording
92587	Evoked otoacoustic emissions; limited (single stimulus level, either transient or distortion products)
92588	comprehensive or diagnostic evaluation (comparison of transient and/or distortion product otoacoustic emissions at multiple levels and frequencies)
92589	Central auditory function test(s) (specify)

Electronystagmogram

92541	Spontaneous nystagmus test, including gaze and fixation nystagmus, with recording
92542	Positional nystagmus test, minimum of four positions, with recording
92543	Caloric vestibular test, each irrigation (binaural, bithermal stimulation constitutes four tests), with recording
92554	Optokinetic nystagmus test, bidirectional, with recording
92545	Oscillating tracking test, with recording
92547	Vertical electrodes

Miscellaneous Services

92590	Hearing aid examination and selection; monaural
92591	binaural
92594	Electroacoustic evaluation for hearing aid; monaural
92595	binaural
92596	Ear protector attenuation measurements

Appendix C
Audiology ICD-9 Codes
Sample of Commonly Used Diagnosis Codes
Codes marked with an asterisk (*) are nonspecific codes

Acoustic neuroma		225.1
Acoustic trauma (explosive)		388.11
Bell's palsy		351.0
Cerumen impaction		380.4
Cholesteatoma	Attic (primary)	385.31
	Diffuse	385.35
	External canal	380.21
	General	385.30*
	Middle ear (primary)	385.32
	Middle ear and mastoid	385.33
	Recurrent, post-mastoidectomy cavity	383.32
Dysequilibrium		780.4
Eustachian tube	Dysfunction	381.81
	Patulous	381.7
Exostosis of earcanal		380.81
Foreign body	Earcanal	931
Hearing loss	Abnormal auditory perception, unspecified	388.40*
	Acoustic trauma (explosive)	388.11
	Asymmetrical	389.8*
	Central	389.14
	Conductive unspecified	389.00*
	External ear	389.01
	Tympanic membrane	389.02
	Middle ear	389.03
	Inner ear	389.04
	Combined type	389.08
	Diplacusis	388.41
	Hyperacusis	388.42
	Impaired discrimination	388.43
	Mixed	389.2
	Noise-induced	388.12
	Presbycusis	388.01
	Recruitment	388.44
	Sensorineural unspecified	389.10*
	Sensory	389.11
	Neural	389.12
	Central	389.14
	Combined type	389.18
	Transient ischemic deafness	388.02
	Other specified form	389.8

Herpes zoster auricularis		053.71
Hyperacusis		388.42
Labyrinthitis	Acute viral	386.35
	Focal	386.32
	Serous	386.31
	Suppurative	386.33
	Toxic	386.34
	Unspecified	386.30*
Meniere's disease	Active	386.00
	Cochlear	386.02
	Cochleovestibular	386.01
	Inactive	386.04
	Vestibular	386.03
Microtia		744.23
Mondini's aplasia		744.05
Multiple sclerosis		340
Nystagmus	General	379.50
	Vestibular etiology	379.54
Ossicles	Discontinuity/dislocation	385.23
Osteoma of earcanal		380.81
Otalgia	General	388.70*
	Otogenic	388.71
	Referred	388.72
Otitis media	Acute: allergic hemorrhagic	381.06
	Mucoid otitis media	381.05
	Serous otitis media	381.04
	With effusion	381.00*
	Hemorrhagic	381.03
	Mucoid (seromucinous, blue drum syndrome, etc.)	381.02
	Serous otitis media	381.01
	Suppurative	382.00
	With tympanic membrane rupture	382.01
	Chronic: adhesive, unspecified Location	385.10
	Drum to incus	385.11
	Drum to stapes	385.12
	Drum to promontory	385.13
	Other	385.19
	With effusion	381.3*
	Mucoid, simple or unspecified	381.20

REFERENCES

AMERICAN MEDICAL ASSOCIATION. (1997). *Physician's current procedural terminology* (4th Ed.). *CPT '98* Revised 1997. Chicago: American Medical Association.

AMERICAN MEDICAL NEWS. (1998). *Editorial: Do it right.* Chicago: August 10, p. 27.

CLINTON, H.R. (1993). *Remarks to the American Medical Association.* Chicago, IL: June 13, 1993.

EMPLOYEE RETIREMENT INCOME SECURITY ACT OF 1974 (ERISA). Federal Statute: 29 U.S.C. §§ 1001 et seq.

FEDERAL TRADE COMMISSION ACT of September 26, 1914, ch. 311, § 5, 38 Stat. 717, 719 (codified as amended at 15 U.S.C. §§ 41–58 [1994]).

HEALTH CARE FINANCING ADMINISTRATION. (1997). *1998 Medicare fee schedule database.* Washington, DC: HCFA, Oct. 17, 1997.

HEALTH CARE SERVICES CORPORATION. (1997). *National provider identifier; Info-Session bulletin.* Chicago, IL: HCSC, 1/22/97, p. 3.

HSIAO, W.C., Braun, P., Dunn, D., Becker, E., De Nico, M., & Ketcham, T.R. (1988). Results and policy implications of the resource-based relative value study. *New England Journal of Medicine, 319*(13);881–888.

SEGAL, M.J. (Ed.). (1995). *Medicare RBRVS: The physicians' guide.* (pp. 60–62). Chicago, IL: American Medical Association.

TITLE XVIII, enacted by the 89th Congress, 1964–65.

WORLD HEALTH ORGANIZATION. (1977). *International classification of diseases. (9th Rev.). Clinical modification (ICD-9-CM).* Geneva, Switzerland: World Health Organization.

Chapter 18

Proposing Audiology Services and Responding to Requests for Proposals (RFPs) for Managed Care Contracting

James A. Benson and Gail Gudmundsen

Outline

ESTABLISHING AN INDEPENDENT IDENTITY AS HEALTHCARE PROFESSIONALS

A fundamental component of the audiologist's identity as an independent professional is the ability to negotiate reimbursement from third-party payers. The managed care organization (MCO) is emerging as the primary provider of healthcare in the United States and offers audiologists an opportunity to ensure their inclusion in reimbursement, define their scope of practice, and secure their role as independent caregivers to those with hearing loss. It is imperative that audiologists incorporate managed care strategies into their day-to-day practice management as logically and professionally as possible.

Inclusion in MCO contracts is not only desirable but may be essential in many cases because the vitality of any healthcare practice depends on its economic viability over time. Audiologists in private practice or clinical settings will at some point in their careers be called on to participate in an analysis of their contribution to revenue—as a point of survival for the private practice or to justify the cost center of a clinic or hospital audiology department. Fundamental to this analysis will be the audiologist's ability to point to successful managed care contracts that provide positive cash-flow and access to the patients who are members of the MCO.

In many urban settings the future existence of the audiology clinic will be determined by its success in negotiating managed care contracts and establishing audiology practitioners as an integral component of the healthcare professions. Furthermore, inclusion in local MCO contracts also prevents the attrition of established patients who join a new health plan or are directed by their MCO to a competing practice or vendor for audiology services. However well established a practice may be in

Audiology: Practice Management. Edited by Hosford-Dunn, Roeser, and Valente. Thieme Medical Publishers, Inc., New York © 2000

a community, inclusion in an MCO is a wise defensive strategy for retaining an established patient base over time.

This chapter will provide an understanding of how to approach and respond to a contract with an MCO to arrive at mutually satisfying agreements. Readers who are unfamiliar with the topic will want to refer to a Glossary of Managed Care Terms (see following pages in this chapter) and to Chapter 17 in this volume.

DEVELOPING RESOURCES

One of the most important components in preparation for proposing audiology benefits to an MCO is the development of resources required to fulfill the needs of the MCO and successfully present a case for participation.

Knowledge of MCO in the Community

Populations that are served by the MCO (i.e., Medicare, Medicaid, and commercial populations) and their enrollment (number of members served) for each respective population served need to be determined. The American Association of Health Plans publishes annual profiles of member MCOs, and most state departments of insurance or departments of corporations will also have this information available (see Table 18–1).

The greatest resource for audiologists contracting with any MCO is their peers in the healthcare community. Collaboration with other healthcare professionals ensures a more complete understanding of the nuances of MCO contracting and can be the best resource for payment history, information about negotiation strategies (both successful and failed), and the biases that the MCO will bring to the table. Such information is critical in preparation for the negotiation. It enables the audiologist to build a proposal that meets the needs of the MCO and the practice, which will produce a positive outcome for their common constituent, the patient.

PEARL

Managed care issues challenge every healthcare professional. Several national resources are available that can provide directories of MCOs and administrators for future reference.

Administrative Resources

Many MCOs require that claims be filed on a HCFA 1500 form. Some MCOs want their providers to use electronic access to claims processing by means of a modem or centralized billing. These requirements may make it necessary for an individual provider or a provider network to contract a third-party administrator (TPA) to process audiology claims and to disburse the MCO's reimbursement to the provider. For this service, the TPA will often charge the provider an administrative charge for processing the claim. TPAs are available in many communities. Locating an established, effective TPA can be accomplished by contacting their national association (see Table 18–1), by referral

from other healthcare providers in the community, or by referral from an accountant. In many instances practice-management firms can provide these services as well.

Analysis of the role and services of a TPA facilitates an accurate assessment of the true costs related to the MCO contract. Before contracting with a TPA, it is essential to evaluate the TPA's reputation, experience, and the length of time the TPA takes to pay providers once payments are received from the MCO. In many instances reimbursement of the audiology provider can be delayed by as much as 90 to 120 days as a result of reimbursement from an MCO through a TPA or practice-management firm. It is also important to establish the TPA's role in follow-up on late claims payment. Many TPAs and most practice-management firms do the follow-up for their clients, producing an administrative efficiency by reducing the time that the audiologist or office manager spends following up on aging claims.

Legal Advice

Legal advice in managed care contracting is an absolute necessity. The practice or provider group should seek advice and a referral from its corporate counsel regarding the nuances of the MCO contract. In most communities an attorney specializing in healthcare practice who has had experience with the MCO offering the contract handles this. Many components of the MCO contract are business oriented and have little to do with the provision of healthcare services. An experienced attorney will save providers an immense amount of time and money by negotiating the contract and pointing out contractual provisions that are extraordinary or unreasonable.

Actuarial Assistance

An actuary develops healthcare fundamentals relevant to the development of costs associated with the inclusion of an audiology benefit into an MCO's plan. In many instances the MCO will have an actuary on staff. Unfortunately, there is not a great deal of actuarial experience with audiology-specific data. It is essential to have an alternative resource for actuarial projections that includes an analysis of the age of the prospective members who will have the audiology services available to them and what percentage of those populations will be likely to seek audiology services.

As an example of variations in anticipated use in two different age groups, the National Center for Health Statistics is projecting that in the year 2000, 2% of persons younger than 15 will have hearing impairment, and 29% of those aged 65 or older will have hearing impairment. The ramifications for not considering the age of an MCO's population by age category when proposing services absolutely will affect practice or clinic economics.

The Academy of Dispensing Audiologists and the American Academy of Audiology jointly produced a guide to managed care contracting, which includes extensive actuarial data for determining costs for use in MCO negotiations. The American Speech, Language and Hearing Association also published several detailed and very understandable resources that include actuarial detail. (See Table 18–1.)

TABLE 18–1 National resources for directories of MCOs

Managed Healthcare Directories

1. Association of Managed Healthcare
   Organizations (AMHO)
   One Bridge Plaza
   Suite 325
   Fort Lee, NJ 07024
   201-947-5545
   Fax: 201-947-3808

2. American Association of Health Plans
   1129 20th Street, NW, Suite 600
   Washington, DC 20036-3421
   202-778-3200

Third-Party Administrators

Society of Professional Benefit Administrators
2 Wisconsin Circle, Suite 670
Chevy Chase, MD 20815-7003
301-718-7722

Actuaries

In local yellow pages

Legal and Accounting

In local yellow pages. Make certain that the firm selected has a specialist in Healthcare law and accounting *as it relates to provider organizations, PPOs, and HMOs* (this is very different from medical practive law and accounting).

Audiology-Specific Managed Care Publications

1. The Academy of Dispensing Audiologists (ADA) and the American Academy of Audiology (AAA) have jointly published a managed care manual that includes worksheets and a diskette for developing capitation rates for managed care contracting. This manual does not replace an actuary for group proposals because actuaries may assist in developing counterproposals and risk sharing agreements with HMOs that limit the groups exposure to losses.
   Contact ADA at 803-252-5646
   Or AAA at 703-524-1923

2. ASHA publishes several managed care publications and a brief actuarial manual that provide useful information in contracting with HMOs.
   Contact ASHA at 301-897-5700

PITFALL
Unfortunately, there is not a great deal of actuarial experience with audiology-specific data.

Increased Use with Funded Plans

Funding of a hearing aid allowance or benefit will increase use of the audiology benefit. MCOs should anticipate increased demand for diagnostic services and hearing aids in a population of members that has not previously had a funded benefit. In general the greater the MCO's contribution to the cost, the higher the use. In addition to actuarial considerations, it is imperative that any increased costs associated with the contract be considered, such as the following:

- Increased administrative expense related to collecting payment and submitting the MCO's bills

- Increased hours of operation
- Higher mandated limits on malpractice liability insurance

PREPARING MATERIALS FOR INSPECTION

Before contracting, an MCO may request inspection of certain materials. It is prudent to have these materials prepared in advance of the negotiation. Not only are they good preparation for the subsequent negotiation, they are also useful in determining the real costs of a managed care contract. Professional and timely presentation of materials requested by an MCO facilitates contracting and enhances the professional image of an audiologist's practice.

Each MCO has various inspection requirements, varying from virtually no materials and documentation required to copies of every protocol and marketing piece a practice has produced. Reasonableness, as defined by the MCO's standard contracting procedure, should be the rule here. If an MCO makes an extraordinary request, review it with peers and an attorney. In many instances unusual requests for documentation may have been taken from contract inspection requirements for a different healthcare profession and may not be applicable or relevant for audiologists.

PEARL

In many instances unusual requests for documentation may have been taken from contract inspection requirements for a different healthcare profession and may not be applicable or relevant for audiologists.

Fee Schedule

Anticipate that the MCO will want to see a list of usual and customary fees for services and hearing aids. Usual-and-customary (or reasonable-and-customary) is the pre-discount price that a fee-for-service patient is charged. The list should be as complete as possible and include all audiology services by Current Procedural Terminology (CPT) code, as well as usual-and-customary pricing for hearing aids. Frequently the MCO will ask for pricing on their application or during a credentialing interview. In some cases they simply have the applicant attach the list separately. In preparing the list, include a separate fee schedule for Medicare, Medicaid, and other MCO contracts for reference purposes during negotiations. It is not prudent to disclose competitive pricing to the MCO. Lists of competing MCO pricing are for internal reference, and this information should be referred to when evaluating the profitability of a prospective contract.

Infection Control Protocol

Some MCOs will want to see an infection control protocol, manual, or plan. Infection control manuals are available from earmold laboratories, audiology specialty-product vendors, and several hearing aid manufacturers. Whatever the resource for an infection control protocol, it must be current, valid, and implemented. Eventually the MCO will perform a site inspection of a prospective provider, and they may well ask to see evidence that documentation of infection control procedures is on file and applied in daily practice. It is a good policy to implement a standard infection control protocol in any healthcare setting, so this should not be viewed as intrusive or bothersome. For further information see Chapter 11 in this volume.

Licenses

Anticipate that the MCO will request a copy of all state licenses required to practice audiology and to dispense hearing aids, where applicable. Copies of academic degrees, any certification, business licenses, Federal Tax ID number, and Medicaid and Medicare provider numbers may be requested. In many instances the MCO will source verify these licenses and credentials, which simply means that they will go to the issuing party (government, association, or university) for

verification. When contracting with providers, MCOs will almost certainly require that an inspection release be signed so that they may investigate responses and verify licenses and credentials at the credentialing source. In most cases the MCO will also require a copy of the individuals' coverage and the practice's complete malpractice insurance policy. Initially, such extensive investigation may feel intrusive and bureaucratic. Most of these inspection criteria are government mandated and are required by the liability or malpractice insurance carrier of the MCO.

Quality Assurance

In many cases MCOs request a practice's quality assurance manual, which provides for patient grievance and satisfaction protocols. Calibration standards for relevant diagnostic or dispensing systems or technologies might be required (refer to Chapter 10 in *Diagnosis*). If a practice does not have a quality assurance protocol, one should be developed and implemented. This manual should exhibit a conscious effort to ensure patient satisfaction with the following:

- The facility (e.g., cleanliness, parking, signage)
- Employees (e.g., courtesy, competence, and professionalism)
- Scheduling (e.g., ability to quickly schedule, wait in office, convenient hours)
- Services (e.g., explanations of price and billing policies, and the audiologist's explanation of the diagnosis, treatment, and recommendations)
- Efficacy of the prescribed hearing aid(s)

For further information, see Chapter 4 in this volume.

The Site Visit

Most MCOs will have site inspection criteria that is completed by the practice in advance of the visit and later verified in a site visit. The site inspection may include a review of policies and procedures at the practice, including calibration records, patient chart notes, patient grievance procedures and complaints, and billing procedures (see sample Site Inspection Checklist in the Appendix). This visit may include an inspection of the site for acceptable signage, parking, cleanliness, compliance with the Americans with Disabilities Act, diagnostic equipment and sound booth, and in some instances familiarity with the MCO's benefit structure.

If the site inspector requests a review of patient files or charts for a patient who is not a member of that particular MCO, it is appropriate to mask the name of the patient to ensure the patient's right to privacy.

It is advisable to have the above-mentioned materials prepared as attachments for use in proposals and when contacting with an MCO to offer audiology services. Many of the site inspection criteria can actually be listed or summarized, acknowledging before the negotiation that a practice already has these procedures and capabilities in place. Preparing a detailed profile of a practice and its policies regarding patient satisfaction, grievance procedures, administrative and billing procedures, quality assurance, and infection control procedures demonstrates an impressive array of proposal and contracting material already developed that will facilitate MCO contracting. This profile serves as an inventory of a practice's managed care capabilities and a complete description of its professional capabilities.

NEGOTIATING

A negotiation can best be described as a set of questions and answers. Every negotiation has several components, and an understanding of these components is essential to a successful conclusion. In *The Complete Negotiator* (Nierenberg, 1986), Gerard I. Nierenberg describes these components as follows:

- Preparation: The development of assumptions (your assumptions and those you believe that the other party holds)
- Techniques of negotiation: An understanding of direct and indirect needs that must be satisfied if both parties are to benefit from the negotiation

Despite the complexity of negotiations, participating in the negotiation should be rewarding and enjoyable. The managed care negotiation defines the profession, describing for other professionals the scope of practice, diagnostic capabilities and technological advancements, as well as the economic realities of providing a successful outcome to the MCO member with hearing loss. Furthermore, MCO negotiations broaden audiologists' professional affiliations and provide an opportunity to share clinical and professional business with other healthcare professionals. Inclusion in managed care contracts broadcasts to a broad public the necessity and viability of the profession of audiology to payers, other healthcare professions, and healthcare consumers in the community.

Negotiating with an MCO is an opportunity to present the audiology profession to the healthcare community. Audiology is not yet a household word, but many MCOs know something about hearing testing and hearing aids. Although MCOs have been around for decades, it was not until the last 5 to 10 years that they have recognized and funded audiology and hearing aid benefits. In 1996 many MCOs began to compete for Medicare and Medicaid patients as the federal government began allowing MCOs to contract in those markets. Audiology services are an attractive addition to supplement an MCO's Medicare offering and are mandated by the government in most Medicaid programs. A current trend exists for MCOs to accelerate products that specifically include audiology and hearing aid benefits in their packages, and

today many MCOs are negotiating with audiologists to provide services and hearing aids for their members.

Three Ways to Initiate Contact

The three ways to begin negotiations with an MCO are by telephone, in writing, and in person. Eventually all these should be done. One approach may be more successful initially, but whichever initial approach is used, the process should eventually include the following.

Contact by Telephone

Contacting an MCO by telephone requires tenacity and patience. MCOs are large administrative entities, and it can be difficult to locate a contact person knowledgeable with the MCO's ancillary benefit contracts, which is typically the classification applied to audiology contracts. It is appropriate to initially contact an MCO's provider relations or provider contracting department. Ask who would handle contracts with audiologists or ancillary providers and who is the manager of that area. Ideal contacts are those persons at the MCO who are empowered to negotiate. In many instances a contract administrator or professional relations telephone personnel are restricted to sending contracting information, describing the current benefit, and performing credentialing activities. Usually the ancillary benefit manager, network development manager, or director of professional relations is authorized to negotiate new benefits, modify fee schedules, or contract with networks of specialty providers. If possible, it is best to negotiate with managerial level employees because they are authorized to negotiate for new providers.

Consider the following scenario:

> You are calling to inquire about contracting with an MCO. Identify yourself as an audiologist, express your knowledge of the MCO's plans offered, and inquire about the current provider(s) contracted for audiology services and hearing aids. If you are familiar with the group or with individual providers currently providing services to that MCO, acknowledge them. Inquire about the MCO contracting with your practice or clinic as an additional provider in your area. It is beneficial to offer letters of recommendation from primary care physicians participating in the MCO's plan.

In many instances a failed first call can still lead to a contract. A thank-you letter with a brochure describing a practice's capabilities can be very effective. A follow-up phone call is appropriate and confirms that the practice still seeks participation in the MCO's plan. An inquiry about recent developments at the MCO might facilitate a contract. As long as the MCO contact perceives the approach as professional and courteous, they will respect continued interest in pursuit of a contract. Many provider contracts are awarded to those professionals who have developed ongoing, professional relationships with their MCO contacts before being contracted as a plan provider.

Contact in Writing

It is imperative that materials presented in written form be informative but concise. All letters and documents should have the same professional tone and appearance. Include a summary of the capabilities discussed in the previous and following sections and offer to supply as much detail as the MCO requests. When submitting a formal proposal, always include a cover letter with a signature and date. The letter should indicate a time and date that a follow-up phone call can be expected for the purpose of discussing the proposal and to set up a meeting with the MCO.

A significant component of this process is education. MCO managers are paid to be aware of developments in healthcare. Supplying them with information from professional journal articles and association publications about the audiology profession's managed care efforts builds audiology awareness and establishes the prospective provider as an invaluable resource for the MCO.

In a Meeting

After thanking the MCO representatives for the opportunity to meet with them, the purpose of the presentation should be clearly stated: To explore the possibility of contracting with that MCO for hearing services. A brief overview of the practice, clinic, audiology group or network, and the cost-effective services that can be provided is given next.

If the MCO representatives have not reviewed the proposal, the following steps may be taken:

- Describe the profession of audiology, its educational requirements, scope of practice, and certification and licensing requirements. List one or two of the national organizations that govern the ethical practices of audiologists, such as the American Academy of Audiology; the American Speech, Language and Hearing Association; or the Academy of Dispensing Audiologists.
- Put the profession in perspective (e.g., 12,000 audiologists are in the United States; 620 licensed audiologists are in the state of Illinois. More ZIP codes are served by audiologists than by any other group of hearing care professionals —hearing instrument specialists and otolaryngologists.)
- When contracting for a network or multioffice practice, review the demographics of the group. Refer to the geographical distribution of the providers' offices. This information is nicely presented in a map format.
- Distinguish audiologists from hearing instrument specialists in terms of education and scope of practice.
- Describe the credentials of the practice, clinic, or group. A good track record with other MCOs is impressive. Emphasize the credentials of the group, the types of practice settings represented, and whether claims are handled independently or have a third-party administrator.
- Inform those present that a mechanism is available for credentialing providers, claims administration, utilization review, quality assurance, and peer review.

- Discuss how contracting with this group is cost-effective for the MCO: primary care physicians (PCPs) can refer directly to audiologists for diagnostic hearing and balance (vestibular) testing and hearing aids. PCPs can also give medical clearance for hearing aids.
- A group that is already capable of credentialing its providers is a plus for an MCO. It is advantageous for the MCO to have a single resource for communicating plan benefits and credentialing requirements to the group. MCO administrators do not have to communicate with every audiology provider, only the spokesperson/administrator.
- Emphasize that your group has a thorough knowledge of Medicare's requirement of physician referral for diagnostic testing, reimbursement rates, policies regarding hearing aids, and procedures for claims processing. Offer to be flexible because the MCO may have a unique claims process. It is important to inform the MCO that the group is also familiar with the reimbursement policies and procedures of state agencies such as Medicaid, Vocational Rehabilitation, and Children's Services.

Follow-Up Strategies

Follow-up with MCO contact persons on a regular basis. Establish a follow-up schedule that seems reasonable. Develop a strategy that encourages easy communications flow, providing an opportunity to mail news and journal articles about managed care and the audiology profession. Updates on what competing MCOs are doing regarding hearing benefits and advertising is useful. Continue to mail practice profile pieces to these contacts and speak with them on the telephone at least quarterly, but more frequently when actively negotiating for inclusion in their plan.

It is of paramount importance to be viewed as an active partner rather than an adversary to managed healthcare when contracting with MCOs. It is usually not a successful strategy to try to force acceptance into an MCO's network. Frequently, this strategy results in outright rejection. Remember that the MCO will view initial contacts and subsequent behavior toward them as indicative of what a partnership will be like. Obviously, collaboration and openness with the MCO will heighten their comfort level with a prospective provider group. Patience and perseverance offers the best opportunity to develop a lasting and beneficial contractual relationship with an MCO.

Being forthright in obtaining a contract that best serves the MCO's referred patients will not always result in an ideal contract; however, it will almost certainly build the MCO's respect for the provider. The best strategic approach is to educate MCOs about the economic realities of individual audiology practice and the audiology profession as a whole.

Avoid an excessively emotional appeal to obtain a contract; balance the economic concerns and arguments in the negotiations with the patient care and quality concerns for the MCO members. Always recognize that the MCO must compete and profit in an increasingly competitive healthcare market. For an MCO to succeed over time it must offer reasonable geographical access to providers for its members; it must write contracts that will sustain its contracted providers over time.

Methods of Contracting

Many varieties of MCOs exist. Not all are large plans with tens of thousands of subscribers. Some large corporations self-insure. Some companies have traditional indemnity insurance with large deductibles supplemented by flexible (medical) spending accounts. Some plans offer discounts through hearing aid or audiology networks but do not fund or reimburse for audiology services or hearing aids. Many insurers and MCOs contract with individual providers, and some medium-to-large sized practices or clinics have exclusive contracts with MCOs.

Two fundamentally different approaches exist to MCO contracting. The first is as an individual practice or clinic, and the second is a group of collaborating audiologists or clinics seeking to collectively contract as an audiology network.

Individual

If providers seek individual contracts, they are competing with their peers in the community. An individual practice's capabilities and geographical location may be critical in determining contract status. It is more difficult for an independent contractor to negotiate reimbursement levels that differ from the MCOs current schedule. It is simply more difficult for the MCO to make any exception or change for an individual provider. It also requires an extraordinary effort to maintain communications with managerial MCO staff; they simply cannot spend much time working with individual providers. However, many successful individual MCO contracts have proven beneficial to audiologists. In negotiating an individual contract, no responsibility for the actions of colleagues exists only for the performance and standards of the individual practice.

Group or Network

In many states audiologists have formed statewide provider networks that contract with MCOs. Some audiology networks have incorporated and registered as independent provider organizations or independent practice associations and must comply with all rules and regulations set forth by laws governing such entities. Compliance with such regulations may entail bonding or depositing funds in a reserve account to pay claims with, annual registration reporting membership and MCO contract specifics, patient and provider grievance procedures, and annual audits. The advantage of a state provider network is to have a collective voice that will advocate for the specific needs of the group and negotiate the inclusion of the network in MCO plans, either locally or nationally.

It is becoming common for state and national audiology networks to secure contracts with MCOs because of their organizational and administrative capabilities. It is desirable for an MCO to contract with an audiology network that already has audiology-specific systems in place for quality assurance, peer review, provider credentialing, use review, claims management, and provider communications.

RESEARCHING THE MCO

Compiling information about the MCO before responding to the RFP will determine how much time to devote to the response. The investment of time and effort that goes into

---

> **PEARL**
>
> Historically, audiology services have been paid by MCOs to physicians, clinics, and hospitals that bill those codes as a component of their scope of practice. Pointing out CPT codes that are commonly filed for reimbursement by audiologists can pay off if the MCO investigates its current costs related to these codes and acknowledges that it is currently providing these services. This approach can circumvent an MCO's response that they are currently not providing these services. This facilitates a negotiation to contract audiologists to provide these services.

responding to the RFP will be influenced by an analysis of the MCO's demographics, reimbursement rates, and the method and timeliness of reimbursement.

Demographics

The MCO will usually give specific details about their members. This includes the number of members by age and sex (the percentage of males with hearing loss is higher than females). By determining how extensive the MCO's membership is in specific geographical areas, it may be possible to predict whether a contract with the MCO will result in a significant increase in patients. If so, will obtaining the contract require a substantial investment in additional staff or administrative capabilities to serve these patients?

Plans Offered by the MCO

Most MCOs offer many types of health plans. MCOs cover commercial populations by contracting with employers to provide care for their employees. In many cases MCOs also provide care for organized labor groups (trade unions), Medicare members, and Medicaid members. Less frequently, MCOs contract to provide services for workers' compensation claimants. To make this mix additionally complex, MCOs provide these services in several ways, as an HMO or PPO or Point of Service Plan.

When negotiating for a contract to provide services for these groups, determine which of the MCO's member populations are under consideration. It is reasonable to anticipate that the reimbursement schedule and methodology will be different for each of these populations, depending on factors such as variable utilization because of more complete funding of the benefit for some populations and the variation in age among different populations. Occasionally an MCO will seek a single schedule for all populations, which is called a single-payer schedule. It is necessary to carefully average all the utilization factors in arriving at a single schedule that will apply to all MCO members.

The MCO's Track Record

In researching the MCO, physicians and other providers who are currently on the panel can add useful information on patient volume and the MCO's promptness in issuing payment for services. If referrals from key physicians in a particular practice area would otherwise be sent to other providers, it may be beneficial to join the plan. Does the MCO have high visibility in the community? Does it advertise extensively? Would a contract with this MCO increase the prestige of the contracted provider(s)?

Cost Considerations

The extent to which an MCO's discount pricing will affect revenue should be determined. Any cost concessions negotiated with the MCO must be balanced, based on research of the MCO. If participation in the MCO's hearing plan provides opportunities for additional patient visits without additional costs in practice overhead, a provider can benefit from additional patients referred by the MCO, even if fees are significantly discounted. However, if an increase in overhead is required to serve those additional patients, these increased costs must be taken into account when negotiating discounted fees with the MCO.

ANALYSIS OF REQUEST FOR PROPOSAL

What Is a Request for Proposal?

An increasing number of MCOs are soliciting specialty providers and provider networks with traditional precontracting invitations to provide details of costs, services, and capabilities. This solicitation is called a request for proposal, or RFP. In most cases the RFP is a legal document that describes the MCO, describes the requirements of participating on their panel, and requests input from providers regarding prospective administrative and quality assurance compliance and competitive pricing details. An RFP is an ideal vehicle to showcase the audiology profession as an individual practice, clinic, or audiology network.

An RFP is unique to each issuing organization. Typically it has been reviewed by the MCO's contracting, legal, and quality assurance management for accuracy and completeness. Unfortunately, many MCOs have little experience with audiology and hearing aids, and the RFP may be medical in its approach. If this is the case, your responses must make the RFP audiology-specific.

Is the Request for Proposal Audiology-Specific?

Evaluate the MCO's RFP to determine whether the RFP is audiology-specific or generically medical in its approach. If the RFP is medical or generic, it will not give audiology-specific questions, and many of the requirements will seem irrelevant. Although responding to a generic or medically oriented RFP is difficult, it presents an opportunity to become an expert on the MCO's behalf by tailoring answers to generic patient-care questions to the practice of audiology. If it specifies that a referral for services is required, the response should address the need for a medical waiver, which augments the answer with an audiology-specific reply. If the proposal discusses "durable medical equipment" generically, discuss hearing aid technology and assistive listening devices in the reply.

Obviously, a knowledge gap exists at the MCO, or they are under a deadline that has required them to issue the generic RFP without investing the time necessary to understand the specialty with whom they are attempting to contract. This is an opportunity to exhibit to the MCO exactly why they should contract audiologists who are trained and licensed in this specialty.

If the RFP is audiology-specific, does it reflect a current understanding of the profession or is it antiquated, requesting details on older less frequently performed diagnostic tests and hearing aid technologies? Examples of such requests are those that discuss body-worn hearing aids or procedures no longer commonly performed, such as electrodermal audiometry, alternate binaural loudness balance, or sensitivity prediction by acoustic-reflex. Structure a reply to offer alternative diagnostic procedures and current hearing aid technology in addition to their request. A phone call to the MCO contact will confirm a desire to be more complete and to include more current diagnostics and hearing aid technology.

An audiology-specific response reflects an investment made by the MCO in learning about the profession. Acknowledge that investment. It is beneficial to determine the resource for the MCO's knowledge about audiology. Do they have a staff audiologist or did they consult with other audiology professionals in the community? In many cases a staff or consulting audiologist has worked to educate the MCO, making inroads on behalf of the profession. If possible, contact that person and acknowledge their effort. It is not unlikely that the same staff or consulting audiologist is a member of the selection committee.

What Is Contained in a Request for Proposal?
Cover Letter and Introduction

The MCO's cover letter accompanying the RFP serves as a style guide in preparing correspondence back to the MCO. Most RFPs are accompanied by a cover letter. The cover letter states critical due dates, meetings dates, and the name of the employee at the MCO who is responsible for the RFP and the address to which the response should be mailed. Often an overview of the MCO is included in the cover letter as well.

The cover letter or RFP introduction indicates how many copies of the formal response should be delivered to the MCO. In many cases the RFP will have a number assigned to it by the MCO, which identifies for their staff all related responses and materials in the selection process. If such a number exists, it should be referenced in all response materials, inquiries to the MCO, and supporting materials that are supplied with the response. The response must be signed and dated.

Overview of the MCO and Need for Services

The first pages of an RFP are typically background information. They describe the MCO's need for services, and their corporate philosophy, and their regard for their membership and their community. Attention to these details is important in formulating a response.

MCO's Plan for Implementation of the Contract

Often the MCO's plan for awarding and implementing the contract is discussed. It is imperative to review this section

PITFALL

A response to an RFP is a formal offer of contract and could be binding. Understand the legal and economic ramifications of what the MCO is requesting. In California, for instance, it is not legal to provide free services simply for the purpose of obtaining a contract to provide healthcare services. If the MCO has a significant Medicaid population that includes Children's Services, the respondent could assume that the increased sales of hearing aids will offset losses from deeply discounted professional services. This assumption could be dangerous. For instance, if the RFP response indicates a bundled diagnostic charge or fails to differentiate charges for pediatric patients, the practice may be inundated with pediatric referrals for which there is no revenue from hearing aid charges or upgrades in hearing aid technology to offset the deeply discounted professional services. In such instances a practice may be forced to increase its staff or decrease its fee-for-service patient scheduling to accommodate the MCO, producing a significant loss or degrading the ability of the practice to serve its patient base.

with intuitive reasoning, gleaning from this discussion the motivations and biases of the MCO. Often it is this section that best determines the real values of the MCO.

- Is it cost or quality centered?
- Does it express a medical bias or does it hit the target in terms of understanding some audiology-specific details?
- Is the MCO formal or informal?
- How would a meeting with this group be structured?

A response should always be professional, but it should be influenced by the style of the RFP.

Terms

In many cases a critical "terms" section is contained in the RFP that explains in some detail the rules of the contract. The content of this section fulfills requirements of both state and federal regulatory agencies that are mandated by the Healthcare Financing Administrative or a credentialing entity, such as the National Committee for Quality Assurance, which audits MCOs and their providers.

This section should also indicate the proposed duration of the contract (typically 1 year) and the degree of exclusivity being offered. Is the plan open to any provider who wishes to contract with the MCO or is there exclusivity available for a select group? It is prudent to understand all these requirements and to identify for the MCO those requirements that may not be relevant to the practice of audiology. In many instances sections of the RFP that are irrelevant to audiology

providers are generic requirements that apply to physicians or hospitals.

RESPONDING TO THE RFP

Give Expanded Answers

In some instances an RFP is a statement of rules and conditions. In responding, treat each statement as a question.

This statement in Table 18–2 actually gives the practice bragging rights. If the practice or the audiology group or network has a quality assurance policy that requires verification of annual renewal or if an administrator verifies this for a practice or group, this is a good opportunity to tell the MCO about that specific protocol or policy. If malpractice policy limits exceed those required, this should be specifically stated in the response.

PEARL

Many respondents to formal proposal requests respond with "yes" and "no" to simplify the response. Avoid the temptation to oversimplify answers and miss the opportunity to show thoroughness or excellence. Answer succinctly but completely, differentiating your response from those who invested little time and effort in attempting to contract with the MCO. Each request for proposal is an opportunity to educate and enhance your image in the healthcare community.

A complete and detailed response exhibits professionalism and eliminates the possibility of future misunderstanding of any statement in the RFP. The example in Table 18–2 shows that the question has been answered, meeting the MCO's criteria, while emphasizing that the practice is already oriented to quality and administrative requirements demanded by MCOs. Rather than a simple affirmation, the MCO review team clearly receives a message of professionalism and compliance.

Educate the MCO

Each statement or question is also an opportunity to educate the MCO about the audiology profession and a specific practice, clinic, or network. An example of this is responding to an unreasonable request: If the section on malpractice requirements states that the policy must also extend to other MCO providers, that would be an unreasonable request probably only applicable to facilities such as hospitals that grant visiting privileges to other MCO providers. The response to a section such as this is to inform the MCO that the request is not applicable to an audiology practice or clinic. As well as stating this in a formal response, such a request merits a telephone call to the MCO contact for clarification, assuring that a responsible party at the MCO shares the view that such a request is unreasonable.

TABLE 18–2 Example of an RFP question and answer

RFP	Response
"Provider shall maintain at all times a general liability and malpractice policy with limits of $1 million per occurrence, and $3 million aggregate."	*"In response to statement No. x: 'provider shall maintain at all times a general liability and malpractice policy with limits of $1 million per occurrence and $3 million aggregate,'* Hearing Professionals, Inc. maintains a malpractice policy issued by XYZ insurance company and renewed annually, with limits of $2 million per occurrence and $6 million aggregate (policy No. 123456, cover page attached as exhibit C). This policy exceeds the requirements of this RFP. In addition, our practice (group) quality assurance protocol requires that confirmation of our policy renewal be placed in our practice records, along with all relevant correspondence 30 days before renewal. Each audiologist and the practice manager will verify such such confirmation. (Please refer to exhibit H, our quality assurance protocol.)"

Sample Questions

Many proposal requests profile the provider, the practice, and the business management capabilities at a practice. Although many of these questions on the surface may seem excessive, redundant, or intrusive, it is important to keep in mind that the MCO is entering into an agreement in which they will be entrusting the practice with their patient referrals and their reimbursement. The MCO is liable if it improperly contracts services. The RFP is the MCO's initial effort to select a business partner. Following are sample questions that are typical of those included on an RFP:

About the Provider

- How long have you been in practice?
- Present a copy of all graduate and undergraduate degrees.
- Where did you serve your internship/clinical fellowship?
- How long have you been at the current practice?
- Have you ever been charged or convicted of a felony?
- What is your malpractice history?
- List and provide details of any malpractice claims filed against you, with dates and status of each claim.
- List and detail any complaints filed against you with any state agency, licensure board, professional association, or better business bureau.
- Have you ever been terminated, suspended, or disciplined by a professional association, licensing authority, review board, or MCO?

About the Practice

- What is the average number of patients seen weekly?
- How many patients are referred to the practice by HMOs and PPOs (list separately)?
- How long at this location?

- What services does the practice provide?
- If this is a network response, list and map the participating location?
- Describe any community service and outreach programs of your group or practice.
- Has the practice ever been in receivership or declared bankruptcy?
- Detail the diagnostic capabilities, equipment, and calibration standards for your practice.
- Does the practice have an infection control protocol in place?
- Describe the patient grievance procedure for the practice.
- Does the practice have a continuing quality assurance program in place?

About the Business

- What are the staffing ratios of providers to administrative personnel at each location?
- Detail the hours of operation at the practice.
- Please list administrative and professional staff for each location.
- Does the practice have electronic claims submission capability?
- Describe the practice policy for coordinating claims and multiple claims submissions.
- Provide copies of the business license and federal and state tax identification numbers for the practice or network.
- Provide a list of services provided, by CPT code, with usual and customary pricing and your bid price.
- Provide a list of hearing aids commonly dispensed at your practice, and list the manufacturer's suggested retail price, your practice's usual and customary price, and your bid price.

UNDERSTANDING ACTUARIAL FACTORS

Cost

In responding to an RFP, cost will be a significant factor in awarding the contract. Respondents must understand their cost factors and charges before offering bids on pricing. This requires an understanding of some basic actuarial principles related to audiology. All managed care contracts entail some degree of risk, and the goal is to minimize that risk (Grimm & Wiehl, 1994).

Inclusion of hearing aids into the managed care contract is the area of highest risk. Many MCO's claims payments are delayed 60 to 120 days from date of service. Most manufacturer or supplier terms for payment for hearing aids are 30 days net. This means that the hearing aid manufacturer is probably owed for the payment of the wholesale cost before reimbursement from the MCO. Many audiology practices and clinics have an established cash-flow, which can finance these purchases, but some do not. Many reasons why an MCO may be late in reimbursing their providers exist, from a change in their claims system to inept administration. It is vital to the economic viability of the audiology practice or clinic that cash-flow and its impact be considered when entering into a contract or proposing pricing to an MCO.

Carve Out

In many instances hearing aid benefits are "carved out" of the MCO's claims pool. Carve outs are payments for services or goods that are separated from any risk because of insufficient actuarial detail or because they are market sensitive. This means that the MCO is paying for audiology services or hearing aids from funds that are separate from those paid to physicians, clinics, and hospitals. This eliminates a medical provider's reluctance to refer to the audiologist for fear of reducing their reimbursement. Basically, if the MCO has set aside these funds in a "carve out," there is no economic impact on the physician, clinic, or hospital for referring patients for audiology services and hearing aids.

PEARL

It is highly advisable to have any funded hearing aid benefit carved out, ensuring that no disincentive exists for the physician to refer MCO members.

If the audiology reimbursement is for professional services only, this is not a significant adjustment to those physician or clinic-capitated reimbursements. But if this includes $500 to $1000 toward hearing aids, this is a significant deduction from a physician or clinic's revenue. The ramifications for this are long term. Physicians will be reluctant to refer patients for services that significantly reduce their reimbursement, and it is increasingly difficult to get referrals for these patients. In some cases after fighting for reimbursement, the patients also become skeptical of the MCO's reimbursement policy, resulting in complaints and lower member satisfaction.

The simplest solution is to ensure that funds for any hearing aid component of the program are handled as a specialty carve out. An additional benefit is that this allows the MCO to develop reliable experience with the hearing aid benefit before forcing their providers to accept the risk for a variable and uncertain use percentage of the MCO's population. Carving out the hearing aid benefit also relieves the provider of the economic consequences when the MCO's marketing department features the hearing aid benefit in their promotions and drives use above the original estimations.

Discounted Fee-for-Service

The simplest method of pricing is a discounted fee-for-service arrangement. With this method a known, prenegotiated reimbursement for each allowed procedure, and precisely what contribution the MCO will make, if any, toward hearing aids is assured. The risk exposure for this contract is limited to the amount that is discounted from the provider's customary fees. Most managed care contracts with audiologists are still written as discounted fee-for-service contracts. As previously mentioned, it is highly advisable to have any funded hearing aid benefit carved out, ensuring that no disincentive for the physician exists to refer MCO members.

In nearly all circumstances the MCO will demand a discount for hearing aids. Sometimes this is brand-specific, but in most instances it is a simple percentage off usual-and-customary charges for the instrument(s). This discount is the incentive the MCO will use to market the hearing benefit to their members. It usually ranges from 15 to 30% off usual-and-customary charges. Less frequently, this is stated as a discount from manufacturers' suggested retail prices (MSRP), in which case the percentage discount will usually reflect 30% savings from MSRP.

Capitation

Capitated payments are an average payment made on a monthly basis to providers for each member in their service area. In established populations of MCO members who have previously received the services that are to be capitated, a great deal of detail is available that tells the MCO and the providers who are negotiating for a capitated payment what percentage of the MCOs population will use the care over a 1-year period. With that number, multiplied by the discounted cost of the services used, the probable cost over a year's period is determined. Divide this by 12, and you have the monthly cost of the benefit.

If the capitated rate is for new services, such as audiology, the MCO has no data to work with and must use averages from other plans or government programs. These data may be wrong, resulting in an overestimation or underestimation of utilization.

Capitation calculations can be complex. A managed care organization calculates capitation by procedure, geography, average malpractice costs (by profession), census data (the ages of their enrolled population), and administrative costs. Each of these impacts the capitation calculation. The costs of procedures vary by geography (some locations are more expensive to lease and pay higher wages), the frequency of use for each procedure also varies by geography. Malpractice rates, although not a significant factor for audiologists, vary dramatically for many healthcare professions. Generally speaking, an MCO will estimate use of a service or incidence of condition by age in 10-year increments. When calculating audiology costs, a population of 30- to 40-year old MCO subscribers will have a far lower use rate than a population of 60- to 70-year old subscribers. Administrative costs are also calculated, averaging administrative staff and overhead costs on a per patient basis. Complex capitation negotiations require the assistance of an actuary familiar with healthcare costs and procedures.

Capitation, however, can be more simply illustrated. If a practice charges a usual and customary rate of $67 for comprehensive audiometry (CPT code 92557) and has agreed to discount services to the MCO by 20%, the discounted rate is $53.60. On referencing a capitation manual it is determined that the anticipated use for the MCO's population for that code is .0103 (or 1.03%). Multiply the discounted rate by the utilization rate ($53.60 x .013) to arrive at the annual cost per MCO subscriber for that code (70 cents). Because capitation is a 12-month average for the annual costs, the annual cost is divided by 12 to arrive at the monthly capitation rate for comprehensive audiometry. In this theoretical population, 5.8 cents per month is the monthly capitation payment. Calculations would then be made for each procedure covered under the capitation agreement.

The obvious ramification for audiologists is that they may have committed to provide services for a population that uses their services at an increased rate, thus they are being paid less for each service provided, deepening the discount to the MCO and jeopardizing the audiologists' profitability. In the case of audiologists obtaining referrals from the MCO's physicians and subject to the demand generated by an aggressive MCO marketing campaign, audiologists have little control over utilization.

Utilization rates for audiology services are low relative to other ancillary benefits such as dental, chiropractic, and vision care as shown in Table 18–3. The lower the utilization rate, the lower any averaged payment structure may be, thus significantly increasing the risk for a provider who accepts an averaged payment, such as capitation. Capitated payments to audiologists are therefore riskier than for those of other more commonly utilized healthcare services, and it is not inappropriate for the audiologist to participate in the development of the actuarial detail required for a successful capitation contract. Every provider has the right to understand

PITFALL

Utilization does not reflect cost, only the frequency at which a service will be demanded within the MCO's population. Although, for instance, in an aging population eyeglasses are demanded at a rate 10 times that of hearing aids, hearing aids cost a great deal more. A hearing aid benefit that allows $500 toward the purchase of hearing aids will usually cost an MCO about 25% of the cost of a vision plan that pays most of the cost of eyeglasses. When presenting costs to an MCO, be certain not to understate the cost by simply reflecting the low utilization rate.

the actuarial assumptions underlying their reimbursement (Grimm & Wiehl, 1994).

PROPOSAL FULFILLMENT

It is unethical and unprofessional to overpromise a provider's ability to deliver the requirements of a proposal or a contract. It is also bad business, resulting in adverse economic expenses related to fulfilling commitments.

Cost Reduction

To use cost reductions as the primary negotiation strategy is naive and may compromise patient care and practice profitability. Always broaden the focus to your common constituent, the patient. Your practice will serve no one if it does not maintain its ability to remain profitable. Today even nonprofit organizations are feeling the pressure to produce profit centers within the organization, which contribute funds to the ongoing operations of the entity. MCOs are corporations, and they too must sustain a positive cash-flow to stay in business, in most cases returning a profit to shareholders. A contract awarded this year is subject to renegotiations next year, and often reasons beyond one's control determine which providers are chosen. If your primary strategy has been cost-centered rather than focused on patient care, quality, and administrative processes, it is much easier for a competitor

TABLE 18–3   Utilization comparison of dental, vision, chiropractic, and hearing care

Dental	Approximately 60%
	(From American Dental Association)
Vision	Approximately 21%
	(From Hewitt and Associates)
Chiropractic	Approximately 7.2%
	(From American Chiropractic Association)
Hearing	Approximately 1.3%
	(From HEAR PO actuarial table)

to take the business. They need only to lower the cost of their services and hearing aids.

Cost Shifting and Its Ramifications for Patient Care

The move to transfer the financial risk for care to the provider is more than just an economic consideration for the MCO. Philosophically it represents the belief that alternative diagnostic and treatment strategies can be performed or ordered by the provider on the basis of need. The economic consequence of that decision is the provider's responsibility. The days of a provider making these decisions without recognition of their consequence to the payer are over. Today, the economics of that decision impact the profitability of the provider and the MCO.

Providers are now faced with the need to initially limit those decisions to the most practical and proven treatments, therapies, and protocols.

CONTROVERSIAL POINT

Acknowledge the rights of the payer. In today's healthcare economy patients anticipate that their needs will be provided by insurance companies and MCOs at a fraction of the actual cost of the services. Understand that the MCO is the party paying for most of the patient's care and has the right to any relevant patient information. If you seek payment from a third-party, that party has a right to fully understand and manage those costs. The economic viability of healthcare reimbursement demands that providers recognize the responsibility that the payer has to be accountable for the cost, quality, and efficacy of patient care.

An incomplete schedule of diagnostic procedures can result in the audiologist being forced to perform a diagnostic procedure for which there is no reimbursement to fully complete an appropriate recommendation or diagnosis of a condition. This is the ethical challenge presented by each MCO contract and negotiation. It is necessary to negotiate a comprehensive enough schedule to perform the services that may be required for a satisfactory patient outcome. Otherwise, providers may find themselves ethically compelled to do so without compensation.

When MCOs offer a hearing aid benefit, there is often an assumption by their members that the dollar amount allotted for the hearing aid(s) is the equivalent of the cost of the instrument(s). That is, if an MCO announces that hearing aids are "paid in full every 3 years," patients may infer that they can have any style, circuitry, or technology they choose. Patients should be informed that the funded amount (e.g., $500 to $750 per ear) may be applied toward the total cost of the instruments, and that they must pay the difference between the benefit and the cost of the instruments that are recommended. If there is no written clarification regarding

---

PITFALL

Do not make an assumption that CPT codes for reimbursement not specified or included in the MCO contract can be charged for. Every code that an audiology practice or clinic will bill for should be specifically discussed with the MCO contracting contact. Frequently, codes that are not included in the contract may be billed to the patient. If they cannot be billed to the patient, the audiologist must determine whether they represent procedures that must be performed to provide adequate patient care. If a practice cannot charge the patient for the service and there is no reimbursement for it, the cost of that service must be factored in to determine the advisability of participating in the MCO's contract.

---

the hearing aid benefit, patients are confused, and providers are put in an awkward position when they discuss amplification options.

Occasionally a patient cannot afford to upgrade to better circuitry. Good patient care and satisfactory outcomes are compromised when a funded hearing aid benefit (or plan discount) is so low that the purchase of appropriate hearing aids is not possible. In these cases audiologists face further ethical challenges. Sometimes they have to accept these compromises when benefits and patient resources are limited.

Sharing Risk with the MCO

It is possible to jointly share economic risk with an MCO, even on a capitated agreement. If the MCO maintains that it anticipates a level of use that appears to be inadequate, the MCO may reconsider capitating, on the basis of a provider's projections, and offer a discounted fee for service contract, which is not impacted by increased utilization. Otherwise, the MCO should be asked to consider a shared-risk agreement on the basis of their forecast. In this scenario the provider agrees to accept capitation on the basis of the MCO's forecast, but if utilization exceeds that forecast by more than 10%, the MCO will increase capitation to cover 50% of the increase in utilization. This limits the provider's loss exposure to 10% and forces the MCO to accept half of the risk above 10%. When faced with this scenario, many MCOs will accept a provider's argument that excessive utilization depends on physician referrals and MCO marketing (factors over which the provider has no control) and re-examine their actuarial assumptions.

Administration

Fulfilling the administrative requirements of a managed care contract requires some degree of flexibility in administrative practices. Providers may be required to complete a standardized voucher, such as the most commonly used HCFA 1500 form, or need to submit additional paperwork that will accompany the HCFA 1500 form. The office staff that processes claims will have to handle variations in claims processing, depending on each MCO's specific requirements. Interestingly, it is often the larger clinics or hospitals that have difficulty with this aspect of administration, having made a significant investment in software and procedures that may require revision to be compliant with the requirements of the new plan.

Administrative personnel must review the administrative requirements of an MCO's RFP or contract. One should not assume that minor changes in administrative procedures or claims submission are easily accomplished. It is advisable to create a flowchart of the administrative requirements of an MCO's contract and submit this flowchart as a component of the proposal or contract. This ensures that the MCO has agreed to the proposed administrative procedures. Patient flow (triage) and paperwork flows are both appropriate components of this flowcharting process.

SPECIAL CONSIDERATION

Once discounting services begins, it will be necessary to run faster not to lose ground.

ONGOING PRACTICE MANAGEMENT ISSUES

Economic Realities

Independent practitioners should analyze their referral base and determine whether it is stable or subject to change as MCOs expand. Managed care can significantly change the economics of a practice. Providers who join active MCOs must be prepared to budget their time to see more patients to maintain their present income level. The fortunate providers will have negotiated appropriately, which will result in increased income. Be flexible but sensible. Try to predict the impact that additional referrals will have on current office space and staff. Physicians are dropping out of some MCOs because reimbursement rates are too low for them to handle the increased volume of patient visits while maintaining their standard of care (Law & Ferguson, 1998; Scott Collins et al, 1997).

Developing Primary Care Referrals

In all probability any amount of negotiation or discounted pricing will not result in significantly increased patient referrals without a campaign to solicit referrals from the MCO's primary care physicians (PCPs). PCPs are deluged with information from MCOs about procedures, administration, and specialists to whom they refer. The materials that audiologists send to primary care physicians must be interesting, informative, and concise. It is likely that the office manager or administrator will actually be the person in the PCP's office who recommends referral sources to the physician.

Initially, a brief letter to physicians should announce a provider's participation in a new MCO contract. With this letter, it is appropriate to enclose a practice brochure, a Rolodex card with the practice information on it, and a professional identity piece describing the profession of audiology and the need for hearing care. Consult professional associations for audiology awareness brochures. Add a handwritten note to the bottom of the letter to PCPs who are already referring, thanking them for their continued referrals. Invite their input regarding managed care contracts; this note can lead to participation as a provider for another MCO on which the physician participates or even develop into a resource for future MCO contracting. Advising audiology peers about a practice or clinic's participation can also result in an increase in referrals. Audiologists who are not participating in the MCO's contract may welcome a peer to whom they can refer those MCO member patients.

PCPs are keenly aware that they also work in a competitive healthcare environment. Acknowledging that concern is professional and appropriate. Follow up a written announcement of MCO participation with a phone call to the PCP's office manager. Determine whether the PCP already refers to any other audiology provider(s), and inquire whether the PCP's office would consider making additional referrals. Keeping in touch on a regular basis is good patient care and good business. Send complete documentation and reports to physicians in a timely manner and make a point when referring PCPs' patients back to their practices for any health condition.

It is also beneficial to meet personally with the PCP's office manager and the physician, if possible. Establishing a personal identity with referring physicians increases the likelihood of receiving their referrals over time. The purpose of this meeting is to establish face-to-face contact that becomes invaluable for future communications with that office. Offer to give a hearing loss workshop at lunch for their staff or to provide point-of-service materials describing hearing loss for the physician to distribute to patients and keep in the waiting room. All materials must be professional.

The final component of developing PCP referrals is maintaining a thorough understanding of the MCO's plan of benefits, administrative procedures, and referral requirements. Knowledge of referral requirements is essential before speaking to primary care physicians. In many cases it is the PCP's lack of familiarity with the referral process for audiology and hearing aid benefits that inhibits referrals. If the hearing aid benefit is carved out, it is advisable to inform the clinic that the referral is revenue-neutral and will not affect the physicians' reimbursement or capitation rate. All information regarding the particulars of the referral process should be summarized in writing and approved by the MCO.

PEARL

PCP's lack of familiarity with various referral processes inhibits referrals. It is advisable to distribute materials that succinctly describe each MCO's referral requirements and a practice's internal administrative procedures to referring physicians' practices. Making the referral process as simple as possible maximizes the potential of any MCO contract.

Practice Promotion

Print Ads, Direct Response, and Patient Recall

Most MCOs require that providers submit any practice promotion materials for approval before distribution. If an MCO contract does not specify guidelines for promotion involving the MCO's name or logo, be certain to inquire about their policy before distributing any material. In yellow pages ads and other print ads, it is often acceptable to list MCO affiliations. To fulfill MCO requirements and to comply with the codes of ethics of professional audiology organizations, always request materials directly from the MCO rather than developing art for a display ad without written permission. Many MCOs will supply logo sheets and window or counter decals.

Listing the names of audiology providers in the MCO provider directory does not guarantee additional referrals, especially in a metropolitan area where there are many providers in the MCO's service area. Each provider or group needs to distinguish itself in the mind of the patient and the PCPs' staffs. Inservices are a good way to establish and keep in contact with referral resources. It is good public relations to send them informational packets, practice brochures, and other materials at regular intervals. An audiology newsletter for physicians is a good way to keep PCPs informed of diagnostic procedures (ABR, ENG, OAEs), new hearing aid technology, and advances in treatment for conditions such as tinnitus.

Consider in advance of open houses and technology demonstrations how MCO members will fit into the promotion scheme. If a discount is offered, will this extend to the MCO member? Have a policy to handle MCO members who respond, so that they understand the limitations of their MCO benefit when considering more advanced hearing aid technology.

The MCO will almost certainly have a policy regarding any patient recall programs. Patient recall letters to MCO subscribers must also receive prior authorization and will probably be restricted to professional services because MCOs have a significant risk exposure from increased utilization, and many do not want their members targeted for hearing aid refits or technology demonstrations.

PITFALL

MCOs have a significant risk from increased utilization. Many do not want their members targeted for hearing aid refits or technology demonstrations.

Announcing and prominently displaying MCO contract identities has a collateral benefit. Existing patients will have acquaintances or family members that belong to an MCO plan that is likely to produce additional referrals. In many cases patients who are considering joining an MCO will make that decision on the basis of the participation of providers they know.

Image

Subjective and objective considerations determine the profile that a practice or clinic will have with an MCO. Subjective considerations are those relating to the "look and feel" of a practice. Objective considerations are those derived from data regarding the MCOs and their members' experience with the audiology providers. For active MCO providers, the "look and feel" of a practice will be reported back to the MCO after a site inspection and by the MCO members who receive services. Establish an "MCO-friendly" office. Protocols should facilitate easy scheduling, patient intake, and processing of authorizations and referrals. Procedures should be streamlined to accommodate the increased office traffic and the accompanying paperwork that will be necessary to process these patients. Not only will this result in good MCO relations, but referring PCPs and their patients will benefit as well.

Is the practice or clinic's focus more on diagnostics or rehabilitation? Does it have a retail atmosphere? Patients want to believe that they are all treated the same, regardless of their insurance plan. Patients feel comfortable when providers are knowledgeable about the policies and procedures unique to their plans. A well-run office has a mechanism for storing the policies and reimbursement schedules of all of its MCO plans. Contracting with an MCO establishes a partnership with that MCO. That perspective also applies in resolving any disputes or problems that arise.

Objective criteria that present a positive image include consistency in pricing and the timely submission of paperwork and claims forms for submission to the MCO. Patient and PCP complaints and feedback are also a component of the MCO's analysis of providers' effectiveness. The best practices adhere to a patient grievance plan that ensures a satisfactory outcome for every patient.

Be prepared for an audit by the MCO. They may seek access to a patient file on the basis of a complaint or on a random statistical audit. In some cases a state agency or other government entity will require an MCO to review a certain percentage of patient files and chart notes. An audit by an MCO does not necessarily mean that a provider's services or policies are suspect; in most cases they are an administrative policy or a quality-assurance requirement.

Educational and In-Service Opportunities

MCO managers who are responsible for contracting ancillary providers are paid, in part, for their knowledge and their ability to bring credible resources to the MCO. Most would welcome the opportunity to assist their claims administrators, marketing staff, and professional relations staff in understanding hearing loss, current diagnostic capabilities in diagnosing hearing loss, and an update on hearing aid technology and associated costs.

A presentation to the MCO's staff or an in-service would be considered desirable by most MCO executives. It is appropriate to offer such services in a formal response to an RFP or after contracting with an MCO. The MCO in-service also offers an opportunity to collaborate with peers in the community in developing the presentation.

Materials recommended for such a presentation are an audiology awareness brochure, an inventory of diagnostic capabilities, demographic detail on hearing loss, a brief overview of the professions that treat hearing loss, and a description of technologies that are available to treat hearing loss and their costs. It is also beneficial to distribute samples of hearing aid types, so that the MCO staff actually has the opportunity to see the comparative size and types of technology that they are making available to their members. It is advisable to present from an outline and to pass out copies of the presentation for note taking. The time allotted for such a presentation varies from 15 minutes to an hour, so these materials are critical for any in-depth understanding by the audience. In-service opportunities often occur in an early morning staff meeting before the start of the workday or in the late afternoon.

In some instances a streamlined version of an MCO in-service can be revised and presented to referring PCPs and their clinical staffs. Usually, clinic and physician practice meetings are early morning or lunch meetings, and a presentation must be abbreviated for this audience. Be sure to leave enough time for questions and answers at any in-service. It is appropriate to add a practice-specific brochure and a business card at a physician in-service.

Ethics

Audiologists are ethically bound to provide the same level of care to all patients. Furthermore, it is discrimination to deny services to any group that the practitioner has agreed to serve. When providers accept the terms and conditions of an MCO contract, they agree to provide services and products at specified rates. It is expected that they will give the same level of care to MCO patients that they give to all other patients, regardless of reimbursement levels. Testing protocols, patient scheduling standards, and follow-up care should not be restricted.

Most audiologists belong to one or more professional organizations. Each organization has a code of ethics that specifies professional conduct and standards that allow for the proper discharge of audiologists' responsibilities to those served and protects the integrity of the profession. A principle that is common to these documents is the statement that "individuals shall not limit the delivery of professional services on any basis that is unjustifiable or irrelevant to the need for the potential benefit from such services" (American Academy of Audiology, 1988).

CONCLUSIONS

Participation in healthcare reimbursement is essential to further establish audiology as an independent healthcare profession. Although it might seem that the process is excessively administrative and tedious, an advantage exists for the participating practice or clinic. It requires a succinct analysis and inventory of a practice's capabilities, both professional and administrative. This inventory defines the profession to others and requires fulfillment of that definition in great detail.

By definition, managed healthcare participation entails risk, and caution must be taken so that negotiated contracts ultimately contribute to the well-being of the practice, the payer, and the profession. Most often there is reward for taking this risk. An independent and economically successful profession ensures the ongoing recruitment of graduate students and new generations of committed audiology professionals who are resourceful in meeting the needs of an aging population with its accelerating rate of hearing loss.

GLOSSARY OF MANAGED CARE TERMS

Capitated Threshold Capitated agreement with a sliding scale or another negotiated rate for services that exceed a projected utilization threshold.

Capitation A per-member, per-month fixed payment to a healthcare provider or health plan for each member enrolled, regardless of the count of care a member requires. The specific services that are covered must be stated. A volume *ceiling* may have been negotiated on the basis of projected utilization.

Capitation, Mixed This is an agreement that excludes specified services from the agreement. These excluded services are paid for on a fee-for-service basis, with discounts, if any, having been previously negotiated.

Carve Outs Those services where excess risk would be assumed if they were included in a capitated payment plan. They include services that lack sufficient historic data to calculate a capitated rate. An example would be a site where there were not sufficient patients treated to statistically predict whether the previous patients were representative of all patients who presented for treatment at that site. The second reason for a carve out would be for those sites that were market sensitive. One example might be breast disease, in which market factors may affect the charge of the treatments for political or marketing purposes.

Coinsurance Percentage of the healthcare bill that the patient is expected to pay, for example, 20% of usual and customary charges.

Community Rating A scale that would set health insurance premiums on the basis of the average cost of medical services in a geographical area, without adjustments for the individual medical history or risk.

Copayments The patient's share of the total medical bill, usually a specific dollar amount.

Deductibles Preset dollar amounts that patients must pay before insurance reimbursement kicks in. Used particularly in traditional indemnity insurance plans to reduce premiums.

EPO (Exclusive Provider Organization) In this arrangement, providers are paid a negotiated fee on an as-used basis rather than being prepaid for their services. Patients usually must see a primary care physician gatekeeper, who will then refer them to specialists if necessary.

ERISA (Employee Retirement Income Security Act) A federal law governing the funding, vesting, and administration of pension and employee welfare and benefit plans.

Fee-for-Service A funding system under which insurers pay medical providers for each service they provide. This has been the most common method in the past and continues today in most situations.

Formulary A list of drugs selected by an MCO as the only drugs the MCO will cover. Typically, the list includes generic drugs that have been found to be safe, efficacious, and cost-effective. The formulary generally excludes expensive brand-name drugs for which there are equal but less expensive substitutes.

Gatekeeper A method to control patient referral by a managed care plan. A patient must see a primary care physician first, who will then refer to a specialist, if necessary.

Group Model HMO Contracts with one independent group of physicians that provide healthcare to the HMO's members, usually in HMO-owned or HMO-managed facilities.

Group Without Walls A formal legal organization that bills under one provider number and provides certain core administrative and management services to physicians who maintain separate, individual offices.

Healthcare Boards Quasi-governmental boards controlled by consumers, doctors, employers, and other healthcare experts charged with setting overall healthcare budgets, designing basic benefit plans, capping charges, and reviewing quality and performance of health networks.

HIPC (Health Insurance Purchasing Cooperative) Large groups of employers banded together to negotiate the best arrangement in the purchase of a healthcare plan.

HMO (Health Maintenance Organization) A managed care health system that controls costs by contracting with specific doctors to provide comprehensive benefits, often in return for a fixed prepaid monthly rate per person. Consumers may pay small fees (copayments) for certain services, but no annual deductibles or additional costs are incurred. Consumers in these plans must use HMO doctors to be covered.

Health Network HMOs, PPOs, or any cooperative system of insurers, doctors, or hospitals that contract with employers to provide medical care.

IPA (Independent Practice Association) An MCO contracts with IPAs, which are groups of medical providers in private practice who have banded together to bid on contracts to provide services. IPA providers typically see private patients and patients from other MCOs.

Managed Care A strategy for reducing or controlling healthcare costs by tightly monitoring and restricting the use and cost of services. An example of a managed care plan is the typical HMO.

Mixed Model A managed care plan that mixes two or more types of delivery systems.

MSO (Management Services Organization) A separate corporation set up to provide management services to a medical group for a fee. It has also been used to refer to a corporation that owns the assets of one or more physician groups.

Network Model HMO Contracts with two or more large, independent group practices or smaller HMOs to provide managed care to its members.

Open Enrollment The annual period, usually occurring for 1 month of the year, when an employee may change health plans.

PHO (Physician-Hospital Organization) Physicians and a hospital form a joint contracting organization to negotiate contracts with insurers.

PPO (Preferred Provider Organization) A managed care system under which an insurance company or MCO contracts with a wide variety of doctors and hospitals to provide services. Physicians usually are paid on a fee-for-service basis but have agreed to discount charges in return for a projected number of patients. Generally, the patients pay deductibles, coinsurance, or copayments. If plan subscribers do not use the "preferred" providers and go to a doctor or hospital outside of the plan, they generally will have lower benefit coverage, higher deductibles, or coinsurance.

Risk In any payment method other than fee-for-service the audiologist assumes the financial liability for treating patients without a relationship to the amount of the revenue received. In a capitated reimbursement method a specific payment is received (i.e., Per Member Per Month [PMPM]) regardless of the number of patients treated; therefore the audiologist assumes the financial risk to treat however many patients are referred for a set payment.

Risk Corridor This is also called shared risk. It involves the concept that all parties share the risk. In the case of capitated arrangements, an upper and lower limit would be established for the number of treatments or patients treated. If the utilization exceeds the upper limit, the payer agrees to reimburse the audiologist at a higher rate. If the utilization is less than the lower limit, the audiologist agrees to refund to the payer a portion of the capitation payment.

RUC (Relative Value Update Committee) The committee of AMA that has been assigned the task of evaluating requests for adjustments in the relative value of a procedure and recommending the new value to HCFA.

Self-Insured An individual who pays his or her own healthcare costs or an employer-managed and employer-controlled health plan that offers a benefits package to its employees and perhaps dependents and pays providers for services from funds set aside for such purposes.

Staff Model HMO An HMO that directly employs its physicians and medical personnel and either owns or manages its hospitals and health centers.

TPA (Third-Party Administrator) An organization or entity other than the health plan or healthcare provider that collects premiums, pays claims, and provides administrative services. Medicare operations are processed in this system in most cases.

Traditional Indemnity Insurance A system that allows consumers to choose their physician and have greater control over the services they receive in return for agreeing to pay for a portion of the costs, typically 10% to 30% in the form of coinsurance and an annual deductible.

TQM (Total Quality Management) A specific method of continuously improving the quality of healthcare service being rendered.

Underwrite The act of an insurer accepting an application for insurance coverage. The basis for determination varies by insurer and the type of coverage requested, and the premium is based on the associated risk to the insurer.

Utilization A term used to describe how often healthcare and other types of services are used over a given period of time. Usually expressed as number of services per 1,000 or per 100,000 persons Eligible for that service.

Utilization Review A program that examines the medical necessity of non-emergency hospital admissions and medical procedures or tests. *Prospective utilization review* may include pre-admission certification of hospital admissions, assigned lengths of stay and second surgical opinions on elective procedures. *Concurrent review* monitors inpatient stays to make sure they continue to be medically necessary. *Retrospective review* involves an audit to determine whether services that were provided were medically necessary or showed evidence of quality of care problems.

Appendix
Site Inspection Checklist

Forms Manual
Site Inspection
Revision 1
Page 1 of 2
9/1/99

SITE INSPECTION

Practice name: _____

Address: _____

_____

Phone number: _____ Fax number: _____

Date of Inspection: _____

Inspection Team: _____

_____

SITE INSPECTION CHECKLIST

Please indicate applicable achievement scores for each criterion: Y= yes; N= no; NA = not applicable.

Category	Achievement
Access and appearance	
Office is identified with a prominently displayed sign.	_____
Waiting area is neat and clean.	_____
Waiting area has adequate seating.	_____
Waiting time is appropriate.	_____
Handicap parking available.	_____
Facility ADA accessible.	_____
Fire safety	
Extinguishers are visible.	
Fire alarms, detectors, and sprinklers are visible and working.	_____
Smoking is not permitted except in designated areas.	_____
Corridors are clear.	_____
Exit doors are unlocked during business hours.	_____
Infection control policies	
Documented infection control policy available.	
Log book of infection control training available.	_____

Medical records
    Records are centrally located.
    Personnel comply with confidentiality guidelines. _____
    Each patient record is contained in an individual folder. _____

Medical records review
    Number of medical records required: _____
    Number of medical records reviewed: _____

Review	Achievment				
	#1	#2	#3	#4	#5
All pages contain patient ID.	___	___	___	___	___
There is an informed consent process.	___	___	___	___	___
Each entry authenticated by author.	___	___	___	___	___
Each entry is dated.	___	___	___	___	___
Each entry is legible.	___	___	___	___	___
Documented reason for each encounter.	___	___	___	___	___
Problems from previous visit addressed.	___	___	___	___	___
Billing appropriate.	___	___	___	___	___
Discounts appropriately listed.	___	___	___	___	___
Insurance or payer on file.	___	___	___	___	___

Equipment review
    Sound booth.
    Audiometer. _____
    Sound-field system. _____
    Immittance meter. _____
    Probe microphone system. _____
    Evoked potential system. _____
    Electronystagmography system. _____
    Otoacoustic emission system. _____
    Infection control system. _____

Equipment maintenance
    Calibration records.
    Preventative maintenance program. _____
    Calibration standards and procedures. _____
    Calibration log and training records on equipment. _____

REFERENCES

AMERICAN ACADEMY OF AUDIOLOGY. (1988). Bylaws and code of ethics. Washington, DC: American Academy of Audiology.

GRIMM, M., & WIEHL, J. (1994). *The managed care contracting manual: A strategic guide to maximizing opportunities and minimizing risks*. Alexandria, VA: Capitol Publications Inc.

LAW, G., & FERGUSON, T. (1998). Doc's just an employee now. *Forbes*, May 18.

NIERENBERG, G. (1986). *The complete negotiator*. New York: Nierenberg & Zeif Publishers.

SCOTT COLLINS, et al. (1997). *The commonwealth fund survey of physician experiences with managed care*. http\www.cmwf.org\physrvy.html. New York: Commonwealth Fund.

Basic Computer Principles

Michael K. Wynne

technology cannot be separated from other technologies. Technologies act in conjunction with each other. Nowhere is this more evident than in the management of dispensing audiology practice. The computer used to select, fit, and modify digital and digitally programmable instruments may also handle audiograms, produce clinical reports, complete orders for products and product repairs, manage financial accounts and patient files, maintain production statistics, and provide Internet access for the audiologist. With various add-on components, that computer also could be used as an instrument to obtain evoked potentials and generate acoustic stimuli for word recognition testing. With multimedia software, that computer can be used as a patient-education kiosk (e.g., demonstrating the advantages of new hearing instrument technologies).

This chapter introduces the general framework for computer hardware technologies. Operating systems, software applications, and the Internet are covered in detail in Chapter 20 in this volume.* Rapidly changing technology is the foundation for many of the changes seen in audiology in the last decade (Fournier & Margolis, 1992; Hayes, 1992; Heard, 1994; Hosford-Dunn et al, 1995; Mendel et al, 1995; Rauterkus, 1992; Sirianni, 1996; Strom 1994, 1995; Wynne, 1996a). The effectiveness of how audiologists adapt and use these technologies is linked to the skills and behaviors of the audiologists themselves. Responding effectively to changes in technology falls within the purview of every audiologist, regardless of the work setting or patient demographics. The challenge to the audiologist is how to make decisions regarding the integration of new technologies, particularly when the novelty and complexity of rapidly changing technologies cloud the precise nature of the capabilities and pitfalls the new technologies offer.

Making good decisions regarding technology integration requires knowledge, and every knowledge base requires a beginning foundation. The goal of this chapter is to provide an introduction to personal computers (PCs). As with any static description of computer technologies, this chapter was

---

*For further reading on applications software, the Internet, and specific hardware and software system for audiology, see American Speech-Language-Hearing Association, 1997; Amerine, 1992; Bevan et al., 1994; Bloom, 1998; Columbo, 1994; Dybala, 1996; Ginsberg, 1992; Heard, 1994; Kuster & Kuster, 1995; Mendel et al., 1995; Mormer, Mormer, & Robertson, 1992; Mormer & Palmer, 1998; Piccolo, 1994; Sullivan, 1998; Swenson, 1995; Wynne, 1996a,b.

Technology does not work in isolation. Not only can technology not be separated from the activities of the audiologist, but one

Audiology: Practice Management. Edited by Hosford-Dunn, Roeser, and Valente. Thieme Medical Publishers, Inc., New York © 2000

SPECIAL CONSIDERATION

Before buying a new computer, ask the following questions:

Does it have the processor and clock speed for the performance you will need?

Does it have sufficient memory (RAM) to run the programs you want to use? Can it run multiple programs simultaneously?

Is the hard drive big enough to store the software you will be running and still have room to add more later?

Does it come with a monitor?

Is it equipped with a high-speed modem that is compatible with your needs?

Does it come with the operating system and other preloaded software you want?

Does it come with 24-hour, 7-day-a-week technical support?

Is the warranty adequate?

Can you get the features you want and avoid paying for those you do not want?

Will it handle your future needs?

outdated as soon as it went to the publisher. In addition, the breadth and depth of the discussion was limited to provide a general introduction to the basic elements of computer systems to practicing audiologists and students. The chapter is organized in an hierarchical and spatial fashion, starting with a brief description of PC system components, then moving out of the PC to a discussion of connections and communications with peripheral devices, and finishing with a limited glossary of terminology commonly used to describe computers and their applications. More comprehensive computer glossaries and dictionaries are available in hard copy form and on the World Wide Web. Finally, the editors of *PC World* and IDG Books Worldwide provide the Dummies Daily—Nerd Word of the Day that delivers a new computer term by e-mail to any of this listserv's users daily (to subscribe, complete the form at http://www.dummiesdaily.com).

SYSTEM HARDWARE

A computer executes instructions. Each instruction tells the computer to add, subtract, multiply, divide, or compare two numbers to see which is larger. The rest is housekeeping (White, 1998). Even an application that appears to do no arithmetic is still using numbers. Consider the automatic error correction in a word processor. Today, when "teh" is entered on the keyboard, the computer appears to recognize the common misspelling and changes it to "the." What does

this have to do with numbers? Well, every character that is typed, including the space bar, transmits a code to the computer. In American Standard Code for Information Interchange (ASCII), a blank is 32, "a" is 97 and "z" is 122. So the computer sees "teh" as the sequence 32 116 101 104 32. The word processor has been programmed to check for this sequence, and when it sees it, it exchanges the 101 and 104. The CPU chip does not know about spelling, but it is very fast and accurate handing numbers.

If everything is numbers, one might think that the speed of the computer is largely determined by how fast it can add. People expect this because adding large numbers takes a long time. Ask someone how much 2 + 2 is and they will respond immediately 4. Ask how much 154,373 + 382,549 is, and they will stop for a minute and take out a pencil. A computer adds numbers with electronic circuits that work just as fast for large or small numbers. Arithmetic is what computers do best, and they do it almost instantly.

The computer handles any task by physically getting an instruction from memory, decoding it, figuring out what data are being referenced, getting the data from memory, and finally performing the arithmetic (Biow, 1997). Performance is limited by the speed with which the instructions and data can be moved around, not by the final computation. Numerous factors help determine how efficient a computer handles this task. The hardware, although not necessarily the most critical element of the computer system, to a great extent determines what someone can do with the computer and how it is done. Tables 19–1 and 19–2 present an outline to help determine user needs and to help determine when to upgrade or purchase a new system because it fails to meet user needs.

The Case

The cabinet and included power supply constitute the case. All components except the monitor and external items fit inside the case and operate from a power supply inside the case. A fan integrated into the power supply cools the power supply and all internally installed components. A small fan is often mounted on the microprocessor for more cooling.

Several different case styles are available, such as mini, medium, and full tower cases. Many older systems use flat desktop styles. Often, the size of the case can limit the user's options for expanding or upgrading the system. A mini-tower case, for example, will house two floppy drives, a CD-ROM drive, and a tape backup system, and neither will most basic desktop cases.

The power supply inside the case takes the 117 V AC from your wall socket and converts it to the +5 volts, +12 volts, −5 volts, and −12 volts the computer requires. Power consumption is directly related to the number and types of components housed within the case. The larger cases have more drive and accessory bays, so the power supply must provide more power. Generally, system developers take this into consideration when they make the cases. A mini-tower case should be rated at 200 watts minimum. A medium case should be rated at 250 watts, and a full tower should support at least 300 watts of accessories.

TABLE 19–1 Factors to consider to determine computer needs

Factors	Considerations
1. Problem definition	Provide clear and concise statements of the problems.
2. Problem analysis	Who will be affected by these problems? How do these problems impact quality of patient care? What factors are causing the problems? What is the extent of these problems?
3. Possible alternatives	How can the objectives be accomplished? What options are available other than computerization?
4. Evaluate alternatives	a) What are the fiscal considerations? • Cost of installed hardware • Cost of software • Cost of additional personnel, if needed • Cost of training • Cost of consumable supplies • Cost of maintenance • Cost and availability of upgrades • Expected savings b) What are the technical considerations? • Levels of technical knowledge and skills needed for system operation • Integration of system with other technical systems within the practice c) What are the organizational considerations? • Restructuring the information flow and organizational culture • Management's, colleagues', and staff's reactions to technology d) What are the staff considerations? • Effects on staff size • Staff training and cross-training needs • New staffing needs e) What are the legal considerations? • Software piracy issues • Documentation, record maintenance, and patient confidentiality f) What are the security considerations? • System security risks • Costs of risk minimization g) What are the patient considerations? • Quality of care (quality of conformance and perceived quality) • Changes in cost of patient care h) What are the marketing considerations? • Changes in SWOT* analysis • Changes in competitive advantages over other practices
5. Recommendation	What office management system will best complement the short-term and long-term goals of the practice while satisfying the current constraints of the office system?

*SWOT analysis: Strengths, weaknesses, opportunities, threats.

The power supply fan prevents the computer chips and circuits from overheating during their operation. This fan must be kept free of dust and obstructions to airflow, so do not let anything block the part of the case where the fan is mounted. Blocking the air flow through your computer will result in heat damage to one or more of the internal components. This fan is the only source for cooling in most computers. Spending a few dollars more for a case with an extra fan is money well spent because two fans are safer than one. Nothing kills a great computer faster than an uncorrected fan failure.

Motherboard and System Devices

In many ways the motherboard is the most important component in the computer, not the processor, even though the processor gets much more attention. Figure 19–1 illustrates a

TABLE 19–2   Guidelines for upgrade decisions

Decision	Economic Considerations	Organizational Considerations	Performance Considerations	Use Considerations
Retain	No funds are available. Benefits will be less than 33% of actual costs. System displays normal maintenance and repair patterns.	Hardware is less than 3 years old. Software upgrade is a maintenance/interim release. Vendor/developer support is excellent. System is well integrated with office management procedures.	Current system is effective and efficient. Current system's functions and features are usable. Current system's operation is logical and user-friendly. Current hardware and software is compatible.	Current system is preferred by most users. System records show stable level of usage. Users are satisfied with system.
Enhance	Limited funds are available. Benefits will be greater than 33% of actual costs. System requires frequent maintenance and repair patterns.	Hardware is 2 to 3 years old. Software upgrade is at least one major version forward. Vendor/developer support is limited. System is presenting problems with current or future office management procedures.	Current system's effectiveness is diminished. Current system's functions and features are inadequate for some tasks. Current system's operation is cumbersome. Current hardware and software present some incompatibility problems.	Current system is accepted but not preferred by most users. System records show declining level of use. Users are expressing concerns about the system.
Replace	Full funding is available. Benefits will be greater than 50% of actual costs. System requires extensive maintenance and repair.	Hardware is greater than 3 years old. Software is no longer compatible with system or operating system. Vendor/developer support is not available. System is incompatible with current or future office management procedures.	Current system will perform required task. Current system's functions and features are inadequate for most tasks. Current systems operation presents obstacle for successful use. Current hardware and software present significant incompatibility.	Current system is neither accepted or preferred by most users. System is rarely used when other options are available. Users are dissatisfied.

motherboard for a Pentium-based computer system. The motherboard plays an important role in the following important aspects of a computer system (Norton, 1997):

Organization: In one way or another everything is eventually connected to the motherboard. The way that the motherboard is designed and laid out dictates how the entire computer is going to be organized.

Control: The motherboard contains the chipset and Basic Input/Output System (BIOS) program, which between them control most of the data flow within the computer.

Communication: Almost all communication between the PC and its peripherals, other PCs, and the user goes through the motherboard.

Processor support: The motherboard dictates directly your choice of processor for use in the system.

Peripheral support: The motherboard determines, in large part, what types of peripherals can be used in a PC. For example, the type of video card the system will use (Industry Standard Architecture [ISA], VESA Local Bus [VLB], Peripheral Component Interconnect [PCI]) depends on what system buses the motherboard uses.

Performance: The motherboard is a major determining factor in the system's performance for two main reasons. First, the motherboard determines what types of processors, memory, system buses, and hard disk interface speed a system can have, and these components directly dictate the system's performance. Second, the quality of the motherboard circuitry and chipset themselves has an impact on performance.

Ability to upgrade: The capabilities of a motherboard dictate to what extent the system can be upgraded. For example, some motherboards will accept regular Pentiums of up to 133 MHz speed only, whereas others will go to 200 MHz. Obviously, the second one provides more capability to upgrade than the first (Rathbone, 1997).

Obviously, motherboards vary, and the number of chips or devices on the board depends on its age and level of integration.

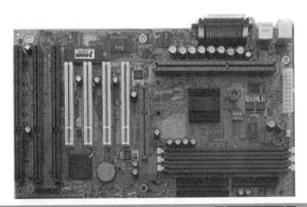

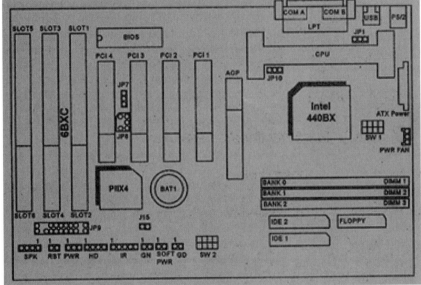

Figure 19–1   The motherboard.

The motherboard has one or more sockets or slots to hold the processor(s). Single-processor motherboards are by far the most common, but dual-processor and even quad-processor boards are not hard to find. (Quad boards often use special, proprietary designs using riser cards.) The type of socket or slot used dictates the type of processor and, in some cases, the speed that can be used by the motherboard. Not surprisingly, the standards for processor sockets and slots have been generally defined by the chip manufacturer. Most older Intel processors, up to the Pentium Pro, use a square-shaped socket for the processor. The newest processors from Intel, starting with the Pentium II, are mounted on a daughterboard, which plugs into an "single-edge connector" (SEC) slot to connect to the motherboard.

Most motherboards today come with between two and eight sockets for the insertion of memory (Minasi, 1996). These are usually either single inline memory modules (SIMMs) or dual inline memory modules (DIMMs). These can come in different sizes. The motherboard usually labels these sockets "SIMM0" through "SIMM7" or "DIMM1" through "DIMM3," and so on. The sockets are almost always filled starting with the lowest numbered socket first. Most Pentium class or higher motherboards require SIMMs to be inserted in pairs, but DIMMs may be inserted individually. Virtually all newer 486 or Pentium class motherboards come with either integrated secondary cache or sockets for secondary cache to be inserted. Also called "Level 2" or "L2" cache, secondary cache is high-speed memory that is used to buffer processor requests to the regular system memory.

Input/Output Bus Slots

All motherboards have one or more system input/output (I/O) buses that are used to expand the computer's capabilities (Gookin, 1997). The slots in the back of the machine are where expansion cards are placed (like the video card, sound card, and network card). These slots allow the capabilities of a system to be expanded in many different ways, and the proliferation of both general purpose and very specific expansion cards is part of the success story of the PC platform.

Most modern PCs have two different types of bus slots. The first is the standard ISA slot; most PCs have three or four of these. These slots have two connected sections and start about a half-inch from the back of the motherboard, extending to around its middle. This is the oldest (and slowest) bus type and is used for cards that do not require a lot of speed; for example, sound cards and modems. Older systems, generally made well before 1990, may have ISA slots with only a single connector piece on each; these are 8-bit ISA slots and will only support 8-bit ISA cards.

PEARL

Chipsets and Controllers

The system chipsets and controllers are the logic circuits that are the intelligence of the motherboard. They are the "traffic cops" of the computer, controlling data transfers between the processor, cache, system buses, peripherals—basically everything inside the computer. Because data flow is such a critical issue in the operation and performance of so many parts of the computer, the chipset is one of the few components that have a truly major impact on a PC's quality, feature set, and speed.

What exactly is a "chipset?" It sounds like something very complex but really is not, although many of the functions it performs are (Gookin, 1997). A chipset is just a set of chips. At one time, most of the functions of the chipset were performed by multiple, smaller controller chips. There was a separate chip (often more than one) for each function: controlling the cache, performing direct memory access (DMA), handling interrupts, transferring data over the I/O bus, and so on. Over time these chips were integrated to form a single set of chips, or chipset, that implements the various control features on the motherboard. This mirrors the evolution of the microprocessor itself: at one time many of the features on a Pentium, for example, were on separate chips.

Pentium systems and newer 486-class motherboards also have PCI bus slots, again, usually three or four. They are distinguished from ISA slots in two ways. First, they are shorter, and second, they are offset from the back edge of the motherboard by about an inch. PCI is a high-speed bus used for devices like video cards, hard disk controllers, and high-speed network cards. Newer PCI motherboards have the connectors for the hard disks coming directly from the motherboard. These connectors are part of the PCI bus, even though the hard disks are not connected to a physical PCI slot.

The newest PCs add another, new connector to the motherboard: an accelerated graphics port (AGP) slot. AGP is not really a bus, but is a single-device port used for high-performance graphics. The AGP slot looks similar to a PCI slot, except that it is offset further from the back edge of the motherboard.

Connectors, Ports, and Headers

Ports are connectors used to connect external cables and devices to the motherboard (Gookin, 1997). In addition to the keyboard and PS/2 mouse connectors, some types of motherboards have on the back edge of the motherboard integrated serial and parallel ports. Motherboards that do not use integrated ports, use headers on the motherboard instead. Headers are groups of pins used to connect devices or ports to the motherboard. A cable runs from the port and is plugged into the header on the board.

The following are the headers that are commonly found on a typical Baby AT-style motherboard (Norton, 1997):

Serial ports: There are usually two serial port headers. Each has 9 or 10 pins, however, only the first 9 are used. Serial ports are the COM ports identified in the system.

Parallel port: This header is used for the external parallel port and has 26 pins (25 are actually used). Parallel ports are frequently abbreviated LPT because they traditionally were used to connect line printer terminals.

PS/2 mouse port: Some good motherboards provide a header for a PS/2 mouse port when this port is not already on the board. The PS/2 mouse header has 5 pins.

USB (universal serial bus): A new technology at the time of this writing, USB is proposed to be the new standard for connecting as many as 127 peripherals such as keyboards, mice, and external modems in a daisy-chain linkage to the PC. Because they are not in common use yet, many motherboards provide a header to run a port for them in the future if needed, instead of an actual port. This header has 10 pins.

Infrared (IR) port: Some motherboards have a header that allows a connection for an infrared communications port, typically used for wireless communication to printers and similar devices. Infrared ports are far more common on laptop computers than desktop machines. These headers have 4 or 5 pins.

Primary and secondary Integrated Drive Electronics (IDE/ATA) hard disk interface: Most newer motherboards have integrated headers for two IDE channels. Each has 40 pins.

Floppy disk interface: Most newer motherboards provide a 34-pin header for the floppy disk cable.

Small computer systems interface (SCSI): Some motherboards have integrated SCSI ports or headers, although they are uncommon. They are either 50 or 68 pins in size, depending on the flavor of SCSI implemented.

Older motherboards that do not have integrated serial, parallel, floppy disk, and IDE hard disk headers or ports use an I/O controller board that plugs into an expansion slot to provide these functions. The connections are almost identical, although in some cases additional jumpers have to be set.

System Bus Functions and Features

The PC has a hierarchy, in a way, of different buses. Most modern PCs have at least four buses as is illustrated in Figure 19–2. Consider them a hierarchy because each bus is to some extent further removed from the processor; each one connects to the level above it, integrating the various parts of the PC together (Chambers, 1998). Each one is also generally slower than the one above it (for the pretty obvious reason that the processor is the fastest device in a modern PC):

The processor bus: This is the highest level bus that the chipset uses to send information to and from the processor.

The cache bus: Higher level architectures, such as those used by the Pentium Pro and Pentium II, use a dedicated bus

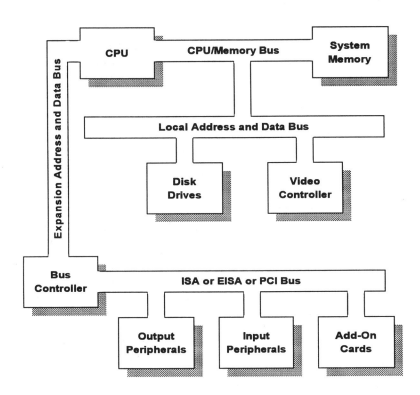

Figure 19–2   The computer bus.

for accessing the system cache. This is sometimes called a backside bus. Conventional processors using fifth-generation motherboards and chipsets have the cache connected to the standard memory bus.

The memory bus: This is a second-level system bus that connects the memory subsystem to the chipset and the processor. In some systems the processor and memory buses are basically the same thing.

The local I/O bus: This is a high-speed I/O bus used for connecting performance-critical peripherals to the memory, chipset, and processor. For example, video cards, disk storage devices, high-speed networks interfaces generally use a bus of this sort. The two most common local I/O buses are the VLB and the PCI.

The standard I/O bus: Connecting to the above three buses is the "good old" standard I/O bus, used for slower peripherals (mice, modems, regular sound cards, low-speed networking) and also for compatibility with older devices. On almost all modern PCs this is the ISA bus.

Some newer PCs actually use an additional "bus" that is specifically designed for graphics communications only. The word "bus" is in quotes because it is not actually a bus, it is a port: the AGP. The distinction between a bus and port is that a bus is generally designed for multiple devices to share the medium, whereas a port is only for two devices (Halliday, 1997). The AGP bus will be described in the section on video cards.

Every bus is composed of two distinct parts: the data bus and the address bus. The data bus is what most people refer to when talking about a bus; these are the lines that actually carry the data being transferred. The address bus is the set of

lines that carry information about where in memory the data are to be transferred to or from.

PITFALL

When purchasing an "Intel Inside" PC, carefully consider limiting the purchase to minimally a Pentium II processor with a clock speed of at least 350 MHz. This is because Intel's 350 MHz or faster processors use an external bus speed of 100 MHz. These chips require the special 440BX chipset. To be upgradeable, slower Pentium II–based systems must use this newer chipset, rather than the lower 66-MHz external bus architecture of the old 440LX chipset. *Therefore insist on the 440BX chipset or realize that you will never be able to upgrade beyond a 333-MHz Pentium II processor.* When purchasing an "AMD Inside" machine, make sure it is the new AMD-K6-2 processor running at least 300 MHz because of its improved performance and lower heat yields.

A bus is a channel over which information flows (Biow, 1997). The wider the bus, the more information can flow over the channel, much as a wider highway can carry more cars than a narrow one. The original ISA bus on the IBM PC was 8 bits wide. The universal ISA bus used now is 16 bits. The other I/O buses (including VLB and PCI) are 32 bits wide.

The memory and processor buses on Pentium and higher PCs are 64 bits wide. The address bus width can be specified independently of the data bus width. The width of the address bus dictates how many different memory locations that bus can transfer information to or from.

The speed of the bus reflects how many bits of information can be sent across each wire each second. This would be analogous to how fast the cars are driving on our analogical highway. Most buses transmit one bit of data per line, per clock cycle, although newer high-performance buses like AGP may actually move two bits of data per clock cycle, doubling performance. Similarly, older buses like the ISA bus may take two clock cycles to move one bit, halving performance.

Bus bandwidth, also called throughput, refers to the total amount of data that can theoretically be transferred on the bus in a given unit of time. Using the highway analogy, if the bus width is the number of lanes and the bus speed is how fast the cars are driving, then the bandwidth is the product of these two and reflects the amount of traffic that the channel can convey per second (Kobler, 1996).

SPECIAL CONSIDERATION

Advantages of the PCI bus

The PCI bus offers more expansion slots than most VLB implementations without the electrical problems that plagued the VESA bus. Most PCI systems support three or four PCI slots, with some going significantly higher than this. The PCI bus offers a great variety of expansion cards compared with VLB. The most commonly found cards are video cards (of course), SCSI host adapters, and high-speed networking cards. (Hard disk drives are also on the PCI bus but are normally connected directly to the motherboard on a PCI system.) However, it should be noted that certain functions cannot be provided on the PCI bus. For example, serial and parallel ports must remain on the ISA bus. Fortunately, the ISA bus still has more than enough speed to handle these devices, even today.

The PCI bus is also part of the Plug and Play standard developed by Intel, with cooperation from Microsoft and many other companies. PCI systems were the first to popularize the use of Plug and Play. The PCI chipset circuitry handles the identification of cards and works with the operating system and BIOS to automatically set resource allocations for compatible peripheral cards.

The most common bus in the PC world, ISA stands for Industry Standard Architecture, and unlike many uses of the word "standard," in this case it actually fits. The ISA bus is still a mainstay in even the newest computers, despite the fact that it is largely unchanged since it was expanded to 16 bits

in 1984. The ISA bus eventually became a bottleneck to performance and was augmented with additional high-speed buses, but ISA persists because of the truly enormous base of existing peripherals using the standard. Also, many devices still exist for which the ISA's speed is more than sufficient and will be for some time to come (standard modems being an example).

Many expansion cards, even modern ones, are still only 8-bit cards. Generally, these are cards for which the lower performance of the ISA bus is not a concern (Norton, 1997). However, access to interrupt request queries (IRQs) 9 through 15 is provided through wires in the 16-bit portion of the bus slots. This is why most modems, for example, cannot be set to the higher number IRQs. IRQs cannot be shared among ISA devices.

Currently by far the most popular local I/O bus, the PCI bus was developed by Intel and introduced in 1993. It is geared specifically to fifth-generation and sixth-generation systems, although the latest generation 486 motherboards use PCI as well (Norton, 1997). The PCI is a 32-bit bus that normally runs at a maximum of 33 MHz. The PCI bus is controlled by special circuitry in the set of chips that is designed to handle it. PCI is also used outside the PC platform, providing a degree of universality and allowing manufacturers to save on design costs.

Table 19–3 shows some of the characteristics of most of the common I/O buses on PCs today (White, 1998). Most buses cannot actually transmit anywhere near these maximum numbers because of command overhead and other factors. Most of these buses can run at many different speeds; the speed listed is the one most commonly used for the bus type.

System BIOS Functions and Operation

When the PC is turned on, the processor is "raring to go," but it needs some instructions to execute. However, because the system was just turned on, the system memory is empty; there are no programs to run. The BIOS sets up the hardware and software addresses, serving as the software interface for the different devices in the system. To make sure that the BIOS program is always available to the processor, even when it is first turned on, it is "hard-wired" into a read-only memory (ROM) chip that is placed on the motherboard.

A uniform standard was created between the makers of processors and the makers of BIOS programs, so that the processor would always look in the same place in memory to find the start of the BIOS program (Bigelow, 1997; Minasi, 1996; Norton, 1997). The processor gets its first instructions from this location, and the BIOS program begins executing. The BIOS program then begins the system boot sequence, which calls other programs, gets the operating system loaded, and gets the PC up and running.

Several components and features are commonly found these days as part of a modern BIOS. The main hardware component of the system BIOS is the system BIOS ROM itself. This is normally located in an electrically erasable read-only memory (EEPROM) chip, which allows it to be updated through software control. This is commonly called a flash BIOS. The BIOS ROM is located in a socket on the motherboard and is relatively easy to locate because it is usually labeled with the name of the BIOS manufacturer (Gookin, 1997) such as Award, American Megatrends (AMI), or

TABLE 19–3 Bus types and characteristics found in most PCs

Bus	Width (bits)	Bus Speed (MHz)	Bandwidth (Mbytes/s)
8-bit ISA	8	8.33	8.3
16-bit ISA	16	8.33	16.6
EISA	32	8.33	33.3
VLB	32	33	133.3
PCI	32	33	133.3
64-bit PCI	2.1	64	66
AGP	32	66	266.6
AGP (×2mode)	32	66×2	533.3
AGP (×4 mode)	32	66×4	1066.6

Phoenix. Often a version number is also on the chip, although the actual BIOS version within the chip may be different from what is labeled because of the ability to flash the BIOS previously mentioned.

The BIOS settings that used to control how the PC works must be saved in nonvolatile memory so that they are preserved even when the machine is off (White, 1998). This is as opposed to regular system memory, which is cleared each time the PC is turned off. A special type of memory is used to store this information, called Complementary Metal Oxide Semiconductor (CMOS) memory, and a very small battery is used to trickle a small charge to it to make sure that the data it holds are always preserved. These memories are very small, typically 64 bytes, and the batteries that they use typically last for years. This nonvolatile memory is sometimes called NVRAM.

PITFALL

Unfortunately, when the battery dies, the CMOS random access memory (RAM) is lost and the computer may not boot up. Always have a hardcopy of the CMOS RAM settings available so that when the battery fails, the system can be recovered. This is particularly important regarding storing information about the hard drives in CMOS. The CMOS RAM settings in most PCs can be accessed by choosing the "Setup" option during the system's boot up (turning the power on). Record the information provided in the "Setup" tables and store this information in a safe place.

The system uses something called a CMOS checksum as an error-detecting code (Chambers, 1998). Each time the BIOS setting is changed, the checksum is generated by adding together all the bytes in the CMOS memory and then storing the lowest byte of the sum. Then, each time the system is booted, the system recomputes the checksum and compares it

with the stored value. If they are different, the system knows that the CMOS has been corrupted somehow and will warn you with an error, typically something like "CMOS Checksum Error." In addition to the standard CMOS memory used to hold system settings, Plug and Play BIOSes use an additional nonvolatile memory to hold extended system configuration data (ESCD). This is used to record the resource configurations of system devices when Plug and Play is used.

BIOS Updates and the Flash BIOS

The quality and the currency of the BIOS determine the features and capabilities of a system to a large degree. The BIOS program in a PC is programmed into a ROM. ROMs are, of course, "read-only" and cannot be altered in the same way RAM is. This presents a problem when a user wants to update BIOS. In "the old days" the manufacturer sent a new BIOS chip, and the user installed the new chip to update BIOS. Although some computers still require the physical upgrade, most newer computers use flash BIOS and can upgrade using special software without having to open the case at all (Minasi, 1996). Machines with flash BIOS capability use a special type of BIOS ROM called an Electrically Erasable Programmable Read-Only Memory. This is a ROM that can be erased and rewritten using a special program.

Plug and Play

The BIOS is one of the four major parts of the system whose cooperation is required to implement Plug and Play features on a PC (Biow, 1997; Meyer, 1998). In short, Plug and Play (also called "PnP" for short) is a system whereby the PC hardware, BIOS, and operating system work together to identify and configure resource use by hardware devices automatically. The intention is to reduce the number of resource conflicts, jumper settings, and manual driver setups required to get the system to work. The BIOS is a key part of this; in fact it does much of the work of identifying and configuring expansion cards and passing configuration information on to the operating system.

The CPU

At the core of every computer is the microprocessor or central processing unit (CPU). It is not the computer's brain (Kobler, 1996). The operating system and software fill that role. The CPU is simply a tiny, fast calculator. The CPU consists of a single integrated circuit that houses hundreds of thousands of transistors. The type of CPU that a system contains determines its processing power or how fast it can execute various instructions. These types are grouped in families that describe their capabilities (Fitch, 1993, Minasi, 1996, Norton, 1997). The family of processors determines to a great extent which software will operate on which computer. The two major families of processors are those that are found in the PC computers (Intel and Intel compatible CPUs) and those that are found in the Macintosh computers. Software written for the PC computer will not work on a Macintosh computer unless either hardware or additional software is added to the Macintosh to make the software compatible. In addition, software written for a more advanced CPU within its own family may not be compatible with an earlier CPU. Regardless of the type of CPU, the power of the processor is generally described by its clock speed. However, several factors actually determine CPU performance. A summary of the characteristics of the PC computer information by processor type is presented in Table 19–4.

Clock Speed

Computer performance is a traffic problem, moving data and instructions from memory and around inside the chip (Minasi, 1996, Norton, 1997). The various parts of a computer hold instructions and data. Periodically they send these data along wires to the next processing station. To coordinate this activity, the computer provides a clock pulse. The clock is a regular pattern of alternating high and low voltages on a wire. The clock speed is measured in megahertz. One megahertz (1 MHz) is a signal that alternates between high and low values 1 million times/s. A 66-MHz PC has a clock that oscillates 66 million times each second. The clock pulse tells some circuits when to start sending data on the bus, whereas it tells other circuits when the data from the previous pulse should have already arrived.

Instructions per Cycle

Each PC instruction carries with it a number of additional operations that would not be obvious to the casual user (White, 1998). First, the computer must locate the next instruction in memory and move it to the CPU. This instruction is coded as a number. The computer must decode the number to determine the operation and the size of the data. Additional information is then moved and decoded to determine the location in memory. Finally, the number is added to the running total. Although a human might take some time to add two eight digit numbers together, the addition is the simplest part of the operation for a computer chip. Decoding the instruction and locating the data take the most time.

Each generation of Intel CPU chip has performed this operation in fewer clock cycles than the previous generation. A 386 CPU required a minimum of six clock ticks to add two numbers. A 486 CPU can generally add two numbers in two clock ticks. A Pentium CPU can add two numbers in a single clock tick. A Pentium II can add three numbers in a single clock tick, and when it discovers that one of the numbers is in slow memory, it will request that number and then skip ahead to add later numbers further down the column coming back to include the missing number when it arrives.

The Pentium chip checks each set of instructions as they are about to execute. If the two instructions are independent (that is, if the second instruction does not use the results of the first instruction), then both can start running at the same time. If the second depends on the previous instruction, it is held up, and in that clock tick only the first instruction begins execution. The next time the clock ticks again, the second instruction (and maybe the one after it) will begin execution, and the previous instruction will advance to the next phase of processing.

Memory

One basic rule exists regarding memory (Gookin, 1998): one never can have too much. The amount of memory depends on two factors: (1) What are the memory requirements of the software you intend to use? and (2) What is the current cost of the memory chips you can use? Memory is measured by the byte (Gookin, 1997; Kraynak, 1998). Think of a "byte" as a

TABLE 19–4 PC system characteristics by the type of CPU

Type of CPU	Clock Speed (MHz)	Bus Width	Addressable Memory	Cache Internal/External (kB)
8088 & 8086 (PC & XT)	4.7–10	8	640 kB	0/0
80286 (AT)	6–25	16	16 MB	0/64
80386	16–40	32	4 GB	0/128
80486 (5×86)	25–133	32	4 GB	8 kB/256
Pentium (6×86)	60–233	64	4 GB	16 Kb/512
Pentium II	233–450	64–100	64 GB	32 kB/512
Pentium III	400–650	100	64 GB	32 kB/512 or 1024

single character. A half page of text is about 1000 bytes or 1 kilobyte (KB). One megabyte (MB) refers to 1 million bytes and 1 gigabyte (GB) refers to 1 billion bytes or 1000 MB. Several different types of memory are in computers today.

Read-Only Memory

One major type of memory that is used in PCs is called ROM. ROM is a type of memory that normally can only be read, as opposed to RAM, which can be both read and written. ROM is used for certain functions within the PC for two main reasons (Bigelow, 1997; Minasi, 1996; Norton, 1997):

Permanence: The values stored in ROM are always there, whether the power is on or not. A ROM can be removed from the PC, stored for an indefinite period of time, and then replaced, and the data it contains will still be there. For this reason, it is called nonvolatile storage.

Security: The fact that ROM cannot easily be modified provides a measure of security against accidental (or malicious) changes to its contents. Computer viruses cannot infect ROM.

ROM is most commonly used to store system-level programs that need to be available to the PC at all times. The most common example is the system BIOS program, which is stored in a ROM called (amazingly enough) the system BIOS ROM. Having this in a permanent ROM means it is available when the power is turned on so that the PC can use it to boot up the system.

Although the whole point of a ROM is supposed to be that the contents cannot be changed, times occur when being able to change the contents of a ROM can be very useful. Several ROM variants can be changed under certain circumstances; these can be thought of as "mostly ROM." Many of these same technologies are used in digital and digitally programmable hearing aids. The different types of ROMs are presented in the following (Bigelow, 1997; Minasi, 1996; Norton, 1997):

ROM: A regular ROM chip is constructed from hard-wired logic much the way that a processor is. It is designed to perform a specific function and cannot be changed. ROM chips are only used for programs that are static (not changing often) and mass produced.

Programmable ROM (PROM): This is a type of ROM that can be programmed using special equipment; it can be written to, but only once.

Erasable Programmable ROM (EPROM): An EPROM is a ROM that can be erased and reprogrammed. A little glass window is installed in the top of the ROM. Ultraviolet light of a specific frequency can be shined through this window for a specified period of time, which will erase the EPROM and allow it to be reprogrammed again. Obviously this is much more useful than a regular PROM, but it does require the erasing light.

EEPROM: EEPROM can be erased under software control. This is the most flexible type of ROM and is now commonly used for holding BIOS programs.

Random Access Memory

The kind of memory used for holding programs and data being executed is called RAM (Gookin, 1997; Kraynak, 1998). RAM differs from ROM in that it can be both read and written. It is considered volatile storage because unlike ROM, the contents of RAM are lost when the power is turned off. RAM is called "random access" because earlier versions of read-write memories were sequential and did not allow random access. The volatility of RAM also means that the user risks losing data unless it is saved frequently. The most common type of RAM is *dynamic RAM*, called DRAM. DRAM must be refreshed often during program execution, or the information stored in it will vanish. Another type of RAM is *static* RAM. SRAM holds data until they are changed, eliminating refresh cycles.

The first 640 KB of RAM is called conventional memory. The name refers to the fact that this is where disk-operating systems (DOS), and DOS programs, conventionally run. Originally, this was the only place that programs could run. Today, despite the availability of much more memory, this 640-KB area remains the most important area for many programs because DOS cannot run programs outside this special area without additional support programs. Why is there a 640-KB "barrier?" The reason is the ill-fated decision by IBM to put the reserved space for system functions above the memory dedicated for user programs, instead of below it. In addition, many of the first processors could not address more than 1 MB of memory. This has caused the conventional memory area to be separated from the rest of the usable memory in the PC (extended memory). The upper memory area is the top 384 KB of the first megabyte of system memory.

In newer operating systems that run in protected mode, which means basically every operating system other than DOS, conventional memory is much less important. These programs are able to make use of extended memory for running programs. Extended memory is also for its hardware drivers in 32-bit operating systems like Windows 98. Certain parts of the code must still run in conventional memory, but because applications are not trying to cram code into the same area, usually no problem exists with limited memory.

All the memory above the first megabyte is called extended memory. This name comes from the fact that this memory was added as an extension to the base 1 MB that represented the address limits of memory of the original 8088 processor. The high memory area (abbreviated HMA) is the first 65,520 bytes (64 KB less 16 bytes) of extended memory. It is special because it is the only part of extended memory that can be used by the

PC while operating in real mode. Normally in real mode, the processor cannot access extended memory at all and must use protected mode or special drivers. This means that under normal DOS operation, extended memory is not available at all; protected mode must be used to access extended memory.

Extended memory is normally used in two ways. A true, full protected mode operating system like Windows NT can access extended memory directly. However, operating systems or applications that run in real mode, including DOS programs that need access to extended memory, Windows 3.1, Windows 95, and also Windows 98, must coordinate their access to extended memory through the use of an extended memory manager. The most commonly used manager is HIMEM.SYS, which sets up extended memory according to the extended memory specification (XMS). XMS is the standard protocol that PC programs use for accessing extended memory. HIMEM.SYS also is used to enable access to the high memory area, which is part of extended memory.

Memory Access and Access Time

Memory access occurs when memory is read or written. A specific procedure is needed and used to control each access to memory, which consists of having the memory controller generate the correct signals to specify which memory location needs to be accessed and then having the data show up on the data bus to be read by the processor or whatever other device requested it (Biow, 1997; White, 1998).

The amount of time that it takes for the memory to produce the data required, from the start of the access until when the valid data are available for use, is called the memory's access time. It is normally measured in nanoseconds (ns). Today's memory normally has access time ranging from 5 to 70 ns. This is the speed of the DRAM memory itself, which is not necessarily the same as the true speed of the overall memory system. Most memory in modern systems is 50, 60, or 70 ns in speed (Bigelow, 1997; Minasi, 1996; Norton, 1997). Systems running with a clock speed of 60 MHz or higher generally require 60 ns or faster memory to function at peak efficiency. SDRAM memory is much faster than conventional asynchronous RAM. It is usually rated at 12, 10, or even 7 ns.

Real and Virtual Memory

Real memory refers to the actual memory chips that are installed in the computer (Underdahl, 1998). All programs actually run in this physical memory. However, it is often useful to allow the computer to think that it has memory that is not actually there, to permit the use of programs that are larger than will physically fit in memory or to allow multitasking (multiple programs running at once). This concept is called virtual memory.

The way virtual memory works is relatively simple (White, 1998). For example, if the operating system needs 80 MB of memory to hold all the programs that are running, but only 32 MB of RAM chips are installed in the computer, the operating system sets up 80 MB of virtual memory and uses a virtual memory manager. A virtual memory manager is a program designed to control virtual memory to manage the 80 MB. The virtual memory manager sets up a file on the hard disk that is 48 MB in size (80 minus 32). The operating system then proceeds to use 80 MB worth of memory addresses. To the operating system, it appears as if 80 MB of memory exists. The virtual memory manager has to handle the fact that the system only has 32 MB of real memory.

Of course, not all of the 80 MB will fit in the physical 32 MB that exist. The other 48 MB reside on the disk in the file controlled by the virtual memory manager. This file is called a swap file. Whenever the operating system needs a part of memory that is currently not in physical memory, the virtual memory manager picks a part of physical memory that has not been used recently, writes it to the swap file, and then reads the part of memory that is needed from the swap file and stores it into real memory in place of the old block. This is called swapping, for obvious reasons. The blocks of memory that are swapped around are called pages.

Virtual memory was a very important invention in computing because it allows multitasking. Without virtual memory, it would be impossible to run a spreadsheet, word processor, and database program at the same time unless sufficient enough memory existed to hold all of them at once. The system would constantly be running out of memory and having to shut down program "A" to open program "B." Most PCs, when running multitasking operating systems like Windows 95, are using virtual memory.

However, virtual memory can also hamper performance (Underdahl, 1998). The larger the virtual memory is compared with the real memory, the more swapping has to occur to the hard disk. The hard disk is much, much slower than the system memory. Trying to use too many programs at once in a system with too little memory will result in constant disk swapping, called thrashing. Thrashing can cause system performance to slow to a crawl. It is caused especially when trying to use an operating system with a lot of system overhead, such as Windows NT, on a computer with insufficient system RAM.

In a real system, it is important to carefully manage how the total memory in the system is used (Chambers, 1998). Some systems try to improve performance through the use of disk caching. As they say, the road to performance hell is often paved with good intentions. In some cases the system will reserve so much of system memory for caching disk accesses that the remaining memory is not enough and thrashing will occur. So you are using part of disk as virtual memory and part of your memory as virtual disk, which seems to be self-defeating.

Cache

About 30 years ago, IBM demonstrated that a mainframe computer could run faster if it had "cache memory." The cache is a high-speed memory area that keeps a copy of the most recently used data in main memory (Kobler, 1996). Most programs go back and reexecute the same instructions, or update the same numbers, and the cache provides better performance.

A modern PC has two levels of cache. A first-level (L1) cache is contained within the CPU chip itself. The Intel 486 family was designed with 8K of L1 cache memory. The original Pentium chip increased this to 16K. The Pentium MMX and Pentium II chips increased it again to 32K. Data in the L1 cache are available immediately without any delay and allow the processor to run at full speed (Bigelow, 1997; Minasi, 1996; Norton, 1997).

An external or second-level (L2) cache is created with a modest amount (256K to 1M) of SRAM memory chips. On a

PITFALL

Some software modules used with NOAH move data to the cache memory in a system. If the system does not have cache memory, it will allocate a specific location in the RAM for storing data. Occasionally, the software will encounter conflicts in the memory allocation and not permit the storage of these data. Although most software modules that have these conflicts have or will have patches to resolve the conflicts, users should avoid these types of conflicts by purchasing systems that have a memory cache. It simply is not a good investment to purchase a system that does not have cache memory.

Pentium motherboard, the L2 cache is soldered to the motherboard. The Pentium CPU chip does not "know" that an L2 cache exists. Any time it needs data that are not in the internal cache, it generates the address on the bus to the memory controller in the motherboard chipset. If the memory controller finds the data in the L2 cache, it routes the request to the SRAM chips and does not generate any wait states. Otherwise, it routes the request to the DRAM and does generate the standard set of wait states.

The Pentium II comes in a package that combines the CPU chip with an integrated set of SRAM L2 cache chips (Bigelow, 1997; Minasi, 1996; Norton, 1997). In the Pentium II, the CPU does know about and manage the L2 cache itself, just as it manages the L1 cache. The CPU has a separate private bus to the L2 SRAM different from the external bus to the motherboard memory controller and therefore to the DRAM. This is quite useful for a CPU chip that can reorder and continue execution of additional instructions. At any moment, it can be block one instruction, fetching a needed unit of data from L2 cache, block a second instruction, fetching a second unit of data from DRAM, and still execute any subsequent instructions not dependent on the two that are blocked using data in the L1 cache.

Hard Disk Drives

Long-term storage is where most of a computer user's data lives (Biow, 1997; Gookin, 1997; Kraynak, 1998). Without some means of long-term storage, the computer is limited to handling only the data it can fit into its memory. Long-term storage is not the same as memory. Just about everything that is stored in "memory" is lost (or goes to data heaven) at one time or another. Computers use a variety of disks to store these data. Perhaps the most important type of long-term storage is the hard disk drive.

The purpose of a hard disk drive is to store computer data and instructions in the form of binary numbers. The source of the data and instructions is any software program that involves the computer's CPU working in conjunction with various peripheral components, including the hard disk drive itself (White, 1998).

Although a hard disk drive is the most complex component in a PC in terms of moving parts, its mechanical operation is actually quite straightforward. In many ways a hard disk drive operates like a music jukebox. Inside the drive's case are one or more constantly spinning aluminum-alloy platters arranged one on top of another in a stack. When a user enters commands through the keyboard or mouse, the hard drive's actuator arm, much like a jukebox's tone arm, responds to these commands and moves to the proper place on the platter. When it arrives, the drive's read/write head, like the needle on the tone arm, locates the information requested. The head reads, or retrieves, the information, transfers it to the CPU, and in short order, the data requested either appear onscreen, are queued up for printing, or are sent whirring across phone lines in the form of a fax or modem message.

Although the jukebox analogy holds for a hard drive's mechanical operation, the way in which hard drives write, store, and read data is more like the way an audio tape recorder works. Audio tape is coated with a thin layer of microscopic metallic particles. Sounds are recorded onto the tape by a recording head. These sounds are played back by a play head. Both the recording and play heads contain a small coil of wire through which electrical currents flow in continuously changing patterns that represent the sounds. As the tape passes under the recording head, it is magnetized by these currents. As it passes under the play head, the magnetic patterns are picked up, translated into audio data, and then passed to the amplifier and loudspeaker.

Data are written to and read from hard drives in much the same way. Like audio tape, hard drive platters are coated with a magnetic material a few millionths of an inch thick. But unlike an audio tape recorder, a disk drive uses a single read/write head to both write and read from the disk. To write information to a hard drive, an electrical current flowing through a coil in the read/write head produces a magnetic pattern in the coating on the media's surface corresponding to the data being written. To read information from a hard drive, the read/write head converts the magnetic patterns recorded on the media to an electrical current that is amplified and processed to reconstruct the stored data pattern.

The platter's surface is organized so the hard drive can easily find data. Concentric rings on the platters, called tracks, are divided into units called sectors. Information is recorded on the outermost track of all platters first. Once the outside track is filled up with data, the heads move inward and begin writing on the next free track. This recording strategy greatly boosts performance because the read/write heads can record more data at one position before having to move to the next track. For example, if the read/write heads in a four-platter drive are positioned on track 15, the drive writes to track 15 on both sides of all four platters before moving the read/write head inward to track 16.

The design of hard disk drives makes them quite fast, much faster than either tape or floppy diskette drives. Unlike floppy drives, hard drives virtually eliminate friction between the disk and read/write head, further speeding performance and reducing wear on the heads and media. When the desktop computer is turned on, the platters in the hard disk drive immediately begin spinning at 3600 rpm or higher. They remain spinning until the computer is turned off or loses power. This rapid spinning creates a tiny cushion of air above each platter, permitting the tiny read/write heads to float, or fly, just above the surface.

PITFALL

All hard disks eventually fail. A basic premise in computer technology is that hardware crashes are inevitable. Eventually, something will happen sometime to a computer system that makes it inoperable or needed information irretrievable. Many risks exist with data stored on a computer system, including hardware failure, software failure, file system corruption, accidental deletion, virus infection, theft, sabotage, and natural disaster. During the development of this chapter, the hard disk on the computer system used by the author to fit hearing aids crashed and the disk could not be accessed without extraordinary effort and costs. Having the NOAH database backed up on a tape drive, saved countless hours and dollars recovering patient data. No one is impervious to these threats and the wise computer user follows the first axiom of computing:

Back Up Back Up Back Up
Routine backup of all data files and all software packages is not an optional task, it is essential to prevent disaster. Although backing up data is in some ways a simple matter—*"just do it!"*—some special techniques that can come into play to make backups more effective and less of a hassle (Wynne, 1996a).

What is remarkable is that the read/write heads are precisely designed to fly just a few microns above the surface of the platters, a space considerably thinner than a shaft of human hair or even a particle of smoke (Bigelow, 1997; Minasi, 1996; Norton, 1997). Despite the speed and tolerances involved, the heads never touch the surface of the platters while the disk is spinning. When the system is turned off, the platters stop spinning, and the read/write heads touch down in a designated landing zone separate from the area on the platters where data are stored. If contamination or severe shock cause the heads to touch the surface or "crash," the heads or data surface can be damaged, data lost, and, in the most extreme cases, the drive can even be rendered inoperable. In the more current and advanced drives, however, crashes are rare because drives are tightly sealed to keep out contaminants and built to withstand shocks in the range of 70 to 100 times the force of gravity (70 to 100 g).

A drive interface is required to provide communication between the computer bus and the hard drive (Kobler, 1996). Among the information specified by drive interfaces is how fast the disk and controller should talk to one another, what kinds of commands they can pass back and forth, the location of data and control lines along the connecting cable, and what level of voltage they should use for data transfer. Thus a drive interface is a standardized combination of connector configuration signal levels and functions, commands, and data transfer protocols.

Two interfaces are commonly in use in today's PCs. Most IBM-compatible PCs use the IDE interface. Also called the AT or ATA (Advanced Technology Attachment) interface, for the PC/AT I/O bus it was designed to work with, IDE can transfer data at a rate of up to 4 MB/s. When connected by means of a bridge to a faster bus (e.g., local bus), AT drives can improve transfer rates up to 13 MB/s. The second most common interface is the SCSI (pronounced "scuzzy"). This higher performance interface, which is used on Apple Macintosh computers and high-performance workstations and servers, can transfer data at a rate of up to 10 MB/s in 8-bit mode and up to 20 MB/s in 16-bit mode.

Floppy Disk Drives

Although floppy disk drives vary in terms of size and the format of data that they hold and the user's convenience to share data across systems, they are all internally similar (Kobler, 1996). In terms of construction and operation, floppy drives are similar to hard disk drives, only simpler. Of course, unlike hard disks, floppy disk drives use removable floppy media instead of integrated storage platters.

The storage capabilities of floppy disks are determined primarily by the disk density. The density of the disk surface refers to the amount of data that can be stored in a given amount of space. This is a function of two basic factors: how many tracks can be fit on the disk (track density) and how many bits can be fit on each track (bit density). The product of these two factors is called area density, normally used to describe the capacity of hard disks. Floppy disks are usually instead specified using the separate terms: track density (measured in tracks per inch or TPI) and bit density (measure in bits per inch or BPI).

Virtually every hard disk has a different set of density characteristics. With floppy disks, the densities are more standardized. In fact, there are two standard types of 5.25" disks, and three standard types of 3.5" disks. These vary solely in terms of their density, which are given specific names. Table 19–5 shows the different density types and their characteristics (Bigelow, 1997; Minasi, 1996; Norton, 1997).

High-density and double-density media are not interchangeable. Always use high-density disks in high-density drives. It is possible to write data to double-density disks in a high-density drive, but you should always use the correct physical media. Although high-density drives are downward compatible with double-density disks, the high-density media are not. If a user wants to use the 720-KB format, the user must use double-density disks, even when using a high-density drive. In addition, the correct media density parameters must be specified when the disk is formatted. Otherwise, critical information can be lost as the disk is used between two or more different systems.

The future of floppy disk drives is difficult to predict (Meyer, 1998). Several different formats may become the new standard. The new formats will be "super floppies" that allow more than 10 MB of storage. One possible format that is emerging is the ZIP drive. This unit can be mounted internally or connect to the system through a parallel (which does not interfere with printing when installed properly) or SCSI port. ZIP disks typically store about 100 MB of data and are faster than a typical floppy drive but slower than a hard

TABLE 19–5   Characteristics of floppy disks

Density characteristic	360 KB (5.25″)	1.2 MB (5.25″)	720 KB (3.5″)	1.44 MB (3.5″)	2.88 MB (3.5″)
Track density (TPI)	48	96	135	135	135
Bit density (BPI)	5876	9869	8717	17,434	34,868
Density name	Double density (DD)	High density (HD)	Double density (DD)	High density (HD)	Extra-high density (ED)

drive. Although less common, Imation's SuperDisk stores 120 MB of data on its diskette and is backward compatible with the 3.5″ 1.44 MB floppy diskette. Both the ZIP disk and the SuperDisk are excellent media for storing large multimedia data files that contain graphics, sound, or video.

Removable Disk and Tape Drives

Removable drives are exactly what the name implies: high-capacity storage units that work like a fixed hard drive but can be removed or exchanged (Gookin, 1997; Kraynak, 1998). They are not fast but the external drives can be connected to different computers, including laptops, and the disks can be exchanged between both external and internal drives across systems. Many companies have developed drives and disks that can hold as much as 2 GB of storage at the time of this writing. The best application of these removable disk drives is hard drive backup.

CD-ROM

In terms of construction and basic components, CD-ROMs, laser disks, and digital video (or versatile) discs (DVDs) are rather similar in most regards to other storage devices that use circular, spinning media, which is not that much of a surprise. The big difference of course is the way the information is recorded on the media and the way that it is read from the media as well.

The middle two letters in "CD-ROM" stand for "read only," so it should not be any surprise that standard CD-ROM drives are read-only devices and cannot be altered. Newer variants of CD-ROMs, CD-R and CD-RW drives, break this long-standing rule of this type of device, and a user can now record or write on the CD disks with these drives (Chambers, 1998; Meyer, 1998).

CD-ROM drives do not use a read head in the conventional sense the way a floppy disk or hard disk does. It is not just that the "head" cannot record, it really is not a single solid head that moves over the surface of CD-ROM media, reading it. The head is a lens, sometimes called a pickup, that moves from the inside to the outside of the surface of the CD-ROM disk, accessing different parts of the disk as it spins. This is just like how a hard disk or floppy disk head works, but the CD-ROM lens is only one part of an assembly of components that together read the information off the surface of the disk.

The actual operation of how the laser beams in a CD-ROM work is quite complicated, but the overall principles are not (White, 1998). A beam of light energy is emitted from an infrared laser diode and aimed toward a reflecting mirror. The mirror is

part of the head assembly, which moves linearly along the surface of the disk. The light reflects off the mirror and through a focusing lens and shines onto a specific point on the disk. A certain amount of light is reflected back from the disk. The amount of light reflected depends on which part of the disk the beam strikes: each position on the disk is encoded as a one or a zero based on the presence or absence of "pits" in the surface of the disk. A series of collectors, mirrors, and lenses accumulates and focuses the reflected light from the surface of the disk and sends it toward a photodetector. The photodetector transforms the light energy into electrical energy. The strength of the signal depends on how much light was reflected from the disk.

Because the read head on a CD-ROM is optical, it avoids many of the problems associated with magnetic heads (Chambers, 1998). No contact occurs with the media as with floppy disks, so there is no wear or dirt buildup problem. No intricate close-to-contact flying height occurs as with a hard disk, so there is no concern about the disk crashing. However, because the mechanism uses light, it is important that the path used by the laser beam be unobstructed. Dirt on the media can cause problems for CD-ROMs, and over time dust can also accumulate on the focus lens of the read head, causing errors as well.

A standard CD has a capacity of about 74 minutes of standard CD audio music. Extended CDs can actually exceed this limit and pack more than 80 minutes on a disk, but these are nonstandard. Regular CD-ROM media hold about 650 MB of data, but the actual storage capacity depends on the particular CD format used.

With CD-ROM drives, the "X" speed (2X, 4X, etc.) is the key metric in determining the rate of information transfer between the drive and the CPU (Bigelow, 1997; Minasi, 1996; Norton, 1997). The first CD-ROMs operated at the same speed as standard audio CD players: roughly 210 to 539 RPM, depending on the location of the heads. This results in a standard transfer rate of 150 KB/s. It was realized fairly quickly that by increasing the speed of the spindle motor and using sufficiently powerful electronics, it would be possible to increase the transfer rate substantially. There is no advantage to reading a music CD at double the normal speed, but there definitely is for data CDs. Thus the double-speed, or 2X, CD-ROM was born. It was followed in short order with 3X, 4X, and even faster drives. Table 19–6 shows a summary of the transfer rates of different types of drives (Bigelow, 1997; Minasi, 1996; Norton, 1997).

The first CD format was of course that which defined the audio CD used in all regular CD players, called CD Digital Audio or CD-DA for short. Data in the CD DA format is encoded by starting with a source sound file, and sampling it to convert it to digital format (White, 1998). CD-DA uses a sample rate of 44.1 kHz. Each sample is 16 bits in size, and the

TABLE 19–6   Transfer rates for CD-ROM drives

Drive	Minimum /Transfer Rate (binary KB/s)	Maximum Transfer Rate (binary KB/s)
1X (CLV)	150	150
2X (CLV)	300	300
4X (CLV)	600	600
6X (CLV)	900	900
8X (CLV)	1200	1200
10X (CLV)	1500	1500
12X (CLV)	1800	1800
16X (CAV)	~930	2400
20X (CAV)	~1170	3000
24X (CAV)	~1400	3600
12X/20X (CLV/CAV)	1800	3600

sampling is done in stereo. Therefore each second of sound requires 176,400 bytes of storage. Audio data are stored on the disk in blocks, which are also sometimes called sectors. Each block holds 2352 bytes of data, with an additional number of bytes used for error detection and correction and control structures. Therefore 75 blocks are required for each second of sound. On a standard 74-minute CD then, the total amount of storage is 783,216,000 bytes or about 747 MB. From this derives the handy rule of thumb that a minute of CD audio takes about 10 MB when it is not compressed.

The data CD or CD-ROM uses two different modes in its standards (Tolliver & Kellogg, 1997). In mode 1, the standard data storage mode used by virtually all standard data CDs, the data is laid out in basically the same way as it is in standard audio CD format, except that the 2352 bytes of data in each block are broken down further; 2048 of these bytes are for "real" data, and the other 304 bytes are used for an additional level of error-detecting and correcting code. This is necessary because data CDs cannot tolerate the loss of a handful of bits now and then the way audio CDs can. Each block on the CD contains 2048 bytes of real data. As with the audio format, there are 75 blocks per "second" of the disk, so on a standard 74-minute CD, this yields a total capacity of 681,984,000 bytes, which is the same as the commonly heard 650 MB (actually 650.39 binary MB). Because the disk is designed to allow the reading of 75 blocks/s, this is the basis for the standard single-speed transfer rate of 150 KB/s. Of course, faster CD-ROM drives transfer at much higher rates.

Mode 2 CDs are the same as mode 1 CDs except that the error-detecting and correcting codes are omitted. Mode 2 format provides a more flexible vehicle for storing types of data that do not require high data integrity; for example, graphics and video can use this format. Furthermore, different kinds can be mixed together; this is the basis for the extensions to the original data CD standards known as CD-ROM Extended Architecture (CD-ROM XA).

Recordable CD (CD-R) drives (once known as Write Once Read Many or WORM drives), and the media they use, allow a regular PC user to create audio or data CDs in various formats that can be read by most normal CD players or CD-ROM drives at a reasonable cost. As "write once" implies, the disks start out blank, can be recorded once, and thereafter are permanent and not re-recordable. The disks created by most CD-R drives are compatible with most CD-ROM and CD audio disks. The keyword, of course, is "most." In particular, some older drives can have problems with the output of some CD-R drives. In general, though, it is not a problem. Some players can actually have more problems with some types of media than with others, because they use different dye and/or reflective metal layers. Changing the type of CD-R blanks used can sometimes fix an incompatibility problem.

A still newer technology, called rewritable CD or CD-RW, ups the ante one more notch by allowing CDs to be both written and rewritten (Bigelow, 1997; Minasi, 1996; Norton, 1997). CD-RW is also sometimes referred to as erasable CD or CD-E. CD-RW media are more similar to CD-R media than they are to regular CD-ROMs. CD-R media replaces the physically molded pits in the surface of the disk with a sensitive dye layer that can be burned to simulate how a standard CD works.

DVD Drives

To provide for the next generation of software, the new DVD format (sometimes this is referred to as the digital versatile disk format), was created. DVD uses the same physical format as CD-ROM but the similarities end there. The physical and logical formats are considerably different. A single side and layer of a DVD-ROM can hold 4.7 GB of data, more than seven times the capacity of a CD-ROM. A second data layer can be built above the first layer, providing an additional 3.8 GB of storage. DVD disks can also be double-sided. With double layers on each side, the disc's total storage can reach

17 GB. The first generation of DVD drives had a transfer rate of 1250 KB/s, which is now referred to as 1X. DVD drives rated at 4.8X work at a remarkably fast speed of 6535 KB/s. Because of the storage and speed capabilities of DVD, it can allow smooth video playback from the computer, even if the computer is busy. The current challenge of DVD technologies is the wide range of video file formats that are stored on DVDs. A future version of DVD called DVD-RAM may in fact even replaced your VCR. This is still quite new technology at the time of this writing and it is changing rapidly.

Sound Card

Some systems such as the Macintosh line of computers were designed with multimedia applications in mind and placed all the necessary components to process sound and graphics on their motherboards. For the PC line of computers, most systems today may take advantage of third-party sound cards and video accelerator cards to enhance multimedia applications and Internet functionality (Tolliver & Kellogg, 1997). Sound cards have a minimum of four tasks (Bigelow, 1997; Minasi, 1996; Norton, 1997). They function as a sound synthesizer, a Musical Instrument Digital Interface (MIDI) interface, an analog/digital converter (A/D) when sound is recorded from a microphone, and a digital/analog converter (D/A) when the digital sounds have to be reproduced in a speaker. The basic characteristics of the signal processing within sound cards are very similar to the signal processing in hearing aids and other digital instruments and will not be addressed in this chapter.

Most sound cards communicate with various peripherals such as microphones, MIDI instruments, and speakers through a variety of connectors. The connectors may look different on different sound cards, but you generally will find a jack for microphone input, a jack for line input, one or more output jacks for speakers, and a DB15 jack for MIDI instruments or a joystick. Sound cards also typically have a 2W built-in amplifier, which is enough to power a set of earphones but provides insufficient power to drive a pair of speakers. That is why speakers connected to a sound card must be self-powered or be driven by an external amplifier.

Video Card

The video card is only one part of the equation that determines what you see on your screen. It is in a way the "middle man," working between the processor and the monitor (Biow, 1997). The monitor, of course, is what actually provides the display that you see. The processor computes and thus determines what you are going to see. A conventional video card does the job of translating what the processor produces into a form that the monitor can display.

Older video cards did this translation only; they were rather dumb in that they could only take what the processor created and send it to the monitor. The processor did all of the work of deciding what would be displayed (White, 1998). This was fine for older environments like DOS and especially for text-based output where the amount of information involved was small. When graphical operating systems like Windows became the norm, suddenly large amounts of data were being shuffled around on the screen, and the CPU was spending a lot of time moving windows around, and drawing boxes, cursors, and frames. As a result, the processor would often get bogged down and performance would decrease dramatically.

To clear this bottleneck, companies began making cards called accelerators. In fact, the Windows graphical user interface drove this effort so much that they were often called Windows accelerators. These were video cards that added processors and memory to enable them to do much of the video calculating work that had been previously done by the processor. With an accelerator, when the system needs to draw a box on the screen, it does not compute where all the pixels need to be and what color, it sends a request to the video card saying "draw a window at these locations," and the video card does it (White, 1998). The processor can then go on to do more useful work. The accelerator, for its part, can be highly customized and tailored to this specific job and therefore it is far more efficient for this task than the CPU.

The screen image that can be seen on a monitor can contain as much as 6 MB of data just for the displayed image alone and not for the data itself that the image represents (Bigelow, 1997; Minasi, 1996; Norton, 1997). A screen of monochrome text, in contrast, needs only about 2 KB of space. In older systems special parts of the upper memory area (UMA) were dedicated to holding this video data. The processor would compute what needed to be displayed, would put it into this area, and then the video card would read it and display it.

As the need for video memory increased into the megabyte range, it began to make more sense to put the memory on the video card itself. The memory that holds the video image is sometimes called the frame buffer. A big advantage of having the memory on the video card is that it can be customized to the task at hand for greater efficiency, instead of using regular system RAM. The memory on the video card comes in many different sizes and flavors, and new technologies to improve performance are being invented all the time (Cambers, 1998). Newer motherboard designs use the new AGP, which lets the video processor access the system memory for doing graphics calculations but keeps a dedicated video memory for the frame buffer. This allows for more flexible memory use without sacrificing performance and is becoming a new standard in the PC world.

The screen image information stored in the video memory (RAM) is of course digital because computers operate on digital numbers. To display the image on the screen, the information in video memory must be converted to analog signals and sent to the monitor. The device that does this is called the RAMDAC, which stands for Random Access Memory Digital-Analog Converter (White, 1998). Many times each second, the RAMDAC reads the contents of video memory, converts the information, and sends it over the video cable to the monitor. The type and speed of the RAMDAC has a direct impact on the quality of the screen image, how often the screen can be refreshed per second, and the maximum resolution and number of colors that can be displayed.

The image that is displayed on the screen is composed of thousands (or millions) of small dots; these are called pixels; the word is a contraction of the phrase "picture element." A pixel represents the smallest piece of the screen that can be controlled individually. Each one can be set to a different color and intensity (brightness). The number of pixels that can be displayed on the screen is referred to as the resolution of the image; this is normally displayed as a pair of numbers, such as 640 × 480. The first is the number of pixels that can be displayed horizontally on the screen, and the second how many can be displayed vertically. The higher the resolution, the more pixels that can be displayed and therefore the more that can be shown on the monitor at once; however, pixels are smaller at high resolution and detail can be hard to make out on smaller screens. Resolutions generally fall into predefined standard sets; only a few different resolutions are used by most PCs (Bigelow, 1997; Minasi, 1996; Norton, 1997).

The aspect ratio of the image is the ratio of the number of X pixels to the number of Y pixels. The standard aspect ratio for PCs is 4:3, but some resolutions use a ratio of 5:4. Monitors are calibrated to this standard so that you can draw a circle and have it appear to be a circle and not an ellipse. Displaying an image that uses an aspect ratio of 5:4 will cause the image to appear somewhat distorted. The only mainstream resolution that currently uses 5:4 is the high-resolution 1280 × 1024.

PEARL

When using the high resolutions on the monitors, try experimenting with the font size settings to improve the screen images. Increasing the font size increases the displayed size of the text on the monitor (not the point size of the printed text in documents) while maintaining a high resolution on the screen.

Some confusion exists regarding the use of the term *resolution* because it can technically mean different things. First, the resolution of the image seen is a function of what the video card outputs and what the monitor is capable of displaying. To see a high-resolution image, such as 1280 × 1024, the system requires both a video card capable of producing an image this large and a monitor capable of displaying it. Second, because each pixel is displayed on the monitor as a set of three individual dots (red, green, and blue), some people use the term *resolution* to refer to the resolution of the monitor, and the term *pixel addressability* to refer to the

number of discrete elements the video card produces. In practical terms most people use resolution to refer to the video image. Table 19–7 lists the most common resolutions used on PCs and the number of pixels each uses (Bigelow, 1997; Minasi, 1996; Norton, 1997).

Each pixel of the screen image is displayed on a monitor using a combination of three different color signals: red, green, and blue. This is similar but not identical to how images are displayed on a television set. Each pixel's appearance is controlled by the intensity of these three beams of light. When all are set to the highest level the result is white; when all are set to zero, the pixel is black, and so on. The amount of information that is stored about a pixel determines its color depth, which controls precisely how the pixel's color can be specified. This is also sometimes called the bit depth because the precision of color depth is specified in bits. The more bits that are used per pixel, the finer the color detail of the image. However, increased color depths also require significantly more memory for storage of the image and also more data for the video card to process, which reduces the possible maximum refresh rate. Table 19–8 shows the color depths used in PCs today (Bigelow, 1997; Minasi, 1996; Norton, 1997).

The refresh rate is the number of times per second that the RAMDAC is able to send a signal to the monitor and the monitor is able to repaint the screen. The refresh rate is important because it directly impacts the ability to view the screen image. Refresh rates that are too low cause annoying flicker that can be distracting to the viewer and can cause fatigue and eye strain. The refresh rate necessary to avoid this varies with the individual, because it is based on the eye's ability to notice the repainting of the image many times per second. Refresh rate is measured in Hertz (Hz), a unit of frequency (Underdahl, 1998).

Because of the variability in video cards, The Video Electronics Standards Association (VESA) was formed to create and define these standards to specify a video card's capabilities. The standards are summarized in the Table 19–9 (Bigelow, 1997; Minasi, 1996; Norton, 1997).

The main problem with playing a movie or TV program on the PC is the sheer volume of data that is involved. Suppose a user wanted to display a 2-hour movie in high-quality, high-resolution graphics. To keep things simple, the user should choose just 640 × 480 in high color (16 bits per pixel) instead of going "all out" to 1024 × 768 in true color. Full-motion video typically means 30 frames/s. To store the data

TABLE 19–7 Factors determining screen resolution

Resolution	Number of Pixels	Aspect Ratio
320 × 200	64,000	8:5
640 × 480	307,200	4:3
800 × 600	480,000	4:3
1024 × 768	786,432	4:3
1280 × 1024	1,310,720	5:4
1600 × 1200	1,920,000	4:3

TABLE 19–8 Color characteristics of video standards

Color Depth	Number of Colors Displayed	Bytes of Storage Colors Per Pixel	Common Name for Color Depth
4-bit	16	0.5	Standard VGA
8-bit	256	1.0	256-color mode
16-bit	65,536	2.0	High color
24-bit	16,777,216	3.0	True color

TABLE 19–9 Characteristics of video adapter standards

Video Adapter	Maximum Resolution/Colors	Character Box Size	Monitors Supported	Graphics Supported?
Monochrome display adapter (MDA)	720 × 350/3	9 × 14	Mono TTL	No
Hercules graphics card (HGC)	720 × 350/3	9 × 14	Mono TTL	Yes
Color graphics adapter (CGA)	640 × 200/2	8 × 8	RGB composite	Yes No
Multicolor graphics array (MCGA)	640 × 200/2	8 × 16	Analog RGB	Yes
Enhanced graphics adapter (EGA)	640 × 350/4	8 × 14	RGB EGA Mono TTL	Yes No No
Video graphics adapter (VGA)	640 × 480/262,144	9 × 16	Analog RGB	Yes
Super VGA (SVGA)	1024 × 768/256	9 × 16	Analog RGB	Yes
8514/A	1024 × 768/262,144	9 × 16	Analog RGB	Yes
Extended graphics array (XGA)	1024 × 768/256	9 × 16	Analog RGB	Yes
Extended graphics array 2 (XGA2)	1024 × 768/262,144	9 × 16	Analog RGB	Yes

required for a full-motion, 2-hour movie at a resolution of 640 × 480 in high color (16 bits per pixel), the system would require approximately 133 GB and it still would not include sound. Also, the data to support this video stream would need to be pumped to the video card at the rate of about 150 million bits/s (Tolliver & Kellogg, 1997). There is a solution to this storage problem: data compression.

The most popular compressed video format is MPEG, which stands for the Motion Pictures Expert Group, the body that defined the standard. MPEG can typically compress as high as 100 to 1, bringing our 2-hour movie down to a much more manageable 1.33 GB. To use MPEG, the video must be encoded using an MPEG encoder and then viewed using an MPEG decoder. The MPEG decoders can either be a dedicated card or use a software application. A high-quality decoder will allow the display of full-screen, smooth video animation while leaving the system CPU free to do other tasks.

Monitors

In simple terms a monitor operates very similarly to how your regular television set works (Biow, 1997). The principle

is based on the use of an electronic screen called a cathode ray tube or CRT, which is the major (and most expensive) part of a monitor (Gookin, 1997). The CRT is lined with a phosphorous material that glows when it is struck by a stream of electrons emitted by guns at the back of the monitor. This material is arranged into an array of millions of tiny cells, usually called dots. These dots are visible on most monitors. To produce a picture on the screen, the electron guns start at the top of the screen and scan very rapidly from left to right. Then, they return to the leftmost position one line down and scan again; this is repeated to cover the entire screen. In performing this scanning or sweeping type motion, the electron guns are controlled by the video data stream coming into the monitor from the video card, which varies the intensity of the electron beam at each position on the screen. This control of the intensity of the electron beam at each dot is what controls the color and brightness of each pixel on the screen. This all happens extremely quickly; in fact, the entire screen is drawn in a small fraction of a second (White, 1998).

Three electron guns (on a color monitor) control the display of red, green, and blue light, respectively. The surface of the CRT is arranged to have these dots placed adjacently in a specific pattern. Separate video streams exist for each color coming from the video card, which allows the different colors to have different intensities at each point on the screen. By varying the intensity of the red, green, and blue streams, the full rainbow of colors is made possible.

Generally, like most things associated with computers, "bigger is better" but this is not always the case. The most popular sizes for monitors are 14 inches, 15 inches, 17 inches, 20 inches, and 21 inches. This number represents the (alleged) diagonal width of the monitor, the distance from one corner of the screen to the opposite corner of the screen, and is the monitor's nominal size. Most monitors use a 4:3 aspect ratio, which means the ratio of their width to their height is 4:3. This corresponds to the ratio used for most of the common video resolution modes such as 640×480, 800×600, and 1024×768 (but not all of them). The maximum resolution of a monitor is roughly related to its size, in that small monitors cannot generally display in very high resolution. However, this is a function of the features and quality (and age) of the monitor, and some 17-inch monitors can handle higher resolution than some 20-inch monitors. Because higher resolutions mean that the pixels become smaller, use of a high-resolution mode on a small monitor can be an exercise in squinting. On the other hand, when large monitors are run in lower resolution modes, the pixels tend to become quite large and "blocky," detracting from the quality of the image.

Most monitors are advertised with a dot pitch specification, usually from 0.25 to 0.40 (Kobler, 1996). Oddly enough, they often do not indicate what the unit is for this measurement; it is millimeters. The CRT's screen is made up of small elements (dots) of red, green, and blue phosphorous material. The dot pitch is the distance between adjacent sets of red, green, and blue elements. The dot pitch of the monitor indicates how fine the dots are that make up the picture. The smaller the dot pitch, the more sharp and detailed the image, all else being equal.

Keyboards

It is simply not enough to have current systems simply rely on the keyboard as the sole input device. However, until voice recognition becomes relatively fast, accurate, and reliable, the keyboard will remain as the primary line of communication between the user and the computer.

Computer keyboards are similar to electric typewriter keyboards but contain additional keys (White, 1998). The keys on computer keyboards are often classified as follows:

Alphanumeric keys—letters and numbers.

Punctuation keys—comma, period, semicolon, and so on.

Special keys—function keys, control keys, arrow keys, Caps Lock key, and so on.

The standard layout of letters, numbers, and punctuation is known as a QWERTY keyboard because the first six keys on the top left row of letters spell QWERTY. The QWERTY keyboard was designed in the 1800s for mechanical typewriters and was actually designed to slow typists down to avoid jamming the keys. The Dvorak Key Layout is an alternative arrangement of the keyboard's alphabetic keys in a layout that more evenly distributes typing among the fingers of both hands—keyboard designed for speed typing. The

Dvorak keyboard was designed in the 1930s by August Dvorak, a professor of education, and his brother-in-law, William Dealy. Unlike the traditional QWERTY keyboard, the Dvorak keyboard is designed so that the middle row of keys includes the most common letters. In addition, common letter combinations are positioned in such a way that they can be typed quickly. It has been estimated that in an average 8-hour day, a typist's hands will travel 16 miles on a QWERTY keyboard, but only 1 mile on a Dvorak keyboard. Although the Dvorak keyboard has been accepted by the American National Standards Institute (ANSI), it has not received widespread use.

No standard computer keyboard exists, although many manufacturers use similar "IBM PC and AT" designs for the keyboards for their systems. Three different PC keyboards actually exist: the original 84-key IBM PC keyboard; the 84-key AT keyboard; and the enhanced keyboard, with 101 keys. The three differ somewhat in the placement of function keys, the Control key, the Return key, and the Shift keys. In addition to these keys, IBM keyboards contain the following keys: Page Up, Page Down, Home, End, Insert, Pause, Num Lock, Scroll Lock, Break, Caps Lock, and Print Screen.

Several different types of keyboards are available for the Apple Macintosh. All of them are called ADB keyboards because they connect to the Apple Desktop bus (ADB). A single ADB port can support as many as 16 simultaneous input devices. The two main varieties of Macintosh keyboards are the standard keyboard and the extended keyboard, which has 15 additional special-function keys.

The Mouse and other Input Devices

Input devices other than the keyboard are sometimes called alternate input devices (Biow, 1997). Mice and pointing devices, such as trackballs, touchpads, and drawing tablets, are all alternate input devices. A mouse is a small object the user rolls along a hard, flat surface. Its name is derived from its shape, which looks a bit like a mouse, its connecting wire that one can imagine to be the mouse's tail, and the fact that one must make it scurry along a surface (Gookin, 1997). Mice contain at least one button and sometimes as many as three, which have different functions depending on what program is running. Many of the newer mice also include a scroll wheel for scrolling through long documents or for surfing the Internet.

The mouse is important for graphical user interfaces because the user can simply point to options and objects and click a mouse button. Such applications are often called point-and-click programs. The mouse is also useful for graphics programs that allow users to draw pictures by using the mouse like a pen, pencil, or paintbrush. Three basic types of mice exist (Bigelow, 1997; Minasi, 1996; Norton, 1997):

Mechanical mouse: This mouse has a rubber or metal ball on its underside that can roll in all directions. Mechanical sensors within the mouse detect the direction the ball is rolling and move the screen pointer accordingly.

Optomechanical mouse: This mouse operates in a similar manner to the mechanical mouse but uses optical sensors to detect the motion of the ball.

Optical mouse: This mouse uses a laser to detect the mouse's movement. The mouse must move along a special mat with a grid so that the optical mechanism has a frame of reference. Optical mice have no mechanical moving parts. They respond more quickly and precisely than mechanical and optomechanical mice, but they are also more expensive and are limited to the resolution of the grid on the mouse pad.

A trackball is a mechanical mouse lying on its back (Kraynak, 1998). The advantage of trackballs over mice is that the trackball is stationary so it does not require much space to use it. In addition, a trackball can be placed on any type of surface, including a lap. For both these reasons, trackballs are popular pointing devices for portable computers. One derivation of the trackball is the fingertip mouse which is nothing but a tiny button about the size of a pencil eraser that sits in the middle of the laptop's keyboard.

Another type of pointing device is the touchpad. This input device is a pressure-sensitive surface that tracks movements and tapping of the user's fingers. They do not require a pen or other stylus and are easily incorporated on laptops. The drawing tablet is simply a larger version of the touchpad but designed specifically for computer art and drafting.

Optical Scanner

With the help of an optical scanner, a user can digitize and store anything that can be copied legally (Johnson, 1998). A scanner works by digitizing an image, dividing it into a grid of boxes, and representing each box with either a zero or a one, depending on whether the box is filled. For color and gray scaling, the same principle applies, but each box is then represented by up to 24 bits. The resulting matrix of bits, called a bit map, can then be stored in a file, displayed on a screen, and manipulated by programs.

Most scanners use charge-coupled device (CCD) arrays, which consist of tightly packed rows of light receptors that can detect variations in light intensity and frequency. The quality of the CCD array is probably the single most important factor affecting the quality of the scanner. Industry-strength drum scanners use a different technology that relies on a photomultiplier tube (PMT), but this type of scanner is much more expensive than the more common CCD-based scanners.

Typically scanners support resolutions of from 72 to 600 dpi (maranGraphics, 1996). The number of bits used to represent each pixel is known as the bit depth. The greater the bit depth, the more colors or gray scales can be represented. For example, a 24-bit color scanner can represent 2 to the 24th power (16.7 million) colors. Note, however, that a large color range is useless if the CCD arrays are capable of detecting only a small number of distinct colors.

PITFALL

It is easy to take advantage of the ease and convenience of scanning or downloading copyrighted material into your own documents without giving appropriate credit. Changes in copyright laws have not kept pace with changes in technologies (Wynne & Hurst, 1995). Plagiarism is wrong. Simply do it; always give credit where credit is due.

Most scanners come bundled with various software programs, which include the image-acquisition software to digitize the image. In addition, nearly all scanners come with a TWAIN driver, which makes them compatible with any TWAIN-supporting software. TWAIN is an acronym for Technology (or Toolkit) Without An Interesting Name, the de facto interface standard for scanners. Unfortunately, optical scanners do not distinguish text from illustrations. All images are represented as bit maps. Therefore to edit text read by an optical scanner, you need optical character recognition (OCR) software to translate the digitized image into ASCII characters. Most optical scanners sold today come with OCR packages.

Digital Cameras

Digital photographs can be produced in a number of ways: (1) by scanning a conventional photograph, (2) by capturing a frame from a video, and (3) directly with a digital camera. A digital camera stores images digitally rather than recording them on film (Meyer, 1998). Once a picture has been taken, it can be downloaded to a computer system, then manipulated with a graphics program, and finally printed. Unlike film photographs, which have an almost infinite resolution, digital photos are limited by the amount of memory in the camera, the optical resolution of the digitizing mechanism, and the resolution of the final output device. Even the best digital cameras connected to the best printers cannot produce film-quality photos.

Printers

For years, computer pundits have been talking about the "paperless" office. Hard copy (printed documents) is far from obsolete, and evidence exists that integration of computer systems into offices and homes has actually increased paper consumption (Albrecht, 1997; Underdahl, 1998). Although printing is the last step in most projects, the hard copy of the project is often the first and only form other individuals will see of that project. Consequently, investing in good quality printers makes sense.

Many different types of printers exist. In terms of the technology used, most printers available at the time of this writing fall into the following categories (Biow, 1997; Underdahl, 1998):

Dot-matrix: Creates characters by striking pins against an ink ribbon. Each pin makes a dot, and combinations of dots form characters and illustrations.

Ink-jet: Sprays ink at a sheet of paper. Ink-jet printers produce high-quality text and graphics.

Laser: Uses the same technology as copy machines. Laser printers produce very high-quality text and graphics.

LCD and LED: Similar to a laser printer, but uses liquid crystals or light-emitting diodes rather than a laser to produce an image on the drum.

Thermal: An inexpensive printer that works by pushing heated pins against heat-sensitive paper. Thermal printers are widely used in calculators and fax machines.

Printers are also classified by their characteristics. The quality of type is an important feature of the printer. The output produced by printers is said to be either letter quality (as good as a typewriter), near-letter quality, or draft quality. Only ink-jet and laser printers produce letter-quality type. Some dot-matrix printers claim letter-quality print, but if you look closely, you can see the difference. The available resolutions in current laser printers range from 300 dpi at the low end to 1200 dpi at the high end. By comparison, offset printing usually prints at 1200 or 2400 dpi. Some laser printers achieve higher resolutions with special techniques known generally as resolution enhancement.

The speed of the printer is measured in characters per second (cps) or pages per minute (ppm); the speed of printers varies widely. Although the line printers connected to mainframe printers are the fastest (up to 3000 lines per minute), laser printers range from about 4 to 20 text pages per minute, which is adequate for most office tasks. An important characteristic of printers for audiology clinics is the difference between impact and nonimpact printers: impact printers are much noisier. However, even nonimpact printers can generate high levels of noise because of their printer engines. The noise of the printer should be assessed before it is used in any clinical operation.

The computer and printer exchange information typically through a parallel interface (Kobler, 1996). Parallel and serial ports differ in the way they transfer data and are not interchangeable. A serial port transfers one bit of data at a time, whereas a parallel port transfers 1 byte (8 bits) of data at a time simultaneously through eight wires in the parallel cable, thus speeding transmission of the data dramatically. The problem with parallel cables is that after about 10 to 12 feet, some interference across the eight channels occurs and data can be lost. Therefore if distant users wish to share printers such as through a network or if the printer is placed at a distant location from the computer, the user will need to use a serial interface for the printer connection.

Modems

A modem converts digital signals from your computer into audible tones that can be transmitted over ordinary analog phone lines. This process is called modulation. On the receiving end, a modem demodulates the analog signals arriving over the phone line into electrical signals, which are then fed to the computer. *Mo*dulation and *Dem*odulation accurately describe what modems do (White, 1998). Modem is a word born out of the combination of these two words: *mo*dulator/*dem*odulator. These words were chosen because they describe the actions a modem takes in the most precise way. Modems are no more than an extension to a computer, designed to use ordinary telephone lines to carry digital computer data (Crumlish, 1997). The particular brand of computer makes no difference; whether it is a PC, Macintosh, laptop, or workstation, the user can send files to other computers. In fact, with the right cable and a little tweaking, a user can use the exact same external modem with an IBM, or a Macintosh, or a Unix workstation. Internal modems must be installed in slots with its specific bus architecture and are not as easy to swap as external modems.

PCMCIA (or "PC Card") modems form a gray area between internal and external modems. Their design is more like an internal modem, but in theory, any computer with a PCMCIA slot of a given type should be able to use a PCMCIA modem of that type. In practice, sufficient variance still exists among different machines to cause occasional compatibility problems, and driver problems often occur between Macintosh and PC machines as well. It is now possible to purchase a PCMCIA modem card that will work on any PC or Macintosh with a type I/type II PCMCIA slot (although it is necessary to buy extra hardware for a desktop machine); however, only a few modems exist for which this is true. At the present, though, PCMCIA modems are really only an option for PC laptops or notebooks and some PowerBooks.

The most important feature in terms of cost is the speed of the modem (Crumlish, 1997). All current modems support the V.34/V.34bis (28,800/33,600 bps) communications standard and typically include error-correction and data compression; in addition, most modems support one of the competing 56,000 bps standards. When a user connects to a service, the connection rate is the highest speed that is mutually supported by both modems so a V.34 (28,800 bps) modem connecting to a 4800 bps BBS access number will only transmit data at 4800 bps.

At present, the V.34bis international standard is the fastest speed available from a large number of vendors. The V.34bis protocol supports connections as high as 33,600 bps over very clean phone lines. V.34bis superseded V.34 (28,800 bps) in mid-1996; many vendors are still producing V.34 modems, and, as mentioned previously, occasional V.32bis 14.4 kbps modems are also available.

In addition to V.34bis, Rockwell and US Robotics have recently released independent protocols (K56flex and X2, respectively) for attaining up to 57,600 bps on standard phone lines (although FCC EMF restrictions have forced them to limit themselves to 56,000 bps; hence the term *56K modems*). Essentially, these protocols take advantage of the phone companies' digital routers to compress and encode data, allowing a provider who has made appropriate arrangements with the local telephone company to push data out at an incredibly high rate of speed.

X2 and K56flex are protocols, not standards. They are also mutually incompatible. If a modem supports the USR's X2 protocol, when the user dials into a provider whose modems use Rockwell's K56flex protocol, the connection will have a default back down to the V.34bis 33.6 kbps connection and not to a 56K connection. Both Rockwell and USR have submitted their protocols to the ITU as a proposed standard, and some kind of 56K standard will probably show up after this book is printed, which will probably be incompatible with one or both of the existing protocols. When purchasing a 56K modem, make sure that the manufacturer will provide an upgrade path to the standard that emerges. Although 56K connections do not require any special phone wiring, they do work much better if the phone lines are "clean" (i.e., they do not have a lot of static). Old or poorly maintained phone lines may prevent making a good 56K connection. If the phone lines are too "dirty" for 56K, try contacting the local telephone company and see if they can be replaced.

ISDN, xDSL, and Cable Modems

Integrated Service Digital Network, or ISDN, is a standard for digital telecommunications (Sapien & Piedmo, 1996). Because ISDN uses an entirely different technology from the existing telephone system, it can achieve two or three times the speed obtained with a "normal" V.34 modem and a much cleaner, more reliable connection. ISDN does not use the same kind of wiring that the "normal" telephone system uses. Just installing ISDN phone lines may run anywhere from $100 to 300 for the local phone company to lay new wiring to a computer in a home or business. This will, in all likelihood, replace any existing phone wiring and may lead to considerably higher phone bills each month. ISDN requires your computer to have special connection hardware frequently called an "ISDN modem" or "digital modem," although technically speaking it is not a modem. Standard modems will not work over ISDN without a special adapter and will not take advantage of ISDN's speed.

A large number of rivals to ISDN for providing high-speed networking at a low cost exist. Most of these rely on "Digital Subscriber Lines" or DSL; and a lot of them exist, each one sticking its own letter in front of "DSL"—hence the collective term for all of them is "xDSL." Only one of the xDSL solutions (HDSL) is in any kind of widespread use at this point, but in general they all provide data-only service (*no* telephone service) over a leased line at speeds higher than ISDN but lower than T1 or T3 (the connections all the major Internet service providers use). The various xDSL systems are all aimed more at corporate or business users and will probably be priced out of the range of private individuals.

The major competitor for "something better showing up," though, is cable modems (Crumlish, 1997). In theory, the cabling used by cable TV companies is a high-grade networking cable capable of transmitting data at speeds that put ISDN to shame; they only need to develop some kind of box that is plugged in at home that will transform data from a computer into something that can be sent back over the cable—the "cable modem" in question. In practice, still a *lot* of bugs need to be worked out, the main one being that all their networking setup assumes data will go only one way from the cable company to a TV. Nonetheless, a number of companies are looking into the possibility of providing this service.

The HI-PRO System

The Hearing Instrument Programming System or HI-PRO is a hardware unit coupled together with a software package that serves as a standardized interface between a PC-compatible computer system and programmable hearing aids and, in some instances, a remote control for programmable hearing aids. It simply provides a common communication interface that a hearing instrument manufacturer can use to program hearing instruments. Because it is a common communication platform, it serves as the linkage between the programmable hearing instrument and the software used to program the instrument. Because it is only an interface, the manufacturer can provide any number of different features in the software and a different interface for specific hearing instruments.

SPECIAL CONSIDERATION

In the future it is feasible, if not likely, that many hearing aid users will have a modified interface for their programmable hearing aids that allows programming the instruments at the user's home without the audiologist leaving the office.

The HI-PRO system connects to a serial (COM) port on the computer system by means of a 9-pin serial data interface (null modem) cable to the RS-232C connector on the rear of the HI-PRO box as is illustrated in Figure 19–3. The hearing instruments connect to the box by means of a cable that has, at one end, a male 6-pin mini-DIN connector that is inserted in the front of the HI-PRO unit.

Unfortunately several issues arise when trying to initially connect the HI-PRO system to the computer. First, if the COM connectors on the PC have a 25-pin connector, a 9- to 25-pin adapter will be required to connect the cable to the PC. Second, the computer must recognize which serial port provides the interface for the HI-PRO unit. Most computers come with a minimum of two serial or COM ports. The computer defaults to recognizing one of a possible four COM ports, numbered sequentially from COM1. Frequently, the mouse or the keyboard may occupy the first COM port. It is critical that the communication protocol for the HI-PRO box is directed to the correct COM port to which it is attached.. The HI-PRO/NOAH software includes a test module to determine whether the COM port selected actually allows communication from the PC to the unit and back again. In addition, because peripherals are only recognized by the operating system when they are connected at the time the system boots up, one should make sure all connections are securely installed before the computer is booted up. If these suggestions do not work and all else fails, contact the support personnel at the hearing instrument manufacturer.

NETWORKS

The first desktop computer systems were stand-alone units (Nunemacher, 1995). Each system had a separate set of applications, its own data, and its own specific profile

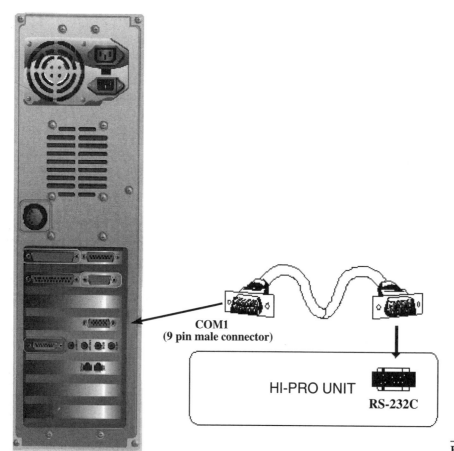

COM1
(9 pin male connector)

HI-PRO UNIT

RS-232C

Figure 19–3   HI-PRO connection to PC

of peripheral equipment. As the capacity of computers increased, the need to share data across systems and the need to share expensive peripherals increased. Connecting computer systems and devices together into a network allow computer users to send and receive information to and from each other. A network allows you to share information without having to carry or mail disks or paper, ensure that your staff has the same software release, communicate with a colleague on another campus, access shared information, and share printers or other devices (Bria & Rydell, 1996; Kreider & Haselton, 1997). Networks even make computer systems work better and more efficiently than when they work alone. Networking is the future for home computing.

Individual workstations (desktop computer systems) are typically connected by cable to a shared computer known as a server (Nunemacher, 1995). Either an ethernet card or token ring board is in each computer that allows it to be connected to the network. Both workstation and server use software that allow the computers to speak the same language. In local area networks (LANs), the server is usually located relatively close to the individual workstations. If the network covers a large geographical area, it is known as a wide area network (WAN). Individual computers can be connected directly to a WAN through a data line from the office or a modem from home without first going through a LAN.

Three components are required to have full access to a network (local or wide) from a workstation. The first component

is hardware. The workstation must have an ethernet card or token ring board installed and a cable running from this card to the data jack in the office. The data jack must be wired from the workstation through the building to the server's backbone. Once this hardware wiring connection is made, the infrastructure is in place to access the network. An introduction to cabling, topologies, routing, bridging, and interfaces is beyond the scope of this chapter, and simple solutions are not readily available for networking more than two or three computers at this time. The second component is network software that recognizes the hardware and will use it. Different software is required, depending on the network access the user wants. For a WAN, software is needed to access the Internet through a computer-to-computer communications protocol such as transmission control protocol/internet protocol (TCP/IP) (Campbell, 1997). Figure 19–4 illustrates the types of Internet connections for both home and business environments. For a LAN, network operating system software such Novell Groupware or Windows NT is needed. If users want to access the WAN and the LAN, both kinds of software are needed. The third component is application software running on the LAN. Examples of these applications would be any network version of word processors, databases, spreadsheets, and so on. These packages are designed to provide multiple access to files and records and to lock files and records so that a particular document can be edited by only one person at a time.

Files are shared by putting them on the server and giving read/write privileges to those who should have access to the

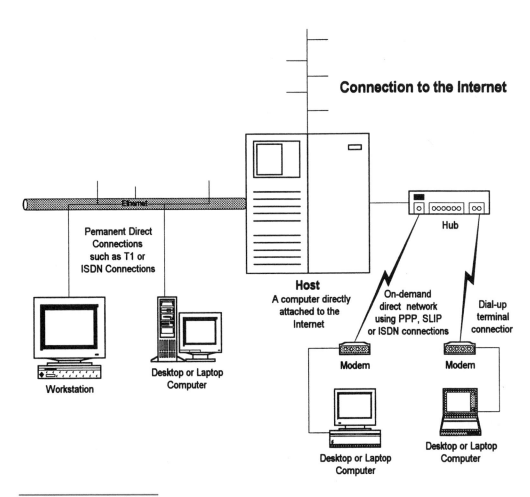

Figure 19–4 Types of Internet connections. (From Wynne [1996a], with permission.)

files. The area on the server is then defined and given a drive letter (i.e., drive G). A user would access these files just as they would files on the hard drive in their own desktop using the appropriate drive letter. Files that need to be available for general access to all users on the network should be stored on the file server. This makes these files easier to access and easier to back up. Personal files would normally be stored on the hard disk on your computer. Occasionally personal space can be allocated to individuals on the server if enough extra space is available.

Open Systems Interconnection

Because the functions and features of a network are quite varied, the International Standard Organization (ISO) has developed the Open Systems Interconnection (OSI) model to organize the functions of a network (Bourke & Grimes, 1995). The OSI model defines the network as a series of layers as defined in Table 19–10. Each layer is responsible for a certain network function and only interacts with the layers immediately above and below it.

Several manufacturers and software developers developed their own conventions before the endorsement of the OSI model. The three examples following represent how vendor models were developed for the mainframe, mainframe, and desktop computers. Systems Network Architecture (SNA) from IBM was designed to support terminals and printers

connected to mainframes through controllers and front-end processors. The user establishes a mutually agreed-on connection with a mainframe, and synchronous communication occurs for the duration of the session. Local Area Transport (LAT) was developed by DEC to route information through an Ethernet connection between user terminals and minicomputer servers. The Novell Internet Packet Exchange/Sequenced Packet Exchange was used for small workgroup LANs and enables program-to-program communication. Most networks today, however, are OSI compatible.

TCP/IP

Transfer Control Protocol (TCP) and Internet Protocol (IP) were developed by a Department of Defense (DOD) research project to connect a number different networks designed by different vendors into a network of networks (the "Internet") (Wynne, 1996b). It was initially successful because it delivered a few basic services that everyone needs (file transfer, electronic mail, remote logon) across a very large number of client and server systems. Several computers in a small department can use TCP/IP (along with other protocols) on a single LAN. The IP component provides routing from the department to the enterprise network, then to regional networks, and finally to the global Internet. On the battlefield a communications network will sustain damage, so the DOD designed TCP/IP to be robust and automatically recover

TABLE 19–10 Network layers by function

Network Layer	Function
Layer 7—Application	Common or generic features of any software application such as e-mail, naming, database assess, file transfer, etc
Layer 6—Presentation	Data formats, syntax, record structure, encryption, and compression
Layer 5—Session	Interface with host operating system that keeps track of the different network sessions
Layer 4—Transport	End-to-end integrity of the message transmitted across the network
Layer 3—Network	Routing of messages across and among networks
Layer 2—Data link	Access to the immediate network
Layer 1—Physical	Electromechangical characteristics of the medium and connectors

from any node or phone line failure. This design allows the construction of very large networks with less central management. However, because of the automatic recovery, network problems can go undiagnosed and uncorrected for long periods of time.

As with all other communications protocol, TCP/IP is composed of the following layers:

Internet protocol: The IP is responsible for moving a packet of data from node to node. IP forwards each packet on the basis of a 4-byte destination address (the IP number). The Internet authorities assign ranges of numbers to different organizations. The organizations assign groups of their numbers to departments. IP operates on gateway machines that move data from department to organization to region and then around the world.

Transfer control protocol: The TCP is responsible for verifying the correct delivery of data from client to server. Data can be lost in the intermediate network. TCP adds support to detect errors or lost data and to trigger retransmission until the data are correctly and completely received.

Sockets: These are packages of subroutines that provide access to TCP/IP on most systems.

Network Nodes

Each computer (also called a node) on the Internet is identified by an individual address, much like a house or apartment is identified by a number and street name. Internet addresses are written as a number in the form 134.68.1.1 and are referred to as IP (Internet Protocol) numbers (Thomas, 1997). IP numbers give information about the node's location on the network and can uniquely identify a workstation to other hosts using TCP/IP.

To make it easier for users to communicate with each other through e-mail, each node has a written name in addition to the numeric IP number. For example, opal.iupui.edu identifies the mail server for the author of this chapter at the time of this writing. The host or node name is the part of an e-mail address that comes after the @ symbol followed by the host's primary domains. There are six primary domains for sites in the United States: com (commercial), edu (educational), gov (government), mil (military), net (network), and org

(organization). The user name then defines the directory location on the node. For example, when e-mail is sent to *mwynne@ iupui.edu*, the message is deposited in the e-mail directory for the user mwynne at the opal.iupui.edu node. The node name is shortened through a mail router at a higher level.

Network Security

Network security involves two areas of concern: theft or vandalism and virus infection. Theft or vandalism can involve either hardware or software/data. Hardware, whether networked or not, can be protected by ensuring that the location is secure. Software and/or data are much more vulnerable on a network because they may be affected by more than one person or workstation. Shared software or data, if damaged or stolen, may hamper the productivity of an entire department (Underdahl, 1998).

Software and/or data can be made more secure by following some simple procedures. First, only authorized persons should have access to the network and network files. All shared resources must have a detailed chain of authorization defining who can read a file, who can write to a file, and who can delete a file. Files and computers should be password protected, and passwords should follow established security guidelines. Backup procedures should be in place and off-site storage of backups should be maintained so that, in the event of a problem, software and data can be restored.

MOBILE COMPUTING

Although laptop computers are easily transported from one location to another, laptop computers are really just small desktop systems. Although Palm PCs, a portable computer that is small enough to be held in a hand (Parker, 1998; Pogue, 1997), have been around for some time, it was only recently that the devices were accepted by general users. Palm PCs are often called handheld computers, Palmtops, pocket computers, and personal digital assistants (PDAs), although this last term is really reserved for those devices that only serve as dedicated personal organizer (Forbes & Ruley, 1998).

Handheld PCs are not intended to be stand-alone computers. They are more like containers for just that slice of desktop you are likely to need on the road. They lack many of the hardware components necessary for desktop systems but offer many advantages over other computer platforms, namely convenience, portability, and functionality. Palm PCs come with built-in connectivity to desktop systems through synchronization hardware and software. Synchronization allows the user to carry and quickly access information that might otherwise stay stored on a desktop system. Most synchronization is accomplished through proprietary software with serial cables, but infrared synchronization between the Palm PC and the desktop but also between Palm PCs is currently available.

Because of their size, Palm PCs use a different operating system than do desktop and laptop computers. A version of Windows was specifically designed for use in many hand-held computers. The Windows CE graphical user interface (GUI) is very similar to Windows 95 so devices running Windows CE should be easy to operate for anyone familiar with Windows 95. Windows CE is not 100% compatible with your desktop Windows applications at this time, but problems are fairly inconsequential. Both the Palm Pilot and the Newton devices come with their own proprietary operating systems. Each operating system presents unique advantages and disadvantages for programmers, but most users will not need to know as much about these operating systems as they do about the operating systems used in the desktop and laptop computers.

OPERATING SYSTEMS

Perhaps the most daunting task facing any new computer user is learning the operating system (Biow, 1997; White, 1998). It is this very task that led to the development of the Macintosh computer and later the Windows-based graphical user interface and operating system. The operating system is the software that controls the overall activity of a computer. It ensures that all components of the computer system are working together smoothly and efficiently. It translates the programming codes present in all application software into instructional sets (command language) and machine language to receive input, organize and store this input, process these data through the CPU to create an output, display the output on the monitor, store the output for later retrieval, and provide a hard copy for the user. It is the operating system that allows the user to sort, copy, move, save, delete, and view files.

Operating systems can be classified according to a number of characteristics (Albrecht, 1998). A multiuser operating system allows two or more users to run programs at the same time. Some operating systems permit hundreds or even thousands of concurrent users. An operating system has multiprocessing capabilities when it supports running a program on more than one CPU, multitasking capabilities when it allows more than one program to run concurrently, and multithreading capabilities when it allows different parts of a single program to run concurrently.

It is the operating system that forces one to ask, "Why doesn't my computer system work like everyone else's?" or "Why can't I use that program on my computer?" Also, it is also the minor moment-to-moment variances in the operating system that often result in crashed systems. Computer hardware crashes caused by mechanical disturbances are uncommon after a 48-hour burn-in. However, because the operating system controls that hardware, a glitch in the commands of the operating system can trigger an irrecoverable hardware crash, either hours of bewildering labor-intensive activity to recover the system, and often several hundred dollars of investment to ensure that the crash will not happen again, and if it does, the user can deal with it effectively and in a timely manner. The good news is that steady changes in operating systems not only have improved how the user can direct the computer but also how to prevent and handle hardware and software errors.

Platforms

To understand what commands the computer will respond to and how that computer collects, stores, retrieves, and passes data, it is first necessary to define the computer platform. A platform refers to the type of operating system used by a computer. Traditionally, programs developed on one platform do not run easily, if at all, on another platform. For example, it is very difficult to run a Macintosh OS program on a computer using the Windows 98 operating system. Incompatibility exists between different versions of an operating system. For example, because Windows for Workgroups 3.11 was developed to assist in connecting to other computers, programs developed for this platform may not have been compatible with the Windows 3.1 operating system. Some programs developed for one platform can be run on another platform, but the computer must be tricked by the operating system. Although Windows 95 and Windows 98 can run most programs developed for Windows 3.1 and MS-DOS, Windows 3.1 and MS-DOS cannot run programs developed specifically for Windows 95 and Windows 98 (these last two operating systems use 32-bit architecture, whereas the other two use a 16-bit architecture, respectively). Windows NT can run most Windows 95 software, but it has more compatibility problems with MS-DOS and Windows 3.1 applications. OS/2 can run most Windows 3.1 and MS-DOS programs but has difficulties with many Windows 95 software programs. Operating systems that were developed relatively early in the desktop computer environment such as CP/M, DOS and ProDOS (Apple II and compatible computers), MS-DOS, and Unix can only run programs written specifically for their respective operating systems (Bigelow, 1997; Minasi, 1996; Norton, 1997). Most Internet servers use Unix, Windows 95 or Windows 98, or Macintosh OS computers and will have difficulty recognizing commands outside their own command language. To make matters worse, users can define which operating system they choose to use on some computers when they power on or boot up their computer systems.

Many aspects of the operating system are common between platforms. All the operating systems are loaded during the boot-up process so that the various devices within the computer can communicate with each other. When the computer hardware first receives electrical power, it performs a hard boot. At this time, the computer will check the locations (direct memory address [DMA] or base address), IRQs, and integrity of the various hardware devices. If a required device is not connected or working properly, the computer will stop the boot-up process and report an error. It is often necessary to look up these errors in a manual or to write them down so that you can discuss them with a repair technician to repair the problem. Hardware devices that are not necessary often will not be registered by the operating system during boot-up unless they are connected and configured properly. If they are not registered, the problem must be corrected and the computer rebooted before that device will work properly (Press, 1997).

A soft-boot occurs when the system is told to reload the operating system from the keyboard. The Macintosh OS, Windows 95, Windows 98, and Windows NT platforms often will perform a soft-boot when a new program is initially loaded onto the system. The soft-boot allows new program extensions or linked file libraries to be accessed by the operating system to run those programs. Because of these extensions and linked file libraries loaded into the operating system at boot-up, it is necessary to remove these extensions and linked file libraries before turning off the computer with these operating systems. Failure to perform this task increases the risk for operating system failure when the system is powered up again.

DOS

DOS is the acronym for disk operating system (Gookin, 1997). The term *DOS* can refer to any operating system, but it is most often used as a shorthand for MS-DOS (Microsoft disk operating system), originally developed by Microsoft for the original IBM-compatible PCs. The initial versions of DOS were very simple and resembled another operating system called CP/M. Subsequent versions have become increasingly sophisticated because they incorporated features of minicomputer operating systems. However, DOS was and remains a 16-bit operating system and cannot support more than 640 K of RAM. It does not support multiple users or multitasking, which makes it more stable and demands less disk storage than Windows, Unix, or OS/2.

For some time, it has been widely acknowledged that DOS is insufficient for modern computer applications. Microsoft Windows helped alleviate some problems, but until Windows 95, it sat on top of DOS and relied on DOS for many services. Newer operating systems, including Windows 95, Windows NT, and OS/2 Warp, do not rely on DOS to the same extent, although they can execute DOS-based programs. It is expected that as these operating systems gain market share, DOS will eventually disappear.

Microsoft Windows

Microsoft developed Windows family of operating systems to provide a graphical user interface for PCs (Underdahl, 1998). Although Microsoft denies that Windows was inspired by the Macintosh operating system, remarkable similarities exist. Like the Macintosh operating environment, Windows provides a GUI, virtual memory management, multitasking, and support for many peripheral devices. The most common versions of Windows is Windows 3.1, Windows 95, and Windows 98.

Although Windows 98 was just introduced, Windows 95 was the dominant operating system at the time of this

writing. It is universally supported, runs both 32-bit and 16-bit software, and includes built-in support for TCP/IP. Windows 98 provides a modest upgrade from the Windows 95 operating system but provides an Internet Explorer interface, support for USB ports, ISDN communication, and DVD drives. It also provides a 32-bit File Allocation Table (FAT) for the hard drives, which allows larger partitions and more efficient data transfer. Both Windows 95 and Windows 98 are memory and drive hogs, requiring rather large amounts of systems resources. Windows 95 and Windows 98 are somewhat more stable than Windows 3.1 but still are prone to instability. It is not known whether Windows 2000 will resolve many of the instability problems associated with multitasking and multithreading found in earlier versions.

In addition to Windows 3.x, Windows 95, and Windows 98, Microsoft also distributes Windows NT, a more advanced operating system that runs on a variety of hardware platforms but requires even larger system resources. Windows NT supports symmetrical multiprocessing and its stability and security features makes it a popular choice as the operating system for networks, Internet Web servers, and intranets (a Web-based company-based network). The difficulties of Windows NT is that it is strictly a 32-bit operating system and does not support 16-bit applications written for Windows 3.x or Windows 95 and DOS.

OS/2 Warp

OS/2 Warp was initially designed by IBM and Microsoft to replace DOS, was introduced by IBM in 1987, and was the first true 32-bit operating system available for PCs (Chambers, 1998). It is a multitasking system running in the protected mode allowing programs to run simultaneously in its own address space. Although it has the same windows, icons, and visual controls as Windows, it is self-contained and does not need DOS or Windows to operate. Yet OS/2 Warp can work with either DOS or Windows 3.1 programs independently or simultaneously. It will not run programs written specifically for Windows 95 or Windows 98. OS/2 Warp can be found in many PCs containing the Nicolet Spirit evoked potential system. Although somewhat more stable than Windows 3.x operating systems, it is no longer adequately supported and, like DOS, will eventually disappear.

Mac OS

Since 1991, Apple's Macintosh operating systems, often termed System x.x, where x.x were the version numbers, have appeared in various and confusing forms. With the release of version 8, the system designator was dropped and Mac OS became the official name of the Macintosh operating system (Tessler, 1997). This operating system was developed with simplicity in mind, and historically Mac users have rightfully gloated when hearing of the difficulties PC users encountered with DOS and Windows. At present, Mac OS is a multithreaded operating system providing integrated Internet support and serves as an excellent platform for multimedia applications. However, even diehard Mac users know that Mac OS is showing its age, and Apple needs to develop a new operating system to replace Mac OS. In 1997, Apple Computer acquired Next, with idea of making NextStep (the operating system for Next computers) the foundation of its new operating system.

Unix

Developed by Bell Labs around 1970 for use on minicomputers, Unix has had a long history of the operating system of choice for minicomputers, workstations, and network systems because of its security, multitasking capabilities, and stability (Chambers, 1998). Unix is actually an operating system chameleon having many forms and flavors that are the result of adapting research and development software to commercial users. Its shell functions both as a command interpreter and a programming language giving capability to function both as an operating system and as a set of mechanisms found in other algorithmic languages used to execute various commands in sequence. Unix was not developed for the uninstructed user, and beginner users have a very difficult time negotiating through its commands. A number of variants of Unix have developed over time to enhance software applications.

Linux

Pronounced /linəks/, Linux is a freely distributable implementation of UNIX that runs on a number of hardware platforms, including Intel and Motorola microprocessors (Chambers, 1998). It was developed mainly by Linus Torvalds. Linux is a complete UNIX clone, capable of running a Windows-based environment, TCP/IP, e-mail, and news software. Almost all major free software packages have been ported to Linux, and commercial software is becoming available. Linux is the one of the most dynamic operating systems to date with several independent users contributing to its code almost daily.

CONCLUSIONS

The information age has led to the age of paradox. As times become more turbulent and the world becomes more complex, there are more paradoxes (Handy, 1994). Many paradoxes or apparent self-contradictions afflict audiology. Paradox has to be accepted, coped with, and understood. Computers both solve and create paradoxes. The application of computer technologies can provide the audiologist with the ability to acquire a wealth of data, organize those data, and summarize those data in a variety of formats. Unfortunately, data processing is not information processing. By collecting meaningful and relevant data, applying structure to these data, integrating the data successfully into appropriate models, and making right decisions in the right way on the basis of these data, data processing becomes information processing. Computers are only tools. Like all other tools, if they are applied correctly to the right task by skilled users, extraordinary outcomes can be achieved.

GLOSSARY

Computer terminology in general and computer-related buzzwords in particular can be confusing, misleading, and even incomprehensible. This glossary of terms and definitions is a good start on the road to computer literacy. It is placed in alphabetical, not historical, order to ease finding selective subjects of interest.

10BaseT This Ethernet standard supports 10 Mbps data throughput by means of the same hardware device in networked systems.

Adapter An adapter connects between two pieces of hardware and translates one form of connection to the other. It can be an interface cable, like a DB25 to parallel printer cable. It can be a 9 to 25 pin adapter for use with a mouse. It can be an add-in card whose purpose is interconnecting the motherboard bus to another device, like a hard disk. The SCSI and IDE hard disk drive controllers are both adapters. So is a video add-in card.

Adapter or Add-on Card Add-on cards connect the motherboard to the devices that operate with the computer. The video card, for example, connects the video monitor to the CPU through the motherboard. The sound card is an adapter that takes digital signals from programs and connects them to your speakers after processing them.

Address Every input or output device connected to the computer by an add-in card has a unique address. This address is how your computer knows where to send data or where to receive information. Memory locations are also addresses. Programs use memory addresses to find stored information to retrieve and process. Addresses can be hardware addresses for a physical device or software data addresses in memory on a computer. The microprocessor treats them the same.

AGP Accelerated Graphics Port video cards use a proprietary bus structure and provide significant improvements on 3-D video performance. They work in hand with the MMX instruction set to provide previously unheard of graphics speed.

ANSI The American National Standards Institute. This group controls specifications for many industrial applications, including the computer industry. The standards for displaying information, screen color, and positioning have designated standards. The ANSI.SYS driver is often loaded as a line in the CONFIG.SYS file. If it is loaded, the computer can respond correctly to ANSI commands in the programs it executes. This DOS command is seldom seen in the Windows 98 platform.

Applet A small program.

Application A program or programs designed to execute a particular operation. For example, a word processor is an application designed to perform writing, editing, spell checking, and publishing functions.

AT Compatible If a peripheral or computer provides the basic functionality of the same product in an original AT computer, it is AT compatible. This is a must for clone devices, so the buyer can have confidence his or her programs and accessories are compatible with the computer or add-on device. IBM compatible is another way of describing compatibility.

Autoexec.bat This is one of the principal DOS configuration files. It is often used by installed programs to set up hardware or allocate memory blocks. The Autoexec.bat file and all lines of code within it are executed in order of appearance. Some applications may be sensitive to the order in which commands appear in this file.

Base Address Everything has a starting point. The first location in memory where a program resides is the base address of the program. Installed hardware devices also have a base address.

Batch Files Like the Autoexec.bat file mentioned previously, DOS recognizes filenames ending in .bat as batch files. These files are normally ASCII files written by the computer user to make life easier.

BBS Bulletin board services exist worldwide for your enjoyment. Not to be confused with the Internet, a bulletin board is normally a single computer or system you can dial up and obtain shareware from or engage in chat groups.

BIOS The Basic Input/Output System is the ROM where your configuration platform resides and is the first code to run when the computer boots up. The BIOS sets up hardware and software addresses and is the software interface between different devices in the computer. BIOS exists on the motherboard, and occasionally video adapters and other add-in cards, and provides interface services to and from the motherboard and these peripherals.

Boot The act of initialization a computer undergoes when it is turned on is called "booting up." The BIOS starts the boot process and performs basic initialization. The CMOS memory then executes configuration information to identify the hardware in the computer and perform basic tests on memory and other components as specified in CMOS setup. Finally, the initialization files Config.sys, Autoexec.bat, and any other configuration files are run to set up components not specified in BIOS or CMOS. Normally, configuration files are modified by programs, so the programs know what hardware exists and can use it. This process occurs as the programs are being installed for the first time. The computer is ready for use after this process is complete.

Bus Unlike the Greyhound or school vehicles, this bus is the pathway that signals and data use to and from the microprocessor and all add-in cards and accessories in the computer. The bus transmits signals to control the video, disk, and I/0 operations, connects the memory and the processor, and is used by programs to control all the above hardware elements. The type of bus is one of the primary reasons some computers are faster than others. An 8-bit bus handles 8 lines of data simultaneously, and a 64-bit bus can handle 8 groups of 8 lines in the same amount of time. Imagine a ribbon cable, like the hard drive interconnecting cable. The more wires in the cable, the more data can be processed simultaneously.

Bus Bandwidth The clock frequency of a bus interface. To calculate the peak bus throughput, multiply the bus frequency by the bus width. If a 100-MHz bus is 64 bits wide, it can transfer 8 bytes per clock cycle 100 million times per second as a maximum throughput.

Bus Width The number of bits the bus allows through the pipeline.

Bit The bit, or BInary digiT, is the building block for all information transmitted to or from any element in a computer. A bit can be a 0 or a 1, where 0 and I are opposite logic states. Computers communicate by building bytes consisting of 8 bits and grouping the bytes in groups of two or more called words.

Byte A byte is a group of 8 bits of computer information. The byte is the most common method to express memory size, hard disk capacity, and file size. A kilobyte is 1024 bytes of information, often called a kB, or kbyte. A megabyte (meg) is 1.024 million bytes of information, often referred to as MB or Mbyte,

the primary measurement unit of hard drive, floppy disk, and memory capacity. The gigabyte (gig) is 1000 megabytes of information or capacity. A terabyte is 1034 gigabytes.

Cache A special bank of memory that holds data, which is often used or which will be required in a few nanoseconds. It speeds up the computer operation because the data does not have to be retrieved from RAM or the hard disk.

CD-R This is a CD-ROM drive that also allows the user to record computer data and audio/video data on compact discs. CD-R drives can only record to the discs once, but CD-RW can rewrite information on recordable discs. CD-RW discs cannot be read on standard CD-ROM drives.

CD-ROM CD-ROM drives are devices that use compact discs to store and retrieve computer data including programs or music programs.

CGA This was the Color Graphics Adapter in the first IBM color systems. The monitor and adapter combination was capable of 320 × 320 resolution and 16 colors, along with rudimentary text support.

Chipset These are the set of chips on the motherboard that help direct instructions from memory and the CPU to the various buses in the computer.

CMOS Complementary Metal Oxide Semiconductor is a process for integrated circuit manufacture. The devices are normally low-power consumption and ideal for battery operation. This makes them usable in portable computers or laptops. Two devices in the computer continue operating even when the power is turned off and the plug is removed from the wall socket. The CMOS clock runs off the small battery on the motherboard, keeping the correct date and time, after they are set correctly. A programmable integrated circuit saves the information entered into the CMOS setup program and reuses it each time the computer is booted up. This device also runs off a small battery.

Command Line and Command Prompt At the DOS level, the screen displays a character or group of characters know as the command prompt, indicating the computer is ready to execute a program. This is the first character string on the command line. When you type, the characters appear after the prompt. The command prompt can be configured.

CompactFlash A portable memory format that is read, by means of an adapter, in PC card drives commonly found in digital cameras.

Config.sys This is the configuration file that is executed after the BIOS and CMOS setup routines are processed. It precedes the Autoexec.bat file in order of execution. The hardware and software device drivers for video, CD-ROM, and sound add-in cards normally reside here. Often several lines are in this file starting with device =. These are device drivers. They control programs like ANSI.SYS, EMM386.EXE, and several hardware drivers.

Coax Standard Ethernet cable, commonly used in networks.

COM Port A designator for a serial port that uses standard hardware settings. PC systems generally default to four COM ports: COM1 through COM4. The COM port must be recognized by the system as being connected to a peripheral device before that device becomes operational.

Controller Cards Controller cards are synonymous with adapter cards. They process data to and from the CPU.

Conventional Memory Often called low memory, this is the first 640 kB of RAM installed in the computer. DOS programs run in this portion of memory. Unfortunately, this area in memory normally houses all the device drivers and Transient Stay-Resident (TSR) programs running around in the computer. This reduces the maximum program size that can run under DOS. Fortunately, Windows 95 and other programs break the 640 kB barrier. Some utility programs also push some of the TSR programs and drivers into upper memory and get some of the 640 kB back.

CPU The Central Processing Unit is the main device on the motherboard. The CPU can be anything from an 8086 through a Pentium III and beyond for the PC environment and the Motorola processors for the Macintosh computers. The CPU determines the bus architecture and system performance and speed. The computer's price is also determined by CPU type.

Current Directory The current directory is the spot in the system path the user is indexed to at the command level. Every operation the user perform runs on files and programs in the current directory or in a directory setup in a path command. The current directory is searched first for commands the user executes, then the path statement is searched until the program executed is found.

Device Hardware connected to or reside within the computer constitutes devices. Most devices are hardware and either accept or transmit data. A video monitor accepts data, a keyboard transmits it. Both are devices. Some software programs set drivers for virtual devices. The virtual device accepts input or gives output but is merely a subprogram and not hardware. This is common in sophisticated graphics programs that swap output and input with other resident programs.

Device Driver Device drivers are software designed to configure hardware in the computer to perform certain tasks. Some of the more common device drivers DOS uses are HIMEM.SYS and ANSI.SYS.

Diagnostic Programs These programs are tools to identify and correct problems. Diagnostic routines range from full blown bum in programs that test all operational parameters of the computer to simple memory test routines.

Directory When DOS is first installed on a blank hard disk, a root directory is created. The root directory is the first place on the hard disk programs where data are stored. The second directory is normally the DOS directory, created by the DOS installation disk to store the DOS program files. As the user installs install other programs, they often create their own directories, or folders, to store the files required to run. A DOS file system is like an upside down tree, with each branch representing a different directory, and the root directory is at the top of this inverted tree. As programs are added, branches grow on the tree. Data files are often lost because users stored them in the wrong directories or forgot which directories the files are located. This can be remedied by using the Browse function in the Windows Explorer programs.

Disk Magnetic medium that rotates on a spindle with read and write heads hovering over it comprises a disk. There are four primary types: hard disks, CD-ROM discs, DVD discs, and floppy disks.

Disk Controller A disk controller is the IDE or SCSI interface between the hard disk and floppy disk drives and the CPU. It can be an add-in card or built-in circuitry on the motherboard.

DLL The dynamic link library files are indispensable little nuggets of software that get deposited surreptitiously on the hard drive that application programs access whenever they need an additional set of instructions not readily available in the executable file. These files cause major headaches if they are unintentionally deleted, are not the right version for the specific application being run, or are located in a subdirectory that cannot be found by the application. When these events happen, the program shuts down and the system could crash.

DMA Direct Memory Access is one way to transfer data between computer memory and a hardware device installed in the computer. DMA does not require CPU involvement, making the process extremely fast.

DOS Disk A DOS disk is one that has been DOS formatted and one that can be used for data storage and retrieval on a DOS-based system.

DOS Memory DOS memory is considered the first 640 kB of addressable memory in the computer. *See* Conventional Memory. It holds boot data, programs, and system information.

DOS The Disk Operating System is software written to perform on a specific type of computer. In the case of MS-DOS, the program was written to operate on IBM and compatible PC systems. Applications unique to the type of hard disk, monitor and adapter, file system, and input/output devices are written and developed into a complete operating system package.

DOS Boot Diskette A floppy diskette with the necessary DOS system files required to launch DOS is called a boot diskette. It may be necessary to have one if something happens to the boot block on the hard drive. A boot disk is an invaluable tool. The DOS manual describes how to make one.

Drive The assembly that transports a floppy diskette, or the entire hard disk drive assembly, is often referred to as a drive. A CD-ROM, DVD, or tape transport system shares the same designation.

Driver The closest layer of software between an operating system and a peripheral.

DVD The digital versatile disc is the next generation CD-ROM that is capable of using multiple layers on both sides of the disk. This provides as much as 17 GB of data, whereas a CD is limited to a maximum of 682 MB. DVD is the preferred means of storing video files.

EDO Standing for extended data output, EDO RAM uses special memory chips that provide more rapid exchange between the RAM and the CPU.

EGA IBM introduced the Enhanced Graphics Adapter to improve graphics display quality in their computers. EGA offered a medium resolution alternative to the existing CGA system. EGA was compatible with both CGA and monochrome display units.

EIDE The Enhanced Integrated Drive Electronics is a motherboard interface for connecting hard drives, CD and DVD drives, and removable storage devices.

EISA The Extended Industry Standard Architecture definition of the internal bus structure on an IBM or compatible PC redefined the existing standard. It offered higher speed and more features than the ISA bus. The real improvement was definition of a 32-bit architecture completely different from the existing and proprietary IBM Micro Channel system and the architecture the clone industry quickly adopted as the 32-bit standard.

EMM The software that controls use and allocation of high memory in a PC is referred to as an Expanded Memory Manager. The specification is sometimes called LIM, for its developers, Lotus, Intel, and Microsoft. The upper memory between the DOS memory (the first 640 kB) and 1 megabyte can be included in the expanded memory. The first 64 kB of upper memory is set aside by the EMM as a map to the extended memory for certain programs to use. Extended memory usually starts at 1 megabyte and runs up to the amount of RAM installed on the motherboard.

EMS Expanded Memory Specification is a standard that governs the hardware and software that comprise expanded memory.

ESDI The Enhanced Small Devices Interface is a definition of the standards applying to the interconnection of a type of high-speed hard disk drive. It joins the currently used SCSI and IDE interface specifications.

Ethernet A network topology in which data are broadcast across the network. It is generally less efficient than other network architecture but it is less complex and less expensive.

Execute When a program is running, it is being executed. A computer executes instruction sets when it runs software programs. An executable file is a file normally having a bat, exe, or com filename extension. In DOS and Unix, files like this can be executed by typing the filename without the extension, then pressing the ENTER key. In Windows, Mac OS, and Linux, the executable file is typically called an application file.

Expanded Memory Expanded memory is the portion of RAM set aside and managed by the EMM. This memory is normally used as a scratch pad for database and spreadsheet programs. The expanded memory manager sets aside a 64-kB portion of upper memory between the DOS memory and IMB. This 64 kB of memory serves as an index to the larger portion of expanded memory above 1 MB. The expanded memory size is limited only by the motherboard capacity and the amount of RAM you have installed on the system. It can be up to 1 terabyte in current Pentium II systems.

Extended Memory In a 286 or higher computer, memory above 1 meg is referred to as extended memory. Disk caching is a principal use for this memory.

File Allocation Table The FAT is an operating system component that tracks where the data is stored on a hard disk. The 16-bit version supports hard drive capacity up to 2 GB and the 32-bit version supports hard drive capacity up to 2 TB.

File A file is a portion of a program or data occupying space in memory or on a disk. Some files are complete programs, but most files are data resulting from program execution. A file stored on a disk is identified in the file archive table, or FAT, by its starting location and size. This way the file can be accessed, modified, or deleted as required by you or program execution.

Filename The filename is a group of ASCII characters you assign to a file to identify it. In a DOS and Windows 3.1 system, a filename can be up to 8 characters with a three-character extension identifying the type of file. In the Windows 95, Windows 98, Mac OS, Linux, and Unix operating systems, the user is not restricted to an eight-character limit, leading to more flexibility when naming files. Filenames must be unique in the same directory, lest they be overwritten by another application.

Filename Extension A string of one to three characters after the period in a filename is the filename extension. The extension normally describes the type of file, so applications can use it.

Firewall A program or device designated to protect network data from being retrieved by an unauthorized user or hacker.

Floppy Disk Floppy diskettes are removable storage media that consist of a single magnetically coated vinyl platter installed in a jacket. The drive for a floppy disk has a spindle that spins the floppy disk, and read/write heads to transfer data to and from the floppy diskette. Floppy diskettes were the most common way to transfer data between computers at the time of this writing.

Gigabyte 1024 megabytes of memory, storage, or information is a gigabyte also referred to as 1 gig.

Hard Disk Hard disks, also known as fixed disks, are multiple magnetic platters, with numerous read and write heads added, all sealed up in an enclosure with a circuit board for cache and sector translation attached. This is an oversimplification, but a good analogy. The reason hard disks are sealed in a very clean medium is the small amount of area between the heads and platters. The smallest dust particle would jam between a head and one disk platter surface, destroying valuable data and crashing the system.

Hardware Interrupt Hardware interrupts alert the CPU of events requiring action. Hardware interrupts are asserted by a keyboard, mouse, hard disk, and so on to inform the microprocessor that software interaction is requested. The action may be to open or close a file on the hard disk, accept movement information from a mouse, or input from the keyboard.

Hexadecimal Unlike the standard base 10 counting system most humans use, computers often use a base 16 system called hexadecimal notation. Four bits of information, represented by 1, 2, 4, and 8 make up the base 16 number system. The 15 numbers that comprise the system are 0 through 9 and A through F. An 8-bit byte, represented by (8 4 2 1) (8 4 2 1) represents 255 different items, 00 through FF.

High Memory HMA, or the high memory area, is the 64-kB area above the 1-MB address range that HIMEM.SYS creates. This area can be used by programs for storage of intermediate results during program execution. When this process occurs, the user has more free DOS memory available for other applications.

Host Adapter Add-in cards that interface between a hardware device, like a hard disk or video monitor, are referred to as host adapters. They process data to and from these devices and the memory, allowing the CPU to expend effort elsewhere. This speeds up execution of programs.

IBM-Compatible If a computer or component provides the same function as the original component in an IBM computer, the device or computer is IBM compatible. This means the software and hardware devices will behave the same in the clone and the original IBM machine.

IDE The Integrated Drive Electronics standard for hard disk control is the most popular today. It regulates the definition of a high-speed integrated drive and controller assembly, hence the name. An adapter to transfer data to and from the hard disk is normally integrated into the motherboard but is also available as an add-on card. The IDE specification is part of the ATA standard. AT-Attachments is the specification used in the interface for hard disk drives to the IBM PC/AT bus.

Interlaced An interlaced monitor is redrawn every other line, often resulting in a noticeable flicker if the refresh rate is not sufficiently fast.

I/O Input/output is the ability of a computer to transfer data to and from internal and external devices. This capability can be inherent in both hardware and software. I/O often refers to a special add-in card or function embedded in the motherboard. This function controls data transfer among devices inside the computer and outside and includes interaction with other computers through a modem or external port.

IRQ Interrupt requests are signals transferred over the bus between add-in cards and the CPU. They instruct the CPU to perform immediate action. Normally IRQ lines are asserted to request the CPU coordinate transfer of data between add-in devices and memory. In current systems the IRQ-dependent devices vie for interrupt priority among 16 different IRQ slots.

IrDA An infrared data-transfer protocol that allows wireless communications between conforming hardware. This protocol is often found in portable and palm PCs.

ISA The 8- and 16-bit bus used by IBM and compatible computers is the Industry Standard Architecture bus. It can accompany a VESA or PCI system. Most computers have up to three ISA connectors, to ensure compatibility with older add-in cards.

ISDN An integrated services digital network line provides a true digital connection between two computers, offering faster connections than conventional modems using standard telephone lines. Transfer rates can be as high as 512 kbps.

Java An object-oriented programming language that functions as if it is a virtual platform. As a result, programs written in Java can run on many different computers without porting or recompiling the code for the operating system. This allows applets to be downloaded from the Internet to run on individual users computers, regardless of the operating system the user has loaded on the system.

Level 2 Cache This secondary cache is the second fastest memory available to the CPU (second only to the level 1 cache). It usually consists of SRAM chips near the CPU, although some processors have on-chip L2 caches.

LoadHigh This statement describes the action of setting an executable file or device driver in the upper memory area or in high memory. With this command in the config.sys or autoexec.bat file, the user can specify the start memory address the command must use.

Local Area Network A series of networked computers that lie close to one another.

Local Bus The VESA standard set down by the Video Electronics Standard Association is a high-speed I/O-to-CPU interface that maintains compatibility with the ISA standard interface.

Logical Devices Partitioning a large hard drive into smaller ones creates a logical device for each partition. DOS treats each partition as a physical device, not as a portion of one drive. A logical drive is a partition as mentioned earlier. Other logical devices are RAM drives created in RAM and maintained by software control. Network drives are considered to be logical devices by the user's desktop computer.

Loopback Adapter This is a special connector wired to allow the user to test communications ports without actually going online.

Math Coprocessor The math coprocessor is integrated into 486DX and all faster microprocessors for IBM and compatible computers. The 486SX, 386, and earlier computers had an expansion slot to accommodate one if required. The math coprocessor performs all the complex math operations, allowing the CPU to perform other tasks.

MCA Micro Channel Architecture is the standard used in the IBM PS/2 computer line. It is an IBM trademark and is incompatible with all other architectures past and present in any other system. MCA systems use different adapters and add-on cards, none of which will work in anything else.

MCGA This is the Multi-Color Graphics Array system implemented in IBM PS/2 computers. It was noted for great gray scale and improved resolution over CGA.

MD The first IBM computers had the Monochrome Display Adapter. The display was either green or amber.

Megabyte 1024 kilobytes of information, storage, or memory is a megabyte or 1 meg.

Megahertz This measure of frequency is in millions of cycles per second. Clock speeds are measured in megahertz.

Memory Memory is any form of storage area for program use that resides in your computer. RAM, hard disks, floppies, and CMOS are types of memory. So are tape cartridges or CD-ROMs. The cache memory is the fastest memory in the system, and the floppy disk is the slowest.

MIDI The Musical Instrument Device Interface is the industry standard driving the computer interface for musical devices. It specifies connections, hardware, and software protocol.

MMX This term refers to the first significant extension to the 1985 era instruction set inside the CISC processor family. The addition of 57 new instructions accelerates calculations in graphics and audio applications, including 2D and 3D graphics, speech recognition and synthesis, and video processing and types of compression. The performance expectations are an increase of 50 to 100% in speed while using multimedia programs and equipment. Intel upgraded its entire product line to MMX in 1997 and introduced a cost-reduced Pentium Pro microprocessor later that year that included the MMX technology.

Modem This name is an abbreviation for the actual function of the device. The *Mo*dulator *Dem*odulator is an analog-to-digital and digital-to-analog converter. The modem converts digital information from a computer-to-analog signals that can travel through the phone lines. It accomplishes the reverse on receiving signals from another computer.

Motherboard The heart and soul of a computer is the motherboard. Everything plugs into it, and the motherboard serves as the information pathway to and from the CPU and each device connected to it. A motherboard typically has the CPU, RAM, cache, and IDE I/O function installed. Add-on functionality in the form of video support, hard and floppy disks, keyboards, and mice complete the computer.

MPEG MPEG, or the moving pictures expert group, is a popular digital video format and compression scheme.

Multitasking Performing more than one operation at once is multitasking. This is normally a software process, where programs and data are quickly swapped between a reserved portion of memory and the active memory a microprocessor is using. In a process like this, the software determines how long each operation remains on hold in reserved memory and how long the operation gets

CPU attention. If the user has a sufficiently fast computer, the user normally will never notice any slowdown in operation while the computer is performing multitasking operations. The foreground process, the one the user can see on the screen, is typically the one getting most of the CPU's attention.

Native Platform The underlying CPU and operating system of a computer. It determines what kind of software can run on the system.

Network A series of computers connected to each other. Each computer can share data with other computers in the network, and all computers connected to the network can use resources like shared printers, shared hard drives, or shared modems.

Network Interface An add-in card to interface between the computer and a network communications hub is called a network interface card. This add-in card processes digital signals from the computer and sends them to a common node all other users share with you.

Online Services Online services are pay for use BBSs with advertisements. They do, however, offer connectivity to a large number of useful and enjoyable sites. Shareware is available, and electronic mail, software support, online games, and chat groups frequently are included. America Online, CompuServe, Prodigy, and the Microsoft Network are examples of online services.

Page Frame On a DOS system, the location in memory between DOS memory and 1 MB, where expanded memory is indexed is called page frame memory.

Parallel I/O Transferring data using the parallel port is extremely fast. Eight or more bits of information can be sent simultaneously using the parallel I/O port on the computer. Data transfer rates of 100 kB are not unusual using this technique. Most desktop computer's printer port (such as LPT1) uses a parallel port.

PC The first model designation IBM gave to its personal computer family was PC. The term has been adopted by all personal computer manufacturers who make IBM compatible computers and accessories. The base IBM machine had 64 kB of memory, an optional tape drive instead of hard drives, and a monochrome display.

PCI The Peripheral Component Interconnect standard developed by Intel specifies a very fast interface between I/O devices and the CPU. The PCI bus slots can hold 32-bit adapter cards and are the primary interfaces for current video adapters and fast IDE I/O cards.

PCMCIA Card The Personal Computer Memory Card International Association device is inserted into a computer, typically notebook computers, to provide specific instructions that are stored in ROM on these cards.

Peer-to-peer A network where every computer is connected to every other computer and no server is required to operate the network.

Pentium This 64-bit microprocessor is capable of operating beyond 233 MHz and contains 16 kB of instruction cache and an internal floating point processor.

Pentium II The replacement for the Pentium Pro, this CPU has MMX instruction sets included, and the capabilities of both the Pentium and Pentium Pro. It is packaged more like an add-on card than a processor. Current versions run at speeds beyond 400 MHz and have an L2 cache of 512 kB.

Pentium III The replacement of the Pentium II, this CPU has a new graphics instruction set and is capable of very fast clock speeds, in excess of 500 MHz.

Pentium Pro The first of the sixth-generation x86 microprocessor chip. It was designed by Intel for use on network computers and high-powered workstation PCs dedicated to computation-intensive tasks such as computer-aided drafting (CAD) or 3-D artwork.

Peripheral A device, like a scanner or printer, that is not necessary for the computer to operate. An internal tape drive or CD-ROM is a peripheral device, as are the external versions.

Physical Drive The hard disk drive containing the user's partitions is a physical drive. The system's floppy drives, tape drive, and CD-ROM drive also are physical drives. The partitions on the system's hard drive, if any, are not physical drives. A physical drive is hardware, not a software-managed partition on the (hardware) disk drive.

Pixel A single dot on the computer monitor. The number of pixels on the screen measured as a function between the horizontal by vertical gives the degree of resolution the screen provides.

Port Address The address in memory through which any hardware device allows access is its port address.

POST When the computer is booted up, the first thing it does is a Power On Self-Test or POST. It runs diagnostic routines on various hardware components as specified in BIOS or CMOS setup. If errors are encountered, the test provides error messages, beep codes, or both.

PS/2 An abbreviation of the Personal System/2 computers, incorporating the MCA bus and specific video adapters.

RAM Random Access Memory is the primary storage computers use to store intermediate results. When a program is executed, data flows into and out of RAM during the processing portion of the program. Only after all operations are performed are the data stored on a hard disk or floppy drive. RAM is identified by its storage capacity and speed. Dynamic RAM (DRAM) must be refreshed or repeatedly written to with the same data to retain information. Cache memory is also RAM. Cache is extremely fast Static RAM (SRAM), which requires no refreshing, hence the speed. Eight nanoseconds is the average pipeline cache RAM's speed.

RAMDAC The random access memory digital-to-analog converter is the chip on the videocard that converts the bits of a digital image into an analog signal. It maintains the color palette and determines the refresh rates. The faster the RAMDAC, the higher the refresh rate the system can handle.

Registry The Windows' mass database of hardware and environmental configuration information. Keep this clean and up to date.

ROM ROM stands for Read Only Memory, and it cannot easily be altered or erased. The ROM in the computer consists of one or more applications programmed into the computer by burning in a memory trace into the chip. EPROMS with setup information specific to your computer. The programs in ROM execute when the computer is booted up. ROM BIOS is the set of programs loaded in the ROM. Often, certain video adapters and add-in cards may have their own ROM BIOS. Some computers today come with FLASH BIOS. This EPROM memory can be changed by running a software program. This is ideal as new BIOS is released to support more hardware devices and faster CPUs.

Root Directory The first directory on a hard disk or floppy diskette is the root directory.

RS-232 A protocol that allows the computer to exchange data with a peripheral through a serial connection.

SCSI The Small Computer System Interface defined by these initials was the fastest thing around until the high-speed IDE drives became a reality. SCSI drives still hold the size record, with drives in the 10 gigabyte range commonplace. SCSI hard drives require a special interface to run in a PC. The interface supports many more drives than are possible with any other drive architecture.

SDRAM Synchronous Dynamic Read-Only Memory is the current standard for fast computer memory. It is nearly as fast as pipeline burst cache, at 10 ns access speed.

SGRAM A cousin of SDRAM, this is a type of single-ported memory often used for videocards that synchronizes with the CPU and uses techniques to optimize graphics processing.

Serial I/O Serial data transfer occurs one bit at a time, unlike parallel I/O, which transfers 1 byte, or 8 bits simultaneously. The good side of serial transfer is compatibility with modems and existing data transfer protocol. Although it is fairly slow at 115 kB/s, it is the most common method of interconnection between computers for data transfer. Communication occurs through one of the serial (or COM) ports in your computer. The other ports can be used by a mouse or other serial device.

Shadow RAM Many computers map BIOS information into faster RAM devices to speed up various operations. The RAM locations specified in CMOS setup as Shadow RAM are where this information is stored and executed.

SIMM The single inline memory module provides a specific shape of the RAM chipset used by the computer system.

Software Interrupt An interrupt command from a program that requires CPU attention is a software interrupt. These can occur on completion of part of a program or when device drivers are invoked. Keyboard operations, drive access, and certain timing services are available to programs as software interrupts.

Subdirectory Any directory within another directory is a subdirectory. Therefore all directories other than the root directory are subdirectories. Subdirectories allow programs to organize data and files by the application with which they are associated.

SVGA The super video graphics array standard is the most common graphics standard for video adapter cards and allows for more than 16 million colors (24-bit or true color).

S-Video The Super-Video standard that divides the signal to carry brightness and color information separately that permits better picture quality.

Swap File When an application runs out of system memory, it begins using the hard drive as virtual memory to save application and documentation data. The hidden temporary files written to the hard drive are called swap files. Unfortunately, the more swap files or virtual memory used, the slower the system operates.

System Bus The pipe that sends data back and forth between main memory on the CPU.

T1 T1 is a high-speed, dedicated phone line for digital communications that can reach a speed of 1.5 megabits/s.

TCP/IP The Transmission Control Protocol/Internet Protocol is a suite of Internet communication protocols. The IP routes data packets across the Internet, whereas TCP makes sure that all of the packets arrive correctly on the receiving end.

TSR Terminate and Stay Resident programs are programs that remain in memory, so the user can easily call up applications within them with a hot key or other command. Some device drivers fall into this category like mouse drivers and the DOS Server command.

Twisted Pair Cable A form of network cable that has the appearance of a telephone cord and is commonly used in Ethernet networks. One wire carries data while the other wire absorbs interference.

UAR/T These initials refer to the device commonly referred to as a Universal Asynchronous Receiver/Transmitter. This device converts parallel bus information into serial data for transfer using a modem. The device reverses the process on receipt of serial data from a modem.

Ultra DMA The ultradirect memory access is the fastest IDE protocol for connecting hard drives and removable storage devices.

UMB Upper Memory Blocks are made available by memory manager programs. They reside in the addressable memory area between DOS memory and 1 MB. TSR programs and part of DOS can be placed in upper memory to free up conventional memory for applications.

USB The Universal Serial Bus is a faster digital I/O port that can act as a serial, parallel, mouse, keyboard, joystick, and even speaker interface. Up to 127 devices can be daisy-chained through the USB port.

Utilities Proograms that help with routine operations like backups, virus testing, file and hard disk testing are normally referred to as either utilities or diagnostic programs.

VGA Video Graphics Array is a high-resolution graphics and text system that supports the previous IBM standards. It uses an analog video monitor as a display unit.

Video Adapter Card The add-on card that interfaces the video monitor to the CPU is the video adapter card. Video adapters come in a wide range of performance and price ranges and support all bus types.

Video Memory Video memory speeds up graphics applications by taking the CPU out of the loop when processing video information. It is often fast memory. Video memory can be DRAM or the faster VRAM.

XMS The Extended Memory Specification is the standard that defines control of any memory above DOS memory. When you load the HIMEM.SYS driver in the Config.sys file, XMS is set up. Other memory management programs and utilities can also set up XMS.

ZIF Socket The zero insertion force socket uses a level to unlatch the CPU from the socket where it can be easily removed and replaced with an upgraded microprocessor chip.

Zip Drive A Zip drive uses a removable cartridge that is about the size of a floppy disk but stores at least 100 MB of data.

REFERENCES

ALBRECHT, M.C. (1997). *Computerizing your business*. Englewood Cliffs, NJ: Prentice-Hall.

AMERICAN SPEECH-LANGUAGE-HEARING ASSOCIATION. (1997). *Technology 2000: Clinical applications for speech-language pathology*. Rockville, MD: American Speech-Language-Hearing Association.

AMERINE, K.L. (1992). Choosing office management software. *Audiology Today, 4*(5);21–23.

APPLETON, E.L. (1998). 1998 state of the industry report. *Inside Technical Training, 2*(6);12–18.

BEVAN, M.A., PIKE, B.F., SALANT, S.G., et al. (1994). *Business practices: Laying the foundation for successful service delivery in communication disorders* (1st ed.). Rockville Pike, MD: American Speech-Language-Hearing Association.

BIGELOW, S.J. (1997). *PC Hardware FAT FAQs*. New York: McGraw-Hill.

BIOW, L. (1997). *How to use computers*. Emeryville, CA: ZD Press.

BOURKE, M., & GRIMES, S. (1995). *Networks*. Redman, WA: SpaceLabs Medical Inc.

BRIA, W.F., & RYDELL, R.L. (1996). *The physician-computer connection*. Chicago, IL: American Hospital Publishing, Inc.

BLOOM, S. (1998). Hearing healthcare practitioners take a practical look at the Internet. *Hearing Journal, 51*(6); 19–28.

CAMPBELL, P. (1997). *Networking the small office*. San Francisco, CA: Sybex.

CHAMBERS, M.L. (1998). *Building a PC for dummies.*® Foster City, CA: IDG Books Worldwide.

COLOMBO, D. (1994). Computerizing your office. *Hearing Review, 1*(6);23,25.

CRUMLISH, C. (1997). *The ABCs of the Internet*. San Francisco: Sybex.

DYBALA, P. (1996). Touring the Web: A read-made hot-list for hearing care providers. *Hearing Review, 3*(10):31–34.

FITCH, J.L. (1993). Computer technology: History and overview. *ASHA, 35*(8);36–37.

FORBES, J., & RULEY, J.D. (1998). Palm PCs go hand in hand. *Windows Magazine, 9*(8);194–206.

FOURNIER, E.M., & MARGOLIS, R.H. (1992). Computers and complexity in the audiologist's clinical life. *Audiology Today, 4*(5);18–21.

GINSBERG, M. (1992). Finding and keeping a quality computer consultant. *Audiology Today, 4*(5);32–37.

GOOKIN, D. (1997). *PCs for dummies,*® (5th ed.). Foster City, CA: IDG Books Worldwide.

GOOKIN, D. (1998). *Buying a computer for dummies*® (5th ed.). Foster City, CA: IDG Books Worldwide.

HALLIDAY, C.M. (1997). *PC SECRETS*® (2nd ed.). Foster City, CA: IDG Books Worldwide.

HANDY, C. (1994). *The empty raincoat: Making sense of the future*. London: Hutchinson Press.

HAYES, D.E. (1992). Computer connections and compatibility: A real life story. *Audiology Today, 4*(5);P30–32.

HEARD, K. (1994). Computerized information system. In: Trudeau, M.D. & Rizzo, S.R. *Clinical administration in audiology and speech-language pathology*. San Diego, CA: Singular Publishing Company, Inc.

HOSFORD-DUNN, H., DUNN, D.R., & HARFORD, E.R. (1995). *Audiology business and practice management*. San Diego, CA: Singular Publishing Group, Inc.

JOHNSON, D. (1998). The skinny on scanning. *Small Business Computers and Communication, 3*(4);108–113.

KOBLER, R. (1996). *PC novice guide to computing basics*. Lincoln, NE: Peed Corporation.

KRAYNAK, J. (1998). *Complete idiot's guide to PCs* (6th ed.). Indianapolis, IN: Que.

KREIDER, N.A., & HASELTON, B.J. (1997). *The systems challenge: Getting the clinical information support you need to improve patient care*. Chicago, IL: American Hospital Publishing, Inc.

KUSTER, J.M., & KUSTER T.A. (1995). Finding treasures on the Internet. *ASHA, 37*(2);43–47.

MARANGRAPHICS, (1996). *Teach yourself computers and the internet visually*. Foster City, CA: IDG Books Worldwide.

MENDEL, L.L., & WYNNE, M.K., ENGLISH K., et al. (1995). Computer applications in educational audiology. *Language Speech, and Hearing Services in the Schools, 26*;232–240.

MEYER, M. (1998). *Computers today and tomorrow*. Indianapolis, IN: Que.

MINASI, M. (1996). *The complete PC upgrade & maintenance guide* (8th ed.). San Francisco, CA: Sybex.

MORMER, K.J., MORMER, E.A., & ROBERTSON. P. (1992). Communications and networks in the audiology practice. *Audiology Today, 4*(5);23–28.

MORMER, E.A., & PALMER, C.V. (1998). A guide to the Internet: It could change the way you work. *Hearing Journal, 51*(6); 29–30,32.

NORTON, P. (1997). *Peter Norton's inside the PC* (7th ed.). Indianapolis, IN: SAMS Publishing, Inc.

NUNEMACHER, G. (1995). *LAN primer* (3rd ed.). Foster City, CA: IDG Books Worldwide.

PARKER, C.O. (1998). *The complete PalmPilot guide*. New York: MIS:Press.

PICCOLO, J. (1994). Choosing an office management system. *Hearing Review, 1*(6);24–25.

POGUE, D. (1997). Top pocket organizers. *Macworld, 14*(9);137–140.

PRESS, B. (1997). *PC upgrade and repair bible*. Foster City, CA: IDG Books Worldwide.

RATHBONE, A. (1997). *Upgrading & fixing PCs For dummies*® (3rd ed.). Foster City, CA: IDG Books Worldwide.

RAUTERKUS, M.F. (1992). Computer compatibility: Possibilities. *Audiology Today, 4*(5);28–30.

SAPIEN, M., & PIEDMO, G. (1996). *Mastering ISDN*. San Fransisco, CA: Sybex.

SIRIANNI, J. (1996). Using the Internet for better hearing healthcare. *Hearing Review, 3*(10);28.

STROM, K.E. (1994). Computers for the hearing care professional. *Hearing Review, 1*(6);22.

STROM, K.E. (1995). A survey of business management software. *Hearing Review, 2*(9);16–21.

SULLIVAN, R.F. (1998). Searching for information on the World Wide Web: Has an infinitude of monkeys created <www.kinglear.com>? *Hearing Journal, 51*(6);34,36,38–39.

SWENSON, C. (1995). Marketing on your PC. *Hearing Review, 2*(9);26, 28, 30.

TESSLER, F.N. (1997). Mac OS 8 arrives. *Macworld, 14*(9); 121–129.

THOMAS, R.M. (1997). *Introduction to local area networks.* San Francisco, CA: Sybex.

TOLLIVER, P.R, & KELLOGG, C. (1997). *PCs for teachers*™ (2nd ed.). Foster City, CA: IDG Books Worldwide.

UNDERDAHL, B. (1998). *Small business computing for dummies.*® Foster City, CA: IDG Books Worldwide.

WHITE, R. (1998). *How computers work, third edition with interactive CD-ROM.* Indianapolis, IN: Que.

WYNNE, M.K. (1996a). Computer technology & office management: New business strategies. In: L. Zingeser, S.T. Stram, J. Langsam, et al. (Eds.), *Guide to successful private practice in speech-language pathology.* Rockville, MD: American Speech-Language-Hearing Association.

WYNNE, M.K. (1996b). Page Ten: You cannot surf the Web without having your Hands On the 'net. *Hearing Journal, 49*(7);10,61–65.

WYNNE, M.K, & HURST, D.S. (1995). Legal issues and computer use by school-based audiologists and speech-language pathologists. *Language, Speech, and Hearing Services in the Schools, 26*;251–259.

Chapter 20

Computer Applications for Audiology and Dispensing

Robert R. de Jonge

INTRODUCTION

The past two decades have been exciting times for people interested in microcomputers. Originally, computers were large, arcane devices housed in their own special rooms and attended to by professionals trained in a highly technical field. These large computers were mysterious, vaguely distrusted, and portrayed by science fiction writers as dark foreboding devices designed to dominate and control the world. Then in the 1970s small computers were sold, at first in kit form to hobbyists who controlled them by writing their own programs in the BASIC programming language. Virtually no commercial software was available. Microcomputers, personal computers (PCs), home computers—no one was quite sure what to call them or even what niche they would occupy. Some envisioned the computer as a device for controlling the home environment: turning lights on and off, adjusting the ambient temperature, and making appliances "intelligent." Soon, pre-assembled computers were marketed by such companies as Apple, Commodore, and Atari. People used these computers for scientific investigation and playing games. Early business systems were powerful for their time having dual floppy drives, 64 kB RAM powered by the 2 MHz Z80 processor. The

success of word processing software helped define the PC as something more than a game machine or household appliance. In the mid-1980s, IBM introduced its own PC and now the microcomputer was viewed as a legitimate, serious tool for businesspeople. A number of workalikes (IBM PC compatible) soon entered the market. Shortly after IBM's entry, Apple introduced the Macintosh (Mac); its graphical interface set a new standard for how the user could easily interact with the machine. Improvements in hardware occurred at a remarkable pace as each new generation of microprocessor replaced the previous—computers with 300+ MHz processors, 128 MB of RAM, and 8 GB hard drives make the most sophisticated computers of only a few years ago seem quaint and underpowered. The increased computing power allowed more sophisticated programs to be developed with an ever-increasing array of useful features. Meanwhile, a global network of computers, the Internet, was being developed. E-mail was replacing the standard mail service, software was being downloaded, and people were getting instant access to information from their homes through telephone lines. Attitudes about computers were changing. Although some people were, and still are, intimidated, many more became excited about the possibilities for working smarter and more efficiently, and new markets opened. Computers filled schools, businesses, government offices, hospitals, and clinics.

The issue of interest in this chapter is what is available for audiology and how the practice of our profession might be enhanced by computer applications? The general focus of this chapter is to identify programs written specifically for audiology and to describe their features. When used in a computing context, the term *application* is a synonym for *computer program*. But *application* can be considered in a broader context (i.e., how can computers facilitate work that is typically performed by audiologists?). Programs (e.g., Microsoft Office 97) are designed for the general computing public that have useful features for audiologists. So these applications, generally referred to as "integrated office suites," will be briefly described.

The purpose of this chapter is to make audiologists and students in training to be audiologists aware of how computers might be integrated into their present and future practice. Toward that end, the chapter is structured with the following guidelines:

- Emphasis is on general, guiding principles that help readers better understand computing and its relevance to audiology. Material covered in this chapter is expected to still be

443

relevant five years hence. This chapter is not a review of the most current versions of applications and software specifics.

- The prevailing attitude is nonjudgmental, intent on informing readers about useful features offered by applications, without providing a critical review of different software packages or recommending one program over another. I developed some of the software applications described, I retain some bias.

- The range of applications to be covered is large and the coverage is broad. Because an audiologist's scope of practice tends to be defined by his or her specific employment setting, no individual audiologist will find use for all the categories of software or be familiar with every program. Consequently, the chapter does not include user-manual–type descriptions of each program. Nor does the mention of a program imply an endorsement of its features or its appropriateness for a particular task.

PEARL

Software is constantly evolving. What is true about a program one day may change entirely the next. Be skeptical about "expert advice." Before buying, ask questions to make sure the software is compatible with your hardware and the programs you run.

GENERAL COMPUTER ISSUES AND APPLICATIONS

The following sections briefly describe important issues for understanding how programs run, what are the major computer applications, and how these programs may be used by audiologists. Computers are often sold with bundled software. Frequently, new users are unfamiliar with these software packages and their potential professional application. Many references are readily available for those seeking additional information. Microcomputing is a popular subject, with many magazines devoted to the topic. Major bookstores have a large section devoted to microcomputing. IDG Books Worldwide, Inc., publishes the "Dummies" series (e.g., Networking for Dummies, Windows 3.1 for Dummies, QuickBooks for Dummies). These books are a very practical, no-nonsense introduction to virtually every application that is described in the following (visit the Web sites at www.idgbooks.com and www.dummies.com for more information). In addition to printed material, another useful source of information is the online manuals that accompany each application. Typically, their help screens explain in detail how each feature of the program works.

Running Computer Programs

To have an overall appreciation of what computers do, it's extremely useful to have a good understanding of exactly what a computer program is. The only activity computers perform is running programs ("executing" is a synonym). To understand what the computer is doing at any time, know the program(s) the computer is running, identify the features those programs have to offer, and learn how to control those features. From the user's perspective, the program appears as a file stored on a disk drive. From a programmers perspective, the program exists as a series of statements that are written according to the syntax of a programming language. Many programming languages (BASIC, FORTRAN, C++, Pascal, HyperTalk, Pearl, etc.) exist and each language can have variations, like Microsoft's version of Visual BASIC. Each language has a highly structured set of rules (syntax) for expressing statements. Program users do not need to know anything about the details of the programming language to use programs effectively. Usually, programs have a main event loop; the program continuously cycles through this main loop looking for an event to react to: a key being pressed, a button being clicked, or an event from a piece of hardware attached to the computer (e.g., modem, printer, HI-Pro box). When an event is detected, the program branches to a subroutine designed to respond to the event, like calculating and displaying a target real-ear insertion gain (REIG) curve when the "NAL" menu item is selected. Collectively, the features that the program offers are the sum of all the subroutines and events the programmer has built into the program—and nothing more.

Programs, Microprocessors, Software Emulation

Once the computer program is written, it must be converted into a format that the microprocessor (Motorola PowerPC, Intel Pentium II, etc.) of the computer understands. Other programs, called compilers or interpreters, convert the (usually) English-like syntax of the programmer's statement into a series numbers that set switches in the microprocessor, which allow the computer to perform the actions requested by the program. Although it is fortunate that neither the user nor the programmer need be concerned with this level of detail, some consequences should be appreciated. The main one is that programs will run only on a particular platform, Mac or PC, because the coding is specific to the particular family of microprocessor (e.g., Intel 386, 486, Pentium). Although it is possible for a program to be cross-platform, that requires the development of different versions of the program. In larger markets developers often produce software that runs on both the Mac and PC or different developers will produce equivalent products for each platform. Software manufactures in small, vertical markets (like audiology), usually focus on a single platform. In the hearing health care industry, almost all software is developed only for the PC.

An exception to the rule that software developed for the PC only runs on PC compatibles is SoftWindows, a program that runs on Macintosh computers, emulating an Intel processor in software. This emulation process allows code developed for a PC to run on a Mac. The main drawback to this emulation is loss of processing speed: programs run very slowly under SoftWindows. An older DOS program may run acceptably on a fast Macintosh, but performance is unacceptably slow for most software. Another alternative for running PC programs on a Mac is an add-in board. This is a PC on a card that fits into a slot inside the Mac. Performance is comparable to a stand-alone PC. Advantages are that desk space is saved, and it is easier to transfer files between the Mac and PC environment. However, the PC cards are only marginally less expensive than a complete stand-alone PC. Also, some PC cards may have fewer serial ports than a real PC and some cards may not have a parallel port available.

Programs developed for an earlier processor (e.g., 386) will run on a later processor (e.g., 586 or Pentium). The newer processor usually has all the features of the previous generations plus additional features that enable the processor to perform calculations more rapidly and more efficiently. The Pentium is backward compatible with previous generations. It is possible that a program written to take advantage of new features in a processor might not run on previous processors lacking those features. However, a well-written program will check to determine which processor is available and adapt accordingly.

Operating Systems, Program Versions, and File Formats

The computer's operating system (OS) is a significant factor influencing whether a program will execute on a computer. The operating system itself is a sophisticated program that controls the computer's basic hardware (monitor, keyboard, disk drives, etc.) and provides an environment within which the user's applications run. The operating system also catalogs and allows the user to manipulate files stored on the computer's hard drive(s) or floppy disk drives. Microsoft developed an early disk operating system (DOS) for the PC. By today's standards, DOS is fairly primitive; the user is presented with a blank screen and commands are typed, one line at a time, with a very specific syntax. The user needed to memorize quite a few commands to control the computer effectively. From the programmer's perspective, DOS did very little to help him or her develop a user interface. Each programmer built the user interface from scratch and each program was likely to have a unique method for controlling how it worked. Learning how to use one program often did not carry over to helping one use another. By contrast, the Macintosh's OS provided a rich "toolbox" to help the programmer develop the user interface: menus, windows, buttons, and so on provide a consistent look and feel from one program to another. This trend was repeated for the PC platform in Windows 3.x, Windows 95, and Windows NT (Cowart, 1995; Jennings, 1997). The important point to realize is that modern programs are not self-contained. Significant portions of the code needed to run a program are part of the OS. As with microprocessors, OSs are often backwardly compatible, but not always. A DOS program likely will run under Windows 3.1 (without the look and feel of Windows) or Windows 95, but a program designed to take advantage of the new features in Windows 95 will not run under Windows 3.1. Also, many DOS programs will not run under Windows NT, especially if the DOS program tries to directly control the hardware. No guarantee exists that a Windows 95 program will run under NT, although most will. So, when the audiologist is contemplating the purchase of a program, the OS environment is a consideration. Microsoft's plans for the future are eventually to migrate to a single OS, Windows NT.

> ### PEARL
>
> **The computing requirements for running audiology software are not too demanding. A computer with resources (hard drive, microprocessor speed, memory, etc.) for running Windows 95 is more than adequate.**

The version number of a program is also important. Many programs, especially popular ones, are constantly evolving. New features make the program more useful, but compatibility issues can arise. The format of the document file often is the problem. Word processing programs are good examples of this. The program (e.g., Microsoft Word version 4.0 for the Mac) is used to create a document, which may be a letter to a physician or an audiological report. The document is saved to disk, and the file has a specific format dictated by the program. The file format becomes more complex as new features are added to the program as it evolves to Word 5.1, then 6.0.1a, and so on. Typically, the more recent versions can read old file formats, but the older programs cannot read the newer formats. For example, a student uses version 5.1 to begin a report in the clinic, saves the file to disk, takes the file to the computer laboratory, updates the file using version 6.0.1a, saves it to disk, returns to the clinic to finish and print the report, but finds that he or she gets an error message indicating that the file cannot be read. This is very frustrating unless one realizes the source of the problem. Often, programs allow document file storage in different formats, such as earlier versions of Word, versions for a different platform (PC), or in a format compatible with a different word processing program (e.g., WordPerfect). A welcome trend in popular cross-platform programs, like Microsoft Word, is that documents are saved in a format that can be read on either platform. A document created on the Mac can be saved on a PC-formatted disk, the file can be edited by Word running on a PC, saved back to disk, read on the Mac, and so forth.

Major Productivity Tools

The major applications for office management are word processing, spreadsheet, database, presentation, and scheduling. These applications are generic, not developed specifically for any one profession, and many programs fall into this category: Microsoft Office, Corel Office, and Lotus SmartSuite are currently the most popular, with Microsoft Office controlling about 85% of the market (Moseley & Boodey, 1996). Microsoft Works is a "lite" version of Office and ClarisWorks has been popular on the Mac. New computers often are sold with these or similar applications bundled. A tendency exists for many users to learn only the basic features of one program, like a word processor, and use that tool to solve all problems, even when creating a database or spreadsheet would be much easier and more efficient. Many different productivity tools are available, and the scope of this chapter permits only a superficial introduction to their main features. However, a general understanding or awareness may encourage audiologists to learn and implement more of these programs in their own practice setting.

The following are some examples of how these productivity tools can be adapted to audiology. Zapala (1998) is using Quattro Pro to develop The Virtual Audiogram shareware that is in a "beta" stage of development (i.e., software that is functional but does not have all the bugs worked out). Air and bone conduction thresholds can be plotted on an audiogram along with the "speech banana" for counseling. The pure tone average and percentage hearing loss is calculated. Tympanograms are plotted along with normative data for immittance parameters, such as peak admittance and acoustic reflex thresholds. The articulation index (AI) is used to derive performance-intensity functions to which the patient's actual intelligibility can be compared (ANSI, 1969; 1993). Hearing aid prescriptions are made for real-ear and coupler gain, and patient information can be stored in a database. Another example is described by Margolis and Thornton (1991) who used spreadsheet programs for tracking audiology patients. Valente et al (1990) use a spreadsheet to calculate prescriptive targets for hearing aid fitting. Real-ear insertion gain, coupler gain, and output are determined. The AI is used to determine the effect on speech intelligibility. The *Educational Audiology Handbook* (Johnson et al, 1997) comes with a disk that contains a variety of forms, checklists, profiles, letters, and fact sheets for use with word processing programs for the Mac and PC (Marttila, 1998). Mendel et al (1995) describe other computer-based technologies for educational audiologists. Newman et al (1997) explain how to use macro statements (described later in this chapter) with a word processor for rapidly generating hearing disability and handicap profiles.

Word Processing

Word processing is one of the most popular activities, and most computer users are familiar with at least one program. Word processors have evolved to the point where even less popular programs are very feature laden and effective. So many features are offered that few people manage to learn them all. A tendency exists to achieve a basic level of competency and a resistence to exploring more complicated features. The main purpose of a word processor is to facilitate the creation, editing, formatting, and printing of documents. Word processors, however, do more than just manipulate text. They can create tables and combine text with graphics in a variety of useful layouts or templates. "Wizards" assist users in creating basic forms, reports, brochures, receipts, contracts, and newsletter-style documents. Blocks of frequently used phrases can be defined and automatically inserted. Similarly, a short sequence of keystrokes can be associated with a complex graphic, such as an audiogram, tympanogram, or letterhead logo. A fairly complicated clinical report can be built easily and rapidly. Word processors frequently have some capability as drawing programs. It is possible to create detailed drawings that can be stored and recalled with a few keystrokes. Colored audiometric symbols can be drawn on a graphic of an audiogram, and the symbols connected. Charting capability allows easy conversion of numerical data into a number of different types of graphs, such as line or bar graphs, scatterplots, or pie charts. Even a spreadsheet can be added to a word processing document for entering numerical data and performing calculations (see the next section). As an example, a template could be created for a monthly report that automatically added and summarized hearing aid–related expenses.

A word processor's mail merge function is used to create form letters that are personalized for each recipient. This is a common form of marketing for dispensers. Most of the letter is the same for each person, but certain segments of the letter, such as the person's name, title and address, are inserted automatically by the program. Usually the inserted information is exported from a database, but it could be entered from the word processing program, too. In this way marketing activities are enhanced by making correspondence more specific and meaningful to the individual by using, for example, the actual warranty expiration date or hearing aid make and model. Mailing labels can be printed for envelopes, or labels can be made for any other purpose, such as labeling drawers for bins containing parts, such as tubing or loaner hearing aids.

Spreadsheet

The main purpose of a spreadsheet is to perform calculations on numerical data. A spreadsheet, as seen on the computer screen, is a matrix of horizontal rows and vertical columns. The rows are numbered sequentially from top to bottom (1, 2, 3, etc.), and the columns are indicated by letters from left to right (A, B, C, etc.). A rectangular cell appears at the intersection of each row and column and is referenced by a letter-number combination. For example, the cell forming the intersection between the third row and third column would be A3. Each cell usually contains three types of entries: text, numbers, or mathematical/logical formulas. Text is usually entered as a label, to identify the values in a row or column. Numerical data entered by the user is used to perform calculations. When a cell contains a formula, the spreadsheet uses the numerical data in the rows and columns to calculate a value, which is displayed in the cell. Spreadsheet programs were originally developed to simulate the pencil and paper spreadsheets that were used to display business-related calculations. However, spreadsheets are useful for displaying and performing calculations on any type of data that fits into the rows and columns tabular type of format. Another feature that makes spreadsheets useful is their ability to help the user visualize data by quickly creating charts. A chart is created by selecting a block of cells containing text, data entered, or the results of calculations. After a format for the chart is

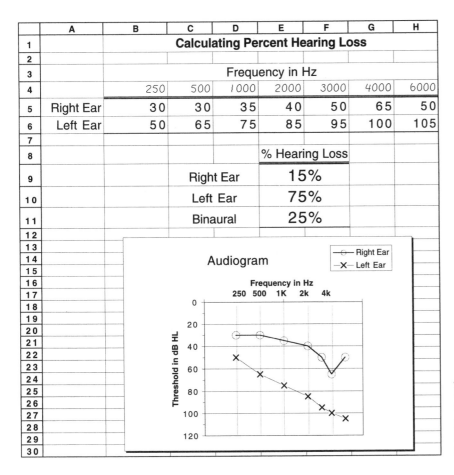

	A	B	C	D	E	F	G	H
1		**Calculating Percent Hearing Loss**						
2								
3		Frequency in Hz						
4		250	500	1000	2000	3000	4000	6000
5	Right Ear	30	30	35	40	50	65	50
6	Left Ear	50	65	75	85	95	100	105
7								
8					% Hearing Loss			
9			Right Ear		15%			
10			Left Ear		75%			
11			Binaural		25%			
12								

Figure 20–1   Example of how an Excel spreadsheet can be used to calculate percent hearing loss. The audiogram is illustrated by a chart that is automatically drawn from the threshold data.

selected (pie chart, bar graph, scatterplot, etc.), the chart is drawn, complete with legends and title.

Figure 20–1 is a simple illustration of how an Excel spreadsheet might be used by an audiologist. The percentage hearing loss is calculated from the pure tone average (500, 1000, and 2000 Hz) using a 25 dB fence and a 1.5% increase in hearing loss for each dB the pure tone average exceeds the fence. The percent binaural hearing loss is calculated by weighting the better ear to the poorer ear using a 5:1 ratio. Audiogram thresholds are entered in cells B5 to H6, and the percentage hearing loss is automatically calculated according to formulas entered in E10 to E12. Note that the text can be styled with different fonts, sizes, justification (centering, left, or right), and borders and single and double lines can be added to ranges of cells. Formatting is flexible and only a few possibilities are shown here. A chart, showing the audiogram, is displayed at the bottom of the spreadsheet. The chart was created in only a few minutes by highlighting the proper range of cells, answering a few questions posed by the "Wizard," and then performing a few modifications (e.g., choosing circles for the right ear, selecting blue for the left ear). When numerical values in the audiogram are changed, the percentage hearing loss is automatically recalculated, and the audiogram is automatically redrawn. The proportions of the audiogram (aspect ratio) are roughly accurate. Excel provided a proper "X" symbol for the left ear. The default circle was too small, so a larger circle was created by using the drawing

tools, and the program was instructed to use the new symbol to plot the audiogram. Creating different audiometric symbols (e.g., bone conduction, no response) proceeds in similar fashion.

Database

Database applications are the major tools for storing, sorting, organizing, cataloging, and retrieving information. A generalized database application can be purchased, but creating a custom database allows great flexibility for managing data unique to a practice. Martin (1991) suggests that audiologists consider including special information about their patients, such as interests or hobbies, difficulties in certain environments, or primary method of communication (oral or sign). Fausti et al (1993) describe how database software was used to store and collect data from a multisite study of ototoxicity.

A database is essentially a collection of records. Each record contains fields, and fields are the objects within which the information is stored. Fields can store text or numeric data, the results of calculations (like the cell in a spreadsheet), or even graphic objects or sounds. For example, each record could store information related to a patient. Typical fields would include the patient's first name, last name, street address, city, state, ZIP code, insurance carrier, and so on. Additional audiometric information could include audiogram thresholds (air and bone, separately for each ear), speech thresholds, word recognition scores, peak admittance, auditory brain stem response (ABR) waveforms, otoacoustic emissions (OAEs), images from video otoscopy. When one stops to consider the potential amount of data that can be generated from an audiological evaluation, the quantity seems endless. Hearing aid information includes date of purchase, purchase price, balance due, make and model, serial number, ear(s) fitted, warranty expiration date, battery club membership, programmable hearing aid session data, and journal entries. Databases can contain all information in a single file (flat file database) or the information can be split into different files (relational database). As the amount of information increases, it is usually easier to manage data if they are divided into smaller logical units. As an example, patient demographic data could be stored in one file, audiometrics in another, hearing aid information in a third. The master file could organize and display a subset of the information.

Databases usually allow display of information in each record to be (on a computer screen) according to a number of different layouts or formats. Each layout is analogous to a report on a subset of the data. Layouts can arrange the data in different orders and incorporate graphical backgrounds to achieve the desired appearance. For example, the audiometric data could be used to automatically generate a standard audiological report. Another use for a custom layout is to produce cells of demographic information to fit on a standard sheet of mailing labels. Yet another layout could be similar to a mail merge form letter. The database could sort the information according to whether patients have pure tone averages greater than a particular value or have a hearing aid older than a particular value, and a mailing could go out describing the features of a new power aid.

Databases generally allow data import or export so that different applications can share data. Data from a word processor or spreadsheet can be imported into the database. Information from the database could be exported to another application. This means that data are not locked into a particular database. If a newer, more useful database program appears on the market, the old data could be exported to it. A database program may reside on a computer connected to a network, and the program may allow users at other computers on the network to run the program remotely, accessing data or entering information. Managing all data from the same database guards against information being fragmented over a number of different computers.

Presentation Software

The purpose of this class of software is to help the presenter convey ideas and images to one or more people in an organized way. Sometimes ideas are best expressed in writing. At other times pictures, diagrams, charts, or a line drawing are more useful. Short video clips, animations, and sound can help to get points across. Presentation software facilitates the creation of multimedia. Many individuals find themselves in the role of presenter. Some examples are classroom instructors giving lectures and trying to stimulate discussion, sales people trying to present a product, members of work groups attempting to persuade managers or inform about the level of progress being made. Audiologists need to explain results of

diagnostic evaluations, counsel and enable patients to understand their impairment and disability, create motivation for patients to try hearing aids or assistive devices, and explain what those devices are and how they work. Audiologists sometimes need to persuade an employer to purchase equipment. Or the audiologist may be explaining the profession to a community group. Although putting a presentation together is never an easy task, this software is very useful for quickly creating professional looking results.

PEARL

Presentation software is not only for groups. Counseling patients, explaining a product line, or unattended waiting room viewing are other uses.

Microsoft PowerPoint is a popular presentation program. Most of the computer-assisted presentations shown at conventions and workshops use PowerPoint. The familiar slide show is a useful metaphor for understanding this application. At its simplest, PowerPoint creates a computerized version of a slide show, each computer screen being analogous to a slide. Slides can have different backgrounds with different colors and shading. Layouts define different formats for how text and graphics appear on the slides, and a number of templates come with the program to help design an attractive display. Different presentations have different purposes, for example, recommending a strategy, selling a product, or training in the use of a technique. A setup Wizard helps create a sample presentation on the basis of the purpose. A variety of media can be incorporated on the slide. Charts can be created from numerical data entered in a spreadsheetlike display and automatically placed on the slide. Pictures, photographic images, or clip art can be imported from other applications. Movies and sounds can be played from within the slide. Slide transitions and other special effects animate the presentation and help hold audience interest. Lecture notes help the speaker remember main points, and handouts can be made for the audience that contain thumbnails (miniature pictures) of the slides and room for written notes. The presentation can be printed on paper, overhead transparencies, or sent to a processing laboratory for 35-mm slides. A presentation can be made to only one or two individuals watching the computer monitor, or the computer's video can be connected to an LCD (liquid crystal display) projector and displayed in large format for larger audiences.

The slides can be advanced manually by the presenter or in a timed mode suitable for unattended viewing, for instance in a waiting room. Such presentations could be useful for common tasks like explaining how to insert a battery, put on a hearing aid, clean wax from a receiver tube, or helpful hints about communicating with persons who are hearing impaired. People tend to become bored with repetitive tasks or move quickly through an explanation that has been given hundreds of times. Computers are patient, do not inadvertently leave out important points, and can serve as documentation that a particular point (e.g., battery ingestion) was covered before the patient left the office.

Scheduling

Contact and information managers are a category of software usually intended to help sales people track and manage data pertinent to their contacts. As part of this software, scheduling can help audiologists manage their appointments. Some schedulers are designed to manage only one individual, others can display appointments for many individuals. It may be possible to use the software over a network and access others' appointment books, schedule appointments for them, or automatically arrange group meetings. Microsoft Outlook 97 is a typical example of this type of software. It is part of Microsoft Office and replaces the previous program, Schedule+. Appointments are viewed on a daily, weekly, or monthly basis. Normal appointment hours can be set, and times not available for appointments can be blocked out. Recurring appointments will appear automatically without manually re-entry. The default length of time for an appointment can be varied (e.g., 15 minutes, half hour), and an appointment can be set to overlap adjacent time slots (i.e., a hearing aid fitting or electronystagmagram could be set to cover more than one time slot). Changes in appointments can be arranged by "dragging" the patient (figuratively) to a new location on either the same or different day. A description of the required services can be entered, along with any notes about the meeting. The appointment can include other personnel or resources, and the scheduler will automatically check to ensure their availability. The scheduler can maintain a "To Do" list, and alarms can be set to act as reminders.

Macros, Object Linking and Embedding, Visual Basic

Although each of the different programs in an office suite possess a great deal of versatility, other features expand their flexibility. For example, the "AutoText" feature of a word processor allows blocks of text (or graphics) to be inserted by associating the text with a name or keystroke combination. Macros are defined in a similar fashion, or they can be assigned a menu item specified by the user. A macro is created by recording a series of keyboard entries and menu selections. Then, the entire sequence is replayed by invoking the keystrokes or choosing the menu item that defines the macro. Repetitive, but highly detailed, sequences of commands can be automated by assigning them to a macro. Microsoft Office also allows the macro to be edited and commands inserted by the Microsoft Visual Basic for Applications programming language. This greatly increases the power and flexibility of the macro. For example, a macro can be written that selects a range of cells in a spreadsheet that defines the audiogram. The effect of the hearing loss on the ability to hear average conversational level speech could be calculated using Visual Basic code that implements the speech intelligibility index or AI.

Object linking and embedding (OLE) blurs the distinction between one program and another. An application's object, like a portion of a spreadsheet, could be embedded in another

---

> **PEARL**
>
> **Microsoft Office includes Visual Basic for Applications. This is a powerful tool for programming word processors or spreadsheets to perform custom tasks.**

application, like a word processor. All of the functions normally available in the spreadsheet would be available from within the word processor. If the embedded object is linked to the original spreadsheet application, whenever a change is made to the spreadsheet, the portion of the word processor document is automatically updated. With OLE, information created in one application flows automatically into another.

Programming

Word processors, spreadsheets, databases, and the other productivity tools offer quite a bit of flexibility for customizing documents. Inevitably, neither they nor off-the-shelf programs will meet the user's needs exactly. The alternative is to write a program. The advantage is a custom product tailored to one's needs, but major disadvantages exist. Computer languages, even the "easier" ones, like BASIC, still require a lot of effort to master. Even after the language is learned, creating and debugging software is a very time-consuming task. Most professionals, including audiologists, do not have the time or inclination to develop their own software. For those who find programming intrinsically rewarding, satisfaction is associated with the creative process and crafting a useful software tool.

Most commercial grade programs are written by professional programmers in a variation of the C programming language, a very powerful language that enables control of virtually every aspect of the computer. C is difficult to learn, especially in regard to controlling the complex user interface presented by Windows and the Mac OS. On the PC, Visual Basic is a favorite tool for amateur programmers, and it allows for the development of sophisticated programs (e.g., DSL 4.1 for hearing aid selection). HyperCard has been popular with Mac users. HyperCard is the programming environment for the HyperTalk programming language. HyperTalk is a high-level, object-oriented, scripting language with an English-like syntax that is fairly easy to learn (de Jonge, 1992). HyperCard is used to create applications called "stacks." The metaphor is that each screen of information is like a note card, and a collection of cards is a stack. SuperTalk, which also runs on the Mac, is a more sophisticated version of HyperCard. ToolBook and MetaCard are similar programs for the PC. These programs provide objects—cards, buttons, text fields, graphic tools—that can be controlled by fragments of computer code (scripts). It is possible to build fairly sophisticated applications in much less time than would be possible with a traditional language (like C). For example, Palmer (1992) used HyperCard to develop a system for tracking student clinical hours, locating assistive listening device products, and scoring a self-report scale of hearing handicap. Sims et al (1992) used HyperCard to develop a custom application for calculating a popular hearing aid fitting prescription. Many other options are available for people who are interested in writing their own multimedia projects (Lieberth & Martin, 1995).

Business and Financial Management

Clinic directors and private practice audiologists soon find themselves in the role of financial manager. Mueller (1990) describes how personal computers can be used for planning and making business decisions. Hosford-Dunn et al (1995) provide an excellent introduction to the basic concepts involved in bookkeeping and account management. These are important activities, and fortunately powerful yet inexpensive (less than $100) software tools are available to help the new business owner get started. Peachtree software and Quicken and QuickBooks from Intuit are examples of popular software packages for managing the finances of any small business, including an audiology practice (Nelson, 1996). Quicken is designed more for personal and home management, while QuickBooks provides a complete double-entry accounting system for a business. An early consideration in setting up the software is to define the categories of financial transactions. QuickBooks provides examples for different types of small businesses, but an accountant should be consulted when setting up a chart of accounts. Careful attention needs to be paid to these accounts. They provide the basic information from which all reports and summaries will be derived. Some examples are applying for bank loans, paying taxes, and viewing the financial health of the business (i.e., profit-loss statements and cash flow analysis). If one is interested in determining "profit centers" in a practice (e.g., selling programmable versus conventional hearing aids versus providing diagnostic services), accounts must be set up to record transactions in these categories.

PEARL

QuickBooks is an inexpensive yet comprehensive program for managing office finances. Seek the advice of an accountant to help set up a chart of accounts.

The software is easy to use if time is taken to learn the program and develop a basic understanding of accounting procedures. Most entries can be made as if using a checking account (i.e., each check that is written must have money taken out of an account, and income is also credited to certain accounts). All financial transactions are maintained in a single file. The file can be copied to disk (or E-mailed as an attachment) and brought to the accountant for tax preparation. Data can be graphed to help visualize relationships for the different accounts. In addition to accounts payable and receivable, other features include online banking and check writing, payroll, customizable invoices, receipts, and inventory.

Networking

The term *personal* computer aptly describes the major characteristic of the early microcomputers. They were stand-alone machines under the dominion of one person who had total control over the system's resources and did not have to share, and could not share, them with anyone else. This situation has advantages (simplicity, control, and security) and disadvantages. The major disadvantage is the inability to share resources like programs and printers. By connecting computers in a network, data stored in a file on the hard drive of one computer can be accessed from another computer. A program on one computer can be run from another computer. For audiologists this can offer significant advantages in certain situations. For example, imagine a busy dispensing office with four fitting rooms that can be used by different audiologists. Each room has a computer with software used to fit programmable hearing aids. Patient X is initially seen by audiologist A in fitting room 1. Without a network, all patient information is stored on the computer in room 1. On the next visit, patient X sees audiologist B (because audiologist A is at a satellite office) in room 2. But X's records are nowhere to be found, and unless some mechanism is in place to keep track of who is fitted where, the records could be in any one of the four fitting rooms. The situation becomes even more complicated if X decides to occasionally drop in at the satellite office. With a network, all data and fitting programs can be stored in one central location (on one computer), and each audiologist can access patient records from any one of the fitting rooms. Also, current operating systems allow a network to be accessed (a dial-up connection over the phone lines by means of a modem) from a computer at a remote location, such as the satellite office. In the ideal situation all pertinent information is available from any location.

Networking is a complex topic, so only a few basic points can be made here. The original operating system for PCs, DOS, did not permit functional networking. Consequently, early network operating systems, like Novell NetWare and LANtastic evolved to fill this need. Microsoft's later OSs (Windows 3.1, 95, and NT) support networking, and most recent networks will be based on Windows. Older networks may still be running the legacy OSs, like NetWare. Today, a common and fairly easy network to construct uses Windows 95's built-in capability for networking and is based on hardware conforming to the ethernet standard. Ethernet is fast, so even though data are located on a remote computer, the illusion is that they are present on one's own computer. Physically, each computer sends a cable out to a device called a "hub," creating a star topology, which routes the signals out to each computer. With the network hardware in place and the system software properly configured, programs and files that are located on other computers appear on one's own desktop, just as if they were stored locally on the hard drive. This is a basic description of what is referred to as a "local area network," or LAN.

One type of network is referred to as "peer-to-peer," the other uses a "client-server" model. In a client-server model one computer designated as the server is the main repository of programs and data files. The other computers (clients) access its services. Usually, the server is dedicated to supplying files and running programs for other users; the server is not for personal use. In a peer-to-peer network all computers can share the role of client or server. The disadvantage to this arrangement occurs if many users are trying to access a single PC. The user of that PC sees his or her machine's performance slow considerable. On the positive side, a peer-to-peer network is relatively easy to set up using Windows 95 or the MacOS, and each OS works similarly. It is also possible to have PCs coexist on a Mac network and Macs share a Windows network. With Windows NT, a client-server model is common. For a relatively small network (up to five computers) setting up a peer-to-peer network will be most practical.

Running software over a network poses significant challenges to software developers, so do not necessarily assume everything will run smoothly. Problems that exist on a single computer are often multiplied when programs are run over a network. On a network it is common for many applications to be running simultaneously. Those programs might run fine by themselves, but when one attempts to access the same resources running at the same time the system will freeze or crash. Several issues need to be considered when running a program over the network, the first is whether the application will accept multiple users. A multiuser program, such as a database, will permit more than one person to access its information at one time. Another issue is access to individual records. The program may allow only one user access to a record at one time, or it may permit many users to read the information, but only one user (usually the first to access the record) can change the information in the record. Security is another issue, deciding who has privileges to access what information on whose computer in which folders. Some information, such as scheduling, should be available to all, but sensitive financial information about the clinic needs to be restricted. Also, if the network can be accessed through a dial-up connection, it is important to ensure that only authorized personnel have access. Although the Macintosh and Windows 95 networks offer security, Windows NT offers more robust and sophisticated protection schemes.

PITFALL

Networking computers offers great possibilities. However, running software over a network poses significant challenges to software developers, especially as the network becomes more complex. Do not necessarily assume everything will run smoothly. It probably will not.

As networks become more useful, flexible, and larger, it becomes a challenge to keep them running. Once in place, they become indispensable and perhaps some critical revenue-generating services (like programming hearing aids) cannot be performed without them. In large organizations people are hired solely to make sure the networks run smoothly. In a small practice several questions need to be answered, such as: Who will administer and troubleshoot the network? Should a consultant be hired, or should one or more

audiologists attempt to take on the responsibility of learning this new skill? Will these audiologists have the time to devote to this task, or will more employees need to be hired, and is the cost justifiable?

The Internet

Undoubtedly the Internet is becoming a major force affecting how information is stored, made available to users, and accessed. The Internet, and especially the World Wide Web (WWW), is growing at a very rapid pace, and with new developments occurring so quickly, it is difficult to envision what it will be like 5 years from now. However, it is extremely likely that Internet applications will profoundly influence what computers are used for in many professions, including audiology. It is likely that accessing the Internet will become the primary use for computers. Wynne (1996) gives a good introduction to the Internet, with an emphasis for audiological applications. For more technical references to the Internet see Dern (1994) and Gilster (1995). Gralla (1997) provides a very concise description of a broad range of topics relating to the Internet. Table 20–1 illustrates the diversity in audiology-related information by describing a variety of Web sites.

PEARL

In the future the main reason why people use computers may be to access the Internet. It is difficult to overemphasize the significance of this technology and the impact it will have on audiology.

A Brief History

What was destined to be the Internet was created in 1969 by the U.S. Defense Department's Advanced Research Project Agency (DARPA). It was an experimental computer network (ARPAnet) connecting the UCLA campus, Stanford Research Institute, UCSB (Santa Barbara), and the University of Utah. The computers (Honeywell 516 minicomputers) were connected by means of high-speed (56 kbps) leased telephone lines. Researchers exchanged E-mail and data files over the network. The networking software, NCP (network control protocol), was developed by Bolt, Beranek, and Newman (BBN) in Cambridge, Massachusetts. This "packet-switching network" was able to route packets around a damaged line (i.e., the network could survive a bomb attack) and in this respect was like the interstate highway system. For more than a decade the ARPAnet grew slowly by adding a computer every 20 days. In 1983 NCP was changed to TCP/IP (transmission control protocol/internetworking protocol), and this is considered to be the beginning of the Internet. At this time the military portion (Milnet) split off to form a separate network. In 1987 the National Science Foundation (NSF) expanded ARPAnet, creating the NSFnet, a high-speed "backbone" to connect five supercomputer centers across the nation (e.g., from MIT to San Francisco to the University of Illinois). The NSFnet charter supported "research and education" as appropriate uses for the Internet. Commercial use of the

TABLE 20–1   **Examples of Web sites that illustrate the diversity of information available on the Internet about audiology**

Web site/Web page	Description
http://www.audiology.com http://www.asha.org	Web sites for the American Academy of Audiology and the American Speech-Language-Hearing Association contain information regarding issues for professionals and consumers.
http://www.mankato.msus.edu/dept/comdis/kuster2/audiology.html	Judith Kuster has compiled links (262 URLs) to a variety of .audiology sites.
http://www.audiologyinfo.com/	Glen Meier and Paul Dybala's site contains links to Web sites of interest to audiologists and consumers.
http://www.audiologynet.com/	Get links to Web sites that provide information about tinnitus, Meniere's disease, acoustic neuroma, cholesteatoma, and other medical conditions.
http://www.yahoo.com/	Search for Web sites by typing words that might appear on those Web sites.
http://www.boystown.org/cel/cochamp.htm	Boy's Town posts information about genetics and hearing loss and they have simulations illustrating cochlear physiology.
http://www.resound.com http://www.starkey.com http://www.oticonus.com	Get information about hearing aid products and services. Most manufacturers maintain a presence on the Web.
http://www.danavox.com/articles/art6.htm	Read a description of the Madsen Aurical system. See a photograph of the hardware and screen shots of the software.
http://www.nlm.nih.gov/	Do an audiology literature review by searching MEDLINE.
http://www.himsa.com/	Find out which products are NOAH certified. Download a "demo" version of NOAH.
http://www.li.net/~sullivan/ears.htm	Get access to hundreds of video-otoscopy images illustrating pathological conditions of the external and middle ear.
http://www.uwo.ca/hhcru/	Visit the Hearing Health Care Research Unit at the University of Western Ontario. Find out more about the DSL[i/o] procedure and where it was developed.
http://www.gennum.com	Get details of the DynamEQ II chip. Download product information in a publication-quality format.
http://www.hearingoffice.com/	Download Hearing Office Lite, office management freeware written by an audiologist.
http://www.frye.com/	Find out about a manufacturer's products, also download the IHAFF software.
http://www.earmold.com/	See what earmold products are available from Westone. Show the pictures to patients.
http://www.audios.com/	Learn about audiological report generating software from Audiologic Software Inc. Download software.
http://www.bio.net/hypermail/AUDIOLOGY/	Read postings to the bionet.audiology newsgroup.
http://www.asha.org/Asha_Member/listserv.htm	Learn how to join a mailing list like the ASHA-audiology-forum.
http://www.measure.demon.co.uk/Acoustics_Software/h_loss.html	This Java applet is a program that runs in a browser window. It calculates the probability of exceeding a fence (amount of hearing loss) based on patient age and duration and level of noise exposure.
ftp://ftp.the.net/mirrors/ftp.utexas.edu/sound/digital-oscilloscope-21.hqx	Download a program that turns the Mac into a digital oscilloscope.

backbone was forbidden. Meanwhile, commercial organizations were creating similar networks (AlterNet, PSInet, etc.). In 1991 Commercial Internet Exchange (CIX), an interconnection point, was created. It merged the commercial and noncommercial networks. This was a great benefit to audiologists, considering their close interaction with hearing aid manufacturers and equipment vendors.

Tim Berners-Lee and others in 1989 at CERN (European Particle Physics Lab in Geneva, Switzerland) developed hypertext markup language (HTML) and hypertext transfer protocol (HTTP) and the WWW and hypermedia were born. The WWW permits the transfer of rich media (i.e., text, graphics, sound) from a host computer (running Web server software) to a remote computer running client software, a Web browser such as Netscape Navigator or Microsoft Internet Explorer. In 1991 the first Web server and browser went online. In January 1993 50 Web servers were in existence, increasing to 4500 in May of 1994. Since then, growth has been exponential. Although the Internet has been around for some time, the WWW is a fairly recent development. Web access accounts for most of the use of the Internet.

HTML, HTTP, Web Sites, and Web Pages

HTML is a language that describes how Web pages are formatted. HTTP is one of the Internet's software protocols that transport Web pages between computers. A Web site is a collection of files, in directories (folders), on the hard drive of a computer connected to the Internet. The computer "hosts" the Web site and runs a Web server program that "serves" these files to a "client" when requested to do so by the client. The client software (e.g., Netscape Navigator) is a Web browser program running on another computer also connected to the Internet. The client requests a "Web page" from the server and (by means of HTTP) the server sends a text file (HTML document) to the client. The HTML document contains hidden tags (HTML code) that tell the browser how to format the document—font size, centering, bold face, and so on. HTML code can also instruct the browser to request a graphics file from the server. The server downloads the picture and the browser displays it with the text. The Web page can look like any page out of a magazine containing colorful, stylized text and graphics.

But, more significantly, HTML defines "hypertext," which usually appears as blue, underlined text in the Web page. Click on the hypertext and a link is invoked (in the HTML code) to another place on the Web page, another Web page, a movie or sound file (which will download), a Java applet, or ActiveX control (small programs), which will download and run on your computer. HTML and HTTP allow for an interesting, interactive experience. The real possibility exists that the Internet can become a virtual extension of one's own computer. The vast collection of resources that exist on all the computers connected to the Internet will appear as though they are located on each individual's computer.

URLs, DNS, and TCP/IP

The Internet is a vast network of networks, consisting of millions of computers spread out across the world and present in most countries. The domain naming system (DNS) is responsible for keeping track of all the computers. DNS assigns a

value to each computer in the form of four, 8-bit numbers separated by dots. This allows for 256^4 or about 4.3 billion unique addresses. A universal resource locator (URL) is also used to help humans remember domain names. For example, the domain "205.242.230.2" is equivalent to "www.iland.net" and represents the Web server software running a Web site for an Internet service provider (ISP). The Web site could be accessed by the address "http://www.iland.net." URLs are so commonly used that it is useful to be able to decipher them. The "http:" portion of the URL indicates that the hypertext transport protocol is being used to transfer information from a Web site. Other protocols, such as ftp, telnet, gopher, mailto, and news, are also used. The "ftp:" protocol is used for downloading files. The rather long URL "ftp://ftp.the.net/mirrors/ftp.utexas.edu/sound/digital-oscilloscope-21.hqx" references a program for the Mac that emulates a digital oscilloscope. The program "digital-oscilloscope-21.hqx" is located in a directory called "sound," which is inside another directory called "ftp.utexas.edu," which is inside still another directory called "mirrors." The "mirrors" directory is located at the "ftp.the.net" domain. Other protocols have different functions. The "telnet:" protocol is used for running programs on a remote computer, "mailto:" for sending E-mail, and "news:" for accessing a newsgroup. A gopher is a menu-based system developed at University of Minnesota (home of the Golden Gophers) for finding and retrieving information.

The domain portion of the URL is "www.iland.net" and references the Web site. Government Web sites end in ".gov," commercial sites are ".com," organizations are ".org," networks are ".net." Different countries also have unique designations; ".dk" and ".ca" indicate Denmark and Canada, respectively. The URL "http://www.danavox.com/articles/art6.htm" references an HTML document (a Web page) called "art6.htm" located in a directory called "articles" in the Danavox company's Web site. The Madsen Aurical system is described in "art6.htm."

A variety of computers exist on the Internet for different purposes. Host computers run Web server programs that are accessed by client software. Other computers, routers, calculate the best route for the packets of information to reach their destination. Some of these routes are high-speed digital lines (150 mbps), others are slower (e.g., a 28.8 kbps modem line). Use of the Internet, or computers in general, can become tedious when they do not respond quickly to our requests. A brief understanding of the protocols, TCP/IP, helps to understand why this can happen. If a large file is being sent over the Internet, it is disassembled at the source and reassembled at the destination. TCP divides the file into smaller parts, packets of about 1500 bytes each. Each packet has header information, information about where the packet came from and where it's going—like splitting a document into individual pages and placing each page within an addressed envelope. IP is responsible for determining the best route for the packet to reach its destination, and each packet may even take a different route. Packets are analogous to cars moving down highways; heavy rush-hour traffic (a large number of packets) or a slow highway (a low-speed transmission line) causes delays and frustration while waiting. Connecting to the Internet at high speeds is a big advantage.

Connecting to the Internet

The following is a brief explanation of how to connect to the Internet, from the home or office, by means of a dial-up, modem-based connection over the same telephone lines used to place voice calls or send faxes (Kobler, 1997). It is also possible to connect from a network administered by a business, university, or hospital. The basic hardware needs are a multimedia computer (graphics and sound), a modem, and an ordinary telephone line. The modem allows your computer to "speak" and "listen" over telephone lines. Establish an Internet account with a company. Companies that are ISPs, for a monthly fee of roughly $15 to $20, provide a gateway to the Internet, an E-mail account, and often space for a small Web site. Online services (like America Online [AOL] or the Microsoft Network [MSN]) provide this in addition to other services. The ISP, or online service, will supply whatever software its users need to connect to the Internet and access its services. Some of this software may be included with the MacOS, Windows 95, or NT. Dial-up software establishes a connection to the ISP or online service, the TCP/IP stack enables data to be sent over the Internet, an E-mail program (Eudora and Pegasus Mail are free and popular) is used to send and receive messages, and a Web browser (Netscape Navigator or Microsoft Internet Explorer) is used to download Web pages. Although ISPs offer guidance and troubleshooting tips, it always helps to cultivate a relationship with a computer-savvy friend.

E-mail and Mailing Lists

The Internet provides a variety of useful activities. Among the most widely used is E-mail. Other than the monthly fee, typically nothing is charged for each message sent or received. Each ISP sets up an E-mail account for its users and provides an application (e.g., Eudora) that allows E-mail to be sent and received. Each user has an E-mail address (e.g., JaneDoe@iland.net). Sending E-mail is extremely simple. Enter the address of the recipient, type a message, and send it. The message is eventually routed, usually in a manner of minutes, to the mail server of the recipient's ISP, where it waits to be downloaded and read. E-mail can contain styled text or appear like an HTML document. It can have other files attached to it, like a graphics image or word processor document. E-mail can be sent to a single person or a group of people. A message can be forwarded to another person (or group of people). This flexibility allows for virtually instantaneous communication with one or more people all over the world.

Mailing lists use E-mail to allow groups of people with similar interest to engage in the equivalent of a "town hall" meeting. After subscribing to a mailing list, such as ASHA's audiology forum, each E-mail message sent to the forum's E-mail address is copied and sent to each other subscriber. Each member of the mailing list can be an active participant in the discussion (for example, Au.D. issues) or he or she can merely observe. Any topic is possible, and discussions cover a wide range of topics from professional issues to clinical interests. For example, an audiologist could post a message relating to test results obtained on an interesting or difficult case, or it could be a request for help or advice from members of the forum. Another message might be notification of a job opening or publicizing a continuing education activity. Usenet is another network that is dedicated to newsgroups, which are similar to mailing lists. More than 12,000 newsgroups are devoted to a variety of interests, some deal with topics such as audiology, deafness, tinnitus, and so on. Bionet.audiology is the newsgroup devoted specifically to issues relating to audiology.

Web Sites

Figure 20–2 illustrates the appearance of a typical Web site. A number of Web sites provide information pertaining to audiologists. Individuals have searched the Web and created Web pages with links to sites that may be of interest to audiologists. Kuster's Web page (see ASHA's Web site at www.asha.org) catalogs 262 links to URLs covering a wide range of topics such as specialties and specialists dealing with hearing loss; support groups for the hearing impaired; anatomy and physiology of the hearing mechanism; disorders, diagnosis, and treatment relating to hearing loss; acoustic neuromas; Meniere's disease; and inflammatory disease of the ear. The list is almost endless, a virtual library of information that can be anything that someone wishes to make public by means of a Web site. Some Web sites are maintained by professional organizations (such as the American Speech-Language-Hearing Association and the American Academy of Audiology, www.audiology.org) to serve their members. Other Web sites are primarily informative or educational in nature; for example, the Boys Town Web site (www.boystown.org) contains information about many topics including genetic hearing loss and basic anatomy and physiology. Short video clips illustrating phenomena like hair cell motility and basilar membrane motion can be downloaded and played. Roy Sullivan's Web site (www.li.net/~sullivan/ears.htm) is devoted to the topic of video otoscopy and provides numerous images of pathological conditions of the external and middle ear. These images can be downloaded and, for example, shared by an instructor with students or used to educate a patient about his or her otological problems.

Other Web sites are devoted to commercial endeavors, occasionally a mix of marketing and educational material or demonstration software for downloading. Most Web sites provide a way to communicate with the company through E-mail. In general, the Web site has the potential for providing rapid access to up-to-date information that can be accessed at any time, night or day, from the office, home, or another remote location like a hotel room. The *Hearing Journal's* annual directory provides an entire section that lists company URLs. Typically, companies provide product information targeted to either professionals or consumers. For example, Gennum Corporation (www.gennum.com) posts information about circuits like the DynamEQ II chip. Details like the number of channels in the chip or slope of the filter skirts can be obtained. Westone

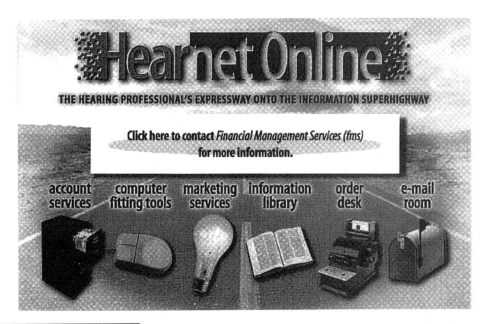

Figure 20–2 Example of a typical, commercial Web site that offers a wide array of online features.

(www.earmold.com) provides images of their swim molds, and most hearing aid manufacturers allow one to browse their product lines. Danavox (www.danavox.com) posts informative articles about loudness scaling procedures, HIMSA (Hearing Industry Manufacturer's Association, www.himsa.com) provides a demonstration version of Noah for downloading, Frye's Web site (www.frye.com) posts the IHAFF (Independent Hearing Aid Fitting Forum) software and user manuals, and Louis DuBrey's Web site (www.hearinginfo.com) offers a free download of Hearing Office Lite, which is database software designed for office management. For a monthly fee, Starkey offers a Web site (www.starkey.com) that is similar to an online service provider like AOL or MSN. Like an ISP, they offer Internet connectivity and an E-mail address. Detailed information about Starkey's hearing aid and software products is available, as well as a number of journal articles, instant access to financial information such as account balances, and the ability to place orders. A useful facility for suggesting appropriate hearing aid fittings is also available. After entering an audiogram, a listing of recent successful fittings is given.

Searching the Internet

No master directory exists for the Internet, but the Web browser has a variety of tools available to help locate information. These are generally referred to as "search engines," like Alta Vista, Excite, or MetaCrawler. Search engines operate by periodically visiting a very large number (perhaps millions) of Web pages, cataloging and indexing their contents, and building a large database about the contents of the Web. Sites of interest are located by searching the database. The browser usually incorporates a direct link to a Web page that is designed specially for searching. Words or phrases are typed into a field, the database is searched, and "hits" are returned (i.e., URLs to pages containing the words). For example, the words "syndromes Treacher-Collins bone conduction hearing aid" might produce a useful Web site. Some

search engines allow boolean search operators like "and" and "or," so hits would be returned on a Web page that contains all the search terms or any of them. Searching the Web can become involved and it is something of an art. The basic idea is to anticipate those words that are likely to appear on a Web page of interest, and then search for those terms. Some search engines offer "intelligent" searches; sophisticated algorithms using artificial intelligence attempt to increase the probability of identifying useful information.

Challenges and Opportunities

An enticing line of reasoning goes along with the question, "Can a computer program be written to do this"? "This" could be any task or activity that a person prefers not to do, perhaps because it is boring, routine, or unattractive in some other respect. Let the computer do it. A computer program is essentially a collection of algorithms. An algorithm is a sequence of steps leading to a desired outcome or the completion of a task. Each step in the process must be entirely explicit. In theory, the following is true:

- If the program has access to all the relevant information needed to achieve an outcome, and
- If the methods necessary to achieving the desired outcome are understood well enough so that each step in the process can be stated explicitly,
- Then it is possible to write a program to accomplish the task.

Most often the answer to the preceding question is, "Yes, but how much in the way of resources is one willing to commit"? The reality is that practical limitations make it unfeasible to implement some solutions. A price always must be paid in time, effort, ingenuity, and computer hardware, which translates to money. Someone needs to become expert in developing computer software and knowledgeable in hardware, or this expertise needs to be purchased. A capable programmer needs to be hired and paid whatever it takes to devote time to the project. Exactly what needs to be accomplished should be explained to the programmer in precise detail. All the staff who are likely to be affected should have input. Make certain that the solution fits efficiently into the "big picture" of how work flows through the office. Purchase the required hardware, spend time troubleshooting the "bugs" in the system. Train employees in using the new system. Continue to train new employees. Be prepared for errors to occur as computers, software, or operating systems need to be upgraded. Computerization offers great opportunities, but be aware of the challenges (Strom, 1997).

PEARL

Do not ask the question, "Can the computer do *this*?" The answer is almost always, "Yes." The real question is, "How much time, money, and effort are you willing to spend?"

Learning the Terminology

The benefit gained from using computers exacts a price, the learning curve. Effective computer use demands familiarity with a whole new set of concepts and ideas. Hardware devices, the OS, and user interface all have names: scroll bars, menus, menu items, combo boxes, tabbed dialogs, control panels, and so on. Take the time to learn the objects' correct names and what the objects do. The benefits become apparent when problems arise that require troubleshooting and the user must explain exactly what happened to an expert. The statement, "I can't 'pull up' my file," is not nearly as informative as "When I click the Start button and go to the Programs folder, I cannot find the Microsoft Word application." Many people do not know even basic information such as the name of their computer, the amount of memory it has, the size of the hard drive, the version number of their application. It is difficult to diagnose the problem without an accurate description of the symptoms. Imagine trying to describe a hearing loss without using the terms "frequency," "decibel," and "threshold" accurately.

PEARL

Make an effort to learn the terminology used to describe the computer and the operating system. When things go wrong, nobody can help unless you can accurately describe the problem.

Attitudes about Computers

Decisions about computer use in the practice are influenced by attitudes about computers. It is helpful for each individual to evaluate one's biases about the technology. Some people are vaguely fearful and mistrust computers, some openly admit to being intimidated. Others embrace the computer with the trusting abandon of a child discovering a new toy. The first group finds many "reasons," which are little more than excuses, for not using computers, even if the benefits are compelling and obvious (Stearns, 1998). The latter group finds computers fascinating devices; computer use is intrinsically rewarding and requires no justification. They may develop a complex, time-consuming, computer-based system even though a manual solution is more efficient. A more appropriate approach is to analyze the practical impact the computer will have on completing the task with the ultimate goal of improving patient service. Will it be accomplished sooner; more efficiently; reduce the number of errors; save money; free personnel from boring or repetitive tasks; allow people to engage in other, more productive activities?

Feasible Solutions?

Is computerization an appropriate solution to a problem? To answer this question, it is necessary to adopt a global perspective to see how this solution fits into the overall work flow in the clinic. Make a detailed analysis of how the job is performed, where it is performed, which steps are taken in what sequence to complete the job, and see whether any major problems exist. Usually they do. For example, the issue may be whether to automate audiological report writing. In most clinics the data used to generate a report come from many sources and separate pieces of equipment, often spread out in different physical locations. Case history information may begin with written comments from the patient (or the patient's chart) entered on a paper form. Answers to additional questions are jotted down by the audiologist on another piece of paper. Or perhaps the computer is located where the case history information is taken, and the patient comments are entered directly into the computer. Data from the audiometer may be manually transferred to a paper audiogram, speech thresholds and word recognition scores written on a form, tympanograms and acoustic reflex data may be printed directly from the tympanometer, OAEs may be stored in a data file and printed on paper, and images from a video otoscope are archived on paper from the video printer. And the list could go on.

It is possible to create a custom database to hold all this information. Fields can be created for demographic information; numerical values for test results; and text describing patient history, impressions, and recommendations. Graphics, like the audiogram, can be created from the numerical data or a scanner can create a digital representation of the paper image for insertion in the database. To search the database for a graphic, a field with a text description could accompany the image. The database would have to be flexible enough to allow for entry of all relevant information, perhaps even a self-report questionnaire on hearing aid satisfaction or the results and accompanying letter from an outside referral source. Otherwise, patient information would have to be maintained in two separate locations, a paper file and an electronic file. If the audiology clinic is part of a larger organization, all information may have to be output to paper anyway.

Such a situation poses significant challenges to creating a comprehensive system of electronic records. Modest goals are more reasonable. Data are generated at different locations, and computers are not located at each location. Most audiometric equipment does not generate information in the proper format. Too much information comes from outside sources, and the format in which the data are received is not controlled. It would take an inordinate amount of time to type or retype information, scan images, and create one's own custom database software, assuming that an off-the-shelf program does not exist to integrate all information. Devising a system that is flexible enough for even present needs and capable of anticipating future needs is a daunting task. Also, it is important to analyze why all this information needs to be collected, to what practical use will it be put? Will there be a future savings in time and efficiency by storing this information, or will the data never be accessed again?

The Ideal Computer-Based System

In the future, it is very likely that a number of computer-based systems will evolve for managing the flow of information through the audiology clinic. The following are some ideas that may prove useful for evaluating programs:

- Consider the amount and type of data the practice generates and how the software will accomodate it. Visualize all the information that appears in the charts and think of how the application will deal with it. Data are the raw material with which computer applications must deal. The amount of information is large and varied. Even something audiologists regard as simple, like an audiogram, is complex when viewed from a programmer's perspective. Sixteen different symbols can be generated for each frequency for air and bone conduction thresholds for each of two ears, masked and unmasked, response and no response. Some testers use mastoid placement of the bone vibrator, others will use the forehead. Sound-field thresholds, aided versus unaided, most comfortable levels (MCLs), loudness discomfort levels (LDLs), acoustic reflex data, ipsilateral versus contralateral will often tax the flexibility of most software. Many possible test procedures can be performed; convention dictates our expectations of how that information will be displayed (e.g., in a table, graph, or narrative form), and the software loses its value if it cannot accommodate data entry for each.

- Automate data entry from external equipment (e.g., audiometers, immittance devices, hearing aid analyzers) into the database application. A considerable time savings can be realized if data can be sent directly to the computer through a network connection or an RS-232 serial communications port. However, a practical limitation exists to the number of devices that can be connected by means of the serial interface. Although PCs can have at most four COM ports, typically they have only two (Kruger & Kruger, 1997).

- Integrate data from different devices or applications. For example, during hearing aid fitting, it is useful to display REIG on the same graph as target gain while the software for adjusting hearing aid parameters is being manipulated. To be effective, sometimes this integration must occur in real time.

- Organization and reporting of data should be flexible. Will the software allow user-defined fields? Can field names

be changed? For example, if a field is labeled "Word Discrimination," can it be changed to "Word Recognition"?

- Consider the scope of the practice in terms of all the procedures that are performed and what software solutions are available for each. Does the software deal with all procedures; does the software integrate well with other packages? For example, maybe one software package does scheduling and another does an exceptional job of accounting. Ideally, these two applications will exchange information. Otherwise, time will be wasted in retyping data. Appendix 10-A in Hosford-Dunn et al (1995) provides a detailed description of procedures that could be automated in a hypothetical audiology practice. The areas they considered relevant were patient and customer care activities (including audiological testing), scheduling, record keeping, planning, correspondence, hearing aid fitting, maintaining product logs and reports, accounting and billing, marketing, and communications.

- The same information should be entered only once. The software should be "smart" enough to find information already stored (like a name and address) so the user does not waste time repeatedly providing the system with "information it already knows." Minimizing redundancy reduces chances for making errors and saves time.

> ### PEARL
>
> **"Smart" software does not waste your time asking for the same information twice. Minimizing redundancy also reduces chances for making errors.**

- The application should automate tasks and not require the audiologist to perform calculations that could be made by the computer, such as pure tone average (PTA); categorizing degree of hearing loss on the basis of PTA; presence or absence of significant air-bone gaps defines type of hearing loss.

- The potential exists for more complex data analysis, the application of artificial intelligence, on the basis of results from the literature. As examples, the likelihood of middle ear effusion is predictable from a combination of the peak admittance and tympanogram slope; the probability that an ABR's wave V latency is outside the normal range can be calculated on the basis of the patient's age.

- The program should also give feedback if unusual or erroneous conditions exist. Audiometry is a repetitive task, and humans tend to make errors. A message could alert the audiologist to a discrepancy between the speech reception threshold (SRT) and the PTA, an interoctave frequency that should be tested, or an air-bone gap that suggests masking.

- Does purchase of the program commit the clinic to a long-term relationship like a "marriage"? Each application often generates a lot of data files, and the format of the files may be proprietary. A significant amount of time and money is invested in creating an informational system that is used to run the clinic. Once a system is running smoothly, people are loath to change for fear the change will cause errors in the system. Updating to a new system always creates glitches, some minor and some major. Companies go out of business, and product support may no longer exist. An application that dominates the market one year may be obsolete a few years later. New products are introduced with valuable features, but one is shackled to the old system by an inability to upgrade. An ideal system allows for exporting and importing data, ability to choose among vendors, and flexibility to purchase new modules without compromising the integrity of the entire system.

DISPENSING AND OFFICE MANAGEMENT

A number of software tools have been developed for assisting dispensing audiologists. The first group of programs is designed to define prescriptive targets and in some cases verification of the selection. These packages are not associated with any particular manufacturer's product (de Jonge, 1996a). They are designed for use with any hearing aid. The second group of programs is provided by hearing aid manufacturers for fitting programmable instruments. Although these applications are specific to each manufacturer's hearing aids, the software is fairly flexible and often works as a general fitting tool for determining prescriptive targets. Office management systems (OMSs) typically are databases tailored to activities that occur in dispensing offices. Most of the early OMSs were not associated with any particular brand of hearing aid. More recently, manufacturers are offering their own OMSs, sometimes by purchasing earlier, independent products.

Software Packages for Hearing Aid Selection/Verification

Converting audiogram thresholds to target insertion gain can be a complicated process, especially for more involved procedures, such as normalizing loudness (Leijon, 1991). For manual calculations, clinically expedient approximations, such as the half-gain rule, made sense. Now, with computers to perform the calculations, complexity of the algorithm is no longer an issue. Also, it is possible to use software to convert from real-ear to 2-cc coupler gain (or output). Applications of CORFIGs and GIFROCs can easily be performed (Killion & Revit, 1993). Table 20–2 summarizes key features of the programs reviewed in this chapter.

PEARL

With computers, the complexity of the algorithm is no longer an issue. Accuracy does not have to be sacrificed for clinical procedures that are simple or easy to remember.

Memphis State University Hearing Aid Prescription

Version 3.1 of the University of Memphis software requires only a PC XT class machine with 256 kB of memory (Cox,

1988). The documentation file can be printed to serve as a user manual. This manual is restricted to an explanation of how to use the program; no information exists about the (considerable) theory or empirical research behind the MSU procedure. However, references are given to several articles that thoroughly explain the rationale and verification of the approach. Additional articles are not only helpful but essential to effectively use and understand the software (Cox, 1983, 1984, 1985; Cox & Alexander, 1990).

This DOS program is text-based, no graphics. A table presents prescriptions for coupler gain, insertion gain, and OSPL90 for 10 frequencies between 250 and 6000 Hz. Features are selected by use of the keyboard with pull-down menus. The user can create, save, and load patient files containing basic information such as name, date, date of birth, clinician, ear tested, and comments. All information relating to the hearing aid prescription and calculations made by the program can be saved. The information is entered, and a table containing the prescription, along with a worksheet for comparing three hearing aids, can be printed.

The principle used for selecting insertion gain is based on the long-term listening range (LTLR). The LTLR is defined by the patient's threshold at the low end and the highest comfortable listening level (HCL) at the high end. Insertion gain can be converted to coupler gain by applying the appropriate corrections for either a behind-the-ear or in-the-ear aid. The OSPL90 curve is selected with consideration given to both the loudness and clarity of speech. OSPL90 can be displayed for either an HA-1 or HA-2 coupler.

The HCL can be measured directly or it can be estimated. The method for measuring HCL uses a descending procedure and stimuli commonly available on standard audiometers. The highest level producing a comfort response is HCL. Because loudness testing can be time consuming and difficult, if not impossible, for some patients to perform, HCL can be estimated with one of two predictive techniques. The first uses regression equations to predict HCL and naturally results in prediction errors. A second procedure was developed to reduce this error and requires that HCLs be measured at only two frequencies, 500 and 4000 Hz. The difference between predicted and measured HCL (called the residual) is calculated by the program and used to adjust HCLs at other frequencies.

Desired Sensation Level (DSL 3.1 to 4.1)

The DSL 3.1 software, like the MSU program, is a DOS program and has very modest hardware requirements. The 137-page DSL manual, "A Computer-Assisted Implementation of the Desired Sensation Level Method for Electroacoustic Selection and Fitting in Children" is clear, well-written, quite comprehensive, and covers both the use of the program and much of the theory behind DSL's procedures (Moodie et al, 1994; Seewald, 1992, 1994; Seewald & Ross, 1988; Seewald et al, 1993a). Client demographic information can be entered, stored, retrieved, or printed. Comments about the type of hearing aid and earmold can be stored with the patient's file, but they are not used in any calculations

The program is focused on the amplification needs of children. For example, the speech spectrum used as the input to the hearing aid is a compromise between adult values for

TABLE 20–2   Programs for hearing aid selection and verification that are not specific to any manufacturer's hearing instrument

Program/System	Author Contact	Key Features
Memphis State University MSU 3.1 DOS PC XT	Robyn Cox 901-678-5831 ausp@memphis.edu/harl	An early, text-based program. Sound is amplified to fit into the long-term listening range. REIG targets are calculated from threshold or loudness measurements, OSPL90 from the highest comfortable listening level. REIG is converted to 2-cc gain for BTE and ITE aids.
Desired sensation level DSL 3.1 PC XT or Mac	Richard Seewald 519-661-3901 dsl@audio.hhcru.uwo.ca	Custom RECDs are calculated for children. REIG is selected so speech is amplified to midpoint of dynamic range. LDLs and RESR are calculated from threshold. Results are visualized on an SPLogram display.
DSL 4.1, DSL[i/o] Windows 3.1 or 95		Level-dependent target REAG curves and i/o functions extend DSL 3.1 for fitting WDRC programmables.
Independent hearing aid fitting forum IHAFF.1.1a PC XT	Dennis Van Vliet 714-579-0717 MBFN77A@prodigy.com	VIOLA uses compression thresholds and ratios to develop target i/o functions for WDRC aids. Targets are based on patients' categorical loudness judgments at selected frequencies. The APHAB is presented, scored, and the results are displayed on graphs.
Fig6, Fig6 for Windows PC XT Windows 3.1 or 95	Etymotic Research 847-228-0006	From audiogram thresholds, target REIG, and coupler gain (BTE, ITE, ITC, CIC aids) are calculated for 40-, 65-, and 95-dB input levels.
Hearing aid selection HAS 2.9 Mac, HyperCard2.2	Support Syndicate for 412-481-2494 rdejong@iland.net	HAS supports many prescriptive procedures and has features of DSL, FIG6, and VIOLA. Speech spectrum audibility is displayed on the audiogram; effects on intelligibility are calculated by the articulation index. Loudness normalization calculates a target i/o function. Tutorial information is included to teach students about hearing aid selection (earmold acoustics, CORFIGs, etc.).
Hearing aid selection program/procedure HASP 2.07 PC AT	Harvey Dillon 612-412-6828 Harvey.dillon@nal.gov.au	NAL-R calculates target REIG. Manufacturer databases are searched to find the hearing aid that most closely matches the prescription. Effects of trim pots and earmold acoustics are considered.

males and females and also considers the spectrum of the child's voice when self-monitoring speech (Cornelisse et al, 1991). Young children tend to have earcanals that are shorter and narrower than adults. A shorter canal will tend to have a real-ear unaided gain (REUG) peaking at a higher frequency. A smaller sized canal will have a larger real-ear coupler difference (RECD). The program calculates prescriptions for young children on the basis of age-specific values for REUG and RECD. Although the program is specifically geared to pediatric fittings, the software is flexible enough to permit adjustment of key parameters to make the hearing aid recommendation applicable to older children and adults.

The theory behind the DSL 3.1 procedure is similar to that of MSUv3.1. An approximate bisecting of the dynamic range is the target level (i.e., desired sensation level re: threshold) for the long-term average conversational speech spectrum (LTASS). Speech should remain audible, above threshold, but not exceed the upper limit of the comfort range, which then becomes the target real-ear saturation response (RESR). The target RESR increases systematically with increases in hearing

loss. The DSL procedure emphasizes the value of measuring, and representing, all variables with a common reference: in-situ earcanal sound pressure levels (SPLs). However, all predictions can be made from audiogram thresholds obtained with conventional earphones, so this is the minimum information that needs to be entered into the program.

Once thresholds are entered, the option is available for supplying additional information about LDLs, REUG, and RECD. Although the program modifies its prescription for changes in REUG and RECD, LDLs are not used to calculate the target RESR. Audiogram thresholds are converted to a minimum audible pressure (MAP) that is the real-ear SPL (RESPL) corresponding to threshold. The target DSL and amplified LTASS are given along with the REAG, REIG, and aided sound-field thresholds needed to verify the insertion gain. The target 2-cc coupler use gain and OSPL90 needed to supply the desired REIG and RESR are given in tabular form.

Logically, the next step in the process is verification of gain and output. The results of this process can be entered and stored. The manual describes how commonly available probe-microphone equipment can be used for verification. Gain can be verified by using real-ear measures or by measuring coupler gain. Output verification involves measuring a RESR to a pure tone sweep at 90 dB or coupler measures of OSPL90.

DSL 3.1 graphically displays selection and verification results on a plot of RESPL (in dB) as a function of frequency. All dB values are represented in RESPLs. For each graph, variables can be added to the display sequentially and can be used in counseling. First, normal thresholds, the thresholds associated with the hearing loss, and LDL are displayed. By adding the LTASS, it can be seen what part of the speech spectrum is audible and what is inaudible. Adding the amplified LTASS and RESR targets can then portray the effect the hearing aid should have on the speech spectrum. The display shows how the measured speech spectrum actually fits into the LTLR and how the measured RESR compares with the target. Overall, this seems like a convenient tool for taking a structured approach to expressing to the parents the purpose and success (or failure) of the hearing aid fitting.

As of this writing, DSL 4.1, also known as DSL[i/o], is the most recent version of the desired DSL, and it has all the essential features of 3.1. Because DSL 4.1 is a Windows program, it provides a consistent, familiar user interface (pull-down menus, toolbars), along with an online help manual. DSL 3.1 was written in an era when most hearing aids were linear. Compression was generally used only as an alternative to peak clipping for output limiting. The new version of

this software deals with wide dynamic range compression (WDRC) hearing aids. The usefulness of version 3.1 is extended by calculating a family of input-level–dependent target frequency response curves (Cornelisse et al, 1994, 1995). Also calculated are target compression ratios and input-output functions. DSL 4.1 is also designed to work with both children and adults, and the software permits the user to define a custom real-ear dial difference (REDD). Figure 20–3 illustrates a typical DSL screen for displaying level-dependent frequency response curves.

The Independent Hearing Aid Fitting Forum Protocol

The IHAFF group met in March of 1993 to begin the process of developing a comprehensive set of protocols for selecting and fitting more advanced hearing aids (i.e., two-channel WDRC). The result of their efforts is a set of software tools that run on modest PCs such as those described for the DSL and MSU procedures. Robyn Cox and associates at the University of Memphis seem primarily responsible for guiding software development, and that university holds the copyright. The program disk is distributed free of charge and contains a comprehensive user manual that can be printed. It can be downloaded from the Frye Electronics Web site (www.frye.com). An overview of the IHAFF protocol can be found in the user manual or in Van Vliet (1995). Valente and Van Vliet (1997) provide a comprehensive review of the procedure. The current version is 1.1a, and it runs under DOS.

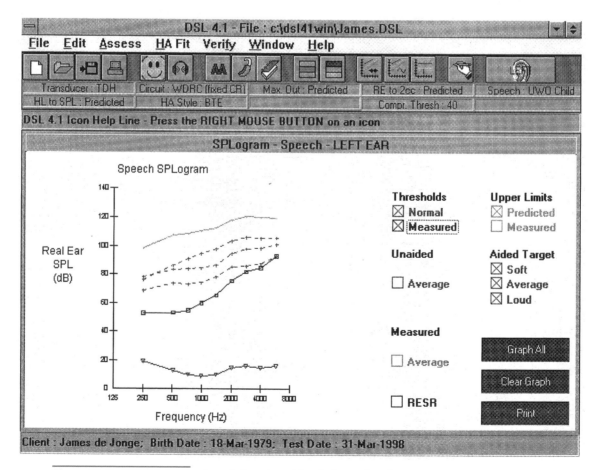

Figure 20–3 DSL[i/o] procedure defines target level–dependent frequency responses.

The IHAFF protocol addresses the issue of targets for hearing aids that have frequency responses that vary as a function of input level (i.e., frequency-dependent, WDRC hearing aids). Generally, IHAFF is based on the guideline that, as with most procedures, speech should be audible but not reach LDL. Also, the aided loudness experience should be comparable to loudness experienced by normal-hearing individuals. Speech that normally sounds soft should, when amplified, also sound soft. Intense speech that is normally experienced as loud should evoke a similar sensation in the hearing aid wearer. The Contour Test and visual input-output locator algorithm (VIOLA) are responsible for converting this theoretical concept into the reality of a 2-cc coupler input-output function for a given hearing aid.

The first step in the process is to enter pure tone thresholds for insert earphones (like the ER-3A) that have been calibrated on an HA-1 coupler. The next step is to perform the contour test, which uses a categorical scaling procedure to measure the individual subject's loudness perception for at least two frequencies (i.e., a low frequency and a high frequency such as 500 and 3000 Hz). These two frequencies would typically be a good choice for a two-channel programmable aid with a crossover frequency of about 1500 Hz. Each frequency is tested by presenting ascending series of pulsed warble tones. At each presentation level the patient chooses which loudness category best describes the stimulus: (0) inaudible, (1) very soft, (2) soft, (3) comfortable but slightly soft, (4) comfortable, (5) comfortable but slightly loud, (6)

loud but Ok, and (7) uncomfortably loud (Hawkins et al, 1987). The data are evaluated to determine the median SPLs corresponding to each of the categories 1 through 7. This information can be gathered manually, but IHAFF contains software to drive a set of common, commercially available audiometers equipped with a serial interface. The computer controls the presentation of stimuli by the audiometer, the operator enters the category number of the subject's response, and the software computes the median SPLs. The next step in the procedure involves relating this loudness data to the perception of speech and creating a target to which a hearing aid's input-output function can be matched.

Three speech spectra associated with differing levels of vocal effort are used to create targets for so-called soft, average, and loud speech: 50-, 65- and 85-dB SPL, respectively. SPLs have been measured for 1/3 octave bands of each speech spectrum. Normal-hearing subjects have rated the loudness of these bands, and these judgments have been equated to the loudness categories associated with warble tones used in the contour test (Cox et al, 1994a,b). Figure 20–4 shows the VIOLA screen for the contour data. Two graphs are shown for the frequencies at which loudness data were generated, 500 and 3000 Hz. Output SPL in a 2-cc coupler is plotted as a function of the SPL input to the hearing aid microphone. Corrections are made for type of hearing aid (BTE, ITE, ITC, or CIC). Targets are shown as asterisks representing levels needed to normalize the loudness of soft, average, and loud speech. The shaded areas represent the soft (1 to 3),

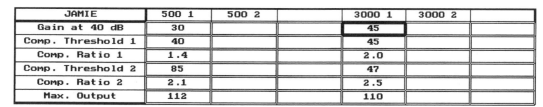

JAMIE	500 1	500 2		3000 1	3000 2	
Gain at 40 dB	30			45		
Comp. Threshold 1	40			45		
Comp. Ratio 1	1.4			2.0		
Comp. Threshold 2	85			47		
Comp. Ratio 2	2.1			2.5		
Max. Output	112			110		

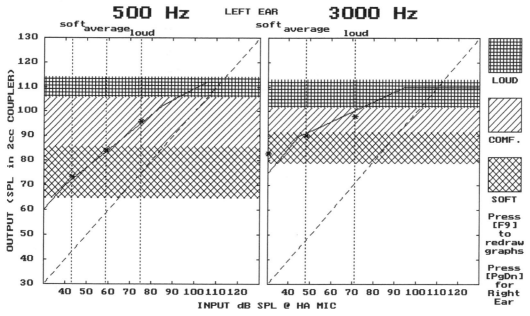

Figure 20–4 VIOLA screen from the IHAFF procedure shows how choosing the correct compression characteristics can match a loudness target.

comfortable (3 to 5), and loud (5 to 7) range of the contour test. At the top of Figure 20–4 are a series of boxes where the user can enter parameters that describe the input-output function of the hearing aid. The user adjusts these kneepoints and compression ratios until an acceptable match is achieved.

The final section of the IHAFF suite is a self-assessment scale, the abbreviated profile of hearing aid benefit (APHAB) as described by Cox and Alexander (1995). The APHAB consists of 24 items drawn from the 66-item profile of hearing aid benefit (PHAB) developed by Cox et al (1991) as a research tool. This shortened version takes approximately 10 minutes to administer and the results can be used to determine how well an individual perceives that he or she is doing with and without the hearing aid, thereby deriving an estimate of benefit. There are six questions related to each of four areas: ease of communication (EC), reverberation (RV), background noise (BN), and aversiveness of sounds (AV). The first three scales evaluate speech communication in quiet, reverberant, and noisy situations. The last scale provides input on perception of intense sounds. Responses to the APHAB have been evaluated on a group of successful listeners with mild-to-moderate hearing loss (Cox & Rivera, 1992). Individual performance on the APHAB can be compared with this reference group. The client can take the APHAB by entering responses to the questions by means of the keyboard. A pencil and paper version can be used for individuals who cannot use the computer, and the clinician can then enter the responses. Once all responses are entered, three graphs are generated that describe the user's performance. The APHAB can be a useful tool for documenting hearing aid benefit.

FIG6

FIG6 was originally a DOS program that had the appearance of a spreadsheet. It is very easy to use. Audiogram thresholds are entered and the program calculates insertion and coupler gain frequency response targets for three input levels (40-, 65-, and 95-dB SPL). These targets are based on empirical research involving loudness perception in groups with varying degrees of sensorineural hearing loss (Hellman & Meiselman, 1993; Lippman et al, 1981; Lyregaard, 1988; Pascoe, 1988; Villchur, 1973). FIG6 is now available as a Windows program from Etymotic Research.

Killion and Fikret-Pasa (1993) describe three types of sensorineural hearing loss, differing mostly in degree of loss. The FIG6 procedure provides input-level–dependent frequency response targets intended to normalize loudness for type I and type II hearing loss (Killion, 1996). The type I hearing loss has a magnitude of up to about 40 dB HL, a type II loss up to 70 dB HL, and type III hearing losses are greater than 70 dB HL and require the patient to listen at levels close to the LDL to understand speech. The FIG6 manual cautions the user to consider a low-distortion aid with compression limiting (variable release time) for hearing losses exceeding 70 dB HL. Figure 6 (from which FIG6 gets its name) of the Killion and Fikret-Pasa (1993) article is a plot of required gain for normal loudness perception as a function of hearing loss. The graph contains three curves; the parameter of the curves is the input level to the hearing aid: 40-, 65-, and 95-dB SPL. From the graph it is possible to read target insertion gain needed to normalize loudness for soft, moderate, and intense inputs for

differing magnitudes of hearing loss. The FIG6 program automatically calculates these targets and uses the appropriate CORFIGs to convert insertion gain to coupler gain for BTE, ITE, ITC, or CIC instruments. FIG6 will display these targets either numerically or as a graph (see Fig. 20–5).

PEARL

By use of DSL or FIG6, level-dependent targets can be quickly estimated from audiogram thresholds. IHAFF takes more time but factors in the patient's loudness perceptions.

Hearing Aid Selection

The current version of Hearing Aid Selection (HAS 2.9) is a HyperCard application (stack). It is based on older programs originally created for the Apple II platform (de Jonge, 1985; 1987). The objective has been to create a structured, scientifically defensible approach to selecting hearing aid characteristics. A primary aim was to introduce graduate audiology students to hearing aid selection, so HAS contains tutorial material about issues such as sound-field transformations and earmold acoustics. The first step in the selection procedure is to enter audiogram thresholds. The AI is used to determine the effect the hearing loss has on the intelligibility of speech (isolated monosyllabic words and words in sentences). The effect is visualized by drawing the audible and inaudible portions of the speech spectrum superimposed on the audiogram. A variety of prescriptive procedures (like POGO, Berger, NAL-R, FIG6, DSL, etc.) are used to target desired output levels (Byrne & Dillon, 1986; Berger et al, 1979; 1989; McCandless & Lyregaard, 1983; Seewald et al, 1993b). For example, average conversational level speech can be used for determining target REIG or REAG for linear aids. Different input levels can be used to develop targets for WDRC aids. Again, the AI is useful for determining the effect of the frequency response (changes in speech spectrum levels) on intelligibility. If speech intelligibility were actually measured, it would be useful to know how much of an improvement in percent correct is needed to produce a statistically significant result. The program gives an estimate for the 95% critical difference (10-, 25-, and 100-item lists) on the basis of the binomial theorem (Thornton & Raffin, 1978).

Target REIG can be converted to 2-cc coupler use-gain for BTE, ITE, ITC, or CIC aids by applying the appropriate corrections for microphone location, RECD (for either HA-1 or HA-2 coupler), and REUG. Target 2-cc use-gain is converted to full-on gain by selecting an appropriate amount of reserve gain. Measured LDLs can be entered directly. Or, LDLs can be calculated from threshold on the basis of the amount of hearing loss, using either Pascoe's data or the prescriptive procedure from DSL 3.1 (Pascoe, 1988; Seewald et al, 1993b). The LDLs are converted to a target RESR using the REDD. Target RESR is converted to an OSPL90 curve using the RECD correction. Also, changes can be made to the RECD, REUG, and REDD to determine the effect of individual variation on the audiogram and the prescriptive targets.

Two procedures can be used to calculate the target input-output function, either DSL[i/o] (Cornelisse et al, 1995) or the

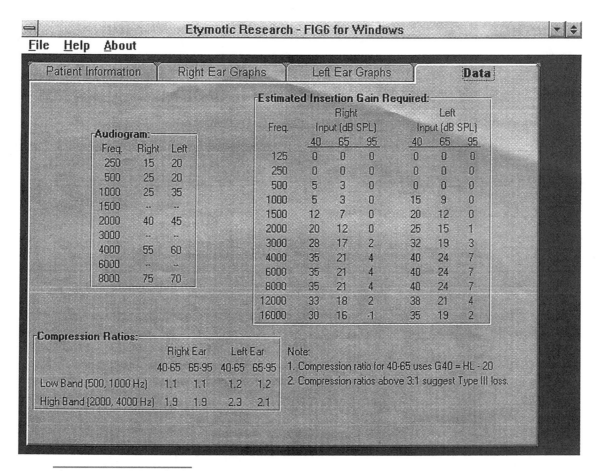

Figure 20–5   FIG6 calculates target level–dependent frequency responses from the audiogram thresholds.

loudness density normalization (LDN) procedure (Leijon, 1991). The DSL procedure defines the target input-output function by setting two points. The first point is based on the amount of residual hearing loss the patient will have. The second is related to the sound-field SPL that will cause the LDL to be reached. The LDN procedures define the input-output function needed to restore normal loudness perception. Similar to VIOLA, the software allows the user to set the maximum output and adjust compression thresholds and ratios for two compressors. Figure 20–6 shows calculation of an input-output function on the basis of a slightly modified version of the DSL approach. Parameters are set so that a residual aided hearing loss of 20 dB exists. A sound-field input causing loudness discomfort for a normal ear will be amplified to a level producing discomfort for the impaired ear.

Hearing Aid Selection Program/Procedure (HASP 2.07)

The previously described hearing aid selection programs emphasize identifying appropriate prescriptions. These prescriptions usually account for differences in REIG and coupler gain, but often they do not account for venting or ear mold acoustics. The Hearing Aid Selection Program (HASP 2.07) does make predictions concerning venting and earmold effects, but it is still left to the dispenser to find an actual hearing aid that will meet the prescription. This is one area where

HASP departs significantly from the previous approaches (Dillon et al, 1992). The program comes with a small core database of hearing aids and, additionally, two large databases of hearing aids from manufacturers (Miracle Ear and Starkey). Once a target prescription is identified, the computer will automatically search the databases to find hearing aids that match. These databases were created by the manufacturers so the dispenser is spared the tedious chore of entering this information manually. However, if desired, the dispenser does have the option of including hearing aids from other manufacturers. HASP is an DOS program that will run on a PC AT compatible computer.

HASP calculates target insertion gain curves using the NAL-R procedure (Byrne & Dillon, 1986; Byrne et al, 1990). The minimum OSPL90 is selected so that 70 dB SPL speech will not saturate the hearing aid. The maximum OSPL90 should not exceed LDL (which is estimated from threshold). HASP allows the user to select vent size, earmold configurations and dampers for BTE instruments. The computer adjusts the frequency response and OSPL90 for sound entering and exiting the vent (Dillon, 1991), considers the occlusion effect, and also can predict the maximum gain available before feedback will occur. The computer "understands" the effect of tone controls and output limiters for the hearing aids within its database, and the program will search for aids that achieve an acceptable match. HASP calculates the root-mean-square deviation, adjusted by AI weights, between the target and the

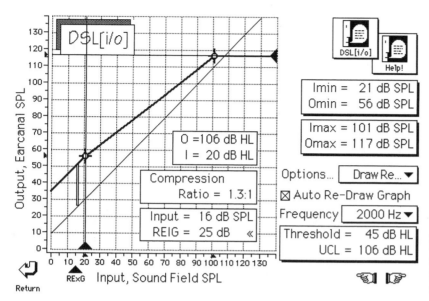

Figure 20–6 HAS 2.9 screen uses a modified DSL approach to defining a target input-output function from two data points related to residual hearing loss and LDL.

hearing aid's response. Acceptable matches can be ranked for "closeness of fit."

The database stores relevant information about the electroacoustic characteristics of the hearing aid. The computer, however, has no knowledge about issues that are important to the fitting but that are difficult to quantify: manipulation skills of the client, years of hearing aid use, and other special needs that the client may have. The dispenser can then combine this factual information with clinical judgment and experience to provide the best instrument.

Programmable Hearing Aids and Office Management

Almost every hearing aid manufacturer offers a programmable product, and each hearing aid requires some programming mechanism. One industry solution is a proprietary, stand-alone, device (i.e., Widex's LP2; ReSound's P3) that connects to individual manufacturers' hearing aids. Micro-Tech programmables interface to a PCMCIA (or simply PC) card (Anderson et al, 1997). This credit-card–sized device inserts into a PC slot on a Newton MessagePad 2000, which is a personal digital assistant (PDA). A PDA is an interesting choice for an interface because it offers so much extra functionality: converting handwritten to typed notes, faxing, drawing, word processing, spreadsheet, address book, appointment calendar, and so on. However, audiologists dispensing from several manufacturers will collect a number of functionally redundant devices. Another approach is for the manufacturer to develop programming software to run on an industry standard PC. An "interface box" connecting the hearing aid to the PC is still required, but the box can be used with many brands of hearing aids.

Even with such a "universal" programming solution, practical problems exist. Hearing aid dispensing happens within a broader context of office management (patient records, scheduling, billing, accounting, marketing, etc.), and audiologists do not want their patient data spread out among a number of different databases. For these reasons it would be burdensome and inefficient for each manufacturer to create a complete suite of applications. NOAH and HI-PRO (hearing

instrument programmer) were developed as solutions to these problems (Anderson & Jelonek, 1994; Jelonek, 1994).

NOAH

NOAH is a software integration platform (Ketchum, 1997), a Windows application developed by HIMSA that runs on standard PCs. NOAH is purchased through the manufacturers who sell NOAH products. Table 20–3 identifies products that are NOAH compatible or in the certification process. HIMSA's Web site (www.himsa.com) maintains a current list of manufacturers, compatible software applications, and instruments. HI-PRO is usually purchased with NOAH. HI-PRO is hardware, a box that connects to the PC's serial port. The programmable hearing aids connect to HI-PRO by means of proprietary cables supplied by manufacturers. The HI-PRO box can be used to program any hearing aid from a NOAH-compatible manufacturer. NOAH provides rudimentary database functions, but it mostly serves as a gateway to software modules written by other manufacturers. These software modules have access to the NOAH database, and NOAH allows the modules from different manufacturers to share information. The software modules fit the general categories of audiological equipment, hearing aid fitting, and office management systems. Most software development has occurred in the hearing aid fitting category, and NOAH is currently functioning primarily as a tool for fitting programmable hearing aids. But it is important to stress that NOAH's potential is not limited to just this function. NOAH software modules can be developed for controlling or communicating with any type of device: clinical audiometer, immittance audiometer, video otoscope, evoked potential, or OAE equipment. Software modules written for comprehensive office management functions can have direct access to data generated by the audiological equipment. A manufacturer would be free to focus on one aspect of audiological management, develop hardware and software for meeting a need, and yet still have their product fit into a broader context of data management.

NOAH has five basic modules. The "client module" (see Fig. 20–7) collects demographic information such as name, address, phone number, birth date, and referral source. The "audiometry module" allows point-and-click entry of audiogram thresholds and entry of numerical values such as speech audiometric and immittance data. Audi-Link permits the installation of audiometer drivers to allow data to be sent directly to NOAH. The "selection of new hearing instrument module" displays a screen showing all the installed manufacturers' software fitting modules. Clicking a manufacturer's logo launches that software. A "NOAH fitting module" is used to collect general information (make, model, battery, ear mold, etc.) from manufacturers who have not developed fitting software. Patients fit with these aids can still be included in the database. The "measurement selection module" is where software is launched for controlling any audiological equipment modules that are installed (audiometers, probemic systems, etc.). Once a client has been selected, the "journal module" provides basic word processing tools for storing written comments.

Open Audiometric Reporting Standard

Open Audiometric Reporting Standard (OARS) is an alternative to the NOAH-compatibility standard. OARS was developed by Qualitone and is used in the Qualitone Prophet hearing aid fitting system and in the dbc-mifco Solo II multimanufacturer hearing aid programmer (Clancy, 1995; Radcliffe, 1996). OARS is currently being studied by an ANSI working group with the idea of developing an open standard for constructing databases of any and all types of audiological information, including both data and graphics. Any database complying with the OARS standard could be accessed by ANSI standard database language (structured query language or SQL). Any third party could develop software without licensing fees or royalties.

Fitting Software

Most conventional equipment has a front end, or control panel, with which the user interacts. Examples are push buttons, dials, knobs, and sliders that control different functions of common appliances like telephones, microwave ovens, radios, and stereo equipment. Windows graphical user interface provides a consistent, easily understood, "virtual control panel" for adjusting programmable hearing aids and their remote controls. A large number of options exist for how this

control panel may appear because so many manufacturers and even more programmable hearing aids exist. Each hearing aid has different physical characteristics, so each instrument has different parameters to adjust. Instruments have varying numbers of bands, channels, and memories. Compression thresholds, compression ratios, attack and release times, overall gain, output, gain in the band or channel, crossover frequency—all of these have the potential for being variable. Virtual controls (push buttons, trim pots, sliders, etc.) are created in software to manipulate these parameters. With well-designed software (Teter & Winthrop, 1994), the function of the control is obvious by its appearance. Frequency responses, input-output functions, conventional audiograms, and SPL audiograms may be used to illustrate the effects of manipulating the controls. The appearance of a typical fitting screen is shown in Figure 20–8.

Robertson (1996) provides a review of manufacturer fitting software. The fitting software may contain an online, comprehensive database of the manufacturer's product line, not just programmables. Selecting a product will often give a picture of the hearing aid and a brief description of its most important features. An audiogram may display the current patient's hearing loss superimposed over the fitting range of the instrument. Some software will suggest a particular model of hearing aid. The software may proceed in a series of ordered steps, helping the dispenser follow a logical sequence. Once a particular aid is selected, usually a number of different prescriptive procedures are available to choose from: NAL-R, DSL[i/o], and FIG6 are popular options, but the manufacturer may have custom algorithms. The target (or level-dependent targets) may be displayed along with the simulated output of the hearing aid, either in 2-cc coupler or real-ear terms. Changing the parameters typically produces a change in the aid's gain, and it is easy to visualize how closely the target is met. An "autofit" option may be present for pressing a button to automatically adjust the aid's parameters to achieve a best match to the target. The manufacturer may provide other tools for visualizing the effect of the chosen frequency response. The audible and inaudible areas of the ACL speech spectrum may overlay the audiogram thresholds, or an AI value could be calculated.

Some fitting software permits loudness scaling so that the patient's subjective preferences are factored into the target (Humes & Houghton, 1992; Humes et al, 1996b). Categorical loudness scaling methods are popular, similar to those used with the IHAFF contour procedure or the LGOB test (Allen et al, 1990). Loudness matching may require a software interface to external hardware that is capable of generating stimuli, such as an audiometer or a real-ear measurement system. But some hearing aids generate their own signals for in-situ measurements. Another option is for calibrated signals to be

TABLE 20–3 NOAH-compatible products for fitting programmable hearing aids (fitting module), office management systems (OMS), drivers for controlling equipment, audiometers (AUD), immitance devices (IMP), hearing instrument testers (HIT), and real-ear probe microphone equipment (REM)

Supplier	Product	Category
Beltone	SelectaFit (3.02) Office Pro*	Fitting module OMS
Bernafon-Maico	OASIS (3.01)	Fitting module
Dahlberg	Merlin (1.00)*	Fitting module
GN Danavox	Danafit (3.80)	Fitting module
Danplex	Danplex Audi-Link Driver (1.5)* for DA73, 74 (AUD)	Driver instrument
Grason-Stadler	GSI Audi-Link Driver (1.0)* GSI 10, 16, 61 (AUD)	Driver instrumet
HCDS	Entity*	OMS
Interacoustics	IA-NOAH-AUD (1.05) for AC30, 33, 40; AD25, 28, 226; AS216; MS40 IA-NOAH-IMP (1.02) for AC40, MS40 IA-NOAH-REM (1.04) for MS25, MS40 Interacoustics Audi-Link Driver (1.03)* for ACS30, 40; AD25, 27; BCA300; MS40	Instrument Driver instrument
Madsen	Hearing Clinic Aurical AUD, REM (2.10), HIT (2.05), Zodiac 901 IMP Zodi-Link* for Zodiac 901 (IMP) Madsen Audi-Link Driver (2.0) for Midimate 622, 602, Orbitor 922, Voyager 502, 522	OMS instrument Driver instrument
Maico	Maico Audi-Link Driver (1.0) for MA52 AUD	Driver instrument
Oticon	OtiSet (3.80) Oticon Office	Fitting module OMS
Philips	Fitting Assistant (4.10a)	Fitting module
Phonak	Phonak Fitting Guide (5.0)	Fitting module
Qualitone	PFS (2.20a)	Fitting module
ReSound	ReSource (5.0)	Fitting module
Rexton	CONNEXX with REXFIT*	Fitting module
Siemens	CONNEXX with SIFIT (3.0) Unity OMS Unity PC Audiometer,* Probe Mic,* Hearing Instrument Analyzer (AUD, REM, HIT) Siemens Audi-Link Driver (1.50)	Fitting module OMS instrument Driver
Sonar	Model 90 (1.4)	Fitting module
Starkey	PFS (2.20a) ProHear* REMware for Rastronics* Starkey Audi-Link Driver (1.03) for AA30	Fitting module OMS Instrument driver
Unitron	UniFit (2.30) Clarity (Total Office Systems)*	Fitting module OMS

*Certification testing in progress.

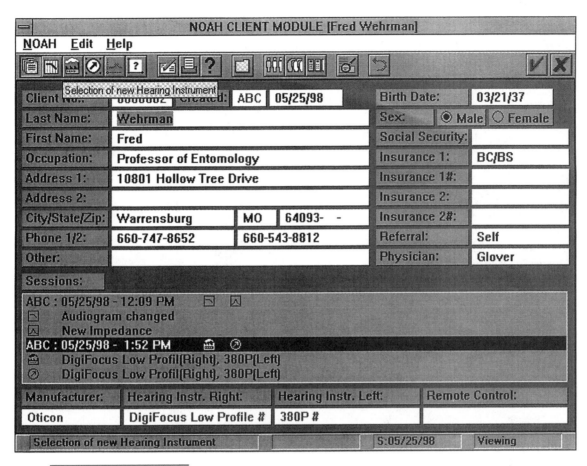

Figure 20–7 Data entry screen from NOAH's client module.

presented in the sound field while the gain (within the channel) of the hearing aid is adjusted to reach an appropriate loudness level relative to normal (Grey & Dyrlund, 1996). If the fitting system is interfaced with a probe-mic system, real-ear verification of targets can be performed. The actual, rather than simulated, effect of manipulating the hearing aid's controls can be visualized directly on the computer screen. Similarly, connecting a hearing aid test box will permit adjusting the aid to 2-cc targets as is recommended for children with the DSL procedure. The software may permit REUG and RECD to be determined for the individual, thereby customizing conversions from coupler to real-ear gain.

Some fitting systems take advantage of the computer's multimedia capability to play digitized sound from a CD-ROM or stored as a data file on the hard drive (Stypulkowski, 1995). Listening environments are simulated using low-level or high-level speech, dishes clattering, traffic noise, or music to help the new hearing aid user judge the appropriateness of the fitting. Other applications provide objective documentation of aided improvement in speech intelligibility. The Hearing in Noise Test for Windows (HINT/Windows) is a PC-based application distributed by Starkey in CD-ROM format. HINT presents sentences in speech-spectrum noise to simulate typical listening in noisy environments where sound is coming from spatially separated sources. The software enables automatic test administration, scoring, and reporting. HINT/Windows, with a proprietary sound-processing card, can also perform audiometry and data management.

Self-report questionnaires, like the APHAB or COSI, can also be part of the fitting software. The computer allows data to be easily collected, archived, analyzed, and displayed. Multimedia computers enable Clear Speech, a training technique for improving intelligibility through modifying speaking style. A fitting program may include software to play recorded materials that demonstrate this technique and print instructions and practice exercises that family members will take home (Schum, 1997). A variety of other material can be printed. Journal entries are maintained in the database or printed for inclusion in a paper file. The patient might take home a printed, custom user manual to reinforce points made during counseling. Even an order form can be printed.

The fitting software may have special features such as an automatic feedback test. The instrument's gain is automatically increased until feedback is present, allowing a hearing aid with an automatic volume control feature to "know" its limits for increasing gain. Troubleshooting user complaints is another process that is automated by some fitting software. A series of multiple-choice questions are asked and the program recommends specific changes in the aid's parameters on the basis of the nature of the complaint (e.g., the silverware sounds too loud). Some software detects unusual or improbable combinations of settings and warns the dispenser. Many other useful features are present. The software may be compatible with another manufacturer's database, allowing those aids to be fitted. Binaural corrections can be applied, automatically reducing gain by a fixed amount (usually 4- to

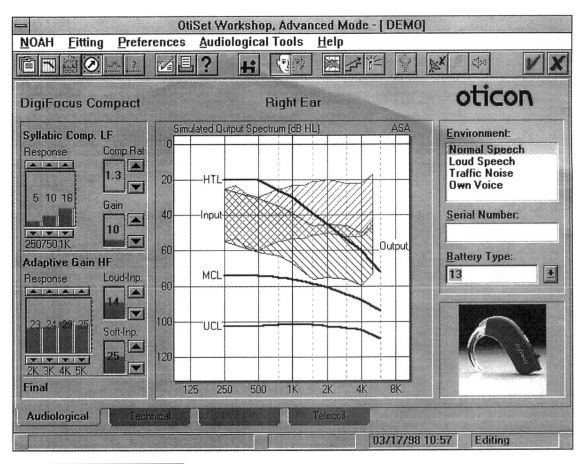

Figure 20–8 Typical screen showing how software can be used as a virtual control panel for programming a digital hearing aid. Effect of the insertion gain on the speech spectrum is displayed.

6-dB). The effect of earmold acoustics may be simulated and entered into the display of the frequency response. Because so many different features are offered by different manufacturers and because these features are likely to change with software updates, it is important for the audiologist to carefully comparison shop to make sure the fitting software offers the right mix of features he or she finds valuable.

Office Management Systems

In addition to the general accounting software described earlier (see QuickBooks in "Business and Financial Management"), a number of programs have been developed specifically for the hearing aid dispensing office. Early systems included Swenson, PC/MacHear, Professional Audiology Manager, Hearcare Software, E-Z Office, and HearWare (Hampton, 1995). Some of the companies have been purchased and their features integrated into hearing aid manufacturer's software. For example Siemen's BOSS (Business Organization Software System) system has been modified by their acquisition of HearWare, which is now the OMS component to Siemen's Unity. Other examples of hearing aid manufacturer's software include Clarity, the OMS offered by Unitron (see Fig. 20–9), ProHear by Starkey, and Hearing Clinic from Madsen. Hearing Office Lite is freeware, developed by a private-practice audiologist, that is based on the FileMaker Pro database software available for Mac and PC

platforms. The program can be downloaded from Louis DuBrey's Web site (www.hearinginfo.com), and support for the program is by means of E-mail.

> ### PITFALL
>
> The client database is the heart of a practice. Before investing time and money in an OMS, be sure that it meets the clinic's needs. Ask specific questions; find out if a "demo" is available. Remember that the "devil is in the details."

A wide range of activities occur in a dispensing office, and plenty of opportunities for automation and support by computer exist. Because a significant number of audiologists operate at more than one location (Skafte, 1997), it is useful for the software to support multiple offices, permit data exchange, and be networkable. Features include scheduling for multiple practitioners, password protection for files and logon, calculating instrument sales commissions and penalties, limiting access to sensitive financial information, creating logs of patient office visits, maintaining detailed records of client information, entering text in client journals, automatic dialing of phone numbers, sending reminders, and flagging a

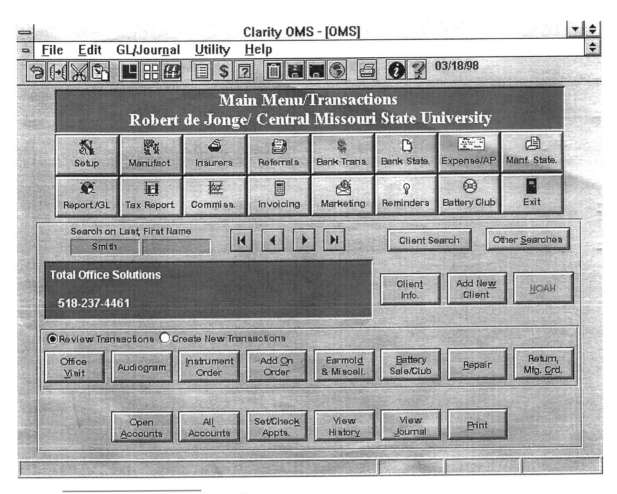

Figure 20–9 Main screen for an office management system.

client with special needs or financial problems. The client database may be able to interface with NOAH or directly support the graphical viewing of audiograms and permit review of testing or fitting information. Some programs offer a general ledger with automatic posting to accounts receivable, computing taxes, generating invoices and sales receipts, generating bills for 30-day (or 60-day or 90-day) open accounts, features for expediting third-party payments, invoicing co-payers, filling out and printing HCFA 1500 forms. Instrument order forms can be linked to battery sales, enrollment in battery clubs, earmold orders, for proper accounting and invoicing. Programs keep track of hearing aid repairs, returns for credit, product inventory, and loaner aids. OMSs deal with managing accounts payable to manufacturers, handle general supplies, automatically print checks with a digital signature, manage bank accounts, and reconcile bank statements. Another important area is marketing. The programs will allow sophisticated sorting of the patient database, generate mail-merge documents (customized form letters), flyers, address envelopes, print labels, include custom letterhead and digital signatures. The program may have templates for generating certain types of documents, such as encouraging an appointment be made for an annual hearing check. The OMS software can also be used to generate reports, charts, and graphs that illustrate the financial health and profitability of the practice. An SQL query, enhanced by

a wizard, may be available to add flexibility to the extraction of information from the entire database. The office software may have integrated facilities for exporting data to other programs, backing up critical data, troubleshooting error messages, and fixing a database corrupted by a system crash.

Integrated Systems

Some manufacturers offer systems containing key hardware and software components needed to handle patient testing, hearing aid fitting, and office management (Gitlin, 1995; Wynne et al, 1993). Madsen Aurical (Grey & Ross, 1995), Siemens Unity, and Starkey ProConnect are three examples. The ultimate goal of these systems is to offer a complete clinic in one package. Hardware usually includes an audiometer, hearing aid test box, a real-ear measurement system, a HI-PRO, perhaps an immittance device, and/or a video otoscope. Other diagnostic equipment (OAE, evoked potential, ENG), unrelated to hearing aid fitting, has not been incorporated. The Aurical is compact, can interface with a notebook computer, and is designed to be portable. Unity is not portable because it requires a desktop computer with slots available to install add-in cards. One advantage these systems offer is a high degree of compatibility between hardware and software. Data are intended to be shared between the integrated modules. This also permits the development of more sophisticated testing and fitting procedures. Real-ear, combined with in-situ loudness measurements, can be referenced for normalizing loudness by adjusting the programmable hearing aid's parameters. This type of measurement avoids problems with individual acoustic variation and correction factors (REUG and RECD) and can compensate for individual preferences in loudness.

OTHER APPLICATIONS

Many other applications for audiology do not deal with hearing aid fitting or managing the dispensing office. Some do not fit neatly into any major category. The computer-based tinnitus evaluation system is an example (Lay & Nunley, 1996). This system consists of a PC, digital audio board, patient headphones, and a module for mixing, attenuating, and amplifying. It can be used for matching the pitch and loudness of tinnitus and for generating noise bands to mask tinnitus. Initially, computer-assisted audiometry was just an automated system for determining threshold. More recently, Kunov et al (1997) describe a system that combines five devices: a clinical audiometer, immittance, evoked responses, transient, and distortion product OAE equipment. Data generated from the different modules can be stored in a database and shared over a network.

Computer-Assisted Audiometry

Currently, these integrated, computer-based systems are the state of the art. Ironically, they are not new. More than 10 years ago in 1987, as part of Project Phoenix, Nicolet developed the first true digital hearing aid, and the Aurora test system was designed as a necessary component to a comprehensive fitting protocol. Aurora's main modules contained an audiometer, real-ear measurement device, hearing aid analyzer, and a database. A PC-based middle ear analyzer was able to send data to the database by means of a serial port. A PC ran DOS applications. A number of possible reasons exist why the audiological community did not accept the system, but soon after its introduction the project folded. Perhaps rumors of its demise became a self-fulfilling prophecy or, for its time, it was "too far ahead of the curve"—too ambitious a project. A parallel exists between the Phoenix and Virtual Corporation. Virtual marketed a Mac-based system consisting of a clinical audiometer, immittance analyzer, probe-mic system, and distortion product OAEs. Software was convenient to use; the Mac served as a prototype for Windows development, and all files could be stored. Virtual is also out of business, perhaps another victim of a marketplace not yet ready for radical innovation (Heide, 1994)?

Most manufacturers now offer audiometers with a serial interface. Software is available that allows data to be transferred from the audiometer to the computer. An example is DSL/Fonix Link that is software that integrates Frye Electronics products to a standard PC. Thresholds from the audiometer are available to the DSL software, and targets are shared with the hearing aid analyzer and probe mic system. Interacoustics manufactures a whole family of audiometers and a middle ear analyzer that are compatible with NOAH (www.interacoustics.com). The ProDigit 2000 audiometer from Decibel Instruments offers a Windows interface to clinical audiometry, including word recognition testing (Shennib et al, 1994).

Picard et al (1993) demonstrated that computer-assisted audiometry could produce reliable thresholds in children as young as 7.5 years and adults up to age 80. This system had been in use before 1987. Despite its fairly long history, no ANSI standards deal with computerized audiometry, including automated procedures. An ANSI working group, S3:76, is dealing with this issue. The most common protocol to automate is the familiar Hughson-Westlake procedure, "down 10 and up 5 dB." This is a very basic example that computers can be used as more than just a virtual control panel for operating equipment. They also have the possibility of becoming expert systems (Moskal et al, 1989; Tharpe et al, 1993), where intelligent decision making is incorporated into the hardware/software.

The Audiometer Operating System

An excellent example of a system that offers helpful decision support is the audiometer operating system (AOS) developed at the Massachusetts Eye and Ear Infirmary (Thornton et al, 1993). The AOS is software, running on a PC in an DOS environment, that controls all functions of an audiometer through the serial port. AOS supports a number of common, commercially available audiometers. The software is entirely aware of the state of the audiometer (i.e., which stimuli are set to be delivered to which ears). AOS can change the state of the audiometer and deliver signals, much as a human operator could. The AOS, unlike the human operator, has instant access to the relevant audiological literature. AOS knows, for example, actual interaural attenuation values, rather than just the 40-dB value that is easy to remember. Two major areas that are addressed by AOS are masking and word recognition testing (Halpin et al, 1996). Masking has long been recognized as a concept that is both difficult to understand and technically challenging to administer. The AOS turns masking on automatically when it is needed, adjusts levels properly according to available air and bone thresholds, and searches for a plateau. This frees the tester from having to recall the theory and memorize constants. The system records detailed information to prepare accurate reports for the computer-generated audiogram. Thornton (1993) states that this system is so successful that technicians can be employed for routine testing, without sacrificing quality. Audiologists can spend more time using their professional training for patient evaluation and management.

SPECIAL CONSIDERATION

The AOS intelligently assists the audiologist during masking and word recognition testing. AOS "knows" when peripheral hearing loss cannot account for poor speech understanding.

Another unique AOS application is with speech recognition testing. The intelligibility of speech is calculated using the AI. Given the level of the speech (knowing its spectrum) and the amount of hearing loss, it is possible to compute intelligibility.

A predicted performance-intensity function is derived, along with estimates of normal variability. The level where PB-max should occur is calculated, and words are presented at that level. Masking can be delivered to the contralateral ear, taking into account such variables as interaural attenuations for each frequency, air-bone gaps, and band sensation level of speech. A masking level can be selected that is just high enough to drive intelligibility to zero in the contralateral ear. The actual word recognition score can be compared with the predicted to determine whether a statistically significant difference exists. A difference would indicate that some factor, other than the audiogram's effect on audibility, is compromising the auditory system. Further investigation could rule out a possible central auditory processing disorder or retrocochlear lesion.

Automating Special Tests

The Computer-Assisted Speech Recognition Assessment (CASRA) was developed to minimize problems associated with conventional speech testing (Gelfand, 1997). A major problem is that the limited number of words typically used (25 or 50 item lists) affects the ability to interpret small differences in performance (Thornton & Raffin, 1978). For example, 92% correct would require a score less than 72% in the other ear to be significant at the 95% confidence level. CASRA solves this problem by presenting 450 items to the listener (150 words, 3 phonemes per word) in 50 three-word combinations. Each test item is displayed on the computer screen. The examiner simply clicks each incorrectly repeated phoneme, and the computer keeps track of the errors and scores the test.

Bochner et al (1997) described The Speech Sound Pattern Discrimination test as a computerized, adaptive delivery system. A mathematical model is used to select test items that, based on the subject's previous responses, are appropriate in level of difficulty. The system was described as useful for evaluating the auditory capabilities of the deaf. By use of the Virtual audiometer, McCullough et al (1994) described a multimedia approach to assessing word recognition for Spanish speakers. Two monitors were used. In the control room the computer displayed a list of words. The tester initiated a trial by selecting a word. In the test booth a picture, showing four test foils, was drawn on the second monitor. By observing the patient's pointing behavior, the audiologist automatically scored the item by clicking a mouse. Myers et al (1996) used a computer-based system for presenting octave-band filtered sound effects. Such stimuli have been suggested as being more appropriate for testing children. The classification of audiogram by sequential testing is a computer-mediated form of visual reinforcement audiometry (Merer & Gravel, 1997). The technique uses a sophisticated mathematical model to predict the child's audiogram from fewer stimuli than is conventionally required. The technique appears to be useful for testing children in the 6- to 60-month range. Game audiometry is incorporated into the previously mentioned ProDigit 2000.

Using standard software that is part of both Windows and Mac OSs, it is fairly easy to present any type of sound recorded on audio CDs. Standard speech recognition materials and assessment of central auditory processing disorders

(CAPD) can be performed with the CDs produced by the Veteran's Administration (Humes et al, 1996a ; Noffsinger et al, 1994). Sound effects and competing messages can be played from Micro Sound Products Party Noise CD. Auditec will produce custom recordable (CD-R) CDs, potentially containing a wide variety of useful materials. Newby and Popelka (1992) described a system that uses the Mac and HyperCard for presenting speech stimuli. In our clinic speech recognition materials have been digitized and stored on the hard drive of a Mac computer located in our test booth. A custom HyperCard stack was developed to play the words in sequence with a user-selectable time delay between presentations. Or, any test item could be presented at random by clicking on the word. The audio output of the computer was inputted to the audiometer in the same manner as a tape deck for instance. Standardized, recorded speech stimuli can be presented with the flexibility of live voice (de Jonge, 1992). Stach et al (1995) found that when a computer is used to manually present recorded speech, there is about a 22% time savings, compared with delivering speech with a fixed time interval. Another HyperCard stack was developed to facilitate the administration of the Frequency Pattern Test (Musiek, 1994). One of six sequences of tones is randomly selected (hi-hi-lo, lo-hi-lo, lo-lo-hi, etc.). The tester presents the sequence by clicking the mouse button, and correct-incorrect responses are tallied automatically by the software. The HyperCard stack contains material describing the test protocol and its interpretation.

PEARL

Under computer control, digitized words are presented with the flexibility of monitored live voice and the standardization of recorded speech.

The SCAN and SCAN-A (available from Oaktree Products) are screening procedures for detecting CAPD in children and adults. Like many tests for CAPD, the audiologist must remember quite a bit of detail regarding test setup, administration, and norms for scoring. With the SCAN, responses must be tallied, raw scores converted to standard scores (based on the child's age), and then converted to percentiles and age equivalents. Many possibilities exist for mistakes to occur and for results to be misinterpreted. ScanWare is a Windows program that, once raw data are entered, completes the scoring. Tables summarizing patient performance are displayed and a narrative report is generated. The report can be printed directly or stored in a file to be read by a word processing program. Considering the difficulty in administering and interpreting a CAPD test battery, it seems that this is one area ripe for computerization.

Diagnostic Testing: ENG, Evoked Potentials, and OAEs

ENG, a procedure for evaluating portions of the balance system, is an example of a technique that derives major benefits from computer control. Several components make up an ENG evaluation, and each protocol should be followed in a certain sequence. Occasionally, as is the case with the calorics, a minimum time interval must pass before the next test is performed. Properly designed software will guide the audiologist through each step of each procedure. In conventional ENG the major equipment items include a light bar, caloric irrigator, amplifiers, and a strip chart for acquiring and recording nystagmus. The recording of nystagmus must be timed with the activation of both the light bar and the irrigator, and a computer can help to coordinate these events. The computer replaces the paper recorder and ocular movements are displayed on the screen and saved to disk for further analysis and archiving. The software automatically identifies the nystagmus and computes the speed of the slow phase, a procedure that takes a great deal of time to perform manually. Because the image displayed on the light bar is under computer control, the speed and accuracy of eye movements can be automatically computed. The results of the random saccade test, along with other tests in the battery, can be summarized and printed in a standard report format.

Evoked potentials, most commonly the ABR, are routinely measured by use of computer-based systems, and these systems co-evolved with the PC. The basic hardware is under computer control. Presentation of stimuli, collection of waveform data, and averaging are all routinely handled by a PC. Once the underlying theory is mastered, practical details of working with the patient are understood. Learning how to use this equipment is essentially a process of learning how to use a computer program. Some of the programs run under DOS; newer programs may take advantage of the Windows environment. The software controls the instrument parameters (a "virtual control panel"), processing of the data (i.e., smoothing, inverting, adding waveforms), display of information, and its analysis. Data can be stored and entered in a database, and reports generated and printed. Automated procedures are available for ABR screening (i.e., the Algo 2). Algorithms have been developed for recognizing the presence of a valid response, and the software program can respond with a pass or fail. OAEs, especially the transient evoked OAEs closely parallel the ABR in terms of computer control of equipment and software for analyzing and displaying data. Both the ABR and OAEs can be used as diagnostic tools and for infant screening. Additional software has been developed to manage screening programs.

Managing Newborn Screening Programs

Approximately 4 million children are born in this country each year. The goal of universal hearing screening is to test each child with either automated ABR, transient evoked OAEs (TEOAEs), or distortion product OAEs. But "detection is a costly exercise if there is a poor design for follow-up services" (Albright & Finitzo, 1997). Follow-up is essentially a matter of information management, and 4 million children would generate a prodigious amount of information. It is inconceivable for manual systems, paper logbooks, to handle the job. And, in addition to the consequences of lost opportunity for early intervention, unidentified children ("misses") pose a threat of litigation. Computer programs track which babies have been screened and which still need to be screened. Babies must return for rescreen and diagnostic ABRs, behavioral evaluations, and medical evaluation. Appointments can be broken and require rescheduling; some children are overdue for appointments or need to be sent a reminder of an upcoming appointment. Pediatricians and parents

receive letters informing them of the results of the screen and subsequent diagnostic evaluation. People managing the program need data analyzed and reported in a useful manner for monitoring key quality indicators of the program (White, 1996).

The Rhode Island Hearing Assessment Project (RIHAP) used RI-Track, a custom-designed dBase IV database for managing its statewide TEOAE screening program. This information management system had a positive effect on the program. After implementing the computer-tracking application, the percentage of successful rescreens increased from 77% to 94% (Johnson et al, 1993). A demonstration disk is available for those interested in obtaining hands-on experience with the software used for testing and database management. The February 1993 issue of *Seminars in Hearing*, which describes the RIHAP, contains a disk with a copy of the database software, the software for running the ILO88 hardware, and a number of sample files to simulate testing and demonstrate the software.

Finitzo and Diefendorf (1997), reporting the results of a national survey of infant screening programs, indicated that 50% of the programs used a computerized data management system. Of those using software, 47% indicated that it reduced the work load. Some of the programs were custom designed in-house, such as RI-Track. Others used Hi-Track, Hi-Screen, and Hi-Data, which is offered by the National Center for Hearing Assessment and Management (NCHAM). Another program is The Screening and Information Management System (SIMS) sold by the OZ Corporation. Biologic Systems developed another database management program, the Infant Screening Database. A variety of options are available for those wishing to automate.

The Hi-Track software, which runs in a DOS environment, can be downloaded from NCHAM's Web site (www.usu.edu/~ncham/). A user manual is included along with a sample database of 50 infants. Instructions suggest that the best way to become familiar with the software is to assume the role of program coordinator and begin experimenting with Hi-Track. Although the program was developed for use with a TEOAE screen, the software can be used with any screening technology. Hi-Track can be used as part of an integrated system, or it can operate in stand-alone mode. Hi-Track will merge data from the Hi-Screen module or from DataBook. DataBook is data management software used with the Algo 2 automated ABR screener.

Generating Audiological Reports

Audiologic Software, Inc. offers a number of PC-based programs that take information from a variety of tests and integrate them into a report. AUDIOS-Direct is designed to connect, by way of an RS-232 serial port, to audiometers and insertion gain analyzers manufactured by Beltone, Madsen, Frye, and Grason-Stadler). Point 'n Click is a stand-alone program, in which data is entered manually. The manual version also supports reports containing immittance, ABR, and ENG data. The program performs some calculations on the ABR and ENG data, based on numerical entries by the user. The reports are printed or saved to disk. The data are available in a database format that can be accessed over a network. Information can also be used to print mailing labels and generate letters. A module exists for using a keyboard to remotely control an audiometer and another for tracking new issues and repairs of hearing aids. A demonstration program is available from the company's Web site (www.audios.com).

Aural Rehabilitation and Hearing Conservation

Cochlear Implants, Aural Rehabilitation, and CAIV

The measurement and interpretation of an electrically evoked auditory response in the initial selection of candidates for cochlear implants requires the use of computers. The subsequent fitting, and follow-up fine tuning, of the cochlear implant is facilitated by software and hardware very similar in concept to the fitting of programmable hearing aids. The computer screen becomes the control panel used to adjust implant parameters so that a wide range of incoming sound is within the user's dynamic range for as many channels as possible. SCLIN for Windows is software used to fit the Clarion cochlear implant (Zimmerman-Phillips & Osberger, 1997). SCLIN is an example of how software can enhance fitting techniques for young children. The variable cooperation of the pediatric population often provides the audiologist with a limited window of opportunity for obtaining useful information. To program a cochlear implant, ideally, thresholds and MCLs would be obtained for all channels. But this information may be missing from children. SCLIN allows channel settings to be interpolated from data obtained on only one or two other channels. Also, children can have difficulty with the concept of loudness, especially for tonal stimuli, so live-voice stimuli can be used to adjust MCLs. The software also allows limits to be set for the range of the volume control, and the memories of the processor can be programmed for different listening environments.

Aural rehabilitation (AR) after implantation is important for developing auditory skills such as sound detection, discrimination, identification, and comprehension. This is particularly true for children who are active in learning language and acquiring speech skills. Children often do not have the advantage of the extensive "auditory database" enjoyed by postlingually deafened adults. Cochlear corporation is distributing a CD-ROM software program, Foundations in Speech Perception, for children with moderate-to-profound hearing losses, including those using cochlear implants. The program is designed for children ages 3 to 12 years and is designed to help the child with both speechreading and auditory training. However, using video as a tool for teaching speechreading has a long history.

Computer-assisted interactive video (CAIV) was first used with a system, described by Sims et al (1979), called "DAVID" (Dynamic Audio Video Interactive Device). DAVID consisted of a computer-controlled videotape player. The software would find videoclips of sentences that students were supposed to speechread. Responses were typed on the keyboard, or a selection was made in a multiple-choice format. Lessons progressed from easier to more difficult as fewer contextual cues were provided. As videodisc technology emerged, it was incorporated into DAVID, replacing the slower videotape player. A number of systems, generally similar in concept to

DAVID, were developed. See Sims and Gottermeier (1995) for a review. The following is an example of how this technology is being applied. Laser Videodisc technology, as described by Tye-Murray (1996), may help to encourage more time spent in AR activities. The high-quality video (and audio) images, which can be played by means of computer control, make videodiscs a natural medium for developing speechreading and auditory training exercises. A variety of materials are currently available (Sims, 1988). The new digital versatile disc (DVD) format is capable of storing the equivalent of a full-length motion picture on a disk the size of a standard CD-ROM. The DVD players, which will also play standard CDs, will become standard equipment in new PCs. This implies an almost universal medium for this type of therapy, both in the clinic and for practice at home.

A training station includes a videodisc player, a computer, and speakers. A touch screen monitor is valuable because it provides a more natural way for a patient to interact with the computer, avoiding problems with typing commands or learning to use a mouse. The computer determines which items are presented and the sequence. The AR program described by Tye-Murray (1996) focused on training for audiovisual recognition of speech, practice in using conversational repair strategies, and communication strategies for patients' spouses and family members. The program provides a full range of analytic and synthetic activities designed to promote effective communication in a variety of natural listening environments. The therapy experiences can operate with the audiologist present or absent, and the software can track performance and display progress reports. While the hearing aid fitting is taking place, family members can receive instructions on appropriate and inappropriate speaking behaviors. The opportunity for the patient and family members to benefit from unattended practice uses the audiologist's time more effectively.

SPECIAL CONSIDERATION

Audiologists may use their time more productively with computer-assisted interactive video. Unattended aural rehabilitation therapy is possible. While the patient is engaged in a hearing aid fitting, family members receive instruction on appropriate communication behaviors.

Hearing Conservation Programs

The Occupational Safety and Health Administration (OSHA) is the federal agency charged with the responsibility for protecting worker's hearing in industrial environments. The worker is protected by being part of a hearing conservation program (HCP). The Occupational Noise Exposure document (29 CFR 1910.95) is the OSHA standard that defines what is an effective hearing conservation program (OSHA, 1981). Audiologists working in industry must comply with this document. The standard specifies virtually every aspect of an HCP, what measurements need to be made and when, what tests must be given, actions taken, and what records need to be kept. Because noise is so pervasive in industry and millions of workers are in HCPs, the amount of data is very large. OSHA requires that specific records be maintained for each worker. For instance, noise exposure levels must be determined, and appropriate attenuation values for hearing protectors calculated. Calibration records for audiometers must be stored along with ambient noise levels within the test suite. Employees must be scheduled for baseline and annual audiograms. Each year the annual audiogram must be saved and compared with the baseline. Corrections for the effects of aging can be looked up from a table and applied. Standard threshold shifts have to be calculated. Employees found to have hearing loss are rescheduled for follow-up audiometry or scheduled for diagnostic evaluations. The standard requires that employees receive timely, written documentation of changes in their hearing. Letters have to be written to referral sources. An OSHA Form 200 must be filed, depending on whether specific criteria are met. In short, a database

must be maintained. Several programs are commercially available (see Table 20–4).

HCP applications are usually designed to interface directly with an audiometer for direct data transfer and to function in a networked environment. The programs are designed to automate paperwork and purport to lower administrative costs. They can record case history information, generate personalized employee notification letters and retest lists, schedule employee hearing tests, analyze trends in audiometric data, and measure program performance, and create reports—in general handle the requirements dictated by the occupational noise standard. The industrial hygienist is often the person responsible for monitoring and safeguarding the worker from all sorts of hazardous exposures, including noise. Consequently, some applications, such as Occupational Health Manager (OHM), include hearing conservation as only one

TABLE 20–4   Sample hearing conservation software programs and a manufacturer of compatible audiometers

Application	Contact Information
Employee Audiometric Reporting System (EARS) Occupational Health Manager (OHM)	501-925-7700 Unique Software Solutions, Inc. 2975 Broadmoor Valley Rd., Suite 200 Colorado Springs, CO 80906 719-576-7859 www.ussi-colo.com
HEAR/TRAK	The HAWKWA Group, Inc. PO Box 69 Wadsworth, IL 60083 74677.1242@compuserve.com
Audio-Graf	Teck Trak Software 855 - 8th Avenue, Suite 202 Calgary, AB T2P 3P1 800-947-5544 www.tecktrak.com
OHC-K	Savear, Inc. 44 Elm Street Huntington, NY 11743 516-271-6454 HJGARD@ aol.com
SPRINTware	Health & Hygiene, Inc. 420 Gallimore Dairy Road Greensboro, NC 27409 910-655-1818 www.Health-Hygiene.com/sprint.htm
Hearing Conservation Interactive Computer Training Program	Interactive Media Communications 100 5th Avenue Waltham, MA 02154 617-890-7707
Audiometers with serial ports for direct input to hearing conservation software industrial testing.	Micro Audiometrics Corporation 2200 South Ridgewood Ave South Daytona, FL 32119-3018 www.microaud.com

of several components to the program. OHM is designed to maintain information about all areas of each employees health. A key issue in selecting software involves giving the tester access to pertinent information at the time of the test. Ideally, programs should present the individual's baseline, the most recent annual audiogram, and expected thresholds for different gender and race groups (Royster & Royster, personal communication, 1998). Programs should also be able to export data for special evaluations, such as the type of audiometric database analysis specified in ANSI S12.13-1991. This is a draft standard offering guidelines for evaluating the effectiveness of hearing conservation programs. Audiogram thresholds are tracked over time for a large number of employees who are exposed to noise. The standard identifies statistical procedures that can be used to compare the noise-exposed group to a control group. Audiometric variability (the year-to-year variability in a population's thresholds) is a valid indicator of the effectiveness of the HCP. Results for the noise-exposed group should not be greater than the control group.

Simpson (personal communication, 1997), who acts as Ford Motor Company's technical consultant to the National Institute of Occupational Safety and Health (NIOSH) tested the HEAR/TRAK software with a public domain database of more than 5000 people and 150,000 audiograms (over eight serial tests). Ford purchased the software for use in 60 plants in the United States. The system was described as being complete, stable, networked to the company's mainframe, and handles approximately 75,000 hearing tests each year.

Telemedicine and Computer-Aided Instruction

Telemedicine, Telehealth

Telehealth can be as simple as traditional correspondence by mail or speaking over the telephone or as complex as taking advantage of computer technology, video compression, E-mail, and the Web. Even remote surgery using robotics is a possibility. The major benefit is improving access to healthcare, linking up people needing service with those professionals who are qualified to provide it. Telehealth involves removing barriers created by geography and improving the efficient use of a provider's time. Mainly, but not exclusively, these services could benefit those living in remote areas, such as the people of Micronesia and Samoa who lack professionals available for treating middle ear disease (Goldberg, 1997).

Staab et al (1997) describe remote teleprogramming (RTP), a service that could potentially improve patient management. In the future both audiologists and their patients would benefit. Patients could be living in either urban or remote areas. RTP is designed as a method for programming hearing aids. The hearing aid's remote control acts as the instrument's programmer. The remote receives its instructions acoustically (dual tone multifrequency), either from loudspeakers attached to a computer or from a standard telephone. The dispenser can change the aid's programming remotely by sending signals to the patient by means of a modem/telephone connection. Eliminating the need for an office visit could save both the patient and audiologist time and money. Care could be given

to patients who are less ambulatory or experiencing problems while on business trips or vacation. Also, the hearing aid could be programmed while the patient is located in a more realistic environment, either their home or a particularly troublesome listening situation.

PEARL

In the future audiologists may routinely use the telephone to remotely program a patient's hearing aid. Video otoscopic images may be sent to physician's offices as attachments to E-mail.

Video otoscopy is another area where possibilities exist for remote patient management (Sullivan, 1995; 1997). Physicians, whether they are physically present or not, can visualize conditions of the external/middle ear. Images from a video otoscope can be captured by computer, compressed (i.e., using the .jpg format), and transmitted to a remote location by means of a modem. The images could be uploaded to a Web site or they could be sent as attachments to an E-mail message. An audiologist testing in a remote area, using a portable video otoscope, computer, and modem, could consult with a physician either online or off.

Database software is available for storing images. TeleMedRx (MedRx, Inc.) is Windows software for database management: image acquisition from the video otoscope, transmission, archiving, printing, and generating reports. Fields are set up so that comments can be written to define the images. This permits database searches for images with particular characteristics (e.g., middle ear effusion, ventilation tube, exostosis, etc.). Starkey's StarView includes a recordkeeping system. Voice recognition allows the software to be controlled in a "hands-off" mode (see Kay [1998] for a review of voice recognition software). Ear Vision is Windows software that performs similar database functions. Searches can be initiated to find images; images can be resized, rotated, written; or live-voice comments can be stored.

Computer-Aided Instruction

Computers can be used in a number of different ways to facilitate the teaching and learning process. The traditional lecture benefits from the structure imposed by a PowerPoint-type presentation and from the use of appropriate media to explain and illustrate certain concepts. The use of pictures, graphs, sound, and video clips all help to get the images out of the mind of the presenter and in plain view of the student. Bringing the abstract down to a more concrete level generally appeals to students and, perhaps, facilitates learning. De Jonge (1992) describes a multimedia classroom (computer, LCD projector, videocassette recorder, videodisc, cassette audio tape, amplifiers, and speakers) that facilitates computer-aided instruction. HyperCard was used to create all lecture material for all classes taught. HyperCard has a built-in programming language, so it is a more flexible tool than standard presentation software, like PowerPoint. Everything used in a lecture (notes, graphs, pictures, etc.) is in plain view of the class. All this material is also available from a server located in the computer commons. Students have access to all lecture material outside of class. Most all students prefer to make hardcopies of the lecture notes and annotate them during class. They can spend more time listening and less time formulating and writing thoughts. Some students express the opinion that they miss a lot of what is said while they are trying to process and write what they have heard.

PEARL

Providing a copy of lectures is a benefit of computer-aided instruction. Students miss a lot of what is said while they are trying to process and write what they have heard.

Software can be used to create simulations that can be demonstrated in class and used independently by students outside of class. Or, in some cases, the software may be designed for a completely independent learning experience. An example is a simulation of an electrical analog model of the middle ear connected to an earcanal, earmold vent, earmold tubing connecting to an earhook, and ending with a hearing aid receiver. Changes can be made to any part of the model and the effect on REIG can be observed (de Jonge, 1996b). Simulations can also be used to assess student learning. A HyperCard stack, the Audiometric Simulator, is an example. Students use a virtual audiometer to test patients. The patient has a case history and true audiogram thresholds already defined. The program allows the virtual patient to respond or not depending on such variables as subject inconsistency, duration of tone presentation, interaural attenuation, occlusion effect, and masking efficiency. During practice, the instructor can allow students to get feedback about whether their thresholds are correct. During assessment they cannot. The simulation allows the student the opportunity to put theory into practice. An accurate audiogram unambiguously documents their knowledge and skill.

A number of similar applications are available through the Support Syndicate for Audiology. Applications deal with topics related to learning anatomy, middle ear physiology, hearing aid selection, audiometry, tympanometry, acoustics, the decibel, ABR, and so forth. Through Parrot Software, Townsend, occasionally collaborating with Olsen and Weiss, has created a number of useful applications for the PC. Some of these deal with immittance and pure tone (with masking) simulation. Others help the student to learn anatomy and mathematical concepts like the decibel. The Dynamic Acoustics program covers the basics of sound transmission, the sine wave, synthesis of complex waveforms, and allows the student to hear the waveforms they are visualizing on the computer screen. Some of this software is also included with an audiology textbook (Bess & Humes, 1995). Other multimedia authors, Bradley and Christenson, developed the Hearing Loss Simulator. This is a Mac application that uses filtering to simulate how speech would sound to patients with different audiogram configurations.

Applications are available for students developing diagnostic skills. Tharpe and Biswas (1997) describe a program, Simon Says, for investigating problem solving in audiology. Simon Says is a computer-based environment for conducting, interpreting, and using audiological tests to form diagnoses. The user would read case history information and formulate hypotheses that are recorded by the software. Additional tests could be ordered, such as immittance or a simulated ABR (Tharpe et al, 1993). Eventually a final diagnosis would be made. An instructor could use this tool for assessing a student's learning processes. "Audiology: Disorders and Evaluation," is another example of how computers can be used to train and assess audiologists learning to make clinical diagnoses. The program, described as a virtual management process, was developed by the Veteran's Administration, runs on a Windows PC, and is distributed on CD-ROM. A number of tutorials and case studies can be investigated. Patients present with symptoms, they are assessed both behaviorally and electrophysiologically, pathological conditions are identified, and the patient is managed. The emphasis is on applying appropriate diagnostic strategies and treatment decisions. Test tutorials are available for the basic evaluation (pure tone and speech audiometry, tympanometry, acoustic reflexes), otoscopy, and more advanced tests like ABR, electrocochleography, OAEs, and the Stenger and tuning fork tests. There are 21 pathological tutorials on such topics as otosclerosis, Meniere's disease, head trauma, and ototoxicity. Examples of case studies include diabetes, functional hearing loss, brain stem tumor, and so on. The software simulates patient evaluation. Tests are ordered and interpreted. During the process, the software provides feedback about inappropriate decisions. At the end the student can compare his or her performance (tests administered and cost of test) to that of an expert.

CONCLUSIONS

As recently as 1991, computers were not even mentioned as a basic equipment need in audiological practice (Teter & Schweitzer, 1991). In an American Academy of Audiology (AAA) needs survey, more than 65% of AAA members indicate a desire for hands-on training with common computer systems and software (Van Vliet, 1997). The "Guidelines for Education in Audiology Practice Management" include the use of computers for office automation as one of six specific competency areas (ASHA, 1995). Computer use included diagnostic applications, data storage and access, tracking patient outcomes and consumer satisfaction, professional correspondence, scheduling and billing, and marketing applications. Computer use is becoming common in virtually all areas of audiology. The use of well-designed software holds the promise for allowing audiologists to work more effectively and productively. With computers handling more routine tasks, audiologists can spend more time helping their patients, thus making the practice of audiology even more satisfying.

REFERENCES

ALBRIGHT, K., & FINITZO, T. (1997). Texas hospitals' quality control approach to universal infant hearing detection. *American Journal of Audiology, 6*;88–90.

ALLEN, J.B., HALL, J.L., & JENG, P.S. (1990). Loudness growth in 1/2-octave bands (LGOB): A procedure for the assessment of loudness. *Journal of the Acoustical Society of America, 88*;745–753.

AMERICAN NATIONAL STANDARDS INSTITUTE. (1969). American National Standard Methods for Calculation of the Articulation Index. (ANSI S3.5-1969). New York: ANSI.

AMERICAN NATIONAL STANDARDS INSTITUTE. (1993). American National Standard Methods for The Calculation of the Speech Intelligibility Index. (ANSI S3.79-Draft). New York: ANSI.

AMERICAN SPEECH-LANGUAGE-HEARING ASSOCIATION. (1995, March). Guidelines for education in audiology practice management. *ASHA, 37*;20.

ANDERSON, B.A., YANZ, J.L., & HAGEN, L.E. (1997). A PCMCIA card for programmable instrument applications. *Hearing Review, 4*(9);47–48.

ANDERSON, M.B., & JELONEK, S. (1994). An integrated hearing care software system. *Hearing Review, 1*(4);26–27.

BERGER, K.W., HAGBERG, E.N., & RANE, R.L. (1979). Determining hearing aid gain. *Hearing Instruments, 30*;26–28,44.

BERGER, K.W., HAGBERG, E.N., & RANE, R.L. (1989). *Prescription of Hearing Aids: Rationale, Procedures and Results* (5th ed.). Kent, OH: Herald.

BESS, F.H., & HUMES, L.H. (1995). *Audiology: The Fundamentals* (2nd ed.). Baltimore: Williams & Wilkins.

BOCHNER, J., GARRISON, W., PALMER, L., & MACKENZIE, D. (1997). A computerized adaptive testing system for speech discrimination measurement: The speech sound pattern discrimination test. *Journal of the Acoustical Society of America, 101*(4);2289–2298.

BYRNE, D., & DILLON, H. (1986). The national acoustic laboratories new procedure for selecting the gain and frequency response of a hearing aid. *Ear and Hearing, 7*;257–265.

BYRNE, D., PARKINSON, D., NEWALL, P. (1990). Hearing aid gain and frequency response requirements of the severely/profoundly hearing-impaired. *Ear and Hearing, 11*;40–49.

CLANCY, D.A. (1995). Highlighting developments in hearing aids. *Hearing Instruments, 46*(12);18,20.

CORNELISSE, L.E., GAGNÉ, J.P., & SEEWALD, R.C. (1991). Ear level recordings of the long-term average spectrum of speech. *Ear and Hearing, 12*;47–64.

CORNELISSE, L.E., SEEWALD, R.C., & JAMIESON, D.G. (1994). Wide-dynamic-range compression hearing aids: The DSL[i/o] approach. *Hearing Journal, 47*(10);23–29.

CORNELISSE, L.E., SEEWALD, R.C., & JAMIESON, D.G. (1995). The input/output formula: A theoretical approach to the fitting of personal amplification devices. *Journal of the Acoustical Society of America, 97*(3);1854–1864.

COWART, R. (1998). *Mastering Windows 95*. San Francisco: Sybex.

COX, R.M. (1983). Using ULCL measures to find frequency/gain and SSPL90. *Hearing Instruments, 34*(7);17–21,39.

COX, R.M. (1984). Relationship between aided preferred listening level and long-term listening range. *Ear and Hearing, 5*;72–76.

COX, R.M. (1985). A structured approach to hearing aid selection. *Ear and Hearing, 6*;226–239.

COX, R.M. (1988). The MSU hearing instrument procedure. *Hearing Instruments, 39*(1);6–10.

COX, R.M., & ALEXANDER, G.C. (1990). Evaluation of an in-situ output probe-microphone method for hearing aid fitting verification. *Ear and Hearing, 11*;31–39.

COX, R.M., & ALEXANDER, G.C. (1995). The abbreviated profile of hearing aid benefit. *Ear and Hearing, 16*;176–183.

COX, R.M., ALEXANDER, G.C., & GILMORE, C. (1991). Objective and self-report measures of hearing aid benefit. In: G.A. Studebaker, F.H. Bess, & L. Beck (Eds.), *The Vanderbilt hearing aid report II* (pp. 201–213). Parkton, MD: York Press.

COX, R.M., GOFF, C.M., MARTIN, S.E., & McCLOUD, L.L. (1994a). The contour test: Normative data. Presented at the American Academy of Audiology Meeting, Richmond, VA, 1994.

COX, R.M., & RIVERA, I.M. (1992). Predictability and reliability of hearing aid benefit measured using the PHAB. *Journal of the American Academy of Audiology, 3*;242–254.

COX, R.M., TAYLOR, I.M., GRAY, G.A., & BRAINERD, L.E. (1994b). The contour test: Applications to hearing aid selection and fitting. Presented at the American Academy of Audiology Meeting, Richmond, VA, 1994.

DE JONGE, R.R. (1985). A microcomputer-based hearing aid selection strategy. *Journal for Comp Users Speech and Hearing, 1*;117–138.

DE JONGE, R.R. (1987). Hearing aid selection using a microcomputer. *Hearing Instruments, 38*(5);126–130.

DE JONGE, R.R. (1992). HyperCard: A tool for computer-aided instruction in audiology. *Journal for Comp Users Speech and Hearing, 8*;137–147.

DE JONGE, R.R. (1996a). Microcomputer applications for hearing aid selection and fitting. *Trends in Amplification, 1*(3);86–114.

DE JONGE, R.R. (1996b). Real-ear measures: Individual variation and measurement error. In: M. Valente (Ed.), *Hearing aids: Standards, options, and limitations* (pp. 72–125). New York: Thieme Medical Publishers, Inc.

DERN, D.P. (1994). *The internet guide for new users*. New York: McGraw-Hill.

DILLON, H. (1991). Allowing for real-ear venting effects when selecting the coupler gain of hearing aids. *Ear and Hearing, 12*;406–416.

DILLON, H., BYRNE, D., & BATTAGLIA, J. (1992). Hearing instrument selection: By dispenser or by computer? *Hearing Instruments, 43*(8);18–21.

FAUSTI, S.A., SCHAFFER, H.I., OLSON, D.J., FREY, R.H., & HENRY, J.A. (1993). Software for managing multi-site auditory research. *Audiology Today, 5*(3);22–25.

FINITZO, T., & DIEFENDORF, A.O. (1997). The state of the information. *American Journal of Audiology, 6*;91–94.

GELFAND, S.A. (1997). *Essentials of audiology*. (pp. 226–227). New York: Thieme Medical Publishers, Inc.

GILSTER, P. (1995). *The SLIP/PPP connection*. New York: John Wiley & Sons.

GITLIN, R. (1995). Software-driven audiology powers hearing professionals. *Hearing Instruments, 46*(5);11–13.

GOLDBERG, B. (1997). Linking up with telehealth. *ASHA, 39*(4);27–31.

GRALLA, P. (1997). *How the internet works.* Emeryville, CA: Ziff-Davis Press.

GREY, H., & DYRLUND, O. (1996). Putting loudness scaling to work: Moving from theory to practice. *Hearing Journal, 49*(3);49,52–54.

GREY, H., & ROSS, T. (1995). PC-bases system offers greater capabilities with less hardware. *Hearing Journal, 48*(4);27,30–31.

HALPIN, C., THORNTON, A., & HOUSE, Z. (1996). The articulation index in clinical diagnosis and hearing aid fitting. *Current Opinion in Otolaryngology and Head and Neck Surgery, 4;*325–334.

HAMPTON, D. (1995). HearWare (v. 5.0) [Software review]. *Ear and Hearing, 16;*325–326.

HAWKINS, D.M., WALDEN, B.E., MONTGOMERY, A.A., & PROSEK, R.A. (1987). Description and validation of an LDL procedure designed to select SSPL90. *Ear and Hearing, 8;*162–169.

HEIDE, V.H. (1994). Project Phoenix, Inc., 1984–1989: The development of a wearable digital signal processing hearing aid. In: R.E. Sandlin (Ed.), *Understanding digitally programmable hearing aids* (pp. 123–150). Boston: Allyn & Bacon.

HELLMAN, R.P., & MEISELMAN, C.H. (1993). Rate of loudness growth in normal and impaired hearing. *Journal of the Acoustical Society of America, 93;*966–975.

HOSFORD-DUNN, H., DUNN, D.R., & HARFORD, E.R. (1995). *Audiology business and practice management* (pp. 171–195,235–261). San Diego, CA: Singular Publishing Group, Inc.

HUMES, L.E., COUGHLIN, M., & TALLEY, L. (1996a). Evaluation of the use of a new compact disc for auditory perceptual assessment in the elderly. *Journal of the American Academy of Audiology, 7;*419–427.

HUMES, L.E., & HOUGHTON, R. (1992). Beyond insertion gain. *Hearing Instruments, 43*(3);32,34–35.

HUMES, L.E., PAVLOVIC, C., BRAY, V., & BARR, M. (1996b). Real-ear measurement of hearing threshold and loudness. *Trends in Amplification, 1*(4);121–135.

JELONEK, S. (1994). NOAH/HI-PRO system offers industry-wide standard for fitting programmables. *Hearing Journal, 47*(5);21–22.

JENNINGS, R. (1997). *Using Windows NT Server 4.* (2nd ed.). Indianapolis: Que Corporation.

JOHNSON, C.D., BENSON, P.V., & SEATON, J.B. (1997). *Educational audiology handbook.* San Diego: Singular Publishing Group, Inc.

JOHNSON, M.J., MAXON, A.B., WHITE, K.R., & VOHR, B.R. (1993). Operating a hospital-based universal newborn hearing screening program using transient evoked otoacoustic emissions. *Seminars in Hearing, 14*(1);46–55.

KAY, R. (1998). Do you hear what I say? [Software review]. *BYTE, 23*(1);115–116.

KETCHUM, P. (1997). Tips for using computers and programmable software. *Hearing Review, 4*(2);23–24,28.

KILLION, M.C., FIKRET-PASA, S. (1993). The 3 types of sensorineural hearing loss: Loudness and intelligibility considerations. *Hearing Journal, 46*(11);31–34.

KILLION, M.C., & REVIT, L.J. (1993). CORFIG and GIFROC: Real ear to coupler and back again. In: G.A. Studebaker, & I. Hochberg (Eds.), *Acoustical factors affecting hearing aid performance* (2nd ed.) (pp. 65–85). Boston: Allyn & Bacon.

KILLION, M.C. (1996). Talking hair cells: What they have to say about hearing aids. In: C.I. Berlin (Ed.), *Hair cells and hearing aids.* San Diego: Singular Publishing Group, Inc.

KOBLER, R.D. (1997). *PC novice guide to going online.* Lincoln, NE: Sandhills.

KRUGER, F.M., & KRUGER, B. (1997). Any port in a storm? Some solutions to computer problems. *Hearing Journal, 50*(4);5353–54,56,58,61.

KUNOV, H., MADSEN, P.B., & SOKOLOV, Y. (1997). Single system combines 5 audiometric devices. *Hearing Journal, 50*(3);32,34.

LAY, J., & NUNLEY, J. (1996). Computer-based tinnitus evaluation system. *Hearing Instruments, 47*(3);46.

LIEBERT, A.K., & MARTIN, D.R. (1995). Authoring and hypermedia. *Language, Speech, and Hearing Services in Schools, 26;*241.

LEIJON, A. (1991). Hearing aid gain for loudness-density normalization in cochlear hearing losses with impaired frequency resolution. *Ear and Hearing, 12;*242–250.

LIPPMAN, P.R., BRAIDA, L.D., & DURLACH, N.I. (1981). Study of multichannel amplitude compression and linear amplification for persons with sensorineural hearing loss. *Journal of the Acoustical Society of America, 69;*524–534.

LYREGAARD, P.E. (1988). POGO and the theory behind. In: J.H. Jensen (Ed.), *Hearing aid fitting: Proceedings of the 13th Danavox Symposium* (pp. 81–94). Copenhagen: Danavox.

MARGOLIS, R.H., & THORNTON, A.R. (1991). Spreadsheet systems for tracking audiology patients. *Audiology Today, 3;*24–26.

MARTIN, R.L. (1991). What your computer should tell you about your patients. *Hearing Journal, 44*(6);42,44.

MARTTILA, J. (1998). Educational audiology handbook [Book review]. *Ear and Hearing, 19*(1);85–86.

MCCANDLESS, G.A., & LYREGAARD, P.E. (1983). Prescription of gain/output (POGO) for hearing aids. *Hearing Instruments, 35*(1);16–21.

MCCULLOUGH, J.A., WILSON, R.H., BIRCK, J.D., & ANDERSON, L.G. (1994). A multimedia approach for estimating speech recognition of multilingual clients. *American Journal of Audiology, 3*(1);19–22.

MENDEL, L.L., WYNNE, M.K., ENGLISH, K., & SCHMIDT-TROIKE, A. (1995). Computer applications in educational audiology. *Language, Speech and Hearing Service Schools, 26;*232–240.

MERER, D.M., & GRAVEL, J.S. (1997). Screening infants and young children for hearing loss: Examination of the CAST procedure. *Journal of the American Academy of Audiology, 8;*233–242.

MOODIE, K.S., SEEWALD, R.C., & SINCLAIR, S.T. (1994). Procedure for predicting real-ear hearing aid performance in young children. *American Journal of Audiology, 3;*23–31.

MOSELY, L.E., & BOODEY, D.M. (1996). *Mastering Microsoft Office Professional for Windows 95.* San Francisco: Sybex.

MOSKAL, N.L., GOLDSTEIN, D.P., & ANDERSON, J.G. (1989). Expert systems in audiology: An introductory look. *Hearing Journal, 42*(10);27,30–31.

MUELLER, J.H. (1990). Using personal computers for business planning. *Hearing Journal, 43*(5);34–38.

MUSIEK, F.E. (1994). Frequency (pitch) and duration pattern tests. *Journal of the American Academy of Audiology, 5;*265–268.

MYERS, L.L., LETOWSKI, T.R., ABOUCHACRA, K.S., KALB, J.T., & HAAS, E.C. (1996). Detection and recognition of octave-band sound effects. *Journal of the American Academy of Audiology, 7;*346–357.

NELSON, S.L. (1996). *QuickBooks 5 for dummies.* (3rd ed.). Foster City, CA: IDG Books Worldwide, Inc.

NEWBY, H.A., & POPELKA, G.R. (1992). *Audiology* (6th ed.) (pp. 303–305). Englewood Cliffs, NJ: Prentice Hall.

NEWMAN, C.W., JACOBSON, G.P., WEINSTEIN, B.E., & SANDRIDGE, S.A. (1997). Computer-generated hearing disability/handicap profiles. *American Journal of Audiology, 6*(1);17–21.

NOFFSINGER, D., WILSON, R.H., & MUSIEK, F.E. (1994). Department of Veterans Affairs Compact Disk (VA-CD) recording for auditory perceptual assessment: Background and introduction. *Journal of the American Academy of Audiology, 5*;231–235.

OCCUPATIONAL SAFETY AND HEALTH ADMINISTRATION. (1981). Occupational Noise Exposure. *Federal Register, 46*;4078–4179.

PALMER, C.V. (1992). Using the HyperCard/HyperTalk programming environment in the clinical and educational audiology setting. *Journal for Comp Users Speech and Hearing, 8*;130–136.

PASCOE, D.P. (1988). Clinical measurements of the auditory dynamic range and their relation to formulas for hearing aid gain. In: J.H. Jensen (Ed.), *Hearing aid fitting: Proceedings of the 13th Danavox Symposium* (pp. 129–152). Copenhagen: Danavox.

PICARD, M., ILECKI, H.J., & BAXTER, J.D. (1993). Clinical use of BOBCAT: Testing reliability and validity of computerized pure-tone audiometry with noise-exposed workers, children and the aged. *Audiology, 32*;55–67.

RADCLIFFE, D. (1996). The computer-enhanced office and clinic: Fitting technology to consumer needs. *Hearing Journal, 49*(9);15–16,19,22,24,26.

ROBERTSON, P.R. (1996). A guide to NOAH-compatible programmable fitting software. *Hearing Review, 3*(2);12,14,16, 19,28,29–30.

SCHUM, D.J. (1997). The use of advance fitting software in the counseling process. *Hearing Review, 4*(2);57–58,62.

SEEWALD, R.C. (1992). The desired sensation level method for fitting children: Version 3.0. *Hearing Journal, 45*(4);36–41.

SEEWALD, R.C., MOODIE, K.S., & ZELISKO, D.L.C. (1993a). Critique of current approaches to the selection and fitting of hearing aids. *Journal of Speech-Language Pathology and Audiology Monograph Supplement, 1*;29–37.

SEEWALD, R.C., RAMJI, K.V., SINCLAIR, S.T., MOODIE, K.S., & JAMIESON, D.G. (1993b). *A computer-assisted implementation of the Desired Sensation Level method for electroacoustic selection and fitting in children: DSL 3.1 user's manual.* The Hearing Healthcare Research Unit Technical Report 02. The University of Western Ontario. London, Ontario.

SEEWALD, R.C., & ROSS, M. (1988). Amplification for young hearing-impaired children. In: M.C. Pollack (Ed.), *Amplification for the hearing-impaired* (pp. 213–267). New York: Grune and Stratton.

SEEWALD, R.C. (1994). Fitting children with the DSL method. *Hearing Journal, 47*(9);10, 49–51.

SHENNIB, A., LANSER, M., & OMIDVAR, F. (1994). Personal digital audiometry: A new dimension in testing. *Hearing Instruments, 45*(3);17–18,20,39.

SIMS, D.G. (1988). Video methods for speechreading instruction. *The Volta Review, 90*;273–288.

SIMS, D.G., & GOTTERMEIER, L. (1995). Computer-assisted interactive video methods for speechreading instruction: A review. In: G. Plant, & K.E. Spens (Eds.), *Profound deafness and speech communication* (pp. 557–577). London: Whurr Publishers Ltd.

SIMS, D.G., KNIGHT, S., & AUSTIN, A. (1992). Macintosh software for revised NAL hearing-aid fitting prescription. *Journal of Comp Users Speech and Hearing, 8*;8–14.

SIMS, D.G., VON FELDT, J., DOWALIBY, F., HUTCHINSON, K., & MYERS, T. (1979). A pilot experiment in computer assisted speechreading instruction utilizing the data analysis video interactive device (DAVID). *American Annals of the Deaf, 124*;618–623.

SKAFTE, M.D. (1997). The 1996 hearing instrument market: The dispenser's perspective. *Hearing Review, 4*(3);8–36.

STAAB, W.J., EDMONDS, J., & GARCIA, H. (1997). Remote teleprogramming (RTP): Future directions to patient management. *Hearing Review (Supplement), 2*;50–52.

STACH, B.A., DAVIS-THAXTON, M.L., & JERGER, J. (1995). Improving the efficiency of speech audiometry: Computer-based approach. *Journal of the American Academy of Audiology, 6*;330–333.

STEARNS, W.P. (1998). Today's computer: An essential fitting tool. *Hearing Review, 5*(1);28.

STROM, K.E. (1997). Don't smash it to bytes. *Hearing Review, 4*(2):4.

STYPULKOWSKI, P.H. (1995). Applying PC technology to hearing aid fitting. *Hearing Journal, 48*(7);27–28,30,32.

SULLIVAN, R.F. (1995). Video otoscopy: Basic and advanced systems. *Hearing Review, 2*(10);12–16.

SULLIVAN, R.F. (1997). Video otoscopy in audiologic practice. *Journal of the American Academy of Audiology, 8*;447–467.

TETER, D.L., & SCHWEITZER, H.C. (1991). Hearing aid dispensing. *Audiology Today, 3*(5);32–35.

TETER, D.L., & WINTHROP, S.J. (1994). Programmable hearing aids: Some practical considerations for dispensers. *Hearing Journal, 47*(4);35,37–39.

THARPE, A.M., & BISWAS, G. (1997). Characterization of problem solving in audiology: Implications for training. *American Journal of Audiology, 6*(1);31–42.

THARPE, A.M., BISWAS, G., & HALL, J.W. (1993). Development of an expert system for pediatric auditory brainstem response interpretation. *Journal of the American Academy of Audiology, 4*;163–171.

THORNTON, A. (1993). Computer-assisted audiometry and technicians in a high-volume practice. *American Journal of Audiology, 2*(3);11–13.

THORNTON, A.R., HALPIN, C., HAN, Y., & HOU, Z. (1993). The Massachusetts Eye and Ear audiometer operating system. Unpublished manuscript. (pp. 1–7).

THORNTON, A.R., & RAFFIN, M.J.M. (1978). Speech-discrimination scores modeled as a binomial variable. *Journal of Speech and Hearing Research, 21*;507–518.

TYE-MURRAY, N. (1996). Laser videodisc technology in the aural rehabilitation setting: Good news for people with severe and profound hearing impairments. In: R.L. Schow, & M.A. Nerbonne (Eds.), *Introduction to audiologic rehabilitation* (3rd ed.) (pp. 516–521). Boston: Allyn & Bacon.

VALENTE, M., VALENTE, M., & VASS, W. (1990). Selecting an appropriate matrix for ITE/ITC hearing instruments. *Hearing Instruments, 41*(4);21–24.

VALENTE, M., & VAN VLIET, D. (1997). The independent hearing aid fitting forum (IHAFF) protocol. *Trends in Amplification, 2*(1);6–35.

VAN VLIET, D. (1995). A comprehensive hearing aid fitting protocol. *Audiology Today, 7*;11–13.

VAN VLIET, D. (1997). AAA member CE needs survey summary. *Audiology Today, 9*(3);17.

VILLCHUR, E. (1973). Signal processing to improve speech intelligibility in perceptive deafness. *Journal of the Acoustical Society of America, 53*;1646–1657.

WHITE, K.R. (1996). Universal newborn hearing screening using transient evoked otoacoustic emissions: Past, present, and future. *Seminars in Hearing, 17*(2);171–183.

WYNNE, M.K. (1996). You can't surf the Web without having your hands on the net. *Hearing Journal, 49*(7);10,61–62, 64–65.

WYNNE, M.K., SEATON, W.H., & ALLEN, R.L. (1993). Integration into office management. *ASHA, 35*(9):50–51.

ZAPALA, D. (1998). The virtual audiogram [Web site]. http://www.concentric.net/~kellytc/viraud.htm.

ZIMMERMAN-PHILLIPS, G., & OSBERGER, M.J. (1997). Programming the Clarion cochlea implant. (In press). http://www.cochlearimplant.com /candidchild.html [April, 1998].

Chapter 21

The Future of Audiology Practice Management

James F. Jerger, Marjorie D. Skafte, and Lars Kolind

In this final chapter three international leaders from diverse sectors of hearing healthcare care look to the future of the audiology profession, graciously sharing their opinions and predictions about the "state of the profession" now and in the probable future. With millennium fever in the air, it seems entirely appropriate that all three projections echo a common and urgent theme of rapid change in which adaptation, advance planning, and ethical behavior are distinct advantages for practice survival. The changes they forecast are powerful and lie ahead in all directions.

Change is their common theme, but as the adage says, "Change is the only constant." The three contributors offer unique views of the hearing healthcare profession, partly because of their training and work backgrounds, the time and number of years that each has toiled to improve hearing healthcare, and what they define as the goals and objectives of the field as a whole. Indeed, it is hardly an understatement to say that the individual contributions of these three people to the academic, business, and manufacturing components of hearing healthcare have shaped the evolution of audiology practice management. Not surprisingly, their views do not always coincide; sometimes they do not even overlap. "SWOT" analyses are much in evidence: one writer sees Strength, another see Weakness; changes are viewed as Opportunities by some, as Threats by others. Paraphrasing Chapter 1, frictions abound as dynamic tensions move audiology practice management relentlessly toward a future that either looms or beckons.

Dr. James F. Jerger opens the discussion by forecasting a uniform doctoral level training requirement for certification or licensure, accompanied by a two-tiered service delivery system incorporating doctoral-level audiologists and master's-level assistants. His SWOT analysis predicts the demise of some educational training programs and the rebirth of others. In another vein, Dr. Jerger warns against ethical lapses as audiologists continue to shift away from academic endeavors to increase their retail presence. His concerns and hope for the future mirror the words of Helmick (Chapter 3, this volume): "Achieving an appropriate balance between good business practices and ethical conduct is, to be certain, a significant challenge but an achievable one nonetheless."

Marjorie Skafte shares Dr. Jerger's views that doctoral-level practitioners coupled with hearing healthcare assistants are likely in future practice management; also the ethic of "patient-first" professional behavior must prevail in the business environment. But Skafte also champions a more sanguine view of the future, seeing strengths and opportunities manifest in four areas: (1) the increasing number of dispensing audiologists in the United States, (2) a healthier and more "involved" senior market, (3) technological advances in hearing aids, and (4) centralization of practice management to realize economies of scale. Although weaknesses and threats are also present in these areas, Skafte believes that they are best overcome by expanding continuing education efforts to increase knowledge of the discipline, of the products, of the profession, and of business practices. Given her enthusiastic view of audiology's forward momentum, it comes as no surprise that a recent publication rates audiology as the 34th best profession of 250 surveyed, well ahead of other healthcare professions such as dentistry, speech pathology, optometry, chiropractic, and even surgery (Kratz, 1999).

Knowledge is key to the future in the opinion of Lars Kolind. His view is positively effusive about the future of hearing healthcare for those practices and practitioners who generate, attract, transform, and share knowledge. Strength and opportunity go to the "innovators"; weakness and threats are the lot of "followers." Interestingly, of the three opinionators, Kolind's view from the manufacturing sector takes the most audiological view of the future. Like Jerger and Skafte, Kolind foresees a two-tiered service delivery system, but one based on severity of hearing loss rather than provider credentials. He predicts that "the business [of dispensing] will be driven by audiology rather than technology."

481

Audiology: Practice Management. Edited by Hosford-Dunn, Roeser, and Valente. Thieme Medical Publishers, Inc., New York © 2000

Concluding the SWOT analyses, and probably speaking for all three contributors, Lars Kolind anticipates significant challenges but also very significant opportunities for the hearing healthcare business in the next 10 years. In 10 years, perhaps as this volume undergoes revision for a new edition, it will be interesting to see how this chapter has stood the test of time. HHD/RJR/MV

THE FUTURE FROM THE ACADEMIC/CLINICAL POINT OF VIEW

James F. Jerger

Perhaps the most far-reaching trend for audiology in the next decade will be the inexorable movement to a doctoral-level profession. It is virtually certain that, eventually, one will have to have a doctoral degree to be certified or licensed to practice audiology. Still many obstacles must be overcome, and the full changeover is certainly several years away, but the prudent individual, and the prudent education program, will begin to prepare for the day when the doctoral degree will be the standard of practice in the profession.

One still unresolved issue is whether the preferred doctoral-level degree will be the conventional doctor of philosophy (Ph.D.) degree, the more recently conceived doctor of audiology (Au.D.) degree, or some combination of the two. Two relevant current trends can be traced. One has been the gradual shift in the conventional Ph.D. in audiology, over the past several decades, from a narrowly defined exercise in basic research training to a more broadly defined emphasis on clinical/applied research. The second trend has been the implementation, in recent years, of a relatively small number of Au.D. training programs designed to focus intensive training on the clinical and administrative aspects of the profession with a lesser emphasis on research training.

Advocates of the Au.D. argue that if audiology is to be a profession rather than an academic discipline, it must have its own professional degree unhampered by the largely irrelevant emphasis on basic research training so characteristic of typical Ph.D. programs. Proponents of the Ph.D., on the other hand, argue that it is supreme folly to abandon an advanced educational structure that has been in place for half a century, is working reasonably well, and is the goal to which many other health service professions aspire. Moreover, they note that the difference between a technician and a true professional may very well be a certain degree of exposure to the discipline of research. My own view, after some experience with both paths, is that both will play important roles in the future development of the profession, the conventional Ph.D. in the preparation of scientists and educators and the Au.D. in the training of administrators and clinicians, especially those in private practice.

One of the most distressing problems facing the profession in its march to the uniform doctoral level is what to do about the master's degree programs. As long as they exist, they represent a serious obstacle to change. Yet, many educational institutions depend on master's level students for their financial survival. These programs cannot be summarily eliminated but they can be altered. The key, I suspect, is a

fundamental change in orientation to a two-tiered profession. Like many other healthcare professions, two levels of workers will evolve: audiologists and audiometrists. The former will hold a doctoral-level degree and will function at a professional level. The latter will have less formal training and will function as assistants to audiologists. Master's degree programs cannot simply be eliminated, but they can be reoriented toward the goal of training workers at the second tier. These fundamental shifts in orientation will pose serious problems for existing educational training programs. Some will certainly not survive the trauma; others will adapt and, perhaps, become even stronger.

CONTROVERSIAL POINT

We will evolve two levels of workers: audiologists and audiometrists.

By this point in the book series, readers have undoubtedly read more than they want to know about managed care, cost containment, and accountability. But it has to be said that these are trends that must necessarily impact the way in which the clinical evaluation of hearing and hearing disorders is conducted in the future. Like our brethren in other divisions of the health sciences, audiologists are going to find it increasingly difficult to structure diagnostic and rehabilitative evaluations with regard to cost efficiency. Gone, or soon to be gone, are the days when audiologists can administer a broad battery of tests to every interesting patient. More refined analyses of the cost/benefit ratios associated with alternative testing algorithms will be required in the future. Some of these analyses have already revealed surprising data. For example, Silman and Silverman (1991) note that application of the Dobie (1985) cost/benefit model to the problem of differentiating cochlear from retrocochlear disorder yields the following interesting result: the performance versus intensity function for phonetically balanced (PB) words (PI-PB) is more cost effective than the auditory brain stem response (ABR). If this jars your sensibilities, you are not alone. What one learns from such models depends critically on the assumptions underlying the models. Silman and Silverman note, for example, that their particular model seems to be biased toward the false-positive rate of the test but is relatively insensitive to its hit rate. The take home message here is that it is to our advantage to become familiar with the concepts of decision and cost-benefit analyses so that we may guide at the helm rather than follow in the wake of these trends.

One of the clearest trends in our profession, over the past few decades, has been the steady increase in the proportion of audiologists entering private practice. This is a good news/bad news situation. The good news is that such a trend is clearly the mark of a maturing healthcare profession. It especially speaks to the creation of a sound financial foundation less dependent on the currents and cross currents of municipal, state, and federal funding. The bad news is that when one's livelihood is geared to success in the marketplace, the fine line defining professionalism versus commercialism tends, in some individuals, to blur. A few individuals may place profitability above sound scientific principle. Only one way exists in which the profession can meet this future challenge: the definition, promulgation, and rigid enforcement of its codes of ethics. Audiologists can expect an increase in ethical lapses and a concomitant increase in the enforcement of ethical standards over the next decade. However, we can be confident that most audiologists in private practice will continue to be guided by professionalism rather than profit.

CONCLUSIONS

1. The profession is moving slowly but steadily to the doctoral level. The defining degree is likely to depend on one's orientation: the conventional Ph.D. for scientists and educators, the Au.D. for administrators and clinicians.

2. To become leaders rather than followers in the cost-containment revolution, audiologists need to think a good deal harder about cost-benefit analyses of diagnostic and rehabilitative procedures.

3. Professionalism versus profitability will surely challenge the ethical principles of audiology, but a strong commitment to codes of ethics ensures that professionalism will triumph.

FUTURE DIRECTION OF AUDIOLOGY PRACTICE MANAGEMENT FROM A BUSINESS POINT OF VIEW

Marjorie D. Skafte

One of the definitions of the word change in *Webster's New World Dictionary of the American Language* (1970) is "passing from one phase to another." This definition appropriately defines what is, and has been for the last three decades of the twentieth century, taking place in healthcare and in hearing healthcare.

When the decade of the 1970s began, healthcare was a cottage industry with a multitude of individuals, physicians, pharmacists, opticians, hearing aid dealers, hospitals, all offering services on an individual basis. The pressures of new technology, government and social policies, the economy, and an increase in the number of both healthcare providers and facilities all have combined to reshape healthcare into centralized and well-structured organizations. As we are poised to enter the twenty-first century, healthcare is, to a large degree, provided in large clinics and hospitals that offer all medical services under the umbrella of one organization. Managed care organizations of some type and government programs such as Medicare and Medicaid play a major role in determining the who, what, when, and where of medical care in the 1990s.

Hearing healthcare has not moved into centralization of services as rapidly as has healthcare as a whole, but changes definitely have been taking place. Thirty years ago, hearing healthcare had only a limited number of providers, products, and services to offer individuals wiith hearing loss. Research

and new technology have brought new medications, varied types of surgery, and a host of new products. Hearing instruments have moved from body-worn and behind-the-ear instruments to in-the-canal units that encompass the latest digital and directional technologies. In the 1970s and 1980s hearing instruments were primarily dispensed from individual retail offices. In the 1990s varied types of dispensing practices have emerged. Hearing instruments can now be purchased in medical clinics, hospitals, audiological private practices, and some university audiology departments, as well as from traditional retail offices. Cochlear implants, assistive listening devices, and even implantable hearing instruments are now available or in the testing stages.

The number of individuals choosing audiology as a profession increased at a steady pace throughout the 1980s and 1990s. Before the adoption of a change in the American Speech and Hearing Association (ASHA) Code of Ethics in March 1979, which listed ASHA's restriction on the commercial dispensing of products, audiologists worked primarily in schools, clinics, hospitals, and rehabilitation centers. The number of audiologists dispensing hearing instruments grew rapidly throughout the decade of the 1980s until, in the 1990s, more than half of the estimated 10,000+ individuals in the United States engaged in hearing instrument dispensing have degrees in audiology (Skafte, 1990) (Fig. 21–1).

On entering the twenty-first century, the necessary ingredients for centralizing hearing care are all in place. The number of individuals with hearing loss who are not using amplification is at an all-time high, new technology abounds, the economy is booming, and a large pool of individuals qualified to provide hearing care is available. The "move into a new phase" for hearing healthcare has already begun, and audiologists involved in management of audiology practices need to make important decisions in preparing for challenges these practices will meet in the competitive business environment of the twentyfirst century.

In addition to the status of the economy, which is consistently listed in dispenser surveys as the major factor in the success of a practice, practice management decisions in the future will be influenced primarily by four major forces: patients, audiologists, new technology, and the practice itself. Each of these influencing forces will be discussed in relation to the overall business management of a practice.

Patients

In a world filled with noise and an aging population the number of individuals with some degree of hearing loss has steadily increased throughout the twentieth century. This number is expected to increase rapidly in the United States in the first 20 years of the twenty-first century as the segment of the population commonly referred to as the "boomer generation" moves into the senior category. The increase in the senior population is already having an impact on providers of hearing care. Statistics show that the aging patient base in hearing instrument dispensing practices has increased by almost 20% since 1980. In 1980, 48.7% of the patients were 65 years of age or older. In 1997, the 65+ segment had grown to 67% of the patient base (Skafte, 1998) (Fig. 21–2).

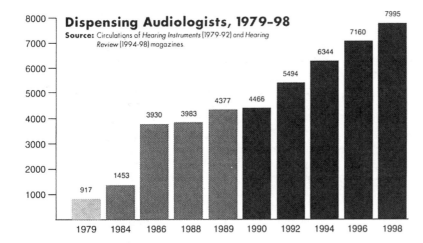

Figure 21–1 Dispensing audiologists. 1979–1998. (From *BPA Publisher Statement of Circulation of Hearing Instruments* [1979–92] and *The Hearing Review* [1994–98].)

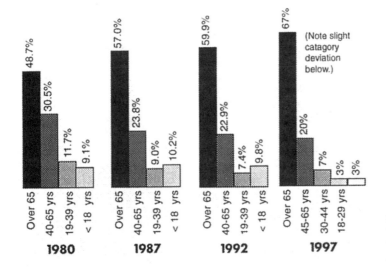

Figure 21–2 An aging client base. Comparison of customers by age groups. 1980–present. (From *The Hearing Review*, 5(6); p. 10, with permission.)

To serve this potential senior market for hearing healthcare appropriately, audiology practices will not only have to be concerned about having appropriate staff numbers, they will also need to acquaint themselves with the changes that have occurred in the lifestyle of the senior population. Retirement today no longer is viewed as a time to "sit back in a rocking chair" and withdraw from the active world. Mature adults of the future are far more apt to be active volunteers in the communities in which they reside. They travel extensively. They enroll in continuing education programs by the thousands. For example, lifelong learning programs in the Elderhostel Institute Network are now in existence on more than 250 college campuses with more than 64,000 members (Network News, 1999). This mature adult population wants to be involved and will be receptive to all types of communication assistance, such as hearing instruments, if those products and services are appropriately presented and if they provide the assistance represented and needed.

If this involved senior market segment is to be reached, hearing care professionals will have to schedule more time for consumer education than ever before. Establishing or increasing the rehabilitation services after the purchase of a

> **SPECIAL CONSIDERATION**
>
> **To reach senior markets of the future, hearing care professionals will have to schedule more time than ever before for consumer education.**

hearing instrument, for example, will be required. Market outreach, such as appropriate newspaper, magazine, TV and radio advertising, and brochures, will have to be developed with a consideration for the changing mind set of the senior population of tomorrow.

A major factor for administrators of audiological practices to consider is that while United States government statistics indicate that the number of individuals with hearing loss increases each year, a comparative increase in the number of first-time users of hearing instruments has not been taking place. Statistics from surveys of hearing instrument dispensers show that in 1983, 75.6% of the individuals who purchased hearing instruments were first-time patients. The number of first-time users steadily declined until 1995 when

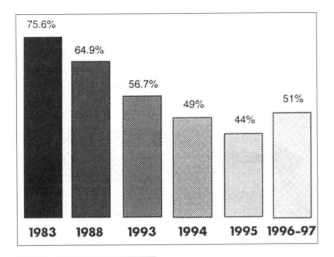

Figure 21–3 Percent of patients who are first-time users of hearing instruments. 1983–present. (From *The Hearing Review*, 5(6); p. 8, with permission.)

only 44% of the customers were first-time patients. In 1996-97, the number of first-time patients rose to 51%, the first increase in 15 years (Skafte, 1998) (Fig. 21–3). A change in the marketing and consumer education programs of the practices/offices engaging in dispensing hearing instruments would seemingly be in order.

Constant surveillance of developing consumer trends is necessary in any profession or business that serves the public and will be particularly imperative as the "boomer generation" becomes an important market segment for an audiology practice. Information will be needed as to their buying practices. Answers will be needed to questions such as: Will they carry over into retirement their preference for banking through ATM machines over face-to-face contact with a bank teller when depositing or withdrawing monies? What will be the marketing preferences of women who have worked at full-time careers while raising families?

Technology

Technological advances literally revolutionized hearing care in the 1980s and 1990s as digital technology and computers were incorporated into both the products used in the provision of hearing care and in the management of audiology practices. What can be expected in the future in new technology in products and how it will impact individuals with hearing loss and the audiologist is discussed in another section of this chapter. Consideration here will focus on two areas where appropriate management decisions relevant to incorporation of new technology into a practice have the potential for major impact on that practice—first, the pace of technological change (PTC) and second, continuing education.

In a period of rapid technological advancements, such as seen in recent years in hearing care, managers of businesses and practices need to plan ahead so reserve capital is available with which to purchase the instrumentation required to add the new technology to a practice. The PTC, the rate at which current technology becomes obsolete, has accelerated rapidly in the past 25 years. In the mid-1970s, for example,

the PTC was considered to be about 25 years and by the early 1990s, it had been shortened to 10 years. Its decline continues today, and it is estimated to be less than 5 years.

Technological Change

The use of computers in hearing instrument dispensing businesses/practices is an example of the rapid pace at which change takes place. In 1984 only 23.3% of hearing instrument dispensing offices used computers. In 1987, that number had increased to 54.5% and in 1997 to 93% (Skafte, 1998).

Conservative administrators may decide to delay purchase of new fitting and testing equipment because they are satisfied with the status quo. When new technologies mature and are available in products and services in other audiology practices, the conservative practices that can not provide new technology will inevitably see sales start to diminish. Practices that have taken reasonable risks and have planned ahead so that capital is available for equipment purchases are in position to take advantage of the initial enthusiasm for a new technology.

Continuing Education

Information on a technological advance is most often available preceding the introduction of products incorporating that technology in manufacturer literature, industry business and professional publications, and at exhibitions and conferences. Regular attendance at industry meetings and allocation of time for reviewing current literature can prepare audiology practice administrators in advance for introduction of relevant technology.

Before a practice begins marketing or using products that incorporate new technology, it is appropriate that all staff members have the necessary training (continuing education) to use the products competently, or in the case of hearing instruments, the necessary background information to fit the instruments to patients properly. Consumer opinion of a new product can suffer irreparable damage as a result of improper application. It should always be remembered that the largest source of patients for any practice is referrals from satisfied customers.

Allocation of capital to enable all staff members to attend continuing education seminars will be an important part of business planning of the future. Whereas it is vital for the owner of a practice or the administrator to be familiar with all new technology, it is often those staff members not involved with administration that provide most of the hands-on care in an audiology practice. Their competency is important to the long-range success of the practice. Insurers and other healthcare purchasers, recognizing a need for quality control in this area, may require certain amounts and types of professional staff continuing education in contractual arrangements for audiology services.

Audiologist

Audiologists dispensing hearing instruments will find themselves filling many roles, from conducting ABR and electronystagmagraphy tests and fitting hearing instruments to ordering product and checking cash flow. At the same time, consolidation of practices into larger entities will call for a clear delineation of the specific tasks to be performed by each staff member. Individual responsibilities will be determined by the demands of the practice and the particular talents and preferences and the number of available staff members. This delineation will enhance both the work flow and the inter-staff relationships within a practice.

Two very basic premises will continue to be requisites for a successful audiological practice just as they are for any type of business or profession that serves the public. Those premises are: (1) the welfare of and the satisfaction of the patient must always be the prime consideration and (2) the degree of success of any profession or business is directly related to the mental attitudes and working relationships of staff members.

Serving as a team member in an audiology dispensing practice will continue to differ greatly from the expectations and experiences of an audiologist in a research laboratory or a public school setting. A private practice is basically a business, a business that serves patients, and like all businesses, it must generate an income with which to pay for products, rent, and taxes as well as provide a source of income for the owner of that practice or the stockholders. Hundreds of articles have been published over the past 40 years relevant to audiologists and their responsibilities in a dispensing practice. One such article, "The Ten Commandments of Hearing Aid Dispensing," although it was published more than 10 years ago, very appropriately describes some of the changes in attitude that are necessary for an audiologist when he or she joins the staff of an audiology practice (Curran, 1986). Some of these "commandments" are:

- Thou shalt heed gravely the message of the bottom line.
- Thou shalt be willing to learn and use fine motor skills.
- Thou shalt develop broad shoulders.
- Thou shalt treat thy competitors with respect.
- Thou shalt be friends with thy customers.

As an audiology practice develops a long-range plan for the future, consideration of the degree level of the audiologists on staff is merited. The requirement of the doctoral degree for audiologists is established for the future. Achieving this degree will require time and monetary investment for audiologists already in a practice, whether attaining the advanced degree comes through distance learning, attending continuing education courses on a part-time basis, or return to college full time. Advance planning can, like preparation for introduction of new technology, move a practice through the challenges of this change more smoothly.

When the number of offices within a practice expands (and with it the number of staff members), it is highly probable that not all the individuals directly involved in testing of hearing and fitting of hearing instruments will have degrees in audiology. In 1997, 21% of the practices owned by a dispensing audiologist reported that both audiologists and hearing instrument specialists were employed by the practice (Skafte, 1998) (Fig. 21–4).

As the number of individuals needing hearing help increases and the centralization of hearing care progresses, a team approach consolidating the talents of physicians, audiologists, and hearing instrument specialists may well become the norm. Perhaps a new team member, the audiologist assistant,

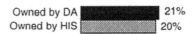

Slightly more than one-fifth of all dispensing offices responding to the *Hearing Review* Dispenser 1998 Survey employ both HISs and DAs, up from 14.5% in the *HR* 1997 survey.

Figure 21–4 Offices employing both hearing instrument specialists (HIS) and dispensing audiologists (DA). (From *The Hearing Review, 5*(6); p. 16, with permission.)

may emerge. In other healthcare professions the use of the services of assistants (i.e., physician assistant, nursing assistant, physical therapy assistant, dental assistant) has become commonplace to alleviate an ever-increasing work load and for reasons of economy that are driven in a large part by managed care demands.

The Practice

Entering the twenty-first century, the centralization of individual audiology private practices into multioffice organizations is already occurring at a relatively rapid pace. The concept of unifying offices under the umbrella of a manufacturer name or the banding together of a number of offices to use joint purchasing power and marketing services is definitely not a new concept. Hearing aid dealer offices of the 1940s, 1950s, and 1960s, for example, were primarily associated with a specific manufacturer and marketed primarily products made by that company. Advertising and marketing support and education of dispensers were chiefly provided by the manufacturer with whom that office was associated.

The centralization movement was accelerated in the 1990s by the expansion of managed care market forces into the hearing care field. These consolidations are taking many forms. In some areas independent audiologists have banded together to form independent practice associations (IPAs). Chains of dispensing offices, often staffed by audiologists, exist in many sections of the United States. Other practices are selling their offices to corporate structures that propose to use the economies of expanded purchasing power and central scheduling, accounting, billing, and marketing services, and so on, to enable them to provide quality service while expanding market share and providing income for the stockholders who finance these corporations. In many cases the seller and staff remain with the practice after the sale.

Other audiology practices contract for management services that allow the staff in these practices to focus on patient care instead of administration. Affiliates of most of these services continue to own their practices and remain independent from corporate entities. A number of practices maintain their independent status through the employment of in-house business managers who are in charge of the administration of the practice.

> ## PITFALL
>
> **Audiologists need to maintain their professional integrity and reputations when they sell to or join corporate, business-oriented audiology management groups.**

The choice of the appropriate management format is one of the major decisions that will face owners of audiology practices in the future. The decision whether to continue to operate an audiology practice as a stand-alone practice or to become a part of a centralized management organization will require careful reflection. For example, before a decision is made to sell a practice, answers are needed to questions such as: Can I cope with change? Am I willing to surrender my right to made independent decisions about practice policies such as determination of the length of time spent with each patient? Who will determine fees for services and products? What rehabilitative services will be offered? What will be the reaction of my staff to decisions in which they had no input? Will recommended or mandatory management decisions differ greatly from those I would personally choose? Is there a possibility that my professional integrity or reputation could be put in question?

On the other side of the coin, owners of audiology practices need to consider the freedom to devote the most of their time and energy to patient care that can result from turning administrative decisions over to someone else. Careful thought needs to be given to questions like: Do I have sufficient education and experience to make the appropriate marketing decisions that will be required in the competitive marketplace of the future? What would I do if several competitors drop product prices to increase their share of the market? Do I have the necessary financial reserve to survive as a practice if a change occurs in the economy? Do I have the marketing know-how to bring more new patients with hearing loss into the practice for hearing healthcare? What is the appropriate decision for the future welfare of my family?

The concept of dispensing practices banding together for economy in management, advertising, and purchasing is certainly not new in hearing instrument marketing. As noted earlier, exclusive franchises with hearing instrument manufacturers were the primary form of marketing in the hearing care field until the 1970s. The emergence of the clinical referral system was a major factor in the changeover by many dispensers to practices/offices that carried several brands of hearing instruments to provide the type and brand of instrument recommended by a clinical referral.

In the 1970s, 1980s, and 1990s, numerous purchasing and marketing groups emerged—some associated with chains of optical products, others specifically focused on hearing care products. Growth of these different types of marketing/purchasing groups has been relatively slow. However, in the mid- and late-1990s, a rapid acceleration took place in the startup of hearing care chains, cooperatives, and management groups. The answers to questions like: "Is bigger better?" and "Are there inherent qualities in hearing instrument testing, fitting, and marketing that do not lend themselves to mass marketing techniques?" will be available only with the passage of time.

CONCLUSIONS

The answers to the questions and the solutions to the problems inherent in marketing of hearing instruments will be individual and will differ from practice to practice, from one section of the country to another. They are problems and questions to which there are no easy answers or solutions. But they are decisions that must be reached before an audiology practice "moves on into that new phase" that will be recorded as history in the twenty-first century.

THE FUTURE OF HEARING HEALTHCARE FROM A MANUFACTURER'S VIEW

Lars Kolind

In the first decade of the twenty-first century we will no longer talk about the postindustrial age. We will talk about the twenty-first century as the *knowledge* age, the *networking* age, or the *information* age. These terms are being used to indicate that the most important factor determining a company's competitive edge is its ability to generate new knowledge, to attract knowledge, to transform knowledge, and to distribute and share knowledge with its customers.

In other words, one hearing aid that may look more or less like another hearing aid may differ tremendously because of the knowledge inside the shell and the knowledge associated with the fitting and aftercare of the instrument. It will no longer be possible to sell the hearing aid because it is digital or because it is small because all hearing aids will be digital and all hearing aids will be small enough. The products that will be sold will be those that satisfy genuine customer needs better than others, and these products will, first and foremost, be different from others because of their content of knowledge (i.e., their content of software instead of hardware).

One important difference between software (knowledge) and hardware is that software can be spread throughout the world at virtually no cost, while a cost will still be associated with movement of physical goods. It is the fact that knowledge can be moved at virtually no cost that will drive competition in society toward becoming fully global and transparent.

These trends will affect healthcare and hearing healthcare as well but other developments will also shape our industry. Forecasts have long indicated that the segment of the population older than 65 is growing. However, this trend will not be the most important one affecting the hearing care system. More important will be the fact that products and services will be far more efficient than today and their benefits will be better documented. Thus the consumption of healthcare will grow, not only because of the increased number of senior citizens but also because the ability to do something to improve quality of life will be much greater.

Government and private providers of managed hearing care will strive to keep costs down but with little success. Hearing healthcare provision is part of the retailing and service

---

PEARL

Consumers will be willing to spend significantly more on healthcare in the future, provided that genuine benefits are present and provided that these benefits are well documented and real.

---

sectors in society. Therefore it will be influenced by some of the general trends affecting these sectors in the years ahead.

Retailing, in general, will come under heavy pressure by trading by means of the Internet. More and more goods and services will be provided by means of the Net. This will drive competition to become fully global. It will put those retailers particularly under pressure who do not add genuine value to the consumer by being physically present, close to where the consumer is. Why should a consumer enter a shop if genuine additional value is not added? This development will put pressure on retailers to apply much more knowledge to what they do and to be able to document the value of what they do to the consumer.

In hearing healthcare such knowledge will deal particularly with diagnostic procedures, hearing aid fitting methods, and aftercare. The retailer must develop and apply a concept for *total patient care*, which includes all phases of the hearing healthcare process, starting with creating realistic expectations and ending with ongoing improvement of the patient's quality of life.

Total patient care starts with developing a general acceptance of a more relevant definition of hearing healthcare quality than the one in use today. Even today, many practices accept real-ear measurements and comparisons between a theoretical target gain curve and a measured gain curve as a relevant criterion for successful hearing care. Hearing care professionals still stick to the real-ear method despite the fact that it works equally well whether the patient is dead or alive. I believe that the only relevant criteria to be used in the future are objective speech recognition data and the subjective satisfaction of the patient (i.e., the customer's perception of quality of life in his or her daily surroundings using the hearing aids). To achieve a significant improvement in customer satisfaction, it is necessary to rethink both the concept of diagnostics and the concept of fitting and fine-tuning hearing aids.

Today, diagnostics for the purpose of hearing aid assessment almost exclusively refer to physical measurements of hearing threshold level (HTL), uncomfortable loudness levels (ULL), and loudness mapping. These measurements are relevant now and will continue to be relevant later. But, if they are not combined with soft data about the relevant sound environments for the patient and the individual priorities of the patient in different sound environments, little hope exists that customer satisfaction will be increased significantly. It is not only necessary to acquire the relevant data, it is also necessary to develop the audiological knowledge needed to select the correct hearing aids and the correct amplification methods to fit the sound environments that are particularly relevant for the patient. The future audiologist will thus work in dialog with a sophisticated expert system, including neural networks,

to help understand the patient's preferences and translate those preferences into amplification strategies.

Such a development will only be possible if computers become an integrated part of the hearing healthcare practice and if hearing aids become fully digital with sophisticated sound processing algorithms built in. This will put tremendous pressure on hearing aid manufacturers. Today, only about five manufacturers worldwide have the technological competence and strength to develop genuinely innovative digital sound-processing technology. Twenty or more manufacturers will market digital solutions, but the basic technology and know-how will come from very few sources. In other words, only five manufacturers will be real innovators, whereas most companies will strive to survive as followers. Those companies that are true innovators will work on a global scale, and they will increasingly develop closer relationships with the most forward-looking retail organizations to leverage their investments and to ensure that the advanced technology is actually used correctly by retailers.

More and more, these collaborations will place the independent hearing healthcare provider under pressure. Individual audiologists and the practices they comprise will be forced to choose whether they want to be innovators or followers. Innovators within retailing will have to team up with innovative manufacturers in strategic alliances that, however, do not necessarily mean joint ownership. It will be more and more difficult for dispensing audiologists to shop around, short-term, between manufacturers for best buys. Such practices will have little long-term future.

Hearing healthcare providers will also be put under tremendous pressure by consumers. Consumers will be significantly better informed, particularly by means of the Internet. It will be very easy to access information that compares different hearing healthcare providers and different manufacturers. Consumers will seek to do business with providers that can document superior quality and performance, and it will be increasingly difficult to base a hearing healthcare practice on aggressive marketing and selling. Hearing healthcare providers will have to base their business on genuine knowledge and proven methods in diagnostics, hearing aid selection, fitting and fine-tuning, and total patient care. This pressure directly from consumers will be reinforced by public authorities and HMOs. Consumers of hearing care (patients and regulators) will be much better informed than today, and they will only be willing to deal with those hearing healthcare providers who can document total patient care. All this leads the hearing healthcare provider to a very important strategic choice: the choice of relationship with quality manufacturers on a long-term basis.

Hearing healthcare providers will also be faced with demands to invest significant amounts in education and technology for their practices. Tomorrow's hearing aid fitting will build on advanced multimedia systems installed in the fitting room, and hearing healthcare providers will be expected to go through training far beyond today's 1-day to 2-day seminars in conjunction with new products. Concepts such as rationales based on average calculations from large numbers of patients will be increasingly obsolete. Such concepts will be replaced by systems that map the individual preferences of users in a variety of listening situations. The business will be driven by audiology rather than technology.

All of this means that the future hearing care practice will be much more knowledge intensive than what we know today. It will probably also mean that hearing healthcare provision will be split into two major segments:

- Provision of hearing healthcare to people with mild and moderate hearing losses
- Provision of hearing healthcare to people with severe and profound hearing losses

People with mild and moderate hearing losses will expect hearing healthcare to be much more like today's optical business (i.e., more commercial, more pleasant, quicker). The traditional audiologist in a first-floor office with modest sign-posting will have only little to do in this segment.

On the other hand, provision of hearing healthcare to patients with severe and profound hearing loss will be much more medical and knowledge intensive than today. Again, the traditional audiologist who is not specialized will have little chance to win competition in this segment.

Here, audiologists must work together with otolaryngologists and other specialists to provide an integrated service with a very high content of knowledge and technology. Hearing healthcare providers of tomorrow will be faced with the choice of whether they want to address one segment or the other. I doubt that many audiologists will be successful in serving both.

CONCLUSIONS

I expect that the hearing healthcare business in the next 10 years will be faced with very significant challenges but also very significant opportunities. The market will grow significantly. Consumers will be willing to pay a very high price for quality hearing, and HMOs and society in general will recognize quality hearing care as an essential part of quality of life for the senior population.

REFERENCES

CURRAN, J.R. (1986). The ten commandments of hearing aid dispensing. *Seminars in Hearing, 7*(2);219–228.

DOBIE, R. (1985). The use of relative cost ratios in choosing a diagnostic test. *Ear and Hearing, 5*;113–116.

GURALNIK, D. (1970). *Webster's new world dictionary of the American language, Second College Edition.* New York: World Publishing Co.

KRATZ, L. (1999). *Jobs rated almanac 1999–2000: The best and worst jobs.* New York: St. Martins Press.

NETWORK NEWS. (1999). Special information sheet. Boston, MA: Elderhostel Institute Network.

SILMAN, S., & SILVERMAN, C. (1991). *Auditory diagnosis.* New York: Academic Press.

SKAFTE, M. (1990). Fifty hears of hearing healthcare—1940–1990. *Hearing Instruments, 41*(9), Supplement; 96.

SKAFTE, M. (1998). The 1997 hearing instrument market—The dispenser's perspective. *Hearing Review, 5*(5);6–22.

Appendix I
ASHA Code of Ethics

Last Revised January 1, 1994

PREAMBLE

The preservation of the highest standards of integrity and ethical principles is vital to the responsible discharge of obligations in the professions of speech-language pathology and audiology. This Code of Ethics sets forth the fundamental principles and rules considered essential to this purpose.

Every individual who is (a) a member of the American Speech-Language-Hearing Association, whether certified or not, (b) a nonmember holding the Certificate of Clinical Competence from the Association, (c) an applicant for membership or certification, or (d) a Clinical Fellow seeking to fulfill standards for certification shall abide by this Code of Ethics.

Any action that violates the spirit and purpose of this Code shall be considered unethical. Failure to specify any particular responsibility or practice in this Code of Ethics shall not be construed as denial of the existence of such responsibilities or practices.

The fundamentals of ethical conduct are described by Principles of Ethics and by Rules of Ethics as they relate to responsibility to persons served, to the public, and to the professions of speech-language pathology and audiology.

Principles of Ethics, aspirational and inspirational in nature, form the underlying moral basis for the Code of Ethics. Individuals shall observe these principles as affirmative obligations under all conditions of professional activity.

Rules of Ethics are specific statements of minimally acceptable professional conduct or of prohibitions and are applicable to all individuals.

PRINCIPLE OF ETHICS I

Individuals shall honor their responsibility to hold paramount the welfare of persons they serve professionally.

RULES OF ETHICS

A. Individuals shall provide all services competently.

B. Individuals shall use every resource, including referral when appropriate, to ensure that high-quality service is provided.

C. Individuals shall not discriminate in the delivery of professional services on the basis of race or ethnicity, gender, age, religion, national origin, sexual orientation, or disability.

D. Individuals shall fully inform the persons they serve of the nature and possible effects of services rendered and products dispensed.

E. Individuals shall evaluate the effectiveness of services rendered and of products dispensed and shall provide services or dispense products only when benefit can reasonably be expected.

F. Individuals shall not guarantee the results of any treatment or procedure, directly or by implication; however, they may make a reasonable statement of prognosis.

G. Individuals shall not evaluate or treat speech, language, or hearing disorders solely by correspondence.

H. Individuals shall maintain adequate records of professional services rendered and products dispensed and shall allow access to these records when appropriately authorized.

I. Individuals shall not reveal, without authorization, any professional or personal information about the person served professionally, unless required by law to do so, or unless doing so is necessary to protect the welfare of the person or of the community.

J. Individuals shall not charge for services not rendered, nor shall they *misrepresent*, in any fashion, services rendered or products dispensed.

K. Individuals shall use persons in research or as subjects of teaching demonstrations only with their informed consent.

L. Individuals whose professional services are adversely affected by substance abuse or other health-related conditions shall seek professional assistance and, where appropriate, withdraw from the affected areas of practice.

For purposes of this Code of Ethics, misrepresentation includes any untrue statements or statements that are likely to mislead. Misrepresentation also includes the failure to state any information that is material and that ought, in fairness, to be considered.

PRINCIPLE OF ETHICS II

Individuals shall honor their responsibility to achieve and maintain the highest level of professional competence.

RULES OF ETHICS

A. Individuals shall engage in the provision of clinical services only when they hold the appropriate Certificate of Clinical Competence or when they are in the certification process and are supervised by an individual who holds the appropriate Certificate of Clinical Competence.

B. Individuals shall engage in only those aspects of the professions that are within the scope of their competence, considering their level of education, training, and experience.

C. Individuals shall continue their professional development throughout their careers.

D. Individuals shall delegate the provision of clinical services only to persons who are certified or to persons in the education or certification process who are appropriately supervised. The provision of support services may be delegated to persons who are neither certified nor in the certification process only when a certificate holder provides appropriate supervision.

E. Individuals shall prohibit any of their professional staff from providing services that exceed the staff member's competence, considering the staff member's level of education, training, and experience.

F. Individuals shall ensure that all equipment used in the provision of services is in proper working order and is properly calibrated.

PRINCIPLE OF ETHICS III

Individuals shall honor their responsibility to the public by promoting public understanding of the professions, by supporting the development of services designed to fulfill the unmet needs of the public, and by providing accurate information in all communications involving any aspect of the professions.

RULES OF ETHICS

A. Individuals shall not misrepresent their credentials, competence, education, training, or experience.

B. Individuals shall not participate in professional activities that constitute a conflict of interest.

C. Individuals shall not misrepresent diagnostic information, services rendered, or products dispensed or engage in any scheme or artifice to defraud in connection with obtaining payment or reimbursement for such services or products.

D. Individuals' statements to the public shall provide accurate information about the nature and management of communication disorders, about the professions, and about professional services.

E. Individuals' statements to the public—advertising, announcing, and marketing their professional services, reporting research results, and promoting product—shall adhere to prevailing professional standards and shall not contain misrepresentations.

PRINCIPLE OF ETHICS IV

Individuals shall honor their responsibilities to the professions and their relationships with colleagues, students, and members of allied professions. Individuals shall uphold the dignity and autonomy of the professions, maintain harmonious interprofessional and intraprofessional relationships, and accept the professions' self-imposed standards.

RULES OF ETHICS

A. Individuals shall prohibit anyone under their supervision from engaging in any practice that violates the Code of Ethics.

B. Individuals shall not engage in dishonesty, fraud, deceit, misrepresentation, or any form of conduct that adversely reflects on the professions or on the individual's fitness to serve persons professionally.

C. Individuals shall assign credit only to those who have contributed to a publication, presentation, or product. Credit shall be assigned in proportion to the contribution and only with the contributor's consent.

D. Individuals' statements to colleagues about professional services, research results, and products shall adhere to prevailing professional standards and shall contain no misrepresentations.

E. Individuals shall not provide professional services without exercising independent professional judgment, regardless of referral source or prescription.

F. Individuals shall not discriminate in their relationships with colleagues, students, and members of allied professions on the basis of race or ethnicity, gender, age, religion, national origin, sexual orientation, or disability.

G. Individuals who have reason to believe that the Code of Ethics has been violated shall inform the Ethical Practice Board.

H. Individuals shall cooperate fully with the Ethical Practice Board in its investigation and adjudication of matters related to this Code of Ethics.

If you have questions about the Code of Ethics, please contact *Jim Jones.*

Search | Index | Professionals | Students | Consumers | Home

AAA Code of Ethics

PREAMBLE

The Code of Ethics of the American Academy of Audiology specifies professional standards that allow for the proper discharge of audiologists responsibilities to those served, and that protect the integrity of the profession. The Code of Ethics consists of two parts. The first part, the Statement of Principles and Rules, presents precepts that members of the Academy agree to uphold. The second part, the Procedures, provides the process which enables enforcement of the Principles and Rules.

PART I: STATEMENT OF PRINCIPLES AND RULES

PRINCIPLE 1: Members shall provide professional services with honesty and compassion, and shall respect the dignity, worth, and rights of those served.

Rule 1a: Individuals shall not limit the delivery of professional services on any basis that is unjustifiable or irrelevant to the need for the potential benefit from such services.

PRINCIPLE 2: Members shall maintain high standards of professional competence in rendering services, providing only those professional services for which they are qualified by education and experience.

Rule 2a: Individuals shall use available resources, including referrals to other specialists, and shall not accept benefits or items of personal value for receiving or making referrals.

Rule 2b: Individuals shall exercise all reasonable precautions to avoid injury to persons in the delivery of professional services.

Rule 2c: Individuals shall not provide services except in a professional relationship, and shall not discriminate in the provision of services to individuals on the basis of sex, race, religion, national origin, sexual orientation, or general health.

Rule 2d: Individuals shall provide appropriate supervision and assume full responsibility for services delegated to supportive personnel. Individuals shall not delegate any service requiring professional competence to unqualified persons.

Rule 2e: Individuals shall not permit personnel to engage in any practice that is a violation of the Code of Ethics.

Rule 2f: Individuals shall maintain professional competence, including participation in continuing education.

PRINCIPLE 3: Members shall maintain the confidentiality of the information and records of those receiving services.

Rule 3a: Individuals shall not reveal to unauthorized persons any professional or personal information obtained from the person served professionally, unless required by law.

PRINCIPLE 4: Members shall provide only services and products that are in the best interest of those served.

Rule 4a: Individuals shall not exploit persons in the delivery of professional services.

Rule 4b: Individuals shall not charge for services not rendered.

Rule 4c: Individuals shall not participate in activities that constitute a conflict of professional interest.

Rule 4d: Individuals shall not accept compensation for supervision or sponsorship beyond reimbursement of expenses.

PRINCIPLE 5: Members shall provide accurate information about the nature and management of communicative disorders and about the services and products offered.

Rule 5a: Individuals shall provide persons served with the information a reasonable person would want to know about the nature and possible effects of services rendered, or products provided.

Rule 5b: Individuals may make a statement of prognosis, but shall not guarantee results, mislead, or misinform persons served.

Rule 5c: Individuals shall not carry out teaching or research activities in a manner that constitutes an invasion of privacy, or that fails to inform persons fully about the nature and possible effects of these activities, affording all persons informed free choice of participation.

Rule 5d: Individuals shall maintain documentation of professional services rendered.

PRINCIPLE 6: Members shall comply with the ethical standards of the Academy with regard to public statements.

Rule 6a: Individuals shall not misrepresent their educational degrees, training, credentials, or competence. Only degrees earned from regionally accredited institutions in which training was obtained in audiology, or a directly related discipline, may be used in public statements concerning professional services.

Rule 6b: Individuals' public statements about professional services and products shall not contain representations or claims that are false, misleading, or deceptive.

PRINCIPLE 7: Members shall honor their responsibilities to the public and to professional colleagues.

Rule 7a: Individuals shall not use professional or commercial affiliations in any way that would mislead or limit services to persons served professionally.

Rule 7b: Individuals shall inform colleagues and the public in a manner consistent with the highest professional standards about products and services they have developed.

PRINCIPLE 8: Members shall uphold the dignity of the profession and freely accept the Academy's self-imposed standards.

Rule 8a: Individuals shall not violate these Principles and Rules, nor attempt to circumvent them.

Rule 8b: Individuals shall not engage in dishonesty or illegal conduct that adversely reflects on the profession.

Rule 8c: Individuals shall inform the Ethical Practice Board when there are reasons to believe that a member of the Academy may have violated the Code of Ethics.

Rule 8d: Individuals shall cooperate with the Ethical Practice Board in any matter related to the Code of Ethics.

Signature: _____Date: _____

PART II: PROCEDURES FOR THE MANAGEMENT OF ALLEGED VIOLATIONS

Approved January 1999

INTRODUCTION

Members of the American Academy of Audiology are obligated to uphold the Code of Ethics of the Academy in their personal conduct and in the performance of their professional duties. To this end it is the responsibility of each Academy member to inform the Ethical Practice Board (EPB) of possible Ethics Code Violations (Principle 8: Rule 8c). The processing of alleged violations of the Code of Ethics will follow the procedures specified below to ensure that violations of ethical conduct by members of the Academy are halted in the shortest time possible.

PROCEDURES

1. Suspected violations of the Code of Ethics should be reported in letter format giving documentation sufficient to support the alleged violation. Letters must be signed and addressed to:
   Chair, Ethical Practice Board
   American Academy of Audiology
   8201 Greensboro Drive, Suite 300, McLean, VA 22102

2. Following receipt of the alleged violation the EPB will request from the complainant a signed Waiver of Confidentiality indicating that the complainant will allow the Ethical Practice Board to disclose his/her name should this become necessary during investigation of the allegation. The EPB may, under special circumstances, act in the absence of a signed Waiver of Confidentiality. The EPB may also act sua sponte (unsolicited) under circumstances where it believes that there has been an ethical violation but no formal complaint by a member has been made. In addition the EPB may convert an action initiated by a member to sua sponte if the complaint is withdrawn. The EPB may also initiate a sua sponte action after it discovers that any of the following have taken place: (a) a felony conviction, (b) a finding of malpractice by a duly authorized tribunal, (c) expulsion or suspension from a state association for unethical conduct, (d) revocation, suspension, or surrender of a license or certificate for ethical violations by a state or local board or similar entity.

3. On receipt of the Waiver of Confidentiality signed by the complainant, or on the decision of the EPB to assume the role of active complainant (sua sponte), the member(s) implicated will be notified by the Chair that an alleged violation of the Code of Ethics has been reported. Circumstances of the alleged violation will be described and the member(s) will be asked to respond fully to the allegation. The members will be given 30 days to comply. All correspondence with the respondents will occur by registered mail.

4. The Chair may communicate with other individuals, agencies, and/or programs for additional information as may be required for EPB review. The Ethical Practice Board will accomplish the accumulation of information as expeditiously as possible to minimize the time between initial notification of possible Code violation and final determination.

5. All information pertaining to the allegation will be reviewed by members of the Ethical Practice Board and a finding reached regarding infractions of the Code. In cases of Code violation, the section(s) of the Code violated will be cited, and a sanction specified when the Ethical Practice Board decision is disseminated.

6. Notification of the actions and decisions of the EPB will be made in writing by registered mail.

7. Resignations of membership may occur at the time of the respondentís initial response to the show cause notice, or following an EPB finding that the respondent has committed a violation of the Code of Ethics, or failed to show good cause why he or she should not be expelled. Voluntary resignations do not allow for reinstatement.

8. Members found to be in violation of the Code may appeal the decision of the Ethical Practice Board. The route of Appeal is by letter format through the Ethical Practice Board to the Board of Directors of the Academy. Requests for Appeal must:
   a. be based upon procedural errors or excessive sanctions not suited to the infraction.
   b. be received by the Chair, Ethical Practice Board within 30 days of the Ethical Practice Board notification of violation.
   c. state the basis for the appeal, and the reason(s) that the Ethical Practice Board decision should be changed.
   d. not offer new documentation.

   The decision of the Board of Directors regarding Appeals will be considered final.

SANCTIONS

1. Reprimand. The minimum level of punishment for a violation consists of a reprimand. Notification of the violation and the sanction is restricted to the member and the complainant.

2. Cease and Desist Order. Violator(s) may be required to sign a Cease and Desist Order, which specifies the non-compliant behavior and the terms of the Order. Notification of the violation and the sanction is made to the member and the complainant, and may on two-thirds vote of the Ethical Practice Board be reported in an official publication.

3. Suspension of Membership. Suspension of membership may range from a minimum of six (6) months to a maximum of twelve (12) months. During the period of suspension the violator may not participate in official Academy functions. Notification of the violation and the sanction is made to the member and the complainant and is reported in official publications of the Academy. Notification of the violation and the sanction will be made to the respondent's state licensing board(s) and may be extended to others as determined by the Ethical Practice Board. No refund of dues or assessments shall accrue to the member. Voluntary resignation of membership during the course of an investigation will not prevent the EPB from notifying state licensing board(s) and possibly others of the infraction and sanction.

4. Revocation of Membership. Revocation of membership will be considered as the maximum punishment for a violation of the Code. Individuals whose membership is revoked are not entitled to a refund of dues or fees. One year following the date of membership revocation the individual may reapply for but is not guaranteed membership through normal channels and must meet the membership qualifications in effect at the time of application. Notification of the violation and the sanction is made to the member and the complainant and is reported in official publications of the Acad-

emy. Notification of the violation and the sanction will be made to the respondent's state licensing board(s) and may be extended to others as determined by the Ethical Practice Board. Voluntary resignation of membership during the course of an investigation will not prevent the EPB from notifying state licensing board(s) and possibly others of the infraction and sanction.

RECORDS

A Central Record Depository shall be maintained by the Ethical Practice Board, which will be kept confidential and maintained with restricted access.

Complete records shall be maintained for a period of five years and then destroyed.

A Book of Precedents shall be maintained by the Ethical Practice Board which shall form the basis for future findings of the EPB.

CONFIDENTIALITY

Confidentiality shall be maintained in all Ethical Practice Board discussion, correspondence, communication, deliberation, and records pertaining to members reviewed by the Ethical Practice Board.

No Ethical Practice Board member shall give access to records, act or speak, independently or on behalf of the EPB, without the expressed permission of the EPB members then active, to impose the sanction of the EPB, or to interpret the findings of the EPB in any manner which may place members of the EPB, collectively or singly, at financial, professional, or personal risk.

Information may be shared with National Office Staff or Legal Council of the Association. The other confidentiality provisions of these procedures bind these persons.

Admin//Bylaws/Code of Ethics I & II 3-99

Appendix II
AAA Scope of Practice in Audiology

Development of a Scope of Practice document began in 1990 with the work of an ad hoc committee on Scope of Practice, chaired by Alison Grimes. The document was put into final format by Robert W. Keith in 1992, and revised again in 1996.

The Scope of Practice document describes the range of interests, capabilities and professional activities of audiologists. It defines audiologists as independent practitioners and provides examples of settings in which they are engaged. It is not intended to exclude the participation in activities outside of those delineated in the document. The overriding principle is that members of the Academy will provide only those services for which they are adequately prepared through their academic and clinical training and their experience, and that their practice is consistent with the Academy Code of Ethics.

As a dynamic and growing profession, the field of audiology will change over time as new information is acquired. This Scope of Practice document will receive regular review for consistency with current knowledge and practice.

POSITION STATEMENT

Audiology: Scope of Practice

I. Purpose

The purpose of this document is to define the profession of audiology by its scope of practice. This document outlines those activities that are within the specialty of the profession. This Scope of Practice statement is intended to be used by audiologists, allied professionals, consumers of audiological services, and the general public. It serves as a reference for issues of service delivery, third-party reimbursement, legislation, consumer education, regulatory action, state and professional licensure, and inter-professional relations. The document is not intended to be an exhaustive list of activities in which audiologists engage. Rather, it is a broad statement of professional practice. Periodic updating of any scope of practice statement is necessary as technologies and perspectives change.

II. Definition of an Audiologist

An audiologist is a person who, by virtue of academic degree, clinical training, and license to practice and/or professional credential, is uniquely qualified to provide a comprehensive array of professional services related to the assessment and habilitation/rehabilitation of persons with auditory and vestibular impairments, and to the prevention of these impairments. Audiologists serve in a number of roles including clinician, therapist, teacher, consultant, researcher and administrator. In addition, the supervising audiologist maintains legal and ethical responsibility for all assigned audiology activities provided by audiology assistants and audiology students.

The central focus of the profession of audiology is concerned with all auditory impairments and their relationship to disorders of communication. Audiologists identify, evaluate, and habilitate/rehabilitate individuals with either peripheral or central auditory impairments, and strive to prevent such impairments. All professional activities related to this central focus fall within the purview of audiology. In addition, professional activities related to assessment and rehabilitation of persons with vestibular disorders are within the scope of practice of audiologists.

Audiologists provide clinical and academic training to students in audiology. Audiologists teach physicians and medical students about the evaluation of hearing, prevention of hearing loss, and habilitation and rehabilitation of persons with hearing impairment. They provide information and training on all aspects of hearing to other professions including psychology, counseling, rehabilitation, education and other related professions. Audiologists provide information on hearing, hearing loss and disability, prevention of hearing loss, and rehabilitation to business and industry. They develop and oversee hearing conservation programs in industry. Further, audiologists serve as expert witnesses within the boundaries of forensic audiology.

The audiologist is an independent practitioner who provides services in hospitals, clinics, schools, private practices and other settings in which audiological services are relevant.

III. Scope of Practice

The scope of practice of audiologists is defined by the training and knowledge base of professionals who are licensed and/or credentialed to practice as audiologists. Areas of practice include assessment and habilitation/rehabilitation of individuals with auditory and vestibular disorders, prevention of hearing loss, and research in normal and disordered auditory and vestibular function. The practice of audiology includes:

A. Identification

Audiologists develop and oversee hearing screening programs to detect individuals with hearing loss of all ages. Individuals licensed as audiologists may perform speech or language screening, or other screening measures, for the purpose of initial identification and referral of persons with other communication disorders.

B. Assessment

Assessment of hearing includes the administration and interpretation of behavioral and electrophysiologic measures of the peripheral and central auditory systems. Assessment of the vestibular system includes administration and interpretation of clinical and electrophysiologic tests of equilibrium. Assessment is accomplished using standardized testing procedures and appropriately calibrated instrumentation.

C. Habilitation and Rehabilitation

The audiologist is the professional who provides the full range of habilitative and rehabilitative services for persons with hearing impairment and disorders of equillibium. The audiologist is responsible for the evaluation and fitting of amplification devices, including assistive listening devices. The audiologist determines the appropriateness of amplification systems for persons with hearing impairment, evaluates benefit, and provides counseling and training regarding their use. Audiologists conduct otoscopic examinations, clean ear canals and remove cerumen, take ear canal impressions, fit, sell, and dispense hearing aids and other amplification systems. Audiologists assess and provide non-medical management for persons with tinnitus using techniques that include, but are not limited to, biofeedback, masking, hearing aids, education, and counseling.

Audiologists are also involved in the rehabilitation of persons with vestibular disorders. They participate as full members of vestibular rehabilitation teams to recommend and carry out goals of vestibular rehabilitation therapy including, for example, habituation exercises, balance retraining exercises, and general conditioning exercises.

Audiologists provide habilitation services for infants and children with hearing impairment and their families. These services may include therapy, home intervention, family support, and case management.

The audiologist is the member of the cochlear implant team who determines candidacy based on auditory and communication information. The audiologist provides pre and post surgical assessment, counseling, auditory training, rehabilitation, implant programming, and maintenance of implant hardware and software.

The audiologist provides habilitation and rehabilitation to persons with hearing impairment, and is a source of information for family members, other professionals and the general public. Counseling regarding hearing loss, the use of amplification systems and strategies for improving speech recognition is within the expertise of the audiologist. Additionally, the audiologist provides counseling regarding the effects of hearing loss on communication and psycho-social status in personal, social, and vocational arenas.

The audiologist administers identification, evaluation, habilitation and rehabilitation programs to children of all ages with hearing impairment from birth and preschool through school age. The audiologist is an integral part of the team within the school system which manages students with hearing impairments and students with central auditory processing disorders. The audiologist participates in the development of Individual Family Service Plans (IFSPs) and Individualized Educational Programs (IEPs), serves as a consultant in matters pertaining to classroom acoustics, assistive listening systems, hearing aids, communication, and psycho-social effects of hearing loss, and maintains both classroom assistive systems as well as students' personal hearing aids. The audiologist administers hearing screening programs in schools, and trains and supervises non audiologists performing hearing screening in the educational setting.

D. Hearing Conservation

The audiologist designs, implements and coordinates industrial and community hearing conservation programs. This includes identification and amelioration of noise-hazardous conditions, identification of hearing loss, recommendation and counseling for use of hearing protection, employee education, and the training and supervision of non audiologists performing hearing screening in the industrial setting.

E. Intraoperative Neurophysiologic Monitoring

Audiologists administer and interpret electrophysiologic measurements of neural function including, but not limited to, sensory and motor evoked potentials, tests of nerve conduction velocity, and electromyography. These measurements are in differential diagnosis, pre- and post-operative evaluation of neural function, and neurophysiologic intraoperative monitoring of central nervous system, spinal cord, and cranial nerve function.

F. Research

Audiologists design, implement, analyze and interpret the results of research related to auditory and vestibular systems.

G. Additional Expertise

Some audiologists, by virtue of education, experience and personal choice choose to specialize in an area of practice not otherwise defined in this document. Nothing in this document shall be construed to limit individual freedom of choice in this regard provided that the activity is consistent with the American Academy of Audiology Code of Ethics.

This document will be reviewed, revised, and updated periodically in order to reflect changing clinical demands of audiologists and in order to keep pace with the changing scope of practice reflected by these changes and innovations in this specialty.

ASHA Scope of Practice in Audiology

Ad Hoc Committee on Scope of Practice in Audiology

This scope of practice in audiology statement is an official policy of the American Speech-Language-Hearing Association (ASHA). The document was developed by the ASHA Ad Hoc Committee on the Scope of Practice in Audiology and approved in 1995 by the Legislative Council (8_95). Members of the ad hoc committee include David Wark (chair), Tamara Adkins, J. Michael Dennis, Dana L. Oviatt, Lori Williams, and Evelyn Cherow (ex officio). Lawrence Higdon, ASHA vice president for professional practices in audiology, served as monitoring vice president. This statement supersedes the Scope of Practice, Speech-Language Pathology and Audiology statement (LC 6-89), ASHA, April 1990, 1–2.

SCOPE OF PRACTICE IN AUDIOLOGY

Preamble

This statement delineates the scope of practice of audiology for the purposes of (a) describing the services offered by qualified audiologists as primary service providers, case managers, and/or members of multidisciplinary and interdisciplinary teams; (b) serving as a reference for healthcare, education, and other professionals, and for consumers, members of the general public, and policy makers concerned with legislation, regulation, licensure, and third party reimbursement; and (c) informing members of ASHA, certificate holders, and students of the activities for which certification in audiology is required in accordance with the ASHA Code of Ethics.

Audiologists provide comprehensive diagnostic and rehabilitative services for all areas of auditory, vestibular, and related disorders. These services are provided to individuals across the entire age span from birth through adulthood; to individuals from diverse language, ethnic, cultural, and socioeconomic backgrounds; and to individuals who have multiple disabilities. This position statement is not intended to be exhaustive; however, the activities described reflect current practice within the profession. Practice activities related to emerging clinical, technological, and scientific developments are not precluded from consideration as part of the scope of practice of an audiologist. Such innovations and advances will result in the periodic revision and updating of this document. It is also recognized that specialty areas identified within the scope of practice will vary among the individual providers. ASHA also recognizes that professionals in related fields may have knowledge, skills, and experience that could be applied to some areas within the scope of audiology practice. Defining the scope of practice of audiologists is not meant to exclude other postgraduate professionals from rendering services in common practice areas.

This scope of practice does not supersede existing state licensure laws or affect the interpretation or implementation of such laws. It may serve, however, as a model for the development or modification of licensure laws.

The schema in Figure AII–1 depicts the relationship of the scope of practice to ASHA's policy documents of the Association that address current and emerging audiology practice areas; that is, preferred practice patterns, guidelines, and position statements. ASHA members and ASHA-certified professionals are bound by the ASHA Code of Ethics to provide services that are consistent with the scope of their competence, education, and experience (ASHA, 1994).

Audiologists serve diverse populations. The client population includes persons of different race, age, gender, religion,

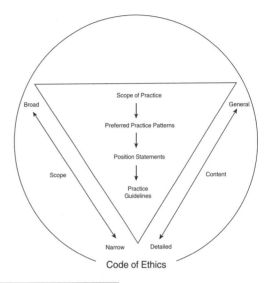

Figure AII–1 Conceptual Framework of ASHA Policy Statements.

The documents depicted in this diagram together serve as a guide to professional practice in audiology.

national origin, and sexual orientation. Audiologists' caseloads include persons from diverse ethnic, cultural, or linguistic backgrounds, and persons with disabilities. Although audiologists are prohibited from discriminating in the provision of professional services based on these factors, in some cases such factors may be relevant to the development of an appropriate treatment plan. These factors may be considered in treatment plans only when firmly grounded in scientific and professional knowledge.

DEFINITION OF AN AUDIOLOGIST

Audiologists are autonomous professionals who identify, assess, and manage disorders of the auditory, balance, and other neural systems. Audiologists provide audiological (aural) rehabilitation to children and adults across the entire age span. Audiologists select, fit, and dispense amplification systems such as hearing aids and related devices. Audiologists prevent hearing loss through the provision and fitting of hearing protective devices, consultation on the effects of noise on hearing, and consumer education. Audiologists are involved in auditory and related research pertinent to the prevention, identification, and management of hearing loss, tinnitus, and balance system dysfunction. Audiologists serve as expert witnesses in litigation related to their areas of expertise.

Audiologists currently hold a master's or doctoral degree in audiology from an accredited university or professional school. ASHA-certified audiologists serve a 9-month postgraduate fellowship and pass a national standardized examination. Where required, audiologists are licensed or registered by the state in which they practice.

Audiologists provide services in private practice; medical settings such as hospitals and physicians' offices; community hearing and speech centers; managed care systems; industry; the military; home health, subacute rehabilitation, long-term care and intermediate-care facilities; and school systems. Audiologists provide academic education in universities to students and practitioners in audiology, to medical and surgical students and residents, and to other related professionals. Such education pertains to the identification, assessment, and nonmedical management of auditory, balance, and related disorders.

SCOPE OF PRACTICE

The practice of audiology includes:

1. Activities that identify, assess, diagnose, manage, and interpret test results related to disorders of human hearing, balance, and other neural systems.

2. Otoscopic examination and external ear canal management for removal of cerumen in order to evaluate hearing or balance, make ear impressions, fit hearing protection or prosthetic devices, and monitor the continuous use of hearing aids.

3. The conduct and interpretation of behavioral, electroacoustic, or electrophysiologic methods used to assess hearing, balance, and neural system function.

4. Evaluation and management of children and adults with central auditory processing disorders.

5. Supervision and conduct of newborn hearing screening programs.

6. Measurement and interpretation of sensory and motor evoked potentials, electromyography, and other electrodiagnostic tests for purposes of neurophysiologic intraoperative monitoring and cranial nerve assessment.

7. Provision of hearing care by selecting, evaluating, fitting, facilitating adjustment to, and dispensing prosthetic devices for hearing lossÑincluding hearing aids, sensory aids, hearing assistive devices, alerting and telecommunication systems, and captioning devices.

8. Assessment of candidacy of persons with hearing loss for cochlear implants and provision of fitting, programming, and audiological rehabilitation to optimize device use.

9. Provision of audiological rehabilitation including speechreading, communication management, language development, auditory skill development, and counseling for psychosocial adjustment to hearing loss for persons with hearing loss and their families/caregivers.

10. Consultation to educators as members of interdisciplinary teams about communication management, educational implications of hearing loss, educational programming, classroom acoustics, and large-area amplification systems for children with hearing loss.

11. Prevention of hearing loss and conservation of hearing function by designing, implementing, and coordinating occupational, school, and community hearing conservation and identification programs.

12. Consultation and provision of rehabilitation to persons with balance disorders using habituation, exercise therapy, and balance retraining.

13. Design and conduct of basic and applied audiologic research to increase the knowledge base, to develop new methods and programs, and to determine the efficacy of assessment and treatment paradigms; dissemination of research findings to other professionals and to the public.

14. Education and administration in audiology graduate and professional education programs.

15. Measurement of functional outcomes, consumer satisfaction, effectiveness, efficiency, and cost- benefit of practices and programs to maintain and improve the quality of audiological services.

16. Administration and supervision of professional and technical personnel who provide support functions to the practice of audiology.

17. Screening of speech-language, use of sign language (e.g., American Sign Language and cued speech), and other factors affecting communication function for the purposes of an audiologic evaluation and/or initial identification of individuals with other communication disorders.

18. Consultation about accessibility for persons with hearing loss in public and private buildings, programs, and services.

19. Assessment and nonmedical management of tinnitus using biofeedback, masking, hearing aids, education, and counseling.

20. Consultation to individuals, public and private agencies, and governmental bodies, or as an expert witness regarding legal interpretations of audiology findings, effects of hearing loss and balance system disorders, and relevant noise-related considerations.

21. Case management and service as a liaison for the consumer, family, and agencies in order to monitor audiologic status and management and to make recommendations about educational and vocational programming.

22. Consultation to industry on the development of products and instrumentation related to the measurement and management of auditory or balance function.

23. Participation in the development of professional and technical standards.

OUTCOMES OF AUDIOLOGY SERVICES

Outcomes of audiology services may be measured to determine treatment effectiveness, efficiency, cost-benefit, and consumer satisfaction. In the future, specific outcome data may assist consumers to make decisions about audiology service delivery. The following listing describes the types of outcomes that consumers may expect to receive from an audiologist:

1. Interpretation of otoscopic examination for appropriate management or referral;
2. Identification of populations and individuals
    a. with or at risk for hearing loss or related auditory disorders,
    b. with normal-hearing or no related auditory disorders,
    c. with communication disorders associated with hearing loss,
    d. with or at risk of balance disorders, and
    e. with tinnitus.
3. Professional interpretation of the results of audiological findings;
4. Referrals to other professions, agencies, and/or consumer organizations;
5. Counseling for personal adjustment and discussion of the effects of hearing loss and the potential benefits to be gained from audiological rehabilitation, sensory aids including hearing and tactile aids, hearing assistive devices, cochlear implants, captioning devices, and signal/warning devices;
6. Counseling regarding the effects of balance system dysfunction;
7. Selection, monitoring, dispensing, and maintenance of hearing aids and large-area amplification systems;
8. Development of a culturally appropriate, audiologic, rehabilitative management plan including, when appropriate:
    a. Fitting and dispensing recommendations, and educating the consumer and family/caregivers in the use of and adjustment to sensory aids, hearing assistive devices, alerting systems, and captioning devices;
    b. Counseling relating to psychosocial aspects of hearing loss and processes to enhance communication competence;
    c. Skills training and consultation concerning environmental modifications to facilitate development of receptive and expressive communication;
    d. Evaluation and modification of the audiologic management plan.
9. Preparation of a report summarizing findings, interpretation, recommendations, and audiologic management plan;
10. Consultation in development of an Individual Education Program (IEP) for school-age children or an Individual Family Service Plan (IFSP) for children from birth to 36 months old;
11. Provision of in-service programs for personnel, and advising school districts in planning educational programs and accessibility for students with hearing loss; and
12. Planning, development, implementation, and evaluation of hearing conservation programs.

REFERENCES

AMERICAN SPEECH-LANGUAGE-HEARING ASSOCIATION. (1995, March). Reference list of position statements, guidelines, definitions, and relevant papers. *ASHA*, 37(Suppl. 14), 36–37.

AMERICAN SPEECH-LANGUAGE-HEARING ASSOCIATION. (1997). Preferred practice patterns for the profession audiology.

AMERICAN SPEECH-LANGUAGE-HEARING ASSOCIATION. (1994, March). Code of ethics. *ASHA*, 36(Suppl. 13), 1–2.

Appendix III
Periodicals in Audiology, Hearing, and Hearing Disorders

The following are the titles of periodicals related to audiology, hearing, and hearing disorders; the name and address of the publisher; and the first year of publication.

Advances in Otolaryngology
Mosby—Year Book
200 N. LaSalle St.
Chicago, IL 60601-1080
1987

ASHA
American Speech-Language-Hearing Association
10801 Rockville Pike
Rockville, MD 20852
1959

Acta Otolaryngological
Scandinavian University Press
Box 3255 S-10365
Stockholm, SWEDEN
1918

Advance for Speech-Language Pathologists and Audiologists
Merion Publications
650 Park Ave. W.
King of Prussia, PA 19406
1991

Advances in Audiology
S. Karger AG
CH - 4009
Allschwilerstr 10
Basel, SWITZERLAND
1983

Advances in Otolaryngology-Rhinology-Laryngology
S. Karger AG
Allschwilerstr 10
Basel, SWITZERLAND
1953

From Roeser, R. (1996). *Roeser's audiology desk reference* (pp. 373–377). New York: Thieme Medical Publishers, Inc.

American Academy of Otolaryngology— Head and Neck Surgery—Bulletin
AA of Otolaryngology—Head and Neck Surgery, Inc.
One Prince St.
Alexandria, VA 22314
1982

American Journal of Audiology: A Journal of Clinical Practice
American Speech-Language-Hearing Association
10801 Rockville Pike
Rockville, MD 20852
1991

American Journal of Otolaryngology— Head and Neck Medicine and Surgery
W.B. Saunders Co.
Curtis Center
Philadelphia, PA 19106
1979

American Annals of the Deaf
Conf of Educ Adm Serv Deaf/Conv Am Inst of Deaf
KDES PAS-6
Washington, DC 20002-3695
1847

American Journal of Audiology
American Speech-Language-Hearing Association
10801 Rockville Pike
Rockville, MD 20852-3279
1991

American Journal of Otology
Thieme Medical Publishers, Inc.
381 Park Avenue South
New York, NY 10016
1979

Annals of Otology, Rhinology and Laryngology
Annal Publishing Co.
4507 Laclede Ave.
St. Louis, MO 63108
1892

Archives of Otolaryngology—Head and Neck Surgery
American Medical Association
515 N. State St.
Chicago, IL 60610
1925

Audecibel
National Hearing Aid Society
20361 Middlebelt
Livonia, MI 48152
1952

Audiology Journal of Auditory Communication—
    Audiology
S. Karger, A.G. Allschwilerstr
26 W. Avon Rd., Box 529
Farmington, CT 06085
1962

Audiology Today
American Academy of Audiology
Georgetown University
Washington, DC 20007-0176

Australian Journal of Audiology
P.O. Box 472
Castle Hill
New South Wales
NLMW1
1979

British Journal of Audiology
Academic Press Ltd.
24-28 Oval Rd.
London, UK NW1 7DX
1967

Clinical Otolaryngology and Allied Science
Blackwell Scientific Publ./Marston Book Service
P.O. Box 88
Oxford, UK OX2 0NW
1976

Deaf American
National Association of the Deaf
814 Thayer Ave.
Silver Spring, MD 10910-4500
1948

Ear Nose and Throat Journal (ENT Journal)
Med Quest Communications Inc.
629 Euclid Ave., #500
Cleveland, OH 44114
1922

Ear and Hearing
Williams & Wilkins
428 E. Preston St.
Baltimore, MD 21202
1975

Electroencephalography and Clinical Neurophysiology
Elsevier Science Ireland Ltd.
P.O. Box 85
Limerick, IRELAND
1956

Hearing Aid Journal
Dr. Narendra Kumar
P.O. Box 2812
110-060 New Delhi, INDIA
1977

Hearing Health
Voice International Publishing Inc.
723 Upr N Brdwy St 522
Corpus Christi, TX 78401
1984

Hearing Instruments
7500 Old Oak Blvd.
Cleveland, OH 44130
1951

Hearing Journal (The)
Williams & Wilkins
428 Preston St.
Baltimore, MD 21202-3993
1983

Hearing Research
Elsevier Science Publishers B.V.
P.O. Box 211 1000 AE
Amsterdam, NETHERLANDS
1978

Hearing Review (The)
Fladmark Publishing Co.
101 West 2nd St.
Duluth, MN 55802
1994

International Journal of Pediatric Otorhinolaryngology
Elsevier Scientific Publishers Ireland Ltd.
Bay 15, Shannon Industrial Estate
Shannon, Co. Clare, IRELAND
1979

Journal of Speech and Hearing Research
American Speech-Language-Hearing Associaiton
10801 Rockville Pike
Rockville, MD 20852
1958

Journal of the Academy of Rehabilitative Audiology (JARA)
Academy of Rehabilitative Audiology
c/o H.L. Beykirch, Ph.D.
Cedar Falls, IA 50614
1969

Journal of the American Deafness
    and Rehabilitative Association
American Deafness and Rehabilitation Association
P.O. Box 251554
Little Rock, AR 72225
1966

Journal of Audiological Medicine
Whurr Publishers Ltd.
196 b Compton Terrace
London, ENGLAND N12UN
1992

Journal of Auditory Research (The)
Groton, CT 06340
1960 (discontinued in about 1990)

Journal of Laryngology and Otology
Headley Bros. Ltd., Ivicta Press
Ashord
Kent, ENGLAND TN24 8HH
1887

Journal of Otolaryngology
Australian Soc. of Oto. Head and Neck Surg. Ltd.
33-35 Atchison Street
St. Leondards, AUSTRALIA NSW 2065
1962

Journal of Sound and Vibration
Academic Press, Ltd.
24-28 Oval Rd.
London, UK, ENGLAND NW1 7DX
1964

Journal of Speech and Hearing Disorders
American Speech-Language-Hearing Association
10801 Rockville Pike
Rockville, MD 20852
1936

Journal of the Acoustical Society of America
American Institute of Physics
335 E. 45th St.
New York, NY 10017
1929

Journal of the American Academy of Audiology
Decker Periodicals
One James St. S
Hamilton, Ontario, CANADA L8N37
1989

Language Speech and Hearing Services in the Schools
American Speech-Language-Hearing Association
10801 Rockville Pike
Rockville, MD 20852
1970

Laryngoscope
10 S. Broadway, #1401
St. Louis, MO 63102-1741
1896

NSSHLA Journal
National Student Speech Language Hearing Association
10801 Rockville Pike
Rockville, MD 20852
1973

Otolaryngologic Clinics of North America
W.B. Saunders Co. (subsid of Harcourt Brace & Co.)
Curtis Center
Philadelphia, PA 19106-3399
1968

Otolaryngology—Head and Neck Surgery
Mosby—Yearbook, Inc.
11830 Westline Industrial Drive
St. Louis, MO 63146
1896

Perspectives in Education and Deafness
Gallaudet University—Pre-College Program
KDES PAS-6
Washington, DC 20002-3695
1982

SHHH Journal
Self Help for Hard of Hearing People, Inc.
7800 Wisconsin Ave.
Bethesda, MD 20814-3524
1980

Scandinavian Audiology
Scandinavian University Press
200 Meacham Ave.
Elmont, NY 11003
1952

Seminars in Hearing
Thieme Medical Publishers, Inc.
381 Park Ave.
New York, NY 10016
1980

Sign Language Studies
Linstok Press Inc.
4020 Blackburn Lane
Burtonsville, MD 20865-1167
1972

Sound
A T Zeitschriftenverlag Bahnhofstr
CH-5001
Aarau, SWITZERLAND
1978

Sound and Vibration (S&V)
Acoustical Publications, Inc.
Box 40416
Bay Village, OH 44140
1967

Tinnitus Today
American Tinnitus Association
Box 5
Portland, OR 97207
1975

Volta Review
Alexander Graham Bell Association for the Deaf
3417 Volta Place NW
Washington, DC 20007
1899

Appendix IV
Organizations Related to Audiology, Hearing, and Hearing Impairment

The following are names of organizations related to audiology, hearing, and hearing disorders, along with the most recent address, phone and fax numbers, and TDD numbers when available.

Academy of Dispensing Audiologists
3008 Millwood Ave.
Columbia, SC 29205-1187
Phone 800-445-8629
FAX 803-765-0860

Academy of Rehabilitative Audiology
Olin E. Teague Veterans Center
1901 S First St.
Audiology Section (126A)
Temple, TX 76504
Phone 817-778-4811 X-4901
FAX 817-771-4563

Acoustic Neuroma Association
P.O. Box 12402
Atlanta, GA 30355
Phone 404-237-8023
FAX 404-237-2704

Acoustical Society of America
500 Sunnyside Blvd.
Woodbury, NY 11797
Phone 516-576-2360
FAX 516-349-7669
TDD 516-576-2360

Alexander Graham Bell Association for the Deaf
3417 Volta Pl. NW
Washington, DC 20007
Phone 202-337-5220
FAX 202-337-8314
TDD 202-337-5220

American Academy of Audiology
1735 N. Lynn St., Suite 950
Arlington, VA 22209-2022
Phone 703-524-2000/800-AAA-2336
FAX 703-524-2303
TDD 703-524-2000

From Roeser, R. (1996). *Roeser's audiology desk reference* (pp. 368–372). New York: Thieme Medical Publishers, Inc.

American Academy of Otolaryngology— Head and Neck Surgery
One Prince St.
Alexandria, VA 22314
Phone 703-836-4444
FAX 703-683-5100
TDD 703-519-1585

American Association of the Deaf-Blind
814 Thayer Ave., 3rd floor
Silver Spring, MD 20910
FAX 301-588-8705
TDD 301-588-6545

American Auditory Society
512 E. Canterbury Lane
Phoenix, AZ 85022
Phone 602-789-0755
FAX 602-942-1486

American Deafness and Rehabilitative Association
P.O. Box 251554
Little Rock, AR 72225
Phone 501-868-8850
FAX 501-868-8812
TDD 501-868-8850

American Hearing Research Foundation
55 E. Washington St., Suite 2022
Chicago, IL 60602
Phone 312-726-9670
FAX 312-726-9695

American Otological Society
Loyola Univ. of Chicago Med. Ctr.
Bldg. 105, Room 1870
2160 South First Avenue
Maywood, IL 60153
Phone 708-216-9183
FAX 708-216-4834

American Professional Society of the Deaf
35 Rainbow Trail
Mountain Lakes, NJ 07046
No phone—use TDD or Relay
 1-800-RELAY-VV

American Society for Deaf Children
2848 Arden Way, Suite 210
Sacramento, CA 95825-1373
Phone 800-942-ASDC
FAX 916-482-0121
TDD 800-942-ASDC

American Speech-Language-Hearing Association
10801 Rockville Pike
Rockville, MD 20852
Phone 301-897-5700
FAX 301-571-0457
TDD 301-897-0157

American Tinnitus Association
P.O. Box 5
Portland, OR 97207-0005
Phone 503-248-9985/800-634-8978
FAX 503-248-0024

Association of Late-Deafened Adults
P.O. Box 641763
Chicago, IL 60664
FAX 708-445-0860
TDD 708-445-0860

Association for Research in Otolaryngology
431 E. Locust St., Suite 202
Des Moines, IA 50209
Phone 515-243-1558
FAX 515-243-2049

Audiological Resource Association
6802 Lee Highway
Chattanooga, TN 37421
Phone 615-894-1133

Audiology Foundation of America
2100 N. Salisbury
West Lafayette, IN 47906
Phone 317-463-5446
FAX 317-497-1136

Auditory Verbal International
2121 Eisenhower Ave., Suite 402
Alexandria, VA 22314
Phone 703-739-1049
FAX 703-739-0395

Better Hearing Institute
5021-B Backlick Rd.
Annandale, VA 22003
Phone 703-642-0580
  800-EAR-WELL
FAX 703-750-9302

The Caption Center
125 Western Ave.
Boston, MA 02134
Phone 617-492-9225
FAX 617-562-0590
TDD 617-492-9225

Cochlear Implant Club International
P.O. Box 464
Buffalo, NY 14223-0464
Phone 716-838-4662
TDD 716-838-4662

Committee on Hearing, Bioacoustics, and Biomechanics
National Academy of Sciences
National Research Council
2101 Constitution Ave., HA178
Washington, DC 20418
Phone 202-334-3026
FAX 202-334-3584

Conference of Educational Administrators Serving the Deaf
1600 South Highway 275
Council Bluffs, IA 51503
Phone 712-366-0571
FAX 712-366-3218

Convention of American Instructors of the Deaf
P.O. Box 377
Bedford, TX 70695
Phone 214-401-3525

Council for Better Hearing and Speech Month
c/o Paige Wesley
10801 Rockville Pike
Rockville, MD 20852
Phone 301-897-5700
FAX 301-571-0457

Council on Education of the Deaf
800 Florida Ave. NE, KDES-PAS12
Washington, DC 20002
Phone 202-651-5020
FAX 202-651-5708

Deafness Research Foundation
9 E. 38th St.
New York, NY 10016
Phone 212-684-6556/800-535-3323
FAX 212-779-2125
TDD 212-684-6559

Dogs for the Deaf, Inc.
10175 Wheeler Rd.
Central Point, OR 97502
Phone 503-826-9220
FAX 503-826-6696

Ear Foundation (The)
2000 Church St., Box 111
Nashville, TN 37236
Phone 800-545-HEAR
FAX 615-329-7935
TDD 615-329-7849

HEAR NOW
9745 East Hampden Avenue, Suite 300
Denver, CO 80321-4923
Phone 303-695-7797
  800-648-HEAR (4923)
FAX 303-695-7789
TDD 800-648-4327

Hearing Aid Foundation
20361 Middlebelt Rd.
Livonia, MI 48152
Phone 810-478-2610
FAX 810-478-4520

Hearing Dog Resource Center
P.O. Box 1080
Renton, WA 98057-9906
Phone 800-869-6898
FAX 206-235-1076
TDD 800-86-6898

Hearing Education and Awareness for Rockers
P.O. Box 460847
San Francisco, CA 94146
Phone 415-441-9081
FAX 415-576-7113
TDD 415-476-7600

Hearing Industries Association
515 King St., Suite 320
Alexandria, VA 22314
Phone 703-684-5574
FAX 703-684-6048

Hearing Loss Link
2600 W. Peterson, Suite 202
Chicago, IL 60659
Phone 312-743-1032

Helen Keller National Center for Deaf-Blind Youths and Adults
111 Middle Neck Rd.
Sands Point, NY 11050
Phone 516-944-8900
FAX 516-944-7302
TDD 516-944-8637

International Hearing Dog, Inc.
5901 E. 89th Ave.
Henderson, CO 80640
Phone 303-287-3425
FAX 303-287-3425

International Hearing Society
20361 Middlebelt Rd.
Livonia, MI 48152
Phone 810-478-2610 800-521-5247
FAX 810-478-4520

National Association of the Deaf
814 Thayer Ave.
Silver Spring, MD 20910
Phone 301-587-1788
FAX 301-587-1791
TDD 301-587-1788

National Association of Earmold Labs
c/o Precision Earmold Labs
830 Sunshine Lane
Altamonte Springs, FL 32714
Phone 407-774-8022/800-327-4792
FAX 407-774-8133

National Board for Certification in Hearing Instrument Sciences
20361 Middlebelt Rd.
Livonia, MI 48152
Phone 810-478-5712
FAX 810-478-4520

National Captioning Institute
5203 Leesburg Pike
Falls Church, VA 22041
Phone 703-998-2400
 800-533-WORD
FAX 810-998-2474
TDD 703-998-2400

National Foundation for Children's Hearing
928 McLean Ave.
Yonkers, NY 10704

National Hearing Conservation Association
431 E. Locust St., Suite 202
Des Moines, IA 50209
Phone 515-243-1558
FAX 515-243-2049

National Information Center on Deafness
Gallaudet University
800 Florida Ave., NE
Washington, DC 20002
Phone 202-651-5051
FAX 202-651-5054
TDD 202-651-50520

National Institute for Hearing Instruments Studies
20361 Middlebelt Rd.
Livonia, MI 48152
Phone 800-521-5247
FAX 810-478-4520

National Institute on Deafness and Other Communication Disorders
9000 Rockville Pike, Bldg., 31, Rm. 3C-35
Bethesda, MD 20892
Phone 301-496-7243
FAX 301-402-0018

New England Assistance Dog Service (NEADS)
P.O. Box 213, 6 Green Street
West Boylston, MA 01583
Phone 508-835-3304
FAX 508-835-2526

New York League for the Hard of Hearing
71 W. 23 St.
New York, NY 10010
Phone 212-741-7650
FAX 212-255-4413

Parents' Section of the Alexander Graham Bell Association for the Deaf
3417 Volta Place NW
Washington, D.C. 20007
Phone 202-337-5220
TDD 202-337-5220

Registry of Interpreters for the Deaf
8719 Colesville Rd., Suite 310
Silver Spring, MD 20910
Phone 301-608-0050
FAX 301-608-0508
TDD 301-608-0050

Self Help for Hard of Hearing People, Inc. (SHHH)
7910 Woodmont Ave., Suite 1200
Bethesda, MD 20814
Phone 301-657-2248
FAX 301-913-9413
TDD 301-657-2249

Sertoma International Foundation
1912 E. Meyer Blvd.
Kansas City, MO 64132-1174
Phone 816-333-8300
FAX 816-333-4320

Service Dog Center
P.O. Box 1080
Renton, WA 98057-9906
Phone 206-226-7357
FAX 206-235-1076

Texas Hearing Dog, Inc.
4803 Rutherglen
Austin, TX 78749
Phone 512-891-9090
TDD 512-891-9090

INDEX